Skin Diseases and Disorders

Edited by Deb Willis

hayle
medical

New York

Hayle Medical,
750 Third Avenue, 9th Floor,
New York, NY 10017, USA

Visit us on the World Wide Web at:
www.haylemedical.com

ISBN: 978-1-63241-518-9

The publisher's policy is to use permanent paper from mills that operate a sustainable forestry policy. Furthermore, the publisher ensures that the text paper and cover boards used have met acceptable environmental accreditation standards.

Printed in China.

Cataloging-in-Publication Data

Skin diseases and disorders / edited by Deb Willis.
p. cm.
Includes bibliographical references and index.
ISBN 978-1-63241-518-9
1. Skin--Diseases. 2. Dermatology. I. Willis, Deb.
RL71 .S55 2018
616.5--dc23

Table of Contents

Preface

Skin diseases and disorders may differ in symptoms and severity. They can be genetic. Some of the common skin diseases and disorders are moles, acne, eczema, rosacea, impetigo, warts and skin cancer. Most of the skin diseases are treatable. The common treatment methods are medicated creams, laser therapy and antibiotics. The topics covered in this extensive book deal with the core aspects of skin diseases and disorders. With state-of-the-art inputs by acclaimed experts of this field, this book targets students and professionals.

The information shared in this book is based on empirical researches made by veterans in this field of study. The elaborative information provided in this book will help the readers further their scope of knowledge leading to advancements in this field.

Finally, I would like to thank my fellow researchers who gave constructive feedback and my family members who supported me at every step of my research.

Editor

1

MiRNA Expression in Psoriatic Skin: Reciprocal Regulation of hsa-miR-99a and IGF-1R

Galya Lerman[1,2], Camila Avivi[3], Corine Mardoukh[3], Aviv Barzilai[4], Ariel Tessone[5], Ben Gradus[6], Felix Pavlotsky[4], Iris Barshack[3], Sylvie Polak-Charcon[3], Arie Orenstein[5], Eran Hornstein[6], Yechezkel Sidi[1,2*¶], Dror Avni[1*¶]

1 Laboratory of Molecular Cell Biology, Center for Cancer Research and Department of Internal Medicine C , Sheba Medical Center, Tel Hashomer, Israel, **2** Sackler School of Medicine, Tel Aviv University, Tel Aviv, Israel, **3** Institute of Pathology Sheba Medical Center, Tel Hashomer, Israel, **4** Department of Dermatology Sheba Medical Center, Tel Hashomer, Israel, **5** Department of Plastic and Reconstructive Surgery and Burns Sheba Medical Center, Tel Hashomer, Israel, **6** Department of Molecular Genetics Weizmann Institute of Science, Rehovot, Israel

Abstract

Background: Psoriasis is a complex disease at the cellular, genomic and genetic levels. The role of microRNAs in skin development was shown in a keratinocyte-specific Dicer knockout mouse model. Considering that two main characteristics of psoriasis are keratinocytes hyperproliferation and abnormal skin differentiation, we hypothesized that aberrant microRNA expression contributes to the psoriatic phenotype. Here, we describe the differential expression of miRNAs in psoriatic involved and uninvolved skin as compared to normal skin, revealing an additional aspect of this complex disorder.

Methodology/Principal Findings: Expression arrays were used to compare microRNA expression in normal skin versus psoriatic involved and uninvolved skin. Fourteen differentially expressed microRNAs were identified, including hsa-miR-99a, hsa-miR-150, hsa-miR-423 and hsa-miR-197. The expression of these microRNAs was reevaluated by qPCR. IGF-1R, which is involved in skin development and the pathogenesis of psoriasis, is a predicted target of hsa-miR-99a. In an *in situ* hybridization assay, we found that IGF-1R and miR-99a are reciprocally expressed in the epidermis. Using a reporter assay, we found that IGF-1R is targeted by hsa-miR-99a. Moreover, over expression of miR-99a in primary keratinocytes down-regulates the expression of the endogenous IGF-1R protein. Over expression of miR-99a also inhibits keratinocyte proliferation and increases Keratin 10 expression. These findings suggest that overexpression of hsa-miR-99a in keratinocytes drives them towards differentiation. In primary keratinocytes grown in high Ca^{++}, miR-99a expression increases over time. Finally, we found that IGF1 increases the expression of miR-99a.

Conclusions/Significance: We identified several microRNAs that are expressed differentially in normal and psoriatic skin. One of these miRNAs is miR-99a that regulates the expression of IGF-1R. Moreover, miR-99a seems to play a role in the differentiation of keratinocytes. We suggest that miR-99a is one of the regulators of the IGF-1R signaling pathway in keratinocytes. Activation of IGF1 signaling results in elevation of miR-99a which represses the expression of IGF-1R.

Editor: Maurizio C. Capogrossi, Istituto Dermopatico dell'Immacolata, Italy

Funding: This research was supported by grants from the Israel Science Foundation (Grant No. 277/07), the Israel Cancer Association (Grant No. 20090085) and the Chief Scientist Office of Israel Ministry of Health, (Grant No. 4898) to D. Avni and Y. Sidi. The funders had no role in study design, data collection and analysis, decision to publish, or preparation of the manuscript.

Competing Interests: The authors have declared that no competing interests exist.

* E-mail: droravni@msn.com (DA); ysidi@sheba.health.gov.il (YS)

¶ These authors contributed equally to this work.

Introduction

Psoriasis is a very common chronic inflammatory skin disorder with an estimated prevalence of 2%. Despite the accessibility, frequency and persistence of this complex disease that involves different cell types and many genes, puzzling questions remain unanswered [1]. Perhaps the most obvious is the lack of major genetic susceptibility determinants, although several psoriatic associated genes have been found (Reviewed in [2]). Susceptibility to psoriasis has been mapped to loci on several chromosomes [3,4,5,6,7,8,9]. This multigenic disease is characterized by abnormally increased keratinocyte proliferation, abnormal differentiation of the epidermis and systemic and local inflammation, which result in the formation of chronic erythematous and scaly lesions [1,10,11]. Psoriatic epidermal hyper proliferation is characterized by over representation of basal keratinocytes, increased number of mitoses and their presence above the basal layer, evenly thickened epidermis with persistence of cell nuclei in the upper cornified layer, and loss of the granular layer. Keratinocyte transit time through the epidermis is accelerated 10-fold compared to normal skin, and differentiated characteristics do not develop [12].

Since the discovery of the first microRNA (miRNA) gene, lin-4, in *Caenorhabditis elegans*, approximately 700 miRNA genes have been identified in humans [13]. MiRNAs play important roles in the regulation of development, proliferation, morphogenesis, apoptosis and differentiation. The role of miRNAs in skin development was demonstrated recently in a mouse model constructed with conditional knockout of Dicer in the skin [14,15]. Yi et al. found more than 100 miRNAs in the skin and showed that epidermis and hair follicles differentially express discrete miRNA families [15]. Loss of keratinocyte-specific Dicer expression produces several distinct defects in the skin that affect both the epithelium and epithelial-mesenchymal signaling. These phenotypes include hyper proliferation in the absence of increased apoptosis [14,15]. Hence, the importance of miRNAs in skin development is evident, although their precise functions in normal skin development and pathogenic conditions are unknown (reviewed in [16]).

The psoriatic phenotype is characterized by keratinocytes hyper proliferation and abnormal skin differentiation. Analysis of keratinocyte-derived miRNAs arrays revealed that hsa-miR-203 is up-regulated in psoriatic plaques [17]. Yet, many of the functions of miRNAs in the skin are largely unknown, and their involvement in the pathogenesis of skin disorders is even less understood. In this study we sought to identify miRNAs involved in the pathogenesis of psoriasis. We compared miRNA expression in normal skin to psoriatic involved and uninvolved skin and revealed 14 novel differentially expressed miRNAs. We further showed that IGF-1R, which has an important role in the psoriatic phenotype, is regulated by hsa-miR-99a.

Results

MiRNA expression analysis

To identify miRNAs involved in psoriasis, we compared miRNA expression in healthy skin to psoriatic involved an uninvolved skin using microarray technology. Full skin biopsies from three patients diagnosed with psoriasis were taken from psoriatic lesions as well as from uninvolved skin near the lesion. Normal skin biopsies were taken from three healthy volunteers. MiRNAs were extracted from the three biopsy types and samples from each type were pooled to reduce genetic variability.

The expression profiles of psoriatic uninvolved skin and lesion skin were compared to that of normal skin (Figure 1A and 1B, table S2 and table S1 respectively). As expected, the expression level of most of the miRNAs was the same. However, several miRNAs exhibited a significant difference in expression in both comparisons. The following differentially expressed miRNAs were specific to the normal versus psoriatic uninvolved skin comparison: hsa-miR-199a*2, hsa-mir-186, hsa-miR-22, hsa-miR-221 hsa-miR-220, hsa-miR-24-1, hsa-miR-296, hsa-miR-331, hsa-miR-324-5p, hsa-miR-329 hsa-miR-423 (hsa-miR-423 is marked as a red square in Fig. 1A). (Figure 1A and Table S3). The comparison between normal and psoriatic lesion skin revealed the following differentially expressed miRNAs: hsa-miR-149, hsa-miR-150, hsa-miR-210, hsa-miR-220, hsa-miR-326, has-miR-324-5p, hsa-miR-342, hsa-miR-326, hsa-miR-328, hsa-miR-345, hsa-miR-346, hsa-miR-197, (hsa-miR-197 is marked in brown in Fig 1B). (Figure 1B and Table S2). Hsa-miR-99a and hsa-miR-150 were found to be differentially expressed, more than a 2-fold difference, in both comparisons (Marked in blue and pink, respectively in Fig 1A and 1B).

In addition, the expression of hsa-miR-423 (Figure 1A) and hsa-miR-197 (Figure 1B) were dramatically changed, exhibiting more than a 2-fold difference in expression. Thus, these four miRNAs were chosen for further investigation. The array results are depicted in Table S1, S2, S3, S4.

Validating the chip results

To verify the results obtained in the chip analysis, we assessed the expression of hsa-miR-99a, hsa-miR-150, hsa-miR-197 and hsa-miR-423 in normal and psoriatic uninvolved and lesion skin using qPCR. RNA was extracted from biopsies taken from 10 healthy volunteers and 16 psoriasis patients. As before, two biopsies were taken from each patient – one from the lesion and one from uninvolved skin. The expression of hsa-miR-99a was ~4.5-fold lower in lesion skin and ~2-fold lower in uninvolved skin as compared to normal skin ($p<0.0001$ P vs. N, using un-paired t-test, Figure 2A). Hsa-miR-150 was under expressed in uninvolved psoriatic skin, ~3-fold less than in normal and psoriatic lesion skin ($p<0.0007$ in P vs. UI, using paired t-test, $P<0.0004$ in UI vs. N, using un-paired t-test, Figure 2B). Hsa-miR-423 was under expressed in uninvolved skin as well as in psoriatic lesion skin, ~2.75 times less than in normal skin, ($P<0.0001$ in P vs. N , $P<0.0003$ in UI vs. N, using un-paired t-test, Figure 2C). Hsa-miR-197 was under expressed in psoriatic lesion skin, ~3-fold less than in normal skin ($P<0.0019$ in P vs. N, using un-paired t-test). Its expression in uninvolved skin was similar to that in normal skin although the results were highly variable (Figure 2D). Not all miRNAs were down regulated in the psoriasis lesion; miR-203 was up regulated in psoriasis lesion samples as compared to normal skin samples (Supporting Information Figure S1) similar to previously published results [17]. Interestingly, we also detected a significant down regulation of miR-203 in the uninvolved psoriatic skin as compared to psoriatic lesion and normal skin ($p<0.009$ and 0.0001, respectively, Supporting Information Figure S1).

Next, we characterized the expression pattern of the four miRNAs in the epidermis. *In situ* hybridizations (ISH) were performed on biopsies of six psoriatic lesion skins, six uninvolved skins and five normal skins using specific LNA probes for hsa-miR-99a, hsa-miR-150, hsa-miR-423 and hsa-miR-197 (Figure 3). The specificity of the probes was confirmed by hybridization with an LNA scrambled-miRNA probe (data not shown). The ISH showed that the four miRNAs are present in keratinocytes and are differentially distributed throughout the epidermis. Hsa-miR-99a was found to be expressed in the upper part of the epidermis and excluded from the basal keratinocyte layer, in normal, uninvolved and psoriatic lesion skin (Figure 3A). Hsa-miR-150 was found to be expressed in the upper part of the epidermis and much less in the basal keratinocytes layer in normal skin. It was completely excluded from uninvolved skin, and appeared to be evenly distributed throughout the psoriatic epidermis (Figure 3B). Hsa-miR-423 appeared to be evenly distributed throughout the normal epidermis, and was hardly detected in the psoriatic lesion and uninvolved skin (Figure 3C). In contrast to miR-99a and miR-150, that were express gradually; higher in the upper epidermis and decreasing until complete absent from the basal layer, miR-197 was excluded from the basal layer of normal, uninvolved and psoriatic lesion skin and also was absent in the upper part of the epidermis in uninvolved and psoriatic lesion skin. At the rest of the epidermis miR-197 seemed to express equally (Figure 3D). The results of the ISH lack quantitative value due to variability in the intensity of staining among the samples. Nevertheless, the distribution of the four miRNAs was successfully demonstrated and the staining pattern was highly reproducible.

Our microarray and qPCR analysis revealed that hsa-miR-150 expression differs significantly between normal, psoriatic lesion and psoriatic uninvolved skin (Figures 1 and 2). Xiao et al. showed that miR-150 is selectively expressed in mature resting B and T cells, but not in their progenitors [18]. Our ISH analysis

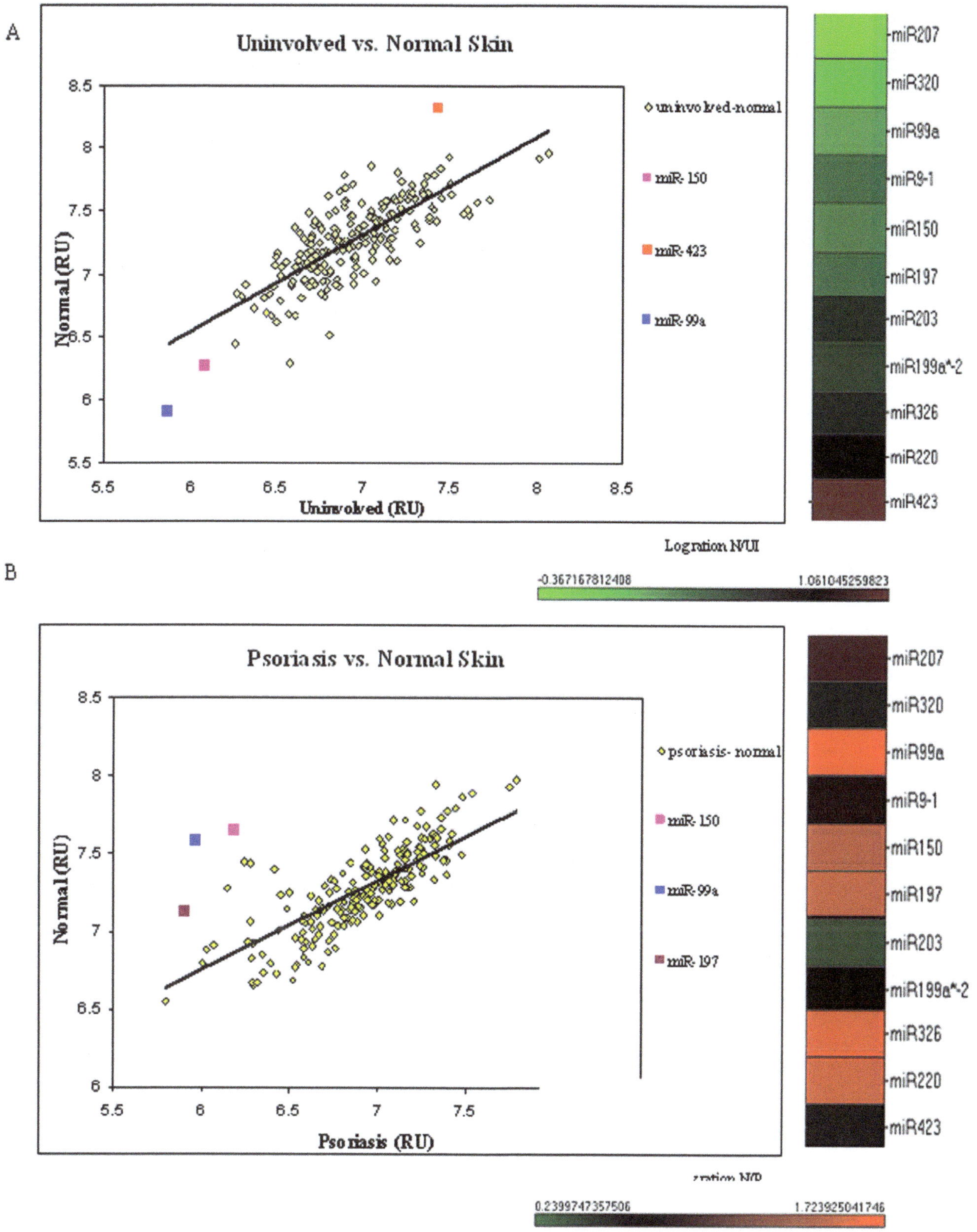

Figure 1. Profiling the expression level of miRNAs in psoriatic involved and uninvolved skin in comparison to normal skin. The expression of individual miRNAs in biopsies of normal skin, and psoriatic uninvolved and lesional skin was determined using miRNA expression array technology. The expression profile of normal skin was compared to uninvolved psoriatic skin (A) and psoriatic lesional skin (B). Abundance of an individual miRNA is shown by its relative position along the scaled y and x axes (arbitrary units). The colored boxes denote miRNAs which were further analyzed. See Table S1 for a detailed calculation of the heat-map.

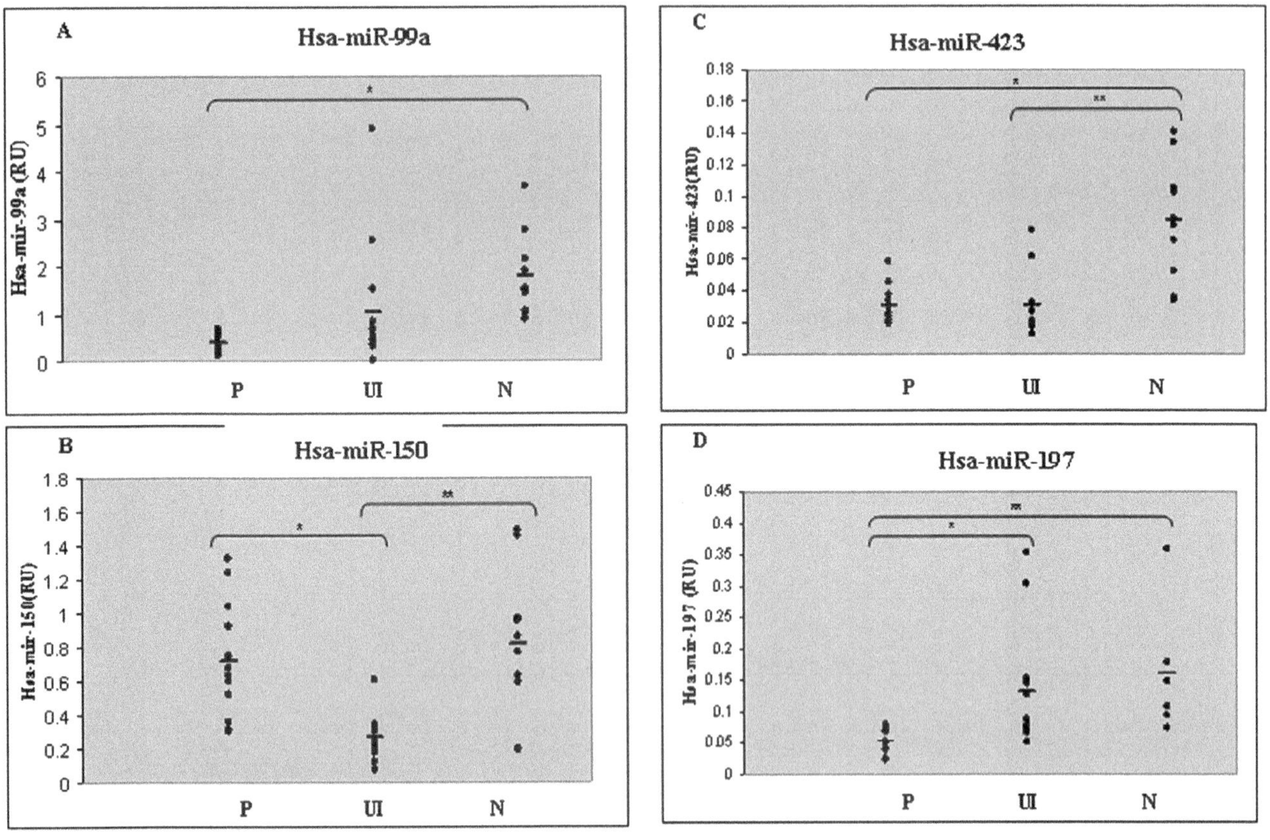

Figure 2. Quantification of miRNAs expression by qRT-PCR. The levels of hsa-miR-99a (A), hsa-miR-150 (B), hsa-miR-423 (C) and hsa-miR-197 (D) in normal skin (N, n = 10), psoriatic lesional skin (P, n = 16), and psoriatic uninvolved skin (UI, n = 16) were quantified by qPCR, and normalized to Rnu48. Each dot represents one sample. The average is denoted by the horizontal line. (A) Hsa-miR-99a (*$p<0.0001$ using un-paired t-test). (B) Hsa-miR-150 (*$p<0.0007$ using paired t-test, **$p<0.0004$ using un-paired t-test). (C) Hsa- miR-423 (*$p<0.0001$, **$p<0.0003$ using un-paired t-test). (D) Hsa-miR-197(**$p<0.009$ **$p<0.0019$ using un-paired t-test).

revealed that miR-150 is expressed in keratinocytes (Figure 3A). In addition we found that hsa-miR-150 is expressed both in HaCaT and PHK, reinforcing the fact that hsa-miR-150 is expressed in keratinocytes. However, miR-150 expression in keratinocytes is much lower than in B or T lymphocyte cell lines (data not shown).

Reciprocal expression of IGF-1R and hsa-miR-99a

To understand the biological role of these differentially expressed miRNAs and their involvement in psoriasis, we sought to identify their possible targets. MiRNAs regulate gene expression mainly through interaction with the 3′UTR of a specific target mRNA. The binding specificity is directed by what is known as the miRNA 'seed' sequence: miRNA seeds are 7 to 8 nucleotides at the 5′ end that serve as the primary determinant of target specificity [19]. Based on this, several algorithms were developed to predict possible miRNA targets. We used these algorithms (miRanda, TargetScan, TargetRank) to predict possible targets for hsa-miR-99a. Between 40–950 predicted target mRNAs were found, one of which was IGF-1R, which was predicted by several algorithms. IGF-1R is known to be involved in the pathogenesis of psoriasis [20,21]. IGF-1R was shown to be up-regulated in psoriasis, specifically in the proliferating basal layer of psoriatic lesions [20,22]. Our ISH analysis revealed that hsa-miR-99a is not found in this layer (Figure 3A). We therefore decided to characterize the distribution of hsa-miR-99a and IGF-1R in the same sample to determine whether their expression pattern is reciprocal. ISH with specific LNA probes to hsa-mir-99a assay was performed on paraffin-embedded psoriatic lesion skin biopsies. Hsa-miR-99a was expressed in the upper part of the epidermis, most pronounced in the stratum spinosum and much less pronounced in the stratum basal layer (Figure 4A) also in normal skin (Figure 4C). The same biopsies were immunostained with anti-IGF-1R antibodies. IGF-1R was indeed up-regulated in the psoriatic lesions as compared to normal skin (Figure 4B and 4D) in agreement with previously published findings [20,22]. Interestingly, IGF-1R was detected mainly in the basal layer of the epidermis, and was absent from the upper epidermal layer (Figure 4B). This reciprocal expression pattern suggests a possible relationship between hsa-miR-99a and IGF-1R.

In order to determine whether IGF-1R is a direct target of hsa-miR-99a, we cloned a fragment of the IGF-1R 3′UTR mRNA downstream to the *Renilla* luciferase reporter gene [23]. Cells were either transfected with IGF-1R 3′UTR-luc alone, or together with increasing amounts of a hsa-miR-99a expression plasmid. The effect of miR-99a on the expression of the luciferase reporter containing the IGF-1R 3′UTR was assessed 72 h later with a standard luciferase reporter assay. Figure 5A (middle panel) shows that luciferase expression dropped to less than 50% in the presence of miR-99a, as compared to the control in the absence of miR-99a, or in the absence of the IGF-1R 3′UTR. These results suggest that hsa-miR-99a regulates the expression of

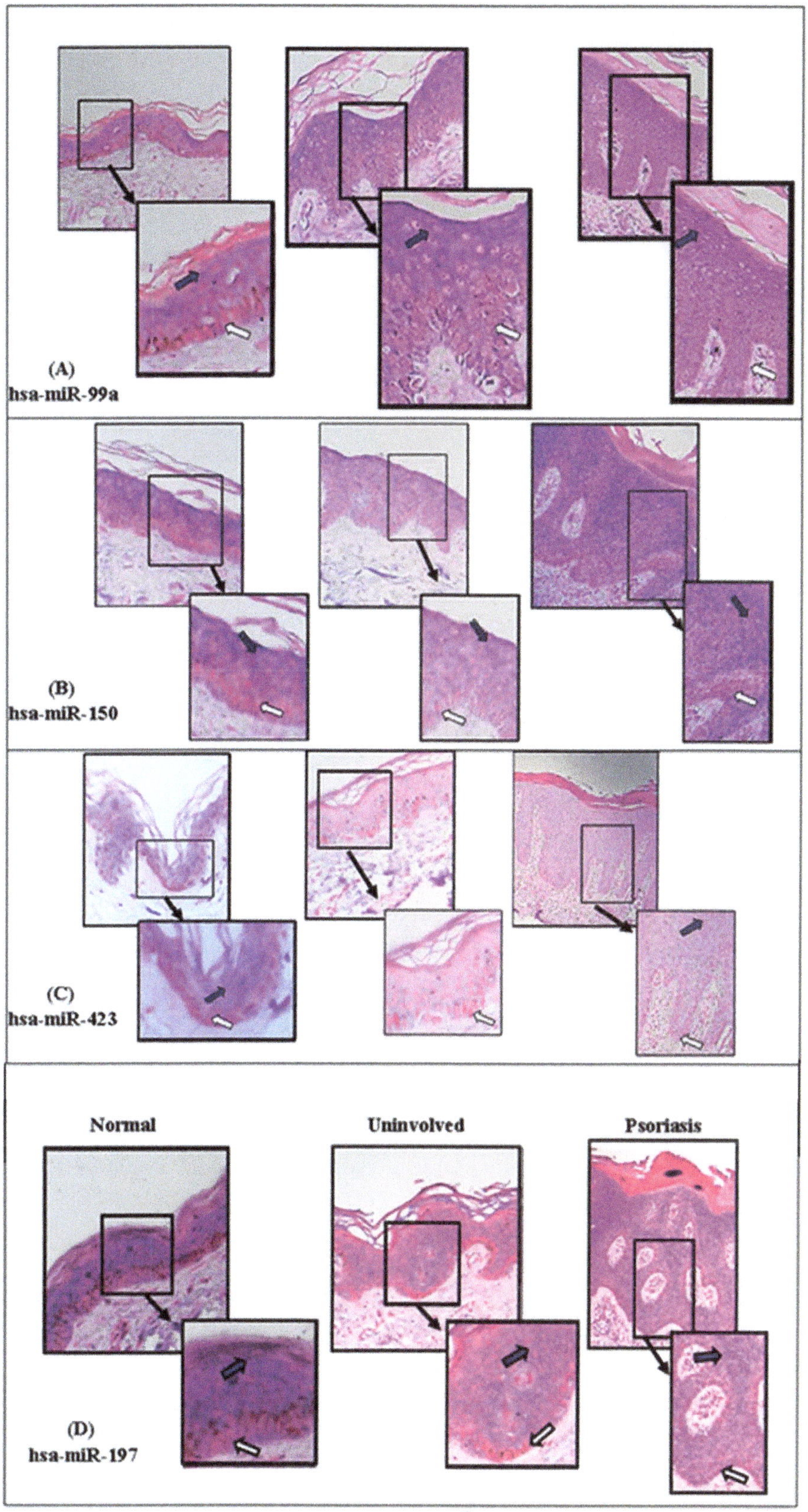

Figure 3. ***in situ hybridization*** **of hsa-mir-99, hsa-mir-150, hsa-mir-423 and hsa-mir-197 in normal, uninvolved and psoriatic skin.** Representative *in-situ* hybridization images showing distribution of hsa-miR-99a (A), hsa-miR-150 (B), hsa-miR-423 (C) and hsa-mir-197 (D) in psoriatic, uninvolved and normal skin. *In-situ* hybridizations were performed on paraffin-embedded sections of the three skin biopsy types. Each section was hybridized with an miRNA-specific LNA probe as indicated. Positive staining appears as a blue-purple color (examples are marked with blue arrows). Samples were co-stained with Nuclear Fast Red counter stain to visualize nuclei that are stained pink (examples are marked with white arrows). All images were captured at 200x magnification.

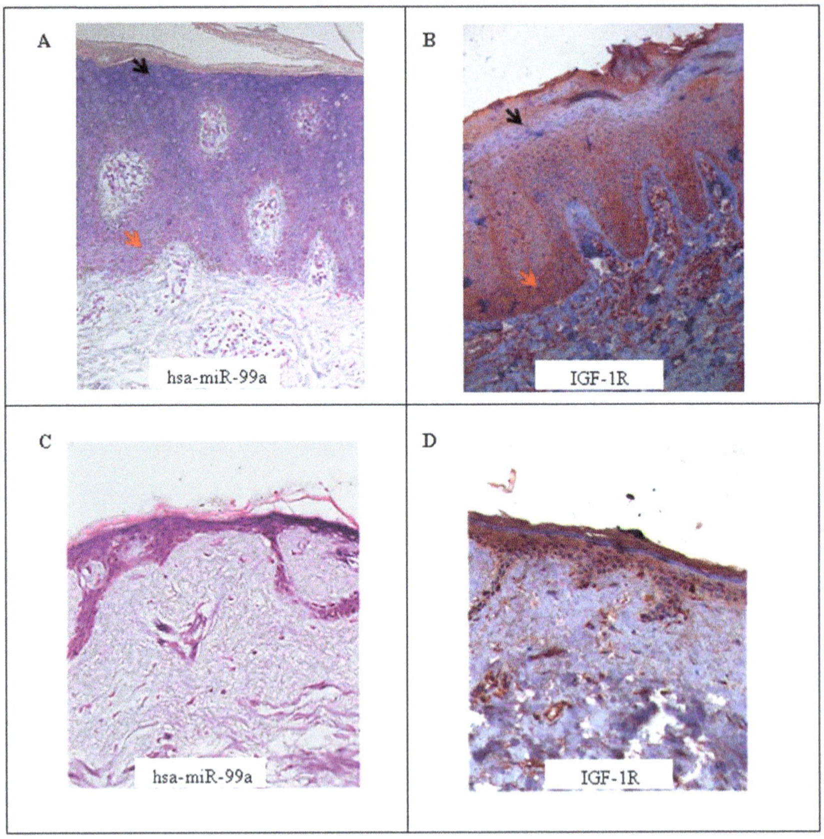

Figure 4. Reciprocal expression of IGF-1R and hsa-miR-99a. The distribution of hsa-miR-99a in psoriatic lesional skin (A) or normal skin (C) was assessed by *in-situ* hybridization. Paraffin-embedded sections of lesional skin biopsies were hybridized with an LNA probe specific to hsa-miR-99a. The cytoplasm of positive cells was stained blue (indicated by black arrows). Nuclei were stained with Nuclear Fast Red counter stain (indicated by red arrows). Magnification, 200x. (B) and (D) The same paraffin-embedded skin biopsy shown in (A and Crespectively;) was immunostained with anti-IGF-1R antibodies. Antibody binding was visualized with the substrate-chromogen AEC. IGF-1R positive cells were stained red (indicted by the red arrow). Nuclei were stained blue with hematoxylin (indicated by the black arrow). Magnification, 200x.

IGF-1R through interaction with its 3′UTR. Next, we verified that the interaction between hsa-miR-99a and its predicted seed response sequence in the IGF-1R 3′UTR is responsible for down-regulating the expression of the reporter gene. We generated an IGF-1R-3′UTR-luc mutant in which four nucleotides in the seed response sequence were changed (TACGGGTA was changed to TA**TAAA**TA). The mutant was co-transfected with the miR-99a expression plasmid as before and luciferase activity was assessed. Figure 5A (left panel) clearly demonstrates that miR-99a has no effect on the mutated IGF-1R-3′UTR, proving that miR-99a seed sequence at the IGF-1R 3′UTR is essential for the regulation of IGF-1R by miR-99a. The effect of hsa-miR-99a on the regulation of IGF-1R was further examined by assessing IGF-1R mRNA and protein levels in primary human keratinocytes (PHK) transfected with RNA pre-miR-99a molecule. A scrambled sequence was used as the control. qPCR analysis showed that the level of IGF-1R mRNA in cells transfected with pre-miR-99a is similar to that in all the controls (untransfected, mock-transfected and scrambled-sequence-transfected cells; Figure 5B and C). In contrast, the level of IGF-1R protein was dramatically reduced in pre-miR-99a expressing cells, as determined by Western blot analysis (Figure 5D). Thus, IGF-1R is regulated at the post transcriptional level. Collectively, these results support our hypothesis that IGF-1R is a direct target of hsa-miR-99a.

Hsa-miR-99a affects proliferation and differentiation of keratinocytes

Thus far, we demonstrated the reciprocal expression pattern of hsa-miR-99a and IGF-1R in the epidermis (Figure 4), and provided evidence for the direct regulation of IGF-1R by hsa-miR-99a (Figure 5). The role of IGF-1R in proliferation of the skin is well established [24]. Our results suggest that miR-99a might be a key regulator of skin homeostasis. We first determined the effect of hsa-miR-99a on keratinocytes proliferation in the human keratinocyte cell line, HaCaT. Stable cell lines were established in HaCaT cells by transfections with an hsa-miR-99a expression plasmid (pMSCV-hsa-miR-99a) or a control plasmid expressing an unrelated small RNA molecule, HTR (pMSCV-HTR) followed by growth in selective medium [23]. The MTT assay was applied and viable cell count was evaluated over time. At 24 h after seeding, the growth rate of cells expressing hsa-mir-99a and HTR was similar. However, with time, the growth rate of the hsa-miR-99a expressing cells slowed down as compared to control cells. By 72 h, the hsa-miR-99a expressing cells had stopped proliferating, whereas the control cells continued to proliferate (Figure 6A). To confirm the effect of hsa-miR-99a on keratinocytes proliferation, we performed a BrdU incorporation assay in the two stable cell lines. The same trend demonstrated by the MTT assay was observed, but with different kinetics (Figure 6B). Thus, both

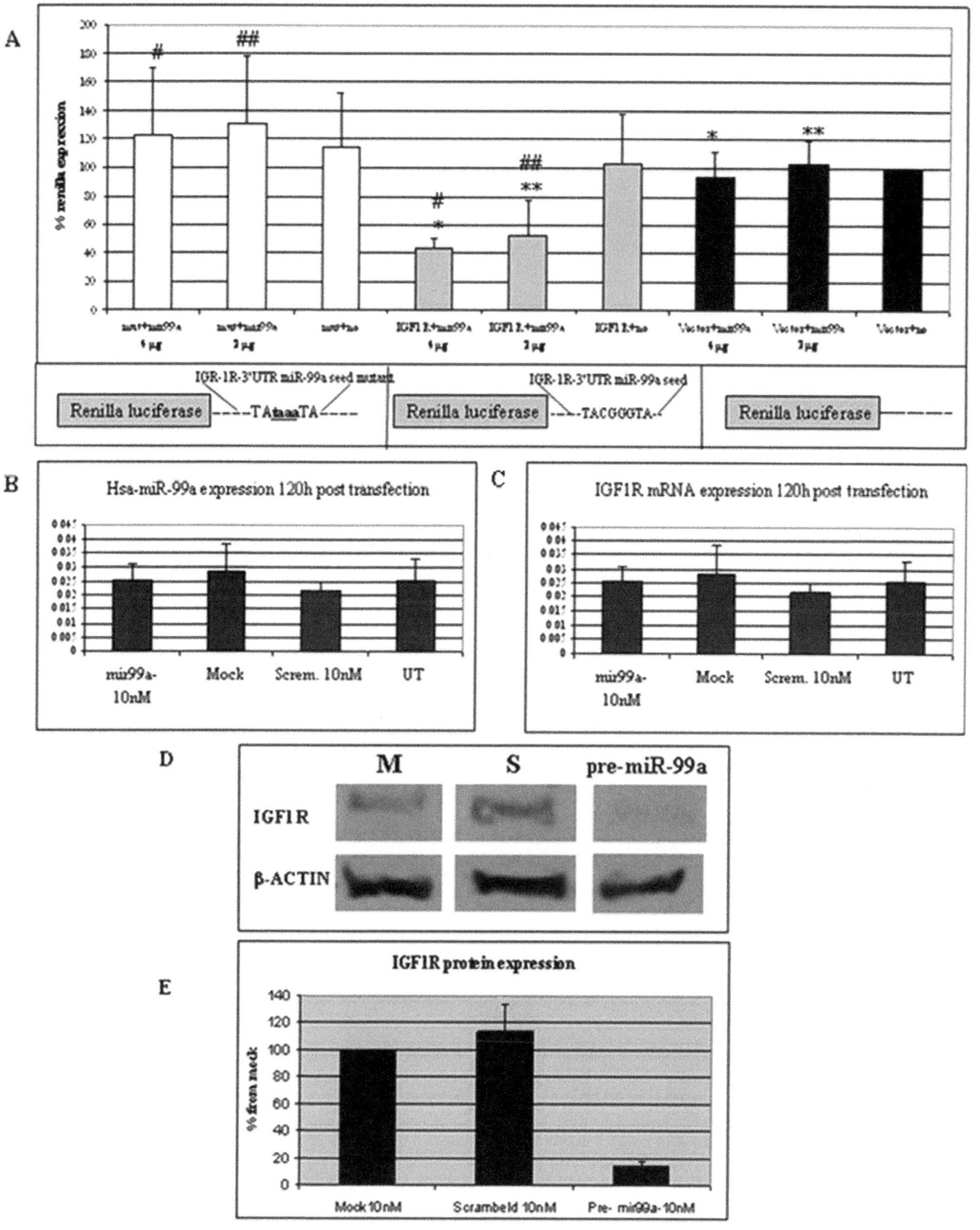

Figure 5. 3′ UTR of IGF-1R is a target of hsa-miR-99a seed sequence. (A) 293T cells were transfected with psi-CHECK2 vectors encoding luciferase (right panel), luciferase fused to the IGF-1R 3′UTR (middle panel), or luciferase fused to a mutated IGF-1R 3′UTR (left panel) together with increasing amounts of an hsa-miR-99a expression plasmid as indicated. A scheme of the reporter vectors is shown under each panel. Luciferase activity was assessed 72 h later, and is depicted relative to that of the control cells transfected with psi-CHECK2 alone (given a value of 100%). Results represent the mean of triplicates. # $p<0.0071$, # # $p<0.0047$, * $p<0.0075$, ** $p<0.0007$. (B–C) PHK cells were transfected with 10 nM pre-miR-99a, a scrambled sequence, mock transfected or left untransfected. RNA was extracted 120 h later, and the level of hsa-miR-99a (B) and IGF-1R mRNA (C)

was quantified by qPCR. Results represent the means of triplicates. Error bars, SD. (D) PHK cells were either mock-transfected or transfected with 10 nM pre-miR-99a, or a scrambled sequence. Cells were processed for Western blotting 120 h later to detect the level of IGF-1R protein. β-actin was used as the loading control. (E). The level of IGF-1R was quantified from the Western blot described in (D) by densitometry (EZQuant-Gel). Results represent the means of triplicate Western blots. Error bars, SD.

proliferation assays demonstrate the inhibitory effect of hsa-miR-99a on keratinocyte proliferation.

Next, we determined the effect of hsa-miR-99a on keratinocyte differentiation. The expression of two keratinocyte differentiation related genes, Keratin14 (K14) and Keratin10 (K10), was evaluated in the two stable cell lines. K14 expression in normal skin is restricted to the basal layer, while K10 is expressed in more differentiated cells [25]. Total RNA was extracted from the two cell lines and RT-PCR was used to amplify K14 and K10 mRNA. Figure 7A shows that K10 expression is elevated and K14 is slightly decreased in the hsa-miR-99a expressing cells as compared to control cells. The same changes in expression were observed by qPCR analysis (Figure 7B and C). Furthermore, primary keratinocytes grown in high Ca^{++} medium, conditions known to induce keratinocyte differentiation [26], exhibited an increase in hsa-miR-99a expression over time, as determined by qPCR (Figure 7D).

We next determined the effect of hsa-miR-99a depletion on keratinocyte proliferation. A knockdown of miR-99a using antagomir did not significantly change the growth rate or proliferation in PHK cells (data not shown). In addition, we used a sponge system

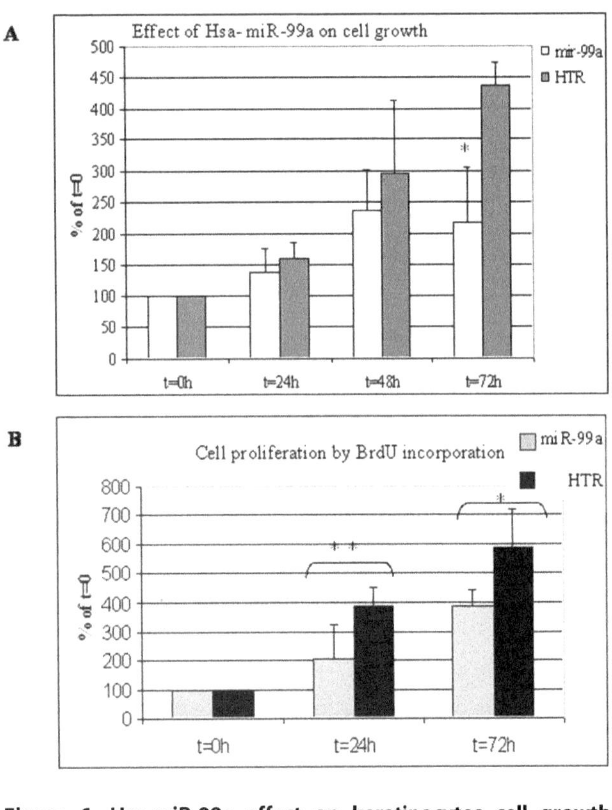

Figure 6. Hsa-miR-99a effect on keratinocytes cell growth. Proliferation of HaCaT cells stably expressing hsa-miR-99a or the HTR control RNA was assessed by MTT (A) and BrdU incorporation (B) assays. Proliferation was calculated as the percentage of the reading at seeding time ($t=0$) given a value of 100%. Mean and standard deviation were calculated from 3 independent experiments. $^*P=0.0037$ in (A) and $^*P<0.0211$ $^{**}P<0.0420$ in (B).

to knockdown hsa-miR-99a in PHK cells [27,28]. In order to verify that the miR-99a sponge is active, we co-transfected 293 cells with luciferase-IGF-1R-3′UTR and hsa-miR-99a expression plasmids together with variable amounts of the sponge expressing plasmid. As expected, luciferase expression was reduced to about 50% in cells transfected with the 3′UTR of IGF-1R and hsa-miR-99a as compared to control cells expressing hsa-miR-99a and the empty luciferase reporter plasmid. However, in the presence of the miR-99a sponge, the miR-99a-induced repression was released; the luciferase level in cells transfected with 4 μg of sponge plasmid was almost completely restored to that of the control (Supporting Information Figure S2). We generated cell lines of HaCaT cells stably expressing the miR-99a sponge or the empty vector control and assessed their proliferation rate using the MTT assay. No significant difference in proliferation rate was observed between the miR-99a sponge expressing and control cell lines (Supporting Information Figure S2). However, a minor but not significant enhancement of IGF-1R protein level was detected in the miR-99a sponge expressing cell line as compared to the control cell line (Supporting Information Figure S2), in agreement with our results demonstrating that IGF-1R is a target of miR-99a (Figure 5). We also determined whether the miR-99a sponge has an effect on keratinocyte differentiation. As shown in Supporting Information Figure S2, there is no change in expression of keratin-10 or keratin-14.

These results indicate that the over-expression of hsa-miR-99a slows keratinocyte growth rate and directs them towards differentiation. As shown in Figure 5, miR-99a regulates the expression of IGF-1R. IGF-1R was shown to have a major role in keratinocyte differentiation [24]. Considering these two facts, we thought that the expression of miR-99a and IGF-1R might be correlated. To further investigate the relationship between miR-99a and IGF-1R, we assessed miR-99a expression in serum-starved PHK cells treated with increasing concentrations of IGF1. Total RNA was extracted 72 h after IGF1 addition, and the miR-99a level was determined by qPCR. The expression of miR-99a was significantly increased in cells treated with 1–25 nM of IGF1 as compared to untreated cells (Figure 8A). Collectively, our results suggest that miR-99a and IGF-1R are co-regulated, functioning together to maintain the balance between keratinocyte proliferation and differentiation.

Discussion

MiRNAs are major regulatory molecules that govern many essential cellular functions, including proliferation, differentiation, cell cycle control and apoptosis. The significance of miRNAs in skin development was demonstrated by Yi et al., who showed that skin formation is impaired in keratinocyte-specific Dicer knockout mice [14,15]. A recent comparison of miRNA expression profiles of psoriatic and normal or atopic dermatitis skins revealed several leukocyte-derived miRNAs and one keratinocyte-derived miRNA, miR-203, which were up-regulated in psoriatic skin [17]. The functions of miR-203 seem to be related to keratinocyte stem cell differentiation [29]. Furthermore, the transcription factor p63, which plays an essential role in epidermis formation, is a target of miR-203 [29]. Our qPCR analysis of miR-203 expression demonstrated that it was up regulated in psoriatic skin compared

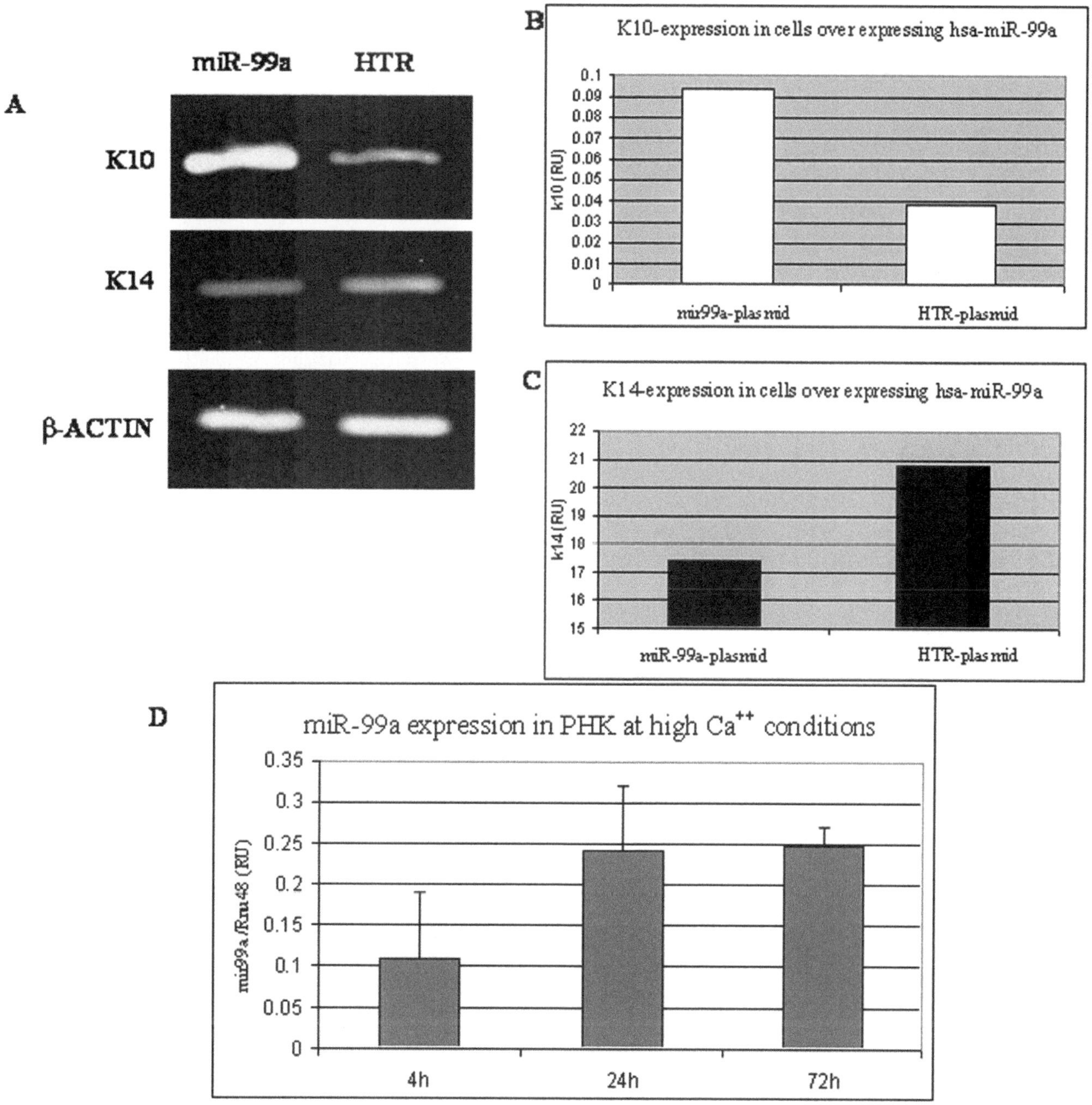

Figure 7. Hsa-miR-99a effect on differentiation of keratinocytes. (A–C) The levels of K10 and K14 differentiation markers were assessed in HaCaT cells stably expressing hsa-miR-99a or the HTR control RNA by RT-PCR (A) and qPCR (B–C) analysis. (D) PHK cells were seeded in high, 1.5 mM Ca^{++} medium. Cells were harvested at the indicated time points and the level of endogenous miR-99a was determined by qPCR.

to normal skin in agreement with previously published findings [17]. Unpredictably, hsa-miR-203 was significantly down regulated in uninvolved psoriatic skin compared to normal as well as psoriatic skin (Supporting Information Figure S1). This result implies that down regulation of miR-203 in uninvolved psoriatic skin may predispose psoriatic uninvolved keratinocytes to hyper proliferation and should be investigated in further studies.

Our comparison of miRNA expression profiles in normal, psoriatic lesion and uninvolved skin revealed several novel candidate miRNAs that might be involved in the pathogenesis of psoriasis (Figure 1). We focused our investigation on hsa-miR-99a, hsa-miR-150, hsa-miR-197 and hsa-miR-423, as they exhibited a significant difference in expression (more than 2-fold) (Figure 1 and Supporting Information Table S1). We verified the expression of these four miRNAs as well as miR-203 in skin biopsy types using qPCR, confirming their differential expression in normal and psoriatic skin (Figure 2 and Supporting Information Figure S1). Interestingly, miR-203 and miR-150 were down-regulated in uninvolved skin as compared to normal skin or lesional skin (Figure 2B and Supporting Information Figure S1), suggesting that in uninvolved skin of psoriasis patients down regulation of these two miRNAs predisposes them to the psoriatic phenotype. The

A

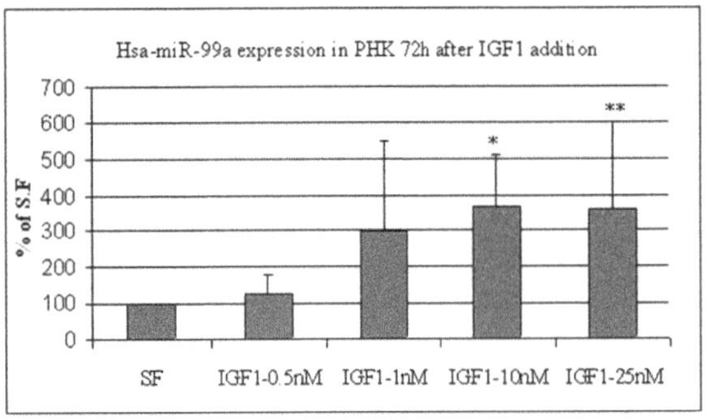

B

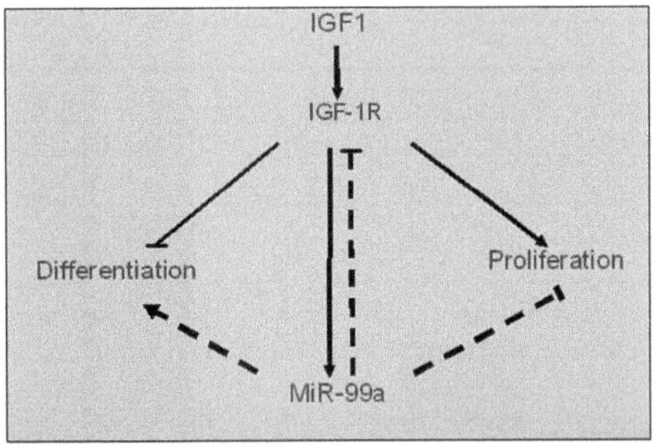

Figure 8. hsa-miR-99a expression in primary human keratinocytes 72 h after IGF1 addition. (A) Serum-starved PHK cells were treated with increasing concentrations of IGF-1 as indicated. The cells were harvested 72 h later and the level of endogenous miR-99a was determined by qPCR (*p = 0.0027 **p = 0.04510). (B) Proposed model describing the relationship between IGF-1R and miR-99a. IGF1 activation of IGF-1R inhibits differentiation and promotes proliferation of keratinocytes [24]. IGF-1R signaling enhances the expression of miR-99a that in turn inhibits IGF-1R expression. This negative feedback loop maintains the balance between proliferation and differentiation in the skin.

expression of hsa-miR-99a, hsa-miR-423 and hsa-miR-197 in the psoriasis lesion were down-regulated compared to normal skin. However, their average expression in the uninvolved skin of psoriasis patients differed; average expression of miR-99a was somewhere between normal and lesion expression levels (Figure 2A), expression of miR-423 was down regulated in uninvolved skin as in the lesion skin in comparison to normal skin (Figure 2C) and miR-197 expression in uninvolved skin was similar to that in normal skin (Figure 2D). This might suggest a biochemical hierarchy in the development of the psoriatic lesion.

We characterized the distribution of the four miRNAs in the epidermis by performing ISH on skin biopsies. This analysis revealed that the four miRNAs are expressed in keratinocytes. In addition, all four miRNAs were either absent or weakly expressed in the basal keratinocyte layer, whereas only hsa-miR-99a, hsa-miR-150 and hsa-miR-423 were present in the upper part of the epidermis (Figure 3). This distribution suggests that these miRNAs have the potential to regulate keratinocyte proliferation and differentiation.

Hsa-miR-150 was shown to be involved in immune cell function. It is selectively expressed in mature resting B and T cells, controlling B-cell differentiation by targeting the transcription factor c-Myb [18]. The involvement of the immune system in psoriasis is well established [10,30,31,32], so it is possible that hsa-miR-150 targets immune system regulators in the skin. A possible target of hsa-mir-150 is IL-7 that is expressed in keratinocytes [33] and is up-regulated in psoriatic lesions [34]. Another possible target is IRAK2 encoding the interleukin-1 receptor-associated kinase 2 that was reported to participate in the IL1-induced up-regulation of NF-kappaB, a pathway known to be involved in the pathogenesis of psoriasis [35]. In addition to a possible role in immune system regulation, hsa-miR-150 might regulate keratinocyte proliferation. Indeed, Wu et al. found that miR-150 promotes gastric cancer proliferation by negatively regulating the pro-apoptotic gene EGR2 [36]. Further investigation is required to identify the targets of hsa-miR-150 in keratinocytes.

We focused on identifying the targets of hsa-miR-99a, the miRNA exhibiting the strongest down-regulation in psoriatic skin (Figure 2A). We used bioinformatics tools to predict possible targets of hsa-miR-99a, and decided to focus on one predicted target, IGF-1R, that is known to be involved in the pathogenesis of psoriasis [20,21]. ISH revealed that both hsa-mir-99a and IGF-1R are expressed in the psoriatic lesion. However, the distribution of their expression is reciprocal, with a high expression of IGF-1R in the basal epidermis layers, from which hsa-miR-99a is absent, and a high expression of hsa-miR-99a in the upper epidermis, from which IGF-1R is absent (Figure 4). Furthermore, we used a standard luciferase reporter assay to demonstrate that the 3′UTR of IGF-1R is regulated by hsa-miR-99a and that this regulation is dependent on the interaction between the hsa-miR-99a seed and the IGF-1R mRNA 3′UTR (Figure 5A). Moreover, we showed that over expression of hsa-miR-99a reduces endogenous IGF-1R protein levels without affecting its transcript levels, demonstrating post-transcriptional regulation of IGF-1R (Figure 5C and D). Thus, we provide strong evidence for the direct regulation of IGF-1R by hsa-miR-99a.

MiRNAs are highly expressed in embryonic tissues [37] and are known to have a key role in differentiation and development. Two main characteristics of psoriasis are keratinocyte hyper proliferation and abnormal differentiation. IGF-1R plays an important role in keratinocyte differentiation by actively inhibiting the differentiation process [24]. Ablation of IGF-1R expression eliminates this inhibition, resulting in facilitated differentiation [24]. Our results suggest that hsa-miR-99a contributes to the homeostasis of IGF-1R expression. We hypothesize that the elevation of IGF-1R in the psoriatic lesion drives the tissue towards proliferation. One of the possible physiological responses to such a situation is up-regulation of hsa-miR-99a expression which may slow keratinocyte proliferation and induce their differentiation. Indeed, HaCaT cells transfected with hsa-miR-99a expression plasmid exhibited a decreased proliferation rate and an increase in expression of a late differentiation marker as compared to control cells (Figures 6 and 7A–C). Moreover, miR-99a expression was up regulated in differentiating PHK cells grown in high calcium medium (Figure 7D). We also examined the effect of down regulating hsa-miR-99a in HaCaT cells. Using a sponge system, we demonstrated that IGF-1R expression is up-regulated in hsa-miR-99a-depleted cells (Supporting Information Figure S2), however the proliferation rate was unchanged (Supporting Information Figure S2). It is possible that the combined effect of several regulators is required to achieve the hyper proliferation phenotype. Lastly, the relationship between hsa-miR-99a and IGF-1R was further demonstrated by an increase in endogenous hsa-miR-99a expression in PHK cells treated with IGF-1 (Figure 8A). We propose a model to describe how hsa-miR-99a and IGF-1R work together to achieve a balance between proliferation and differentiation in the skin (Figure 8B). Activation of IGF-1R in skin enhances proliferation and inhibits differentiation. Over time, IGF-1R signaling up-regulates the expression of miR-99a that in turn down-regulates the expression of IGF-1R, driving the cells toward differentiation. Is the entire effect of miR-99a on keratinocyte differentiation mediated through its effect on IGF-1R? It is possible; however, it is not probable, since miRNAs usually have more than one target. Our model fits well with the work of Yi et al in which miR-203 was given a comparable role in restricting proliferation and inducing differentiation of keratinocytes [38]. Based on our results and previous studies, we suggest that keratinocytes in the psoriatic lesion are prompted to proliferation, possibly by mediators produced by immune system cells. These mediators may either directly or through the involvement of stromal cells, enhance over proliferation of keratinocytes in the basal layer. During the passage of these cells from the basal layer into the stratum spinosum, differentiation signals are activated; our study describes one such signal, involving hsa-miR-99a-mediated suppression of IGF-1R expression.

In addition we found that some of the miRNAs we analyzed are expressed differentially in the uninvolved skin compared to normal skin. These results prove that the uninvolved skin of psoriasis patients differs from normal skin. This fact suggests that the regulation of miRNA expression plays a major role in the pathogenesis of psoriasis. Are the psoriatic uninvolved keratinocytes more susceptible to inflammatory mediators? It is interesting to further investigate if these differences can be used as diagnostic markers or as therapeutic agents.

This study raises additional questions: Is the activation of these miRNAs specific to the psoriasis lesion? The process by which proliferating keratinocytes eventually differentiate is common to several additional inflammatory skin disorders and wound healing. Are the same miRNAs involved in all these biological processes, or do specific miRNAs act in specific processes? The answers to these questions will shed light on our understanding of the differences between these disorders.

Materials and Methods

Patients

All skin donors were of Caucasian origin aged 18 to 85 years (Table S5). All patients were clinically diagnosed with Psoriasis Vulgaris, and did not receive systemic immunosuppressive treatment, phototherapy (Psoralen and UVA (PUVA)/solarium/UVB), or topical therapy for at least 3 weeks prior to skin biopsy (for further details see, Table S5). Three mm punches were taken mostly from upper and lower limbs. The uninvolved samples were taken from the same area, about 5 cm away from the lesion biopsy. Normal skin biopsies were taken from full thickness skin remaining after plastic surgery. All the biopsies were evaluated by a dermatopathologist for histological diagnosis. Half of each biopsy was snap-frozen and the other half was embedded in paraffin. The study was approved by both the Tel Aviv University and Sheba Medical Center Helsinki Ethics Committees. All participants provided written informed consent.

MiRNA array

Total RNA including miRNAs from normal skin (n = 3), psoriatic lesion (n = 3), or psoriatic patient uninvolved skin (n = 3), was isolated using Ambion mirVana™ miRNA Isolation Kit. Total RNA (2 µg) from each sample was labeled with the mirVana miRNA Labeling Kit (Applied Biosystems/AmbionUSA). The fluorescently-labeled RNA samples were hybridized to an expression array as previously described [39]. The array was scanned and analyzed using Genepix pro 4000b Axon and JMP statistic software.

Cells cultures

293T and HaCaT cells were grown in DMEM and MEM medium, respectively, supplemented with glutamine, antibiotics and 10% fetal bovine serum (Biological Industries, Israel) in a 5–8% CO_2 incubator at 37°C.

PHK cells were grown in an 8% CO_2 incubator at 37°C, in high Ca^{++} (1.5 mM) medium: DMEM / HAM (Biological Industries, Israel) /10%FBS (Gibco). Keratinocytes were harvested from mashed skin (left over from plastic surgery) and grown on a feeder layer of 5000 rad γ irradiated 3T3 mice fibroblast cells.[40].

Cell growth and proliferation assays

Cell growth was assessed by seeding 3000 HaCaT cells per well in 96-well plates. Viable cell counts were monitored from seeding time (t = 0) to 72 h. Cell counts were determined using the MTT (3-[4, 5-dimethylthiazol-2-yl]-2, 5-diphenyl tetrazolium bromide)-based Cell Growth Determination Kit TOX-1 (Sigma-Aldrich, Israel Ltd. Rehovot 76100 ISRAEL) and the BrdU colorimetric kit (cat. 11 647 229001Roche), according to the manufacturer's instructions Each experiment was performed in triplicate.

Quantitative real time PCR (qPCR)

Total RNA of skin biopsies and cells was extracted using Ambion *mirVana*™ miRNA Isolation Kit. Quantification of miRNAs by *TaqManH* Real-Time PCR was performed on 10 ng RNA using the ABI 7900HT thermocycler (Applied Biosystems) for 40 cycles. Target miR/ gene expression was normalized between different samples based on the values of RNU48/Rplpo expression respectively.

In situ hybridization

In situ transcriptional levels of the different miRNAs were evaluated on paraffin-embedded skin biopsy specimens from 3 healthy skins and 5 psoriasis patients volunteers. Formalin-fixed tissues were dehydrated, embedded in paraffin and sectioned at 4 µm. A section of a healthy volunteer skin biopsy and 2 sections of involved and uninvolved skin from a psoriatic patient were placed on each slide. The slides were warmed up to 60°C for 1 h, de-waxed in xylene and rehydrated. Sections were hybridized overnight with digoxygenin-labeled miRCURY LNA probes (Exiqon, Denmark), and incubated with anti-digoxygenin antibody conjugated with alkaline phosphatase for 1 h. The color reaction was performed at 1–48 h. Counter staining was done by Nuclear Fast Red counter stain. The stained sections were reviewed with a light microscope and analyzed by a dermato pathologist who was blind to the tissue origin.

IGF-1R immunostaining

The formalin-fixed tissues were treated in the same manner as the ISH slides. Antigen retrieval was performed using a pressure cooker (Milestone, Microwave Laboratory Systems) at 120°C for 5 min in 0.1 M citrate buffer pH 6. The slides were blocked in 3% H2O2/MeOH and then incubated with primary antibody to IGF-1R (Abcam, ab54274, 1:750). Detection was performed with the Histostain SP Broad Spectrum kit (Zymed Laboratories, Inc. USA). The antibody binding was visualized with the substrate-chromogen AEC, counterstained with hematoxylin.

Cloning and plasmids

The plasmids pMSCV-miR-99a and pMSCV-HTR were kindly provided by Agami, R.[23].

A genomic fragment containing 1070 bp of the 3′UTR of IGF-1R mRNA (NCBI Reference Sequence: NM_000875.3) from position 9251 to 10320 was amplified by PCR using the following primers:

1-5′-ACAGGTCAGAGGGTTTC-3′; 2- 5′-CAGTCAAGT-CTTCCCATGT-3′.

PCR fragments were cloned into pCRII-TOPO plasmid (Invitrogen,USA). The XhoI fill-in KpnI fragment was cloned into psiCHECK-2 plasmid (Promega,USA) digested with XhoI and PmeI.

An IGF-1R 3′UTR mutant for the hsa-mir-99a seed sequence was created using the Megaprimer Mutagenesis assay [41,42] using primer 1 and primer 3: 5′-TAGAT**TATAAATA**GT-CAGTT-3′.

The hsa-miR-99a over expression oligo, Pre-miR miRNA precursor, was purchased from Ambion- Applied Biosystems. The miR-99a sponge expression plasmid was generated as follows: two complementary oligo nucleotides of ~120 bases were synthesized and annealed generating double stranded DNA containing four hsa-mir-99a "sponge" sequences with XhoI and XmaI restriction sites on either end. The double stranded DNA was cloned into XhoI and XmaI sites of pTurbofp635-c plasmid (Evroege, Russia). DNA synthesis and the cloning was performed by GenScript USA.

Determination of mRNA levels by RT-PCR

Total RNA was extracted using *mirVana*™ isolation kit (Applied Biosystems/Ambion, USA). RT-PCR was performed using the Verso thermo-scientific kit using the following primers:

krt14: 5′-AGCAGCAGAACCAGGAGTAACAAG-3′
5′-GGCGTAGGTGGCGATCT-3′
krt10: 5′- GCTGACATCAACGGCCT-3′
5′- AGCATTCATTTCCACATTCAC-3′
β-actin: 5′- CCTGGCACCCAGCACAAT -3′
5′- GCCGATCCACACGGAGTACT -3′

Transfections

293T cells were seeded at 0.5–1×10^5 cells per well and transfected by calcium phosphate in HEPES buffer method, as described [43].

HaCaT cells were transfected using Lipofectamine™ 2000 Reagent (Invitrogen,USA).

Luciferase Assay

Luciferase assay was performed 72 h post transfection using the The Dual-Luciferase® Reporter (DLR) Assay System (Promega,USA).

Determination of protein expression level by Western blotting (WB)

WB was performed as described previously [44], using primary specific antibody (IGF-1Rβ c20 CS-713 Santa Cruz Biotechnology, USA)/ (Beta Actin AC-15 (Abcam UK).

Supporting Information

Figure S1 The level of hsa-miR-203 in normal skin (N, n = 10), psoriatic lesional skin (P, n = 16), or psoriatic uninvolved skin (UI, n = 16) was determined by qPCR and normalized to Rnu48. Y bars are arbitrary units that define fold change. Each dot represents one sample. Average is denoted by the horizontal line. *P<0.009,**p<0.0001.

Figure S2 A) 293T cells were co-transfected with 10 ng psiCheck vector, or psiCheck-IGF-1R-3′UTR plasmid, together with 2 μg of hsa-miR-99a expressing plasmid. In addition cells were transfected with 0 μg, 2 μg, or 4 μg of miR-99a sponge expressing plasmid. 48 hours post transfection cells were harvested and subject to Dual-Luciferase Reporter assay. Each experiment was done in triplicates. The average of 3 wells transfected with vector lacking the IGF-1R 3′UTR and without miR-99a sponge expressing plasmid (vector+0) was valued as 100%. The average is of 4 independent experiments. Paired *t* test results; # p<0.0044, * p<0.0052. B) HaCaT cells were stably transfected with plasmid expressing miR-99a sponge, or with the vector plasmid. After, almost two months of G418 selection, the same amount of cells from each plate were harvested and subjected to Western blot analysis, using either IGF1R or actin antibodies, the graph is average of three experiments; densitometry and calculation were done with ImageJ. C) MTT assay of HaCaT cells expressing the miR-99a sponge plasmid (sponge) or the empty vector (vector). 4000 cells were seeded in each well of 96 well plates. 4 h after seeding MTT was added and counted as time 0. The graph represents an average of three experiments, in each experiment every time point is an average of three wells. D) Total RNA was extracted form vector expressing or miR-99a sponge expressing cells, and was subject to RT-PCR using specific primers as indicated, the graph is average of three experiments; densitometry and calculation were done with ImageJ.

Table S1 Summary of miRNAs that were change in each of the comparisons also marked whether these miRNAs were up regulated, or down regulated, or unchanged. In each miRNA the fold change is noted, marked in yellow these miRNAs that were chosen for further analysis. In the comparison of normal to psoriatic skin also added miRNAs that were shown to change by Sonkoly et. al.[2]. Among these miR-133a was marked as miRNA that did change in there work by 1.76 fold, and in our screening miR-133a did change by 1.8 fold (marked in blue), however, we defined as change two fold or more.

Table S2 Comparison of normal versus psoriatic lesional skin. Total RNA from normal skin (n = 3), psoriatic lesional (n = 3), was isolated using Ambion mirVana™ miRNA Isolation Kit. Two μg of total RNA from each sample were labeled with the mirVana miRNA Labeling Kit (Applied Biosystems/Ambion Austin, TX 78744-1832, USA). The normal was labeled red and the psoriasis green. The fluorescently-labeled RNA samples were hybridized to an expression array as previously described [1]. The array was scanned and analyzed using Genepix pro 4000 b Axon and JMP statistic software. After background-subtracted, normalized spot intensities presented as $\log_e$ of the scanned value, ratio calculated of N to P for individual spot is note (Each miRNA is represented on the CHIP either 4 or 8 times; the value is an average of all spots of the same miRNA). MiRNAs that were found to change more than two fold are highlighted as well as miRNAs that were further analysis.

Table S3 Comparison of normal versus uninvolved psoriatic skin. Total RNA from normal skin (n = 3), or psoriatic uninvolved skin (n = 3) was isolated using Ambion mirVana™ miRNA Isolation Kit. Two μg of total RNA from each sample were labeled with the mirVana miRNA Labeling Kit (Applied Biosystems/Ambion Austin, TX 78744-1832, USA). The normal was labeled green and uninvolved red. The fluorescently-labeled RNA samples were hybridized to an expression array as previously described [1]. The array was scanned and analyzed using Genepix pro 4000 b Axon and JMP statistic software. After background-subtracted, normalized spot intensities presented as $\log_e$ of the scanned value, ratio calculated of N to UI or for individual spot is note (Each miRNA is represented on the CHIP either 4 or 8 times; the value is an average of all spots of the same miRNA). MiRNAs that were found to change more than two fold are highlighted as well as miRNAs that were further analysis.

Table S4 Comparison of psoriatic versus uninvolved psoriatic skin. Calculation were taken from tables S2 and table S3 After background-subtracted, normalized spot intensities presented as $\log_e$ of the scanned value, ratio calculated of UI to P for individual spot is note (Each miRNA is represented on the CHIP either 4 or 8 times; the value is an average of all spots of the same miRNA). MiRNAs that were found to change more than two fold are highlighted as well as miRNAs that were further analysis.

Table S5 Patient characteristics.

Acknowledgments

We thank Nir Gefen and the entire laboratory of Prof. Izraeli at the Center for Cancer Research Sheba Medical Center Tel Hashomer, for fruitful discussions and valuable assistance throughout this study.

Author Contributions

Conceived and designed the experiments: GL YS DA. Performed the experiments: GL CA DA. Analyzed the data: GL AB EH YS DA. Contributed reagents/materials/analysis tools: AT BG FP EH. Wrote the paper: GL YS DA. Helped prepare the paraffin embedded blocks and helped perform the in situ hybridization assay: CM SP-C IB. Helped collect normal skin samples: AO.

References

1. Galadari I, Sharif MO, Galadari H (2005) Psoriasis: a fresh look. Clin Dermatol 23: 491–502.
2. Nestle FO, Kaplan DH, Barker J (2009) Psoriasis. N Engl J Med 361: 496–509.
3. Hwu WL, Yang CF, Fann CS, Chen CL, Tsai TF, et al. (2005) Mapping of psoriasis to 17q terminus. J Med Genet 42: 152–158.
4. Barker JN (2001) Genetic aspects of psoriasis. Clin Exp Dermatol 26: 321–325.
5. Elder JT, Nair RP, Henseler T, Jenisch S, Stuart P, et al. (2001) The genetics of psoriasis 2001: the odyssey continues. Arch Dermatol 137: 1447–1454.
6. Bowcock AM (2005) The genetics of psoriasis and autoimmunity. Annu Rev Genomics Hum Genet 6: 93–122.
7. Sagoo GS, Cork MJ, Patel R, Tazi-Ahnini R (2004) Genome-wide studies of psoriasis susceptibility loci: a review. J Dermatol Sci 35: 171–179.
8. Giardina E, Sinibaldi C, Novelli G (2004) The psoriasis genetics as a model of complex disease. Curr Drug Targets Inflamm Allergy 3: 129–136.
9. Bowcock AM, Shannon W, Du F, Duncan J, Cao K, et al. (2001) Insights into psoriasis and other inflammatory diseases from large-scale gene expression studies. Hum Mol Genet 10: 1793–1805.
10. Bowcock AM, Krueger JG (2005) Getting under the skin: the immunogenetics of psoriasis. Nat Rev Immunol 5: 699–711.
11. Schon MP, Boehncke WH (2005) Psoriasis. N Engl J Med 352: 1899–1912.
12. Jiang WY, Chattedee AD, Raychaudhuri SP, Raychaudhuri SK, Farber EM (2001) Mast cell density and IL-8 expression in nonlesional and lesional psoriatic skin. Int J Dermatol 40: 699–703.
13. Olsen PH, Ambros V (1999) The lin-4 regulatory RNA controls developmental timing in Caenorhabditis elegans by blocking LIN-14 protein synthesis after the initiation of translation. Dev Biol 216: 671–680.
14. Andl T, Murchison EP, Liu F, Zhang Y, Yunta-Gonzalez M, et al. (2006) The miRNA-processing enzyme dicer is essential for the morphogenesis and maintenance of hair follicles. Curr Biol 16: 1041–1049.
15. Yi R, O'Carroll D, Pasolli HA, Zhang Z, Dietrich FS, et al. (2006) Morphogenesis in skin is governed by discrete sets of differentially expressed microRNAs. Nat Genet 38: 356–362.
16. Lowes MA, Bowcock AM, Krueger JG (2007) Pathogenesis and therapy of psoriasis. Nature 445: 866–873.
17. Sonkoly E, Wei T, Janson PC, Saaf A, Lundeberg L, et al. (2007) MicroRNAs: Novel Regulators Involved in the Pathogenesis of Psoriasis? PLoS ONE 2: e610.
18. Xiao C, Calado DP, Galler G, Thai TH, Patterson HC, et al. (2007) MiR-150 controls B cell differentiation by targeting the transcription factor c-Myb. Cell 131: 146–159.
19. Grimson A, Farh KK, Johnston WK, Garrett-Engele P, Lim LP, et al. (2007) MicroRNA targeting specificity in mammals: determinants beyond seed pairing. Mol Cell 27: 91–105.
20. Hodak E, Gottlieb AB, Anzilotti M, Krueger JG (1996) The insulin-like growth factor 1 receptor is expressed by epithelial cells with proliferative potential in human epidermis and skin appendages: correlation of increased expression with epidermal hyperplasia. J Invest Dermatol 106: 564–570.
21. Wraight CJ, White PJ, McKean SC, Fogarty RD, Venables DJ, et al. (2000) Reversal of epidermal hyperproliferation in psoriasis by insulin-like growth factor I receptor antisense oligonucleotides. Nat Biotechnol 18: 521–526.
22. Krane JF, Gottlieb AB, Carter DM, Krueger JG (1992) The insulin-like growth factor I receptor is overexpressed in psoriatic epidermis, but is differentially regulated from the epidermal growth factor receptor. J Exp Med 175: 1081–1090.
23. Voorhoeve PM, le Sage C, Schrier M, Gillis AJ, Stoop H, et al. (2006) A genetic screen implicates miRNA-372 and miRNA-373 as oncogenes in testicular germ cell tumors. Cell 124: 1169–1181.
24. Sadagurski M, Yakar S, Weingarten G, Holzenberger M, Rhodes CJ, et al. (2006) Insulin-like growth factor 1 receptor signaling regulates skin development and inhibits skin keratinocyte differentiation. Mol Cell Biol 26: 2675–2687.
25. Deyrieux AF, Wilson VG (2007) In vitro culture conditions to study keratinocyte differentiation using the HaCaT cell line. Cytotechnology 54: 77–83.
26. Micallef L, Belaubre F, Pinon A, Jayat-Vignoles C, Delage C, et al. (2009) Effects of extracellular calcium on the growth-differentiation switch in immortalized keratinocyte HaCaT cells compared with normal human keratinocytes. Exp Dermatol 18: 143–151.
27. Ebert MS, Sharp PA (2010) MicroRNA sponges: Progress and possibilities. Rna.
28. Ebert MS, Neilson JR, Sharp PA (2007) MicroRNA sponges: competitive inhibitors of small RNAs in mammalian cells. Nat Methods 4: 721–726.
29. Yi R, Poy MN, Stoffel M, Fuchs E (2008) A skin microRNA promotes differentiation by repressing 'stemness'. Nature 452: 225–229.
30. Nickoloff BJ (1999) Skin innate immune system in psoriasis: friend or foe? J Clin Invest 104: 1161–1164.
31. Gudjonsson JE, Johnston A, Sigmundsdottir H, Valdimarsson H (2004) Immunopathogenic mechanisms in psoriasis. Clin Exp Immunol 135: 1–8.
32. Nickoloff BJ, Qin JZ, Nestle FO (2007) Immunopathogenesis of psoriasis. Clin Rev Allergy Immunol 33: 45–56.
33. Wagner LA, Brown T, Gil S, Frank I, Carter W, et al. (1999) The keratinocyte-derived cytokine IL-7 increases adhesion of the epidermal T cell subset to the skin basement membrane protein laminin-5. Eur J Immunol 29: 2530–2538.
34. Bonifati C, Trento E, Cordiali-Fei P, Carducci M, Mussi A, et al. (1997) Increased interleukin-7 concentrations in lesional skin and in the sera of patients with plaque-type psoriasis. Clin Immunol Immunopathol 83: 41–44.
35. Muzio M, Ni J, Feng P, Dixit VM (1997) IRAK (Pelle) family member IRAK-2 and MyD88 as proximal mediators of IL-1 signaling. Science 278: 1612–1615.
36. Wu Q, Jin H, Yang Z, Luo G, Lu Y, et al. MiR-150 promotes gastric cancer proliferation by negatively regulating the pro-apoptotic gene EGR2. Biochem Biophys Res Commun 392: 340–345.
37. Stefani G, Slack FJ (2008) Small non-coding RNAs in animal development. Nat Rev Mol Cell Biol 9: 219–230.
38. Sonkoly E, Wei T, Pavez Lorie E, Suzuki H, Kato M, et al. (2009) Protein Kinase C-Dependent Upregulation of miR-203 Induces the Differentiation of Human Keratinocytes. J Invest Dermatol.
39. Baskerville S, Bartel DP (2005) Microarray profiling of microRNAs reveals frequent coexpression with neighboring miRNAs and host genes. Rna 11: 241–247.
40. Rheinwald JG, Green H (1975) Formation of a keratinizing epithelium in culture by a cloned cell line derived from a teratoma. Cell 6: 317–330.
41. Colosimo A, Xu Z, Novelli G, Dallapiccola B, Gruenert DC (1999) Simple version of "megaprimer" PCR for site-directed mutagenesis. Biotechniques 26: 870–873.
42. Lai R, Bekessy A, Chen CC, Walsh T, Barnard R (2003) Megaprimer mutagenesis using very long primers. Biotechniques 34: 52–54, 56.
43. Ausubel FM, Brent R, Kingston RE, Moore DD, Seidman JG, et al. (1999) Short protocols in molecular biology. New York: Wiley.
44. Lilling G, Hacohen H, Nordenberg J, Livnat T, Rotter V, et al. (2000) Differential sensitivity of MCF-7 and LCC2 cells, to multiple growth inhibitory agents: possible relation to high bcl-2/bax ratio? Cancer Lett 161: 27–34.

Fibromodulin-Deficiency Alters Temporospatial Expression Patterns of Transforming Growth Factor-β Ligands and Receptors during Adult Mouse Skin Wound Healing

Zhong Zheng[1], Kevin S. Lee[1], Xinli Zhang[1], Calvin Nguyen[1], Chingyun Hsu[1], Joyce Z. Wang[2], Todd Matthew Rackohn[1], Dwarak Reddy Enjamuri[3], Maxwell Murphy[1], Kang Ting[1*], Chia Soo[4,5*]

1 Dental and Craniofacial Research Institute and Section of Orthodontics, School of Dentistry, University of California Los Angeles, Los Angeles, California, United States of America, **2** Department of Emergency Medicine, State University of New York Downstate/Kings Country Hospital Center, New York, New York, United States of America, **3** Department of Psychobiology, University of California Los Angeles, Los Angeles, California, United States of America, **4** UCLA and Orthopaedic Hospital Department of Orthopaedic Surgery and the Orthopaedic Hospital Research Center, University of California Los Angeles, Los Angeles, California, United States of America, **5** Division of Plastic and Reconstructive Surgery, Department of Surgery, School of Medicine, University of California Los Angeles, Los Angeles, California, United States of America

Abstract

Fibromodulin (FMOD) is a small leucine-rich proteoglycan required for scarless fetal cutaneous wound repair. Interestingly, increased FMOD levels have been correlated with decreased transforming growth factor (TGF)-β1 expression in multiple fetal and adult rodent models. Our previous studies demonstrated that FMOD-deficiency in adult animals results in delayed wound closure and increased scar size accompanied by loose package collagen fiber networks with increased fibril diameter. In addition, we found that FMOD modulates *in vitro* expression and activities of TGF-β ligands in an *isoform-specific* manner. In this study, temporospatial expression profiles of TGF-β ligands and receptors in FMOD-null and wild-type (WT) mice were compared by immunohistochemical staining and quantitative reverse transcriptase-polymerase chain reaction using a full-thickness, primary intention wound closure model. During the inflammatory stage, elevated inflammatory infiltration accompanied by increased type I TGF-β receptor levels in individual inflammatory cells was observed in FMOD-null wounds. This increased inflammation was correlated with accelerated epithelial migration during the proliferative stage. On the other hand, significantly more robust expression of TGF-β3 and TGF-β receptors in FMOD-null wounds during the proliferative stage was associated with delayed dermal cell migration and proliferation, which led to postponed granulation tissue formation and wound closure and increased scar size. Compared with WT controls, expression of TGF-β ligands and receptors by FMOD-null dermal cells was markedly reduced during the remodeling stage, which may have contributed to the declined collagen synthesis capability and unordinary collagen architecture. Taken together, this study demonstrates that a single missing gene, *FMOD*, leads to conspicuous alternations in TGF-β ligand and receptor expression at all stages of wound repair in various cell types. Therefore, FMOD critically coordinates temporospatial distribution of TGF-β ligands and receptors *in vivo*, suggesting that FMOD modulates TGF-β bioactivity in a complex way beyond simple physical binding to promote proper wound healing.

Editor: Zhongjun Zhou, The University of Hong Kong, Hong Kong

Funding: This study was supported by the Plastic Surgery Research Foundation (2013 National Endowment for Plastic Surgery Research Grant Program) and NIH-NIAMS (SBIR grant 1R43-AR064126). The funders had no role in study design, data collection and analysis, decision to publish, or preparation of the manuscript.

Competing Interests: Drs. Kang Ting, Chia Soo, and Zhong Zheng are inventors on fibromodulin-related patents filed from UCLA, including 'Fibromodulin peptides' (USA, Application No. PCT/US2010/036262; Europe, Application No. WO2010US36262; P. R. China, Application No. 201080023050.1; Korea, Application No. 2011-7030786; and Canada, Application No. CA 2763466), and 'Method and compositions for modulating myofibroblast activities' (Application No. PCT/US12/42517). Drs. Kang Ting, Chia Soo, and Zhong Zheng are founders of Scarless Laboratories Inc. which sublicenses fibromodulin-related patents from the US Regents. Dr. Chia Soo is also an officer of Scarless Laboratories, Inc.

* E-mail: kting@dentistry.ucla.edu (KT); bsoo@ucla.edu (CS)

These authors contributed equally to this work.

Introduction

Wound healing is a highly ordered and well-coordinated process involving inflammation, proliferation, and remodeling orchestrated by a myriad of cytokines and growth factors [1–3]. Transforming growth factor (TGF)-β, which is like a cytokine owing to its small molecular weight and selective effect on multiple inflammatory processes, is one of the most crucial modulators in wound healing [1–6]. TGF-β is produced by several cell types that are present in wound site including activated macrophages, neutrophils, platelets, fibroblasts, and keratinocytes [3,5,7]. Three mammalian TGF-β isoforms (TGF-β1, β2, and β3), which share 64–86% amino acid sequence homology, are all essential for wound healing regulation [5,8,9]. Interestingly, although all three TGF-β isoforms exert their effects by binding to transmembrane type II receptor (TβRII), which activates type I receptor (TβRI) to initiate signal transduction [10] they exhibit different and even opposite functions. For example, compared with TGF-β1 and β2, TGF-β3 presents more potent inhibition on DNA synthesis in keratinocytes [11]. Moreover, TGF-β1 significantly promotes migration of dermal fibroblasts, while TGF-β3 exerts remarkable anti-migratory effects on these cells [12–14]. In addition, TGF-β1 and β2 are known to promote fibroplasia, while TGF-β3 may or may not reduce scar [15–20]. It is worthy of note that TGF-βs can bind to a variety of extracellular matrix (ECM) proteins and regulate their expression and activities [21–26], and these ECM molecules in turn can modulate TGF-β expression and activities [21,27–29]. For instance, application of decorin, a small leucine-rich proteoglycan (SLRP) family member, for prevention of TGF-β-mediated fibrosis in various tissues is currently being attempted due to the high-affinity interactions between decorin and TGF-β isoforms [27–31].

To date, 18 SLRP family members have been discovered, which are grouped into five classes based mainly on evolutionary conservation, homology, and chromosomal organization [32]. Regardless of the classification, SLRPs share common functionality including interaction with diverse molecules such as TGF-βs, collagens, and other ECM molecules, and thus have wide-ranging functions from regulation of collagen matrix architecture and mechanical properties to control of cellular proliferation and differentiation [32–34]. Notably, fibromodulin (FMOD), a class II keratin sulphate SLRP, is essential for maintenance of endogenous stem cell niches [35]. In fact, FMOD-deficiency leads to osteogenesis of tendon stem/progenitor cells [35], resulting in a structurally and mechanically abnormal tendon phenotype [36,37]. Moreover, recent studies demonstrated that FMOD can directly reprogram somatic cells to a minimally proliferative, multipotent progenitor state [38], indicating that FMOD regulates intracellular signaling cascade and determines cell fate in addition to carrying out ECM structural functions [39].

In terms of skin wound repair, our previous studies have demonstrated that high expression of FMOD in fetal skin decreases during the transition from scarless fetal-type repair to adult-type repair with scarring [40,41]. Likewise, adult animals with FMOD-deficiency display abnormal wound healing: they exhibit delayed dermal wound closure and increased scar formation with reduced angiogenesis and unordinary collagen architecture [14,42]. Importantly, when we used FMOD to rescue rat fetal wounds at day 19 of gestation (E19) from scar formation, TGF-β1 expression was significantly decreased [40]. We have also found that FMOD modulates expression and activities of TGF-βs in an *isoform-specific* manner [14,40,41]. For example, FMOD potentiates TGF-β1-induced cell migration and reverses TGF-β3 inhibition of migration, governing timely epithelialization and granulation tissue formation. Thus, the relationship among FMOD expression, TGF-β activity, and scarring in both fetal and adult wound repair suggests that FMOD may exert anti-scarring effects by orchestrating TGF-β expression and function.

In this study, we investigated the temporospatial distribution of TGF-β ligands and receptors in both adult FMOD-null and wild-type (WT) mouse wounds to further elucidate how FMOD coordinates TGF-β bioactivity to promote proper cutaneous wound healing.

Materials and Methods

Ethics statement

All animal surgery procedures were performed under institutionally approved protocols provided by the Chancellor's Animal Research Committee at UCLA (protocol number: 2000–058).

Primary intention wound closure model

Three and one-half month old male 129/sv WT and FMOD-null mice [36] were anesthetized, and the dorsal skin was sterilely prepared [14]. Four full-thickness, 10 mm×3 mm skin ellipses with the underlying *panniculus carnosus* muscle were excised on each mouse. Each open wound edge was injected with 25 μl phosphate-buffered saline or 0.4 mg/ml recombinant FMOD solution (25 μl×2 edges = 50 μl total per wound). Wounds were then closed primarily with 4–0 Nylon using two simple interrupted sutures consistently placed at one-third intervals in each 10 mm length wound. All wounds were separated by at least 2 cm to minimize adjacent wound effects [14]. Sutures were removed at day 7 post-injury and wounds were harvested at 0.5, 1, 2, 3, 5, 7 and 14 days after injury. Unwounded skin samples from identical locations in three animals were collected as controls. Tissue for RNA isolation (entire wound +1 mm edge) was immediately frozen in liquid nitrogen and stored at −80°C until RNA extraction [14]. Wound tissue for histology (entire wound +10 mm edge) was bisected centrally between the two 4–0 Nylon sutures, perpendicular to the long axis of each 10 mm length wound, and placed in formalin [14].

Histology and immunohistochemistry

After fixation, skin samples (from 36 wounds of 16 animals per time point) were dehydrated, paraffin-embedded, and cut into 5-μm sections for hematoxylin and eosin (H&E) and immunohistochemical (IHC) staining. To ensure consistent sampling from the center rather than the periphery of the wound, specimens were sectioned starting from the areas of previous wound bisection. Immunohistochemistry staining was performed as previously described [43]. Relative inflammatory infiltration in 8 animals per genotype (2 randomly chosen wound edge fields and 2 randomly chosen wound bed fields per animal) was semi-quantitatively evaluated by three blinded reviewers using the following criteria:

Control: unwounded WT skin tissue ($\leq$2 inflammatory cells per field based on 32 randomly selected fields from 16 unwounded WT animals)

Score 0: <2 times the unwounded skin tissue

Score 1: 2–5 times the unwounded skin tissue

Score 2: 5–10 times the unwounded skin tissue

Score 3: 10–15 times the unwounded skin tissue

Score 4: >15 times the unwounded skin tissue.

All antibodies used in this study were obtained from Santa Cruz Biotech. (Santa Cruz, CA) except for the antibody against lumican that was purchased from Abcam Inc. (Cambridge, MA) (**Table 1**). Computerized immunolocalization intensity analysis was performed using the commercial software Image-Pro® Plus 6.0 (Media Cybernetics Inc., Rockville, MD). Relative dermal protein expression was quantified by the mean optical density of staining signal × percent area positively stained ×100 [14,44].

Quantitative reverse transcriptase-polymerase chain reaction (qRT-PCR)

Total RNA was extracted using TRIzol® Reagent (Invitrogen, Carlsbad, CA) and treated with RNase-Free DNase Set (Qiagen, Valencia, CA) to remove chromosomal DNA contamination. 1 μg total RNA was reverse transcribed into cDNA in a 20-μl reaction mixture with 50 pmol of oligo$(dT)_{20}$ primer and 1 μl (200 U) of SuperScript^{TM} III reverse transcriptase (Invitrogen). Expression of mRNA was measured by qRT-PCR using TaqMan® Gene Expression Assays (**Table 2**) on a 7500 Fast Real-time PCR System (Applied Biosystems, Foster City, CA) [14]. Concomitant

Table 1. Description of Primary Antibodies Used for Indirect Immunostaining.

Antibody	Initial Concentration	Origin	Epitope recognition	Final concentration (diluted in PBS)
TGF-β1 (V)	200 μg/ml	Rabbit polyclonal IgG	Extreme carboxy terminus of TGF-β1 (region of mature peptide)	0.002 g/L (1:100)
TGF-β2 (V)	200 μg/ml	Rabbit polyclonal IgG	Extreme carboxy terminus of TGF-β2 (region of mature peptide)	0.002 g/L (1:100)
TGF-β3 (V)	200 μg/ml	Rabbit polyclonal IgG	Extreme carboxy terminus of TGF-β3 (region of mature peptide)	0.002 g/L (1:100)
TβRI (V-22)	200 μg/ml	Rabbit polyclonal IgG	Carboxy terminus of TβRI (region of mature peptide)	0.002 g/L (1:100)
TβRII (C-16)	200 μg/ml	Rabbit polyclonal IgG	Carboxy terminus of TβRII (region of mature peptide)	0.002 g/L (1:100)
TβRIII (C-20)	200 μg/ml	Goat polyclonal IgG	Carboxy terminus of TβRIII (region of mature peptide)	0.002 g/L (1:100)
Lumican(L-20)	1000 μg/ml	Rabbit monoclonal IgG	Internal region of lumican	0.02 g/L (1:50)

glyceraldehyde-3-phosphate dehydrogenase (GAPDH) was also performed in separate tubes for each RT reaction with TaqMan® Rodent GAPDH control reagents (Applied Biosystems). For each gene, at least three separate sets of qRT-PCR analysis were performed using different complementary DNA templates.

Scratch wound assay

Primary dermal fibroblasts from WT and adult FMOD-null mice were derived and maintained following the published procedure [45]. A scratch wound assay was performed to mimic the scarring process *in vitro* [46]. Briefly, passage 3 dermal fibroblasts were grown in 6-well tissue culture plates until confluence. After 12 h serum starvation, the cell monolayer was scraped to generate a single 1-mm wide gap. The wounded monolayer was washed 3 times with phosphate-buffered saline (PBS) to remove dead cells prior to 24 h incubation in DMEM medium (Invitrogen). 100 pM TGF-β1 or -β3 (Sigma-Aldrich, St. Louis, MO) in PBS was used to regulate fibroblast migration [14], while 10 μM TβRI-specific inhibitor SB-431542 (Sigma-Aldrich) [47] was used to attenuate TβRI-mediated TGF-β bioactivities. Cell migration was documented by photographs taken immediately after scraping, as well as 24 h later. Migration was quantified by measuring the average wound gap between the wound edges before and after the treatment using the commercial software Image-Pro® Plus 6.0, and calculated as: Cell migration (%) = $(Gap_{0h}\text{-}Gap_{24h})/Gap_{0h} \times 100\%$.

Statistical analysis

The results are graphically depicted as the mean ± the standard error of mean. Statistical significance was computed using ANOVA (13.0 for Windows, SPSS, Chicago, IL). Independent-sample *t*-test was used to compare results of two groups. Individual comparisons between two groups were determined using the Mann-Whitney test for non-parametric data. *P* value <0.05 was considered statistically significant.

Table 2. TaqMan® Gene Expression Assay.

Gene	Genbank no.	TaqMan® Gene Expression Assay no.*
TGF-β1	NM_011577.1	Mm00441724_m1
TGF-β2	NM_009367.1	Mm00436952_m1
TGF-β3	NM_009368.1	Mm00436960_m1
TβRI	NM_009370.2	Mm00436971_m1
TβRII	NM_009371.2	Mm00466494_s1
TβRIII	NM_011578.2	Mm00803538_m1

* Commercial TaqMan® Gene Expression Assays were purchased from Applied Biosystems, Foster City, CA, USA.

Results

FMOD-null mice exhibit increased inflammation

Wound inflammatory infiltration was scored from 1 (minimal) to 4 (high) by three independent pathologists using the criteria described in **Materials and Methods** section. At day 0.5 post-injury, WT wounds showed minimal inflammatory cell numbers (score: 1) within the fibrin clot at the wound edge and significant inflammatory infiltrate (score: 3) at the wound base upon H&E staining (**Figure 1A**). At the same locations, FMOD-null wounds showed moderate inflammatory cell numbers (score: 2) at the wound edge and, like WT wounds, significant inflammatory infiltrate (score: 3) at the wound base (**Figure 1A**). For both genotypes, neutrophils comprised the major inflammatory cell type present at day 0.5 post-injury, followed by monocytes (about 10%) and lymphocytes (about 5%). At day 1 post-injury, WT wounds exhibited mildly to moderately elevated inflammatory infiltrate at both the wound edge and wound base (score: 2 to 3) (**Figure 1B**), with a higher lymphocyte proportion at the wound periphery (about 15%). In contrast, highly increased inflammatory infiltrate (score: 4) was observed at both the wound edge and wound base of FMOD-null mice at day 1 post-injury (**Figure 1B**). Macrophages were noted 1 day after injury at the wound base of FMOD-null mice, and not until 2 days after injury in WT mice. Overall, FMOD-null mice demonstrated higher inflammatory infiltration than WT animals before wound closure (**Figure 1C**), and inflammatory cell density was significantly reduced with macrophages as the dominant immune cell type (above 50%) in both genotypes after would closure.

TGF-β1 protein expression is elevated in migrating epidermis and granulation tissue of FMOD-null wounds

To determine how FMOD-deficiency affects wound healing, expression of TGF-β ligands and receptors was documented in adult FMOD-null mice and compared with that in WT controls. Cellular and ECM TGF-β ligand and receptor immunostaining patterns are shown in **Figure 2** (which provides information on global TGF-β ligand and receptor staining and relative cell density), while the dermal protein expression and relative total wound mRNA transcription levels are summarized in **Figure 3** (for TGF-β ligands) and **Figure 4** (for TGF-β receptors). In addition, specific staining intensities for epidermal, dermal,

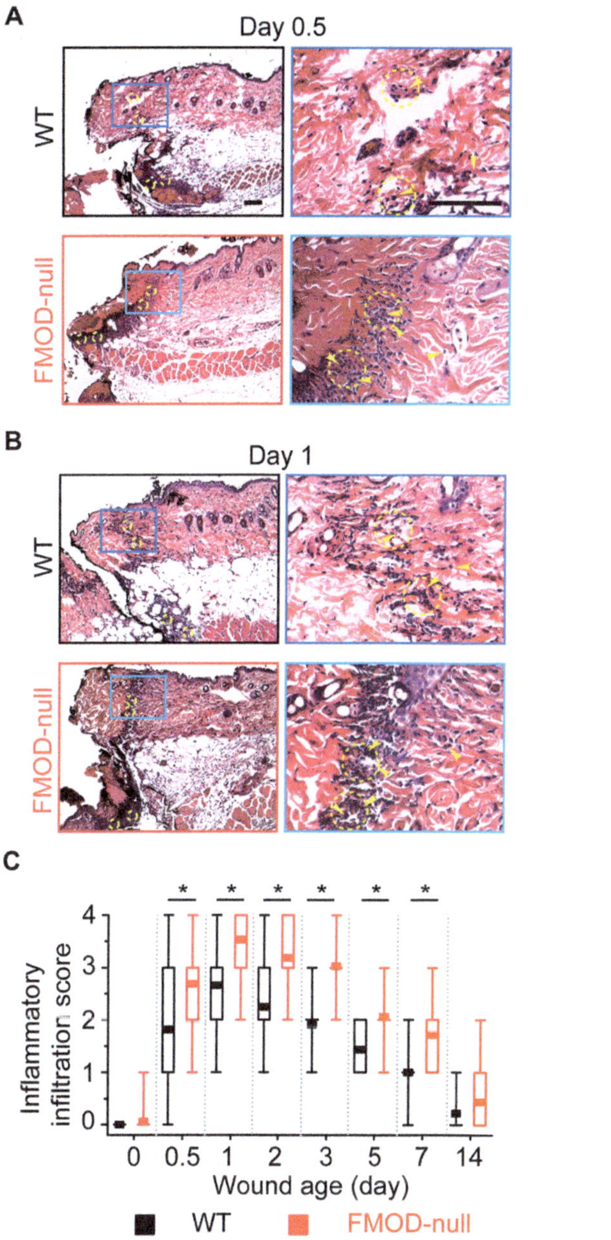

Figure 1. Hematoxylin and eosin (H&E) staining of wounded WT and FMOD-null adult mice skin. (**A**) At day 0.5 post-injury, minimal (score: 1) inflammatory infiltrate was present at the wound edge of WT mice (*upper right*), while significant (score: 3) inflammatory infiltrate was detected at the wound base. On the other hand, moderate (score: 2) and significant inflammatory infiltrates were observed at the wound edge (*lower right*) and base of FMOD-null mice, respectively. (**B**) At day 1 post-injury, moderate and significant inflammatory infiltrates were seen at the wound edge (*upper right*) and base of WT mice, respectively. Meanwhile, high (score: 4) inflammatory infiltrate was observed at both the wound edge (*lower-right*) and base of FMOD-null mice. (**C**) Relative inflammatory infiltration (median, 25–75% quartile, min, max) in 8 animals per genotype (2 randomly chosen wound edge fields and 2 randomly chosen wound bed fields per animal; N = 32) was semi-quantitatively evaluated by three blinded reviewers. Yellow arrowheads: representative inflammatory cells (not all inflammatory cells are indicated); yellow circles: randomly chosen fields for inflammatory infiltration evaluation. Bar = 100 μm. *, significant difference determined by the Mann-Whitney test.

inflammatory, and hair follicle cell types are summarized in **Tables 3** and **4** (which provide information on individual cell TGF-β ligand and receptor staining intensities, respectively).

During the wound healing process, although the relative inflammatory infiltrate (primarily comprised of neutrophils, monocytes, and macrophages) was greater in FMOD-null wounds compared with WT wounds (**Figure 1**), the TGF-β1 staining intensity for the individual inflammatory cells was relatively similar between WT and FMOD-null wounds (**Figure 2A** and **Table 3**). Strong (+++) TGF-β1 staining was observed at the epithelial wound edge in both WT and FMOD-null genotypes (**Table 3**). TGF-β1 staining was detected at the migrating epidermis at day 1 post-injury in FMOD-null mice, while TGF-β1 staining was hardly observed at the migrating epidermis in WT mice at the same wound healing stage (**Figure 2A** and **Table 3**). With respect to fibroblasts, both WT and FMOD-null mice exhibited negligible (−) TGF-β1 staining prior to injury, but TGF-β1 signals were increased to moderate (++) levels in about 10% of FMOD-null fibroblasts at day 1 post-injury and in WT fibroblasts at day 2 (**Table 3** and **Figure 3A**). These observations correlated with the qRT-PCR data demonstrating similar *TGF-β1* expression levels in WT and FMOD-null mice before injury and before wound closure (**Figure 3B**). However, after wound closure (day 3 for WT wounds and day 5 for FMOD-null wounds [14]), TGF-β1 staining intensity in WT and FMOD-null fibroblasts increased to strong levels at days 7 and 14 (**Figure 2A** and **Table 3**). At day 7 post-injury, ECM of WT granulation tissue showed only minimal TGF-β1 signals, while ECM of FMOD-null granulation tissue showed strong TGF-β1 staining that contributed to significantly higher total dermal TGF-β1 protein expression levels in FMOD-null wounds (**Table 3**, **Figures 2A** and **3A**). Peak TGF-β1 ECM staining at day 7 coincided with peak fibroblast density rather than peak inflammatory cell density in FMOD-null wounds – suggesting that the source of elevated ECM TGF-β1 in FMOD-null wounds is likely fibroblasts rather than inflammatory cells. Interestingly, total *TGF-β1* mRNA expression when normalized to *GAPDH* was significantly higher in WT wounds than in FMOD-null wounds during the entire 14-day experimental period (**Figure 3B**), while total dermal TGF-β1 protein expression levels were significantly higher in FMOD-null wounds at day 7 post-injury (**Figure 3A**). The reason for this apparent discrepancy between TGF-β1 mRNA and protein expression profiles at day 7 may be that qRT-PCR results are reflective of gene expression per cell, and thus do not take into account the increased cell density in day 7 FMOD-null granulation tissue (**Figure 2A** and *ref.* [14]). In contrast, IHC results are reflective of total TGF-β1 protein expression quantity in all the cells present within the granulation tissues. Cell density was significantly higher in FMOD-null wounds at day 7 post-injury, but a single WT cell may have had a relatively higher *TGF-β1* mRNA transcriptional activity than a single FMOD-null cell. Thus, the total amount of stained TGF-β1 protein was higher in FMOD-null wounds at day 7 post-injury. Overall, WT and FMOD-null wounds demonstrated similar TGF-β1 staining intensities for inflammatory cells, epidermal cells, hair follicles, and fibroblasts. However, epidermal TGF-β1 staining was significantly more pronounced in FMOD-null mice relative to WT mice at day 1 post-injury, while TGF-β1 staining in ECM of granulation tissue was more prominent in FMOD-null mice at day 7 post-injury.

TGF-β2 expression in FMOD-null wounds is increased at early wound stage but decreased after wound closure

After injury, inflammatory cell TGF-β2 staining intensity was increased to strong levels at day 0.5 post-wounding, but reduced to

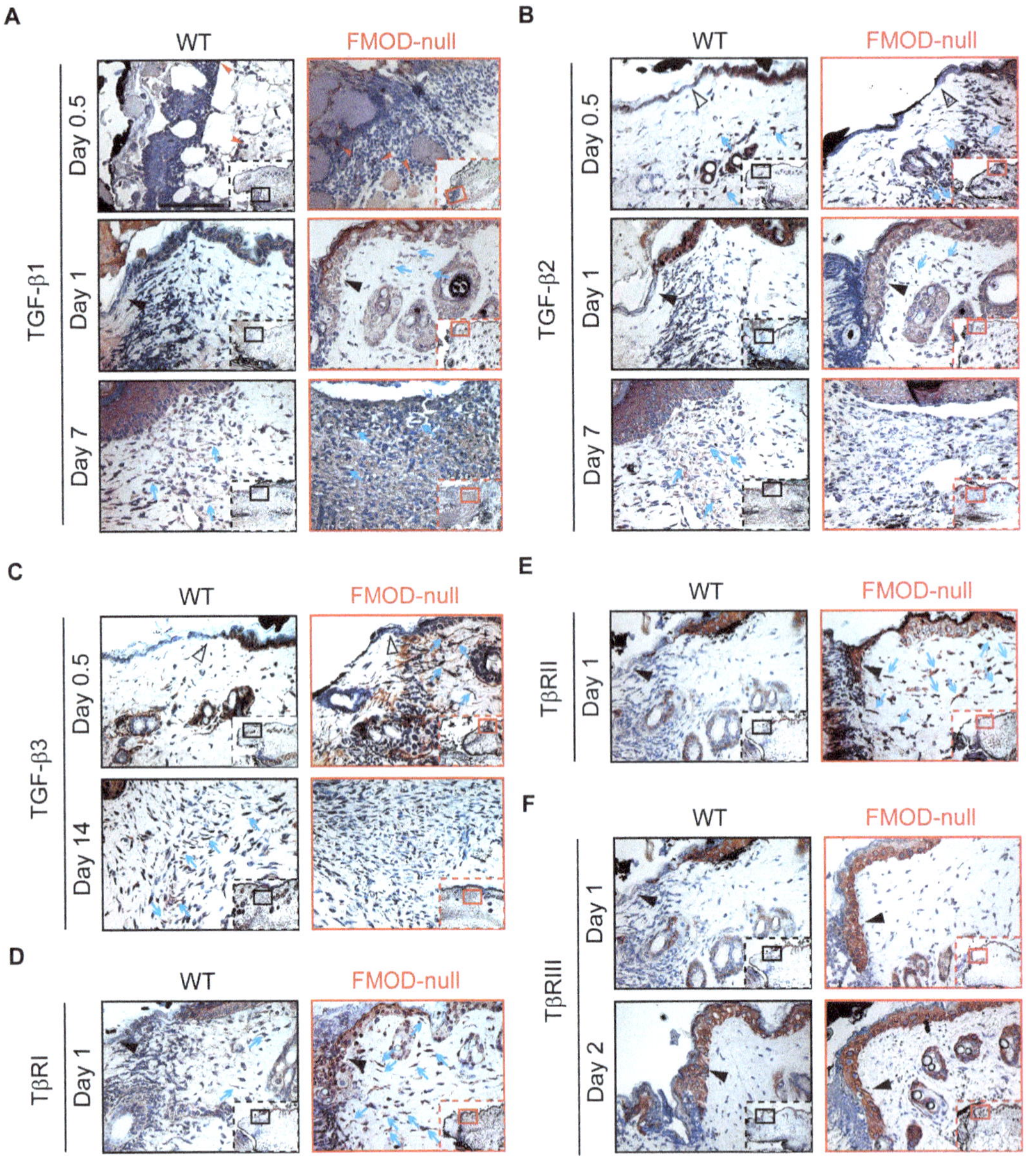

Figure 2. Immunohistochemical (IHC) staining of wounded WT and FMOD-null adult mice skin. (**A**) TGF-β1, (**B**) TGF-β2, (**C**) TGF-β3, (**D**) TβRI, (**E**) TβRII, and (**F**) TβRIII. Inserts show low magnification view. Red arrowheads: inflammatory cells; open black triangles: epidermis at wound edge; solid black triangles: migrating epidermal tongues; blue arrows: dermal fibroblasts. Bar = 100 μm.

negligible levels at days 7 and 14 in WT and FMOD-null mice (**Table 3**). Unwounded skin exhibited strong TGF-β2 staining in epidermis and hair follicles, but TGF-β2 levels in WT and FMOD-null epithelial wound edges dropped to negligible levels without a marked difference between the two genotypes at day 0.5 post-injury (**Table 3**). With respect to fibroblasts, WT displayed strong TGF-β2 staining intensity at day 0.5 post-injury that diminished by day 1 post-injury, followed by an upswing in TGF-β2 expression that peaked at day 7 (**Figure 2B** and **Table 3**). Meanwhile, FMOD-null fibroblasts presented strong TGF-β2 signals during day 0.5 to day 2 post-injury that disappeared after wound closure (**Figure 2B** and **Table 3**). After wound closure, TGF-β2 signals were moderate in WT granulation tissue ECM at day 7 that decreased to minimal levels by day 14 post-injury (**Figure 2B** and **Table 3**), while minimal TGF-β2 staining was observed in FMOD-null granulation tissue ECM at days 7 and 14 (**Figure 2B**, **Table 3**). In addition, total dermal TGF-β2 protein staining (**Figure 3C**) and *TGF-β2* mRNA transcriptional activity (**Figure 3D**) were significantly higher in FMOD-null wounds at day 0.5 post-injury relative to WT wounds. Unlike TGF-β1, both total dermal TGF-β2 staining (**Figure 3C**) and *TGF-β2* mRNA transcription (**Figure 3D**) analyses showed that TGF-β2 levels were significantly decreased in FMOD-null granulation tissue at day 7 post-injury. Overall, TGF-β2 expression in FMOD-null wounds was higher at the early wound edge but lower after wound closure compared with that in WT wounds.

TGF-β3 expression in FMOD-null mice is boosted at day 0.5 post-injury but becomes lower than WT expression at day 14 post-injury

In WT and FMOD-null mice, inflammatory cell TGF-β3 staining was negligible in unwounded tissue, increased during days

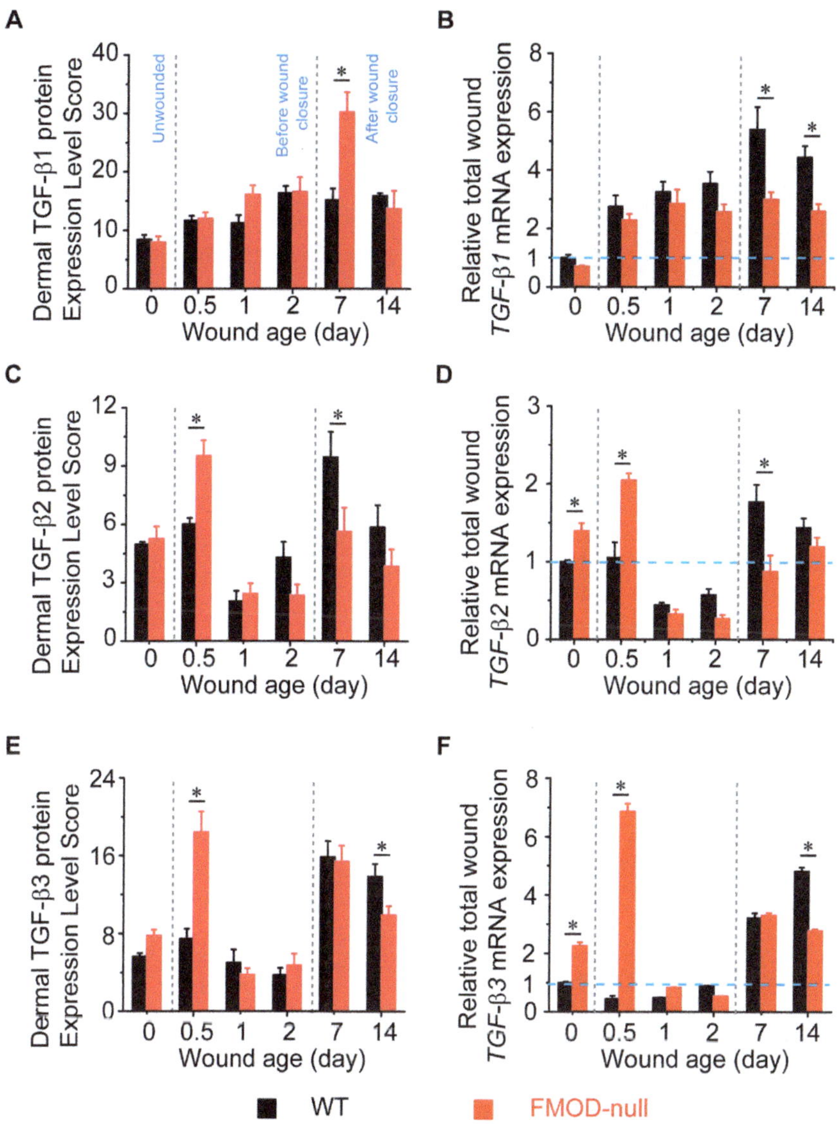

Figure 3. Quantification of dermal protein expression (A, C, E; N = 9) and total wound RNA (B, D, F; N = 4) expression of TGF-β ligands. (**A, B**) TGF-β1, (**C, D**) TGF-β2, and (**E, F**) TGF-β3. RNA expression is normalized to unwounded WT skin (blue dotted line). *, $P<0.05$.

1 and 2 post-injury, and returned to the baseline levels after wound closure (**Table 3**). Similar to TGF-β1 and -β2, unwounded skin showed strong TGF-β3 staining in epidermis and adjacent hair follicles of both WT and FMOD-null groups (**Table 3**), but the TGF-β3 expression dwindled by day 0.5 post-injury (**Table 3**). As described in our previous observation [14], in contrast to WT wounds with negligible ECM and fibroblast TGF-β3 staining, FMOD-null wounds displayed strong TGF-β3 signals in both the ECM and ~25% of dermal fibroblasts at day 0.5 post-injury (**Figure 2C** and **Table 3**). This finding correlated with higher total dermal TGF-β3 protein expression (**Figure 3E**) and mRNA transcription at day 0.5 (**Figure 3F**). At day 14 post-injury, WT fibroblasts displayed strong TGF-β3 staining while FMOD-null fibroblasts only exhibited negligible signals (**Figure 2C** and **Table 3**). Thus, TGF-β3 expression was relatively higher in WT wounds than FMOD-null wounds at day 14 post-injury (**Figure 3E, F**).

Expression of TGF-β receptors is increased in FMOD-null wounds at early stage of wound healing

For WT and FMOD-null mice, individual inflammatory cell TβRI [*aka.* activin receptor-like kinase 5, (ALK5)] staining was negligible in unwounded tissues. At day 0.5 post-injury, inflammatory cells exhibited moderate TβRI staining in FMOD-null wounds but negligible staining in WT wounds (**Table 4**). From days 1 to 2 post-injury, inflammatory cells of both groups presented strong TβRI signals, which returned to negligible levels by day 7 (**Table 4**). Meanwhile, strong TβRI staining was found in the migrating epidermis of FMOD-null mice at day 1 post-injury but not in WT controls (**Figure 2D** and **Table 4**). Interestingly, elevated expression of lumican – another class II SLRP that binds to TβRI and thus promotes epithelial migration [48] – was also found in the FMOD-null migrating epidermis as evidenced by IHC staining (**Figure S1**). As we reported previously [14], more dermal fibroblasts strongly expressing TβRI were found in FMOD-null wounds than in WT wounds, although

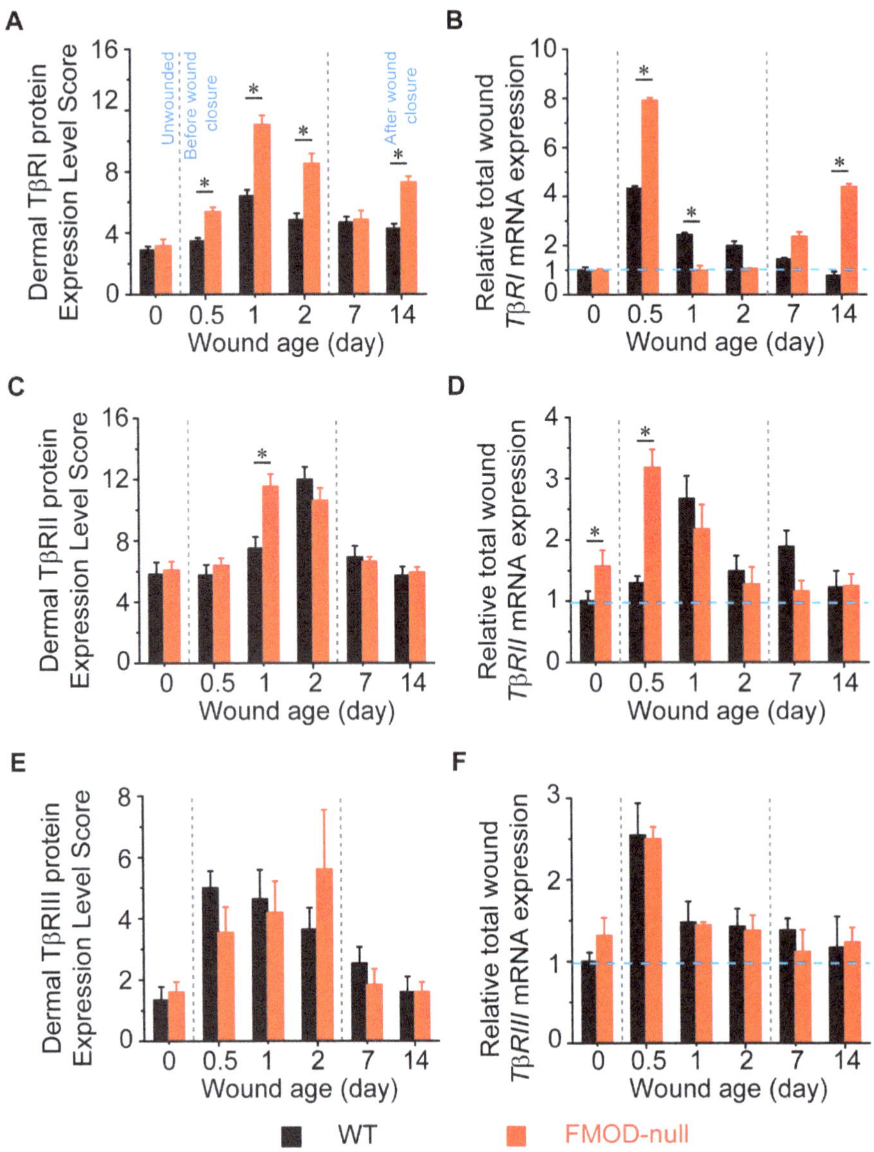

Figure 4. Quantification of dermal protein expression (A, C, E; N = 9) and total wound RNA (B, D, F; N = 4) expression of TGF-β receptors. (**A, B**) TβRI, (**C, D**) TβRII, and (**E, F**) TβRIII. RNA expression is normalized to unwounded WT skin (blue dotted line). *, $P<0.05$.

similar staining density was observed in both wounds (**Figure 2D** and **Table 4**). Unwounded WT and FMOD-null skin tissues had similar total TβRI expression (**Figure 4A, B**). After injury, *TβRI* transcripts of WT mice peaked at day 0.5 post-injury and slowly decreased to baseline levels by day 14 (**Figure 2B**). *TβRI* transcripts of FMOD-null mice also peaked at 0.5 day post-injury, but were ~1.84 times WT *TβRI* transcripts at the same time point (**Figure 4B**). FMOD-null *TβRI* mRNA levels then rapidly declined to baseline by day 1, but rebounded at days 7 and 14 (**Figure 4B**). Generally, the trends in TβRI protein expression paralleled its mRNA transcription pattern, but were relatively delayed and less dramatic in the degree of changes. Overall, total dermal cell TβRI protein was significantly increased in FMOD-null wounds relative to WT wounds at 0.5, 1, 2 and 14 days after injury (**Figure 4A**).

WT and FMOD-null wounds exhibited similar TβRII staining intensities for individual inflammatory cells at all examined time points (**Table 4**). Our previous studies [14] have already demonstrated that TβRII staining in unwounded WT epidermis, hair follicles, and dermal fibroblasts transiently drops to negligible levels at days 0.5 and 1 post-injury before returning to strong levels by day 2 (**Figure 2E** and **Table 4**). On the contrary, the strong TβRII staining in unwounded FMOD-null epidermis and hair follicles persisted at the same levels during the entire 14-day experimental period (**Figure 2E** and **Table 4**). In addition, FMOD-null fibroblasts exhibited strong TβRII signals from days 0.5 to 7 post-injury until receding to minimal levels of unwounded skin at day 14 (**Figure 2E** and **Table 4**). Similar to TβRI (**Figure 4A, B**), there was a lag phase between the peak mRNA transcription and protein expression of TβRII (**Figure 4C, D**). The reason behind the lag between TβRII mRNA and protein expression is unclear, but it has been described in a mouse embryonic model [49]. In sum, these data demonstrated that FMOD-null wounds have higher TβRII expression than WT wounds during the first 24 hours post-injury.

Table 3. Relative Immunostaining Intensity of TGF-β Ligands in Wounded WT and FMOD-null Adult Mice*.

After injury	Unwounded		0.5 day		1 day		2 days		7 days		14 days	
TGF-β1	**WT***	**FN***	**WT**	**FN**	**WT**	**FN**	**WT**	**FN**	**WT**	**FN**	**WT**	**FN**
Epidermis												
Migrating epi.	N/A*	N/A	N/A	N/A	−*	+++*	+++	+++	N/A	N/A	N/A	N/A
Outer layer	+++	+++	+++	+++	+++	+++	+++	+++	+++	+++	+++	+++
Basal layer	+++	+++	+++	+++	+++	+++	+++	+++	+++	+++	+++	+++
Dermis												
ECM	−	−	−	−	−	−	−	−	+*	+++	+	+
Fibroblasts	−	−			−	++*	++	++	+++	+++	+++	+++
Inflammatory cells†	−	−	++	++	++	++	+++	+++	+++	+++	+++	+++
Hair follicles‡	+++	+++	+++	+++	+++	+++	+++	+++	+++	+++	+++	+++
After injury	**Unwounded**		**0.5 day**		**1 day**		**2 days**		**7 days**		**14 days**	
TGF-β2	**WT**	**FN**	**WT**	**FN**	**WT**	**FN**	**WT**	**FN**	**WT**	**FN**	**WT**	**FN**
Epidermis												
Migrating epi.	N/A	N/A	N/A	N/A	−	+++	+++	+++	N/A	N/A	N/A	N/A
Outer layer	+++	+++	−	−	+++	+++	+++	+++	+++	+++	+++	+++
Basal layer	+++	+++	−	−	+++	+++	+++	+++	+++	+++	+++	+++
Dermis												
ECM	−	−	−	−	−	−	−	−	++	+	+	+
Fibroblasts	−	−	+++	+++	−	+++	+	+++	+++	−	−	−
Inflammatory cells	−	−	+++	+++	+++	+++	++	++	−	−	−	−
Hair follicles	+++	+++	+++	+++	+++	+++	+++	+++	+++	+++	+++	+++
After injury	**Unwounded**		**0.5 day**		**1 day**		**2 days**		**7 days**		**14 days**	
TGF-β3	**WT**	**FN**	**WT**	**FN**	**WT**	**FN**	**WT**	**FN**	**WT**	**FN**	**WT**	**FN**
Epidermis												
Migrating epi.	N/A	N/A	N/A	N/A	−	+++	+++	+++	N/A	N/A	N/A	N/A
Outer layer	+++	+++	−	−	+++	+++	+++	+++	++	++	++	++
Basal layer	+++	+++	−	−	+++	+++	+++	+++	+++	+++	+++	+++
Dermis												
ECM	−	−	−	+++	+	++	−	−	+	+	+	−
Fibroblasts	−	−	−	+++	+	++	+	+	++	++	+++	−
Inflammatory cells	−	−	−	−	++	+	−	++	−	−	−	−
Hair follicles	+++	+++	−	−	+++	+++	+++	+++	+++	+++	+++	+++

* WT, wild-type; FN, FMOD-null; N/A, not applicable; −, negligible staining (<5%); +, minimal staining (5%–25%); ++, moderate staining (25%–50%); +++, strong staining (>50%).
†In general, unwounded control skin contained very few inflammatory cells. The chart reflects the intensity of intracellular TGF-β staining and not the actually number of inflammatory cells present.
‡Due to no hair follicle regeneration was detected in the adult skin wounds in this study, the chart reflects the influence of the wounds on adjacent hair follicles.

Table 4. Relative Immunostaining Intensity of TGF-β Receptors in Wounded WT and FMOD-null Adult Mice.

After injury	Unwounded		0.5 day		1 day		2 days		7 days		14 days	
TβRI	**WT***	**FN***	**WT**	**FN**	**WT**	**FN**	**WT**	**FN**	**WT**	**FN**	**WT**	**FN**
Epidermis												
Migrating epi.	N/A*	N/A	−*	−	−	+++*	+++	+++	N/A	N/A	N/A	N/A
Outer layer	+++	+++	−	−	+++	+++	+++	+++	+++	+++	+++	+++
Basal layer	+++	+++	−	−	+++	+++	+++	+++	+++	+++	+++	+++
Dermis												
ECM	−	−	−	−	−	−	−	−	−	−	−	−
Fibroblasts	+++	+++	−	++*	+++	+++	+++	+++	+++	+++	+++	+++
Inflammatory cells†	−	−	−	++	+++	+++	+++	+++	−	−	−	−
Hair follicles‡	+++	+++	−	−	+*	+	+++	+++	+++	+++	+++	+++
After injury	**Unwounded**		**0.5 day**		**1 day**		**2 days**		**7 days**		**14 days**	
TβRII	**WT**	**FN**	**WT**	**FN**	**WT**	**FN**	**WT**	**FN**	**WT**	**FN**	**WT**	**FN**
Epidermis												
Migrating epi.	N/A	N/A	−	+++	−	+++	+++	+++	N/A	N/A	N/A	N/A
Outer layer	+++	+++	−	+++	+++	+++	+++	+++	+++	+++	+++	+++
Basal layer	+++	+++	−	+++	+++	+++	+++	+++	+++	+++	+++	+++
Dermis												
ECM	−	−	−	−	−	−	−	−	−	−	−	−
Fibroblasts	+	+	−	+++	−	+++	+++	+++	+++	+++	+	+
Inflammatory cells	−	−	−	−	+++	+++	+++	+++	++	++	−	−
Hair follicles	+++	+++	−	+++	−	+++	+++	+++	+++	+++	+++	+++
After injury	**Unwounded**		**0.5 day**		**1 day**		**2 days**		**7 days**		**14 days**	
TβRIII	**WT**	**FN**	**WT**	**FN**	**WT**	**FN**	**WT**	**FN**	**WT**	**FN**	**WT**	**FN**
Epidermis												
Migrating epi.	N/A	N/A	−	−	−	+++	+++	+++	N/A	N/A	N/A	N/A
Outer layer	+++	+++	+++	+++	+++	+++	+++	+++	++	+++	+++	++
Basal layer	+++	+++	+++	+++	+++	+++	+++	+++	+++	+++	+++	+++
Dermis												
ECM	−	−	−	−	−	−	−	−	−	−	−	−
Fibroblasts	−	−	−	−	−	−	−	−	−	−	−	−
Inflammatory cells	−	−	−	−	−	−	−	−	−	−	−	−
Hair follicles	+++	+++	−	−	+	+++	++	+++	++	+++	+++	+++

* WT, wild-type; FN, FMOD-null; N/A, not applicable; −, negligible staining (<5%); +, minimal staining (5%–25%); ++, moderate staining (25%–50%); +++, strong staining (>50%).

†In general, unwounded control skin contained very few inflammatory cells. The chart reflects the intensity of intracellular TGF-β receptor staining and not the actually number of inflammatory cells present.

‡Due to no hair follicle regeneration was detected in the adult skin wounds in this study, the chart reflects the influence of the wounds on adjacent hair follicles.

The epidermis and hair follicles of unwounded WT and FMOD-null mice exhibited strong type III TGF-β receptor (TβRIII, *aka.* betaglycan) staining (**Table 4**). Both genotypes lost TβRIII signals in the migrating epidermis at day 0.5 post-injury but re-gained strong baseline levels by day 1 for FMOD-null wounds and day 2 for WT wounds (**Figure 2F** and **Table 4**). WT hair follicles demonstrated minimal (day 1) to strong (day 14) TβRIII staining, while strong TβRIII signals were observed in FMOD-null hair follicles from days 1 to 14 (**Table 4**). No obvious TβRIII staining was detected in dermal inflammatory cells, ECM, or fibroblasts in either genotype during the entire experimental period (**Table 4**). As such, no significant deviation from the baseline for total TβRIII expression was detected (**Figure 4E, F**). Meanwhile, the lack of ECM staining indicated that the majority of TβRIII protein existed in the membrane-anchored form rather than the soluble form [50]. Taken together, all three TβRs were upregulated in FMOD-null wounds in comparison with WT wounds, especially at early wound healing stages.

TβRI is essential in TGF-β modulation of dermal fibroblast migration

Consistent with our previous studies [14], FMOD-null dermal fibroblasts demonstrated significantly less motility in comparison with WT controls (**Figure S2** and **Figure 5**). TGF-β1 restored FMOD-null fibroblast migration to PBS-treated WT levels, while TGF-β1 markedly increased WT dermal fibroblast migration (**Figure S2**). Although TβRI-specific inhibitor SB-431542 reduced WT fibroblast migration, SB-431542 did not considerably influence FMOD-null dermal fibroblast migration (**Figure S2**). However, SB-431542 markedly attenuated the pro-migratory effects of TGF-β1 on both WT and FMOD-null fibroblasts (**Figure S2**). On the other hand, TGF-β3 significantly inhibited WT and FMOD-null dermal fibroblast migration to 50% and 8%, respectively, of PBS control levels (**Figure 5**). Surprisingly, SB-431542 entirely prevented TGF-β3's inhibition on WT and FMOD-null fibroblast migration (**Figure 5**), indicating that the anti-motility effect of TGF-β3 on dermal fibroblasts is dependent on TβRI-mediated signal transduction.

Discussion

In a rat fetal wound model, we previously demonstrated elevated FMOD expression as a potential mechanism for scarless healing in fetal wounds at day 16 of gestation (E16) relative to scarring E19 wounds [41]. Moreover, we restored scarless repair in normally scarring E19 skin wounds by FMOD protein application, while FMOD blockade by anti-FMOD antibodies induced scar in normally scarless E16 wounds [40]. With respect to adult wound repair, the role of FMOD in regulating collagen fibrillogenesis was elucidated in our previous studies using FMOD-null mice, which exhibited loose package collagen fiber networks with increased fibril diameter [42]. We also found that FMOD-deficiency dramatically altered adult mouse wound healing, leading to delayed dermal cell migration, granulation tissue formation and wound closure, decreased vascularity, and increased scar size accompanied by less orderly collagen architecture [14,42]. Based on these findings, adenoviral FMOD administration was used to ameliorate adult rabbit wound healing [51]. In addition, recent studies revealed that FMOD expression is reduced in human post-burn hypertrophic scar [52,53]. These studies indicate that FMOD is profoundly involved in cutaneous wound healing.

Remarkably, FMOD and TGF-β1 levels showed inverse trends in both fetal and adult wound healing processes (as one increases the other decreases and *vice versa*) [40,41,43,53]. Specifically, in adult wounded mice, higher TβRI levels in FMOD-null inflammatory cells indicate that FMOD-deficiency enhanced chemotactic response of these cells towards TGF-β ligands [54,55], which may have contributed to the successively increased inflammatory cell recruitment in FMOD-null animals soon after injury. In addition, TGF-βs could have promoted inflammatory infiltration either directly or by inducing inflammatory cell activation and synthesis of multifunctional cytokines (such as interleukins, tumor necrosis factor-α, and platelet-derived growth factor) [54–56]. Since inflammatory cells that initially infiltrated FMOD-null wounds exhibited higher sensitivity to TGF-βs than those in WT wounds due to the increased TβRI expression, the inflammatory autocrine network may have been strengthened [54,55,57], resulting in the relatively exaggerated inflammatory response in FMOD-deficient animals during the entire wound healing period. It is worthy of note that the infiltrating inflammatory cells not only combat invading pathogens but also participate in tissue degradation and reestablishment [58]. Therefore, alteration of inflammatory infiltration may have profound influence on downstream migration, proliferation, differentiation, and ultimately the quality of the healing response. For instance, inflammatory cytokines induced by TGF-βs during the inflammatory stage initialize epithelialization in cutaneous wound healing [5], which may be one reason for faster epithelial migration in FMOD-null wounds relative to WT controls [14]. Because TGF-β1 stimulates epidermal cell migration [59–62], earlier and increased expression of TGF-β1, TβRI, and TβRII in migrating epidermal tongue may have promoted FMOD-null epithelial migration. Meanwhile, although TβRIII itself has no inherent signaling function, membrane-anchored TβRIII enhances TGF-β signal transduction by presenting TGF-β ligands to TβRII [63]. Thus, expression of membrane-anchored TβRIII in FMOD-null migrating epidermal tongue may also have contributed to the increased epithelial migration. Although FMOD and lumican share 47% amino acid sequence identity and the same collagen-binding region [64], they have inverse expression trends in connective tissues and different functions in the regulation of ECM assembly and cellular behavior [36,65–68]. For instance, we observed increased lumican expression in FMOD-null wound migrating epidermis in our current study. Since lumican promotes epithelial migration *via* binding to TβRI [48], the co-localization and co-elevation of lumican and TβRI could be an additional reason for the accelerated epidermal migration of FMOD-null wounds.

Once epidermal cells begin migrating, epidermal and dermal cells no longer remain adhered to one another, and this disconnection allows the lateral movement of epidermal cells over the wound matrix [3,7,69]. Importantly, during the epithelialization period, ECM proteins such as fibronectin together with type I collagen provide the 'railroad tracks' on top of dermis that facilitate migrating epidermal cells to separate desiccated eschar from viable tissue and reestablish the epithelial layer [3,7,69]. However, our previous studies have shown that expression of both fibronectin and type I collagen is decreased in FMOD-null wounds compared with that in WT wounds before wound closure [14]. Instead of migrating on the ECM layer deposited by dermal cells that have newly moved into the wound area as in WT wounds, epidermal cells migrated more intimately on dermis in FMOD-null wounds, hindering normal establishment of viable epithelial layer into the wounds [14]. Moreover, TGF-β3 selectively halts dermal fibroblast proliferation and migration and leads to retarded dermal cell entry [12–14]. In our current study, we have shown that TβRI plays an essential role in TGF-β3-mediated inhibition of FMOD-null dermal fibroblast migra-

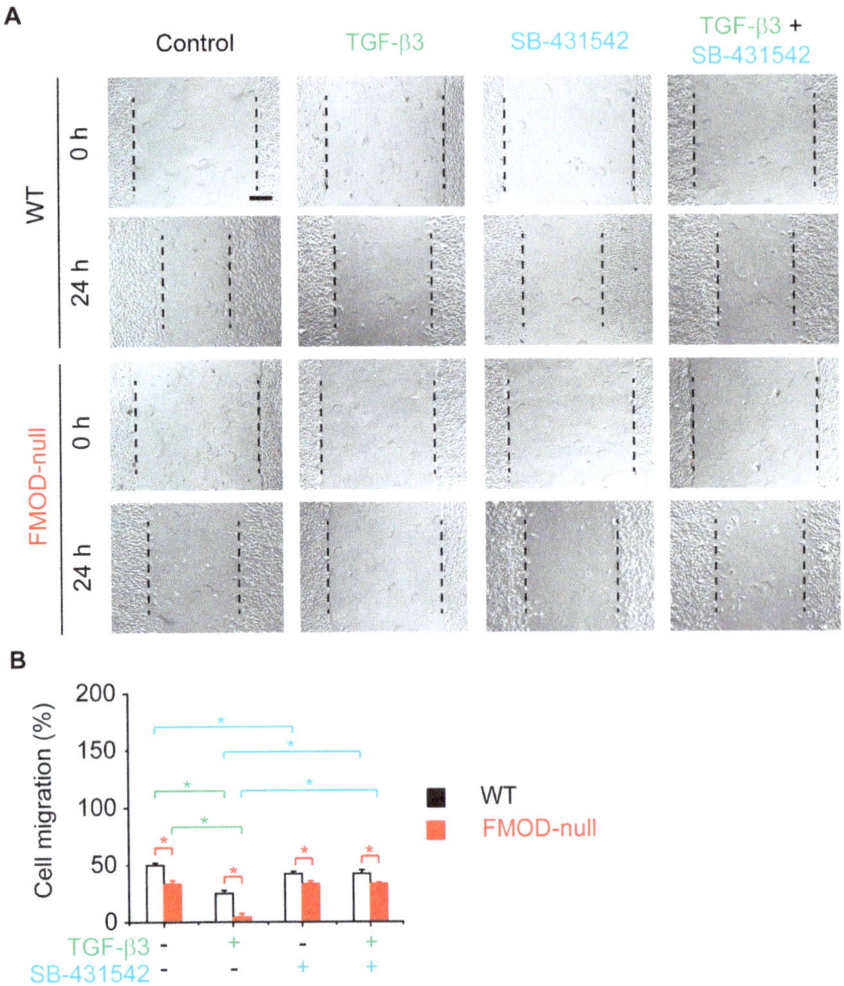

Figure 5. ***In vitro*** **migration assay of primary dermal fibroblasts derived from adult WT and FMOD-null mice skin.** Cell migration was documented by photographs taken immediately after scraping, as well as 24 h later (**A**). Migration was quantified by measuring the average wound gap between the wound edges before and after the treatment, and calculated as: Cell migration (%) = (Gap_{0h}-Gap_{24h})/Gap_{0h} ×100% (**B**). 100 pM TGF-β3 was used to inhibit dermal fibroblast migration *in vitro*, while 10 μM TβRI-specific inhibitor SB-431542 was used to block TβRI-mediated signal transduction. Bar =200 μm. N=6; *, $P<0.05$. Red stars indicate the significance that resulted from FMOD-deficiency; green stars indicate the significance that resulted from TGF-β3 application; and blue stars indicate the significance that resulted from SA-431542 blockage of TβRI.

tion. Additionally, Bandyopadhyay *et al.* demonstrated that the level of TβRII determines the uptake of the anti-motility signal of TGF-β3 on dermal fibroblasts [12]. Hence, high TGF-β3, TβRI, and TβRII levels in FMOD-null dermis resulted in lack of accompanying dermal cell migration and proliferation and subsequently delayed granulation tissue formation, leading to a greater wound surface area requiring epithelialization [12–14]. Taken together, despite that epithelial migration was accelerated in FMOD-null wounds, the need for migration through a large, deep, U-shaped dermal concavity extending from superficial dermis to subcutaneous fat delayed epithelialization and led to an excessively exuberant fibroproliferative response after wound closure to cause extensive scarring [14].

Furthermore, the production capability of all three TGF-β ligands by individual dermal cells was reduced during the remodeling stage in FMOD-null wounds accompanied by a decrease in collagen synthesis, which is predominantly stimulated by TGF-β [14]. Adding to the increased fibrotic cell density, the abnormal TGF-β expression may have further contributed to the disorganized collagen distribution in FMOD-null scars [42]. Meanwhile, previous studies have shown that FMOD activates the classical and the alternative pathways of complement [32,70]. Considering that administration of complement components in acute injury models promotes wound healing by enhancing angiogenesis and wound strength [71,72], it is possible that the weakened activation of the complement cascade caused by FMOD-deficiency led to a less vascularized, less strengthened scar in FMOD-null mice. Therefore, the present study clearly provides valuable insight into the novel and complex role of FMOD in orchestrating TGF-β bioactivity during wound repair and reveals that FMOD critically coordinates temporospatial distribution of TGF-β ligands and receptors in various cell types during the entire adult mouse wound healing process (**Figure 6**).

Since its discovery, TGF-β has been shown to have cell-specific effects on cellular proliferation, differentiation, and metabolism [8,73–76]. In particular, TGF-β is known to regulate wound repair and can be produced by a variety of cells that are active in the wound healing process [5,9,75,77]. In addition, the expression level and pattern of TGF-β ligands and receptors are differentially regulated during normal and impaired wound healing [5,78,79],

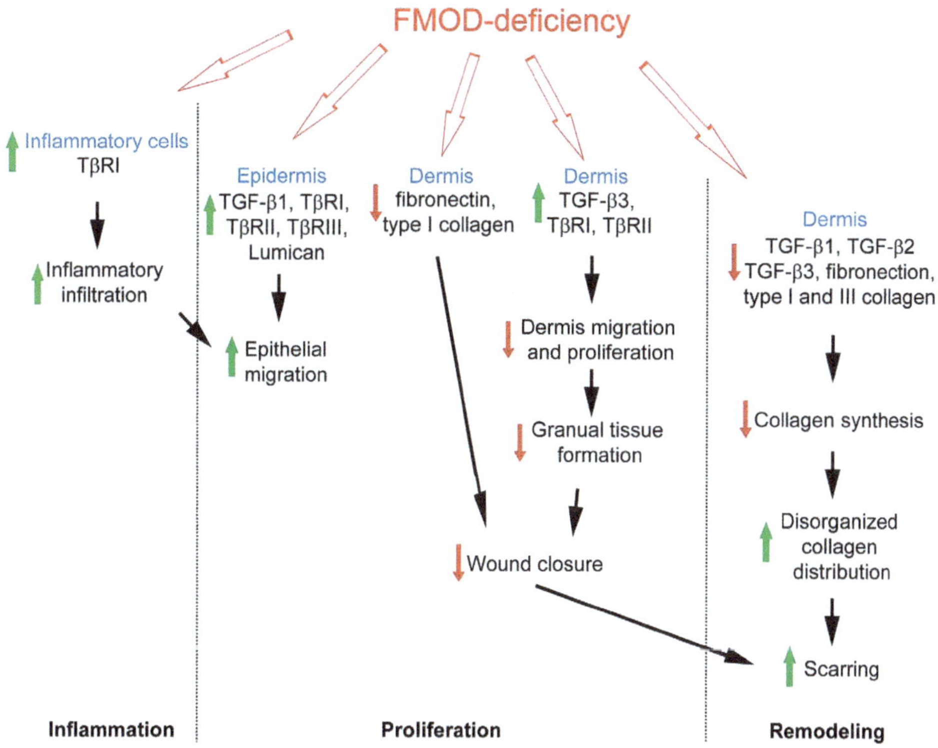

Figure 6. A brief summary of the major effects of FMOD-deficiency on adult mouse wound healing.

which suggests that the concomitant expression of TGF-β isoforms and their signal-transducing receptors govern potential TGF-β activities. In this study, a single missing gene, *FMOD*, leads to marked alterations in wound healing phenotype as well as in temporospatial expression of TGF-β ligands and receptors throughout the wound repair process. The profound alterations in FMOD-null mice demonstrate that TGF-β signaling is contextually dependent on relative ligand, receptor and modulator (e.g., FMOD) ratios, and that the onset, degree, distribution and duration of TGF-βs are crucial to the wound healing process.

As a broadly distributed ECM component, FMOD exerts functions in a variety of biological processes. All SLRP members, including FMOD, have a central protein core made up of 6–10 leucine-rich repeats (LRRs) flanked by cysteine-clusters and substituted with covalently lined glycosaminoglycan (GAG) side chains [32,33]. They are able to bind to various types of collagens, thereby regulating the kinetics, assembly, and special organization of fibrils and protecting collagen fibrils from cleavage by collagenases [32,33]. For instance, FMOD-deficient mice have impaired collagen fibrillogenesis in tendon and predentin in addition to dermis [36,65,80]. However, the biological functions of SLRPs extend far beyond their interactions with collagens since they also interact with various growth factors and cytokines, allowing modulation of their diverse functions [32–34]. For example, in agreement with our previous research [14,40,41], this study demonstrates that FMOD interacts with TGF-βs to modulate the cellular responses in cutaneous wound healing. In addition, our recent studies have revealed that FMOD can promote angiogenesis [68], which is essential in wound healing especially during the remodeling stage. FMOD also offers potential therapeutic benefits in saphenous vein graft failure by reducing associated neointima formation [81]. Thus, FMOD is a potential agent that can aid tissue regeneration. Moreover, Oldberg *et al.* found that FMOD determines carcinoma stroma matrix structure and fluid balance in carcinoma [82]. Other studies revealed FMOD as a novel tumor-associated antigen in leukemia, lymphoma, and leiomyoma [83–85]. Hence, FMOD may additionally play a vital role in cancer diagnosis and treatment. Finally, FMOD has been found to be integral in maintenance of endogenous stem cell niches [35], and we have discovered that continual treatment with FMOD in a serum-free condition is sufficient to reprogram somatic cells to a minimally proliferative, multipotent stage [38]. Thus, FMOD has an extensive function in cell fate determination as well. On the other hand, upregulation of FMOD in inflamed joint and gingival tissues indicates that FMOD is also involved in sustained inflammation, possibly *via* activating the complement cascade [70,86]. Taken together, FMOD as well as other SLRP family members are implicated in diverse biological functions during development and in various pathologies. Future research should aim at translating the rapidly expanding knowledge on SLRPs into the clinical setting by elucidating the detailed mechanisms underlying their functions and defining therapeutic strategies for inflammatory, fibrotic, and malignant disorders.

Supporting Information

Figure S1 IHC staining of lumican in wounded WT and FMOD-null adult mice skin at 1 day post-injury. Inserts show low magnification view. Black triangles: migrating epidermal tongues. Bar = 100 μm.

Figure S2 *In vitro* migration assay of primary dermal fibroblasts derived from adult WT and FMOD-null mice skin. Cell migration was documented by photographs taken immediately after scraping, as well as 24 h later (**A**). Migration was quantified by measuring the average wound gap between the wound edges before and after the treatment, and calculated as: Cell migration (%) = $(Gap_{0h}-Gap_{24h})/Gap_{0h}$ ×100% (**B**). 100 pM TGF-β1 and/or 10 μM TβRI-specific inhibitor SB-431542 were used. Bar = 200 μm. N = 6; *, $P<0.05$. Red stars indicate the significance that resulted from FMOD-deficiency; yellow stars indicate the significance that resulted from TGF-β1 application; and blue stars indicate the significance that resulted from SA-431542 blockage of TβRI.

Acknowledgments

FMOD-null animals were kindly provided by Dr. Ake Oldberg (Lund, Sweden).

Author Contributions

Conceived and designed the experiments: ZZ XZ KT CS. Performed the experiments: ZZ KSL CN CH JW TMR DRE MM. Analyzed the data: ZZ KSL XZ CN. Contributed reagents/materials/analysis tools: KT CS. Wrote the paper: ZZ KSL XZ MM KT CS.

References

1. Clark R (1996) Wound repair: overview and general considerations In: Clark R, editor. The Molecular and Cellular Biology of Wound Repair. New York: Plenum Press. pp. 3–50.
2. Broughton G Jr, Janis JE, Attinger CE (2006) The basic science of wound healing. Plast Reconstr Surg 117: 12S–34S.
3. Lorenz HP, Longaker MT (2008) Wounds: Biology, Pathology, and Management. In: Norton JA, Barie PS, Bollinger RR, Chang AE, Lowry SF et al., editors. Surgery: Springer New York.
4. Clark RAF, Henson PM (1988) The molecular and cellular biology of wound repair. New York: Plenum Press.
5. O'Kane S, Ferguson MW (1997) Transforming growth factor βs and wound healing. International Journal of Biochemistry and Cell Biology 29: 63–78.
6. Henry G, Garner WL (2003) Inflammatory mediators in wound healing. Surg Clin North Am 83: 483–507.
7. Singer AJ, Clark RA (1999) Cutaneous wound healing. N Engl J Med 341: 738–746.
8. Massague J (1990) The transforming growth factor-beta family. Annu Rev Cell Biol 6: 597–641.
9. Penn JW, Grobbelaar AO, Rolfe KJ (2012) The role of the TGF-beta family in wound healing, burns and scarring: a review. Int J Burns Trauma 2: 18–28.
10. Chaudhury A, Howe PH (2009) The Tale of Transforming Growth Factor-Beta (TGF beta) Signaling: A Soigne Enigma. Iubmb Life 61: 929–939.
11. Graycar JL, Miller DA, Arrick BA, Lyons RM, Moses HL, et al. (1989) Human transforming growth factor-beta 3: recombinant expression, purification, and biological activities in comparison with transforming growth factors-beta 1 and -beta 2. Mol Endocrinol 3: 1977–1986.
12. Bandyopadhyay B, Fan J, Guan S, Li Y, Chen M, et al. (2006) A "traffic control" role for TGFβ3: orchestrating dermal and epidermal cell motility during wound healing. The Journal of Cell Biology 172: 1093–1105.
13. Han GW, Li FL, Singh TP, Wolf P, Wang XJ (2012) The Pro-inflammatory Role of TGF beta 1: A Paradox? International Journal Of Biological Sciences 8: 228–235.
14. Zheng Z, Nguyen C, Zhang XL, Khorasani H, Wang JZ, et al. (2011) Delayed Wound Closure in Fibromodulin-Deficient Mice Is Associated with Increased TGF-beta 3 Signaling. Journal of Investigative Dermatology 131: 769–778.
15. Shah M, Foreman DM, Ferguson MW (1995) Neutralisation of TGF-beta 1 and TGF-beta 2 or exogenous addition of TGF-beta 3 to cutaneous rat wounds reduces scarring. J Cell Sci 108: 985–1002.
16. Lin RY, Sullivan KM, Argenta PA, Meuli M, Lorenz HP, et al. (1995) Exogenous transforming growth factor-beta amplifies its own expression and induces scar formation in a model of human fetal skin repair. Annals of Surgery 222: 146–154.
17. Wu LC, Siddiqui A, Morris DE, Cox DA, Roth SI, et al. (1997) Transforming growth factor beta 3 (TGF beta 3) accelerates wound healing without alteration of scar prominence – Histologic and competitive reverse-transcription polymerase chain reaction studies. Archives of Surgery 132: 753–760.
18. Murata H, Zhou L, Ochoa S, Hasan A, Badiavas E, et al. (1997) TGF-beta 3 stimulates and regulates collagen synthesis through TGF-beta 1-dependent and independent. Journal of Investigative Dermatology 108: 258–262.
19. Occleston NL, Laverty HG, O'Kane S, Ferguson MW (2008) Prevention and reduction of scarring in the skin by Transforming Growth Factor beta 3 (TGFbeta3): from laboratory discovery to clinical pharmaceutical. J Biomater Sci Polym Ed 19: 1047–1063.
20. (2011) Juvista Fails Late-Stage Trial. Drug. Discovery & Development (www.ddmag.com).
21. Danielpour D, Sporn MB (1990) Differential inhibition of transforming growth factor beta 1 and beta 2 activity by alpha 2-macroglobulin. J Biol Chem 265: 6973–6977.
22. Paralkar VM, Vukicevic S, Reddi AH (1991) Transforming Growth-Factor-Beta Type-1 Binds to Collagen-Iv of Basement-Membrane Matrix – Implications for Development. Developmental Biology 143: 303–308.
23. Hildebrand A, Romaris M, Rasmussen L, Heinegard D, Twardzik D, et al. (1994) Interaction of the small interstitial proteoglycans biglycan, decorin and fibromodulin with transforming growth factor β. Biochem J 302: 527–534.
24. Grande J, Melder D, Zinsmeister A, Killen P (1993) Transforming growth factor-beta 1 induces collagen IV gene expression in NIH-3T3 cells. Lab Invest 69: 387–395.
25. Li X, McFarland DC, Velleman SG (2006) Effect of transforming growth factor-beta on decorin and beta1 integrin expression during muscle development in chickens. Poult Sci 85: 326–332.
26. Heegaard AM, Xie ZJ, Young MF, Nielsen KL (2004) Transforming growth factor beta stimulation of biglycan gene expression is potentially mediated by Sp1 binding factors. J Cell Biochem 93: 463–475.
27. Kolb M, Margetts PJ, Sime PJ, Gauldie J (2001) Proteoglycans decorin and biglycan differentially modulate TGF-beta-mediated fibrotic responses in the lung. American Journal of Physiology-Lung Cellular and Molecular Physiology 280: L1327–L1334.
28. Zhang Z, Garron TM, Li XJ, Liu Y, Zhang X, et al. (2009) Recombinant human decorin inhibits TGF-beta1-induced contraction of collagen lattice by hypertrophic scar fibroblasts. Burns 35: 527–537.
29. Zhang Z, Li XJ, Liu Y, Zhang X, Li YY, et al. (2007) Recombinant human decorin inhibits cell proliferation and downregulates TGF-beta1 production in hypertrophic scar fibroblasts. Burns 33: 634–641.
30. Isaka Y, Brees DK, Ikegaya K, Kaneda Y, Imai E, et al. (1996) Gene therapy by skeletal muscle expression of decorin prevents fibrotic disease in rat kidney. Nat Med 2: 418–423.
31. Baghy K, Iozzo RV, Kovalszky I (2012) Decorin-TGF beta Axis in Hepatic Fibrosis and Cirrhosis. Journal of Histochemistry & Cytochemistry 60: 262–268.
32. Iozzo RV, Goldoni S, Berendsen AD, Young MF (2011) Small Leucine-Rich Proteoglycans: The Extracellular Matrix: an Overview. In: Mecham RP, editor: Springer Berlin Heidelberg. pp. 197–231.
33. Merline R, Schaefer RM, Schaefer L (2009) The matricellular functions of small leucine-rich proteoglycans (SLRPs). J Cell Commun Signal 3: 323–335.
34. Schaefer L, Schaefer RM (2010) Proteoglycans: from structural compounds to signaling molecules. Cell Tissue Res 339: 237–246.
35. Bi Y, Ehirchiou D, Kilts TM, Inkson CA, Embree MC, et al. (2007) Identification of tendon stem/progenitor cells and the role of the extracellular matrix in their niche. Nat Med 13: 1219–1227.
36. Svensson L, Aszodi A, Reinholt F, Heinegard D, Oldberg A (1999) Fibromodulin-null mice have abnormal collagen fibrils, tissue organization, and altered lumican deposition in tendon. J Biol Chem 274: 9636–9647.
37. Viola M, Bartolini B, Sonaggere M, Giudici C, Tenni R, et al. (2007) Fibromodulin interactions with type I and II collagens. Connect Tissue Res 48: 141–148.
38. Zheng Z, Jian J, Zhang XL, Zara JN, Yin W, et al. (2012) Reprogramming of human fibroblasts into multipotent cells with a single ECM proteoglycan, fibromodulin. Biomaterials 33: 5821–5831.
39. Iozzo RV, Schaefer L (2010) Proteoglycans in health and disease: novel regulatory signaling mechanisms evoked by the small leucine-rich proteoglycans. Febs Journal 277: 3864–3875.
40. Soo C, Beanes S, Dang C, Zhang X, Ting K (2001) Fibromodulin, a TGF-ß modulator, promotes scarless fetal repair. Surgical Forum 578–581.
41. Soo C, Hu FY, Zhang X, Wang Y, Beanes SR, et al. (2000) Differential expression of fibromodulin, a transforming growth factor-beta modulator, in fetal skin development and scarless repair. Am J Pathol 157: 423–433.
42. Khorasani H, Zheng Z, Nguyen C, Zara J, Zhang XL, et al. (2011) A Quantitative Approach to Scar Analysis. American Journal of Pathology 178: 621–628.
43. Soo C, Beanes SR, Hu F-Y, Zhang X, Dang C, et al. (2003) Ontogenetic transition in fetal wound transforming growth factor-β regulation correlates with collagen organization. American Journal of Pathology 163: 2459–2476.
44. Allen A, Southern S (2002) A novel technique of computer-assisted image analysis to quantify molecular stress in cetaceans.
45. Denton CP, Khan K, Hoyles RK, Shiwen X, Leoni P, et al. (2009) Inducible lineage-specific deletion of TbetaRII in fibroblasts defines a pivotal regulatory role during adult skin wound healing. J Invest Dermatol 129: 194–204.
46. Xiao YQ, Liu K, Shen JF, Xu GT, Ye W (2009) SB-431542 inhibition of scar formation after filtration surgery and its potential mechanism. Invest Ophthalmol Vis Sci 50: 1698–1706.
47. Inman GJ, Nicolas FJ, Callahan JF, Harling JD, Gaster LM, et al. (2002) SB-431542 is a potent and specific inhibitor of transforming growth factor-beta superfamily type I activin receptor-like kinase (ALK) receptors ALK4, ALK5, and ALK7. Mol Pharmacol 62: 65–74.

48. Yamanaka O, Yuan Y, Coulson-Thomas VJ, Gesteira TF, Call MK, et al. (2013) Lumican Binds ALK5 to Promote Epithelium Wound Healing. PLoS One 8: e82730.
49. Mariano J, Montuenga L, Prentice M, Cuttitta F, Jakowlew S (1998) Concurrent and distinct transcription and translation of transforming growth factor-β type I and type II receptors in rodent embryogenesis. Int J Dev Biol 42: 1125–1136.
50. Lopez-Casillas F, Cheifetz S, Doody J, Andres J, Lane W, et al. (1991) Structure and expression of the membrane proteoglycan betaglycan, a component of the TGF-beta receptor system. Cell 67: 785–795.
51. Stoff A, Rivera AA, Mathis JM, Moore ST, Banerjee NS, et al. (2007) Effect of adenoviral mediated overexpression of fibromodulin on human dermal fibroblasts and scar formation in full-thickness incisional wounds. J Mol Med 85: 481–496.
52. Honardoust D, Varkey M, Hori K, Ding J, Shankowsky HA, et al. (2011) Small leucine-rich proteoglycans, decorin and fibromodulin, are reduced in postburn hypertrophic scar. Wound Repair and Regeneration 19: 368–378.
53. Honardoust D, Varkey M, Marcoux Y, Shankowsky HA, Tredget EE (2012) Reduced Decorin, Fibromodulin, and Transforming Growth Factor-beta 3 in Deep Dermis Leads to Hypertrophic Scarring. Journal of Burn Care & Research 33: 218–227.
54. Brandes ME, Mai UE, Ohura K, Wahl SM (1991) Type I transforming growth factor-beta receptors on neutrophils mediate chemotaxis to transforming growth factor-beta. J Immunol 147: 1600–1606.
55. Brandes ME, Wakefield LM, Wahl SM (1991) Modulation of monocyte type I transforming growth factor-beta receptors by inflammatory stimuli. J Biol Chem 266: 19697–19703.
56. Lagraoui M, Gagnon L (1997) Enhancement of human neutrophil survival and activation by TGF-beta 1. Cell Mol Biol (Noisy-le-grand) 43: 313–318.
57. Wahl SM, Hunt DA, Wakefield LM, Mccartneyfrancis N, Wahl LM, et al. (1987) Transforming Growth-Factor Type-Beta Induces Monocyte Chemotaxis and Growth-Factor Production. Proc Natl Acad Sci U S A 84: 5788–5792.
58. Eming SA, Krieg T, Davidson JM (2007) Inflammation in wound repair: Molecular and cellular mechanisms. Journal of Investigative Dermatology 127: 514–525.
59. Hebda PA (1988) Stimulatory effects of transforming growth factor-beta and epidermal growth factor on epidermal cell outgrowth from porcine skin explant cultures. Journal of Investigative Dermatology 91: 440–445.
60. Sun T, Adra S, Smallwood R, Holcombe M, MacNeil S (2009) Exploring hypotheses of the actions of TGF-beta1 in epidermal wound healing using a 3D computational multiscale model of the human epidermis. PLoS One 4: e8515.
61. Decline F, Okamoto O, Mallein-Gerin F, Helbert B, Bernaud J, et al. (2003) Keratinocyte motility induced by TGF-beta1 is accompanied by dramatic changes in cellular interactions with laminin 5. Cell Motil Cytoskeleton 54: 64–80.
62. Cui W, Fowlis DJ, Cousins FM, Duffie E, Bryson S, et al. (1995) Concerted action of TGF-beta 1 and its type II receptor in control of epidermal homeostasis in transgenic mice. Genes Dev 9: 945–955.
63. Lopezcasillas F, Payne HM, Andres JL, Massague J (1994) Betaglycan Can Act as a Dual Modulator of Tgf-Beta Access to Signaling Receptors – Mapping of Ligand-Binding and Gag Attachment Sites. Journal of Cell Biology 124: 557–568.
64. Svensson L, Narlid I, Oldberg A (2000) Fibromodulin and lumican bind to the same region on collagen type I fibrils. FEBS Lett 470: 178–182.
65. Ezura Y, Chakravarti S, Oldberg A, Chervoneva I, Birk DE (2000) Differential expression of lumican and fibromodulin regulate collagen fibrillogenesis in developing mouse tendons. Journal of Cell Biology 151: 779–787.
66. Kalamajski S, Oldberg A (2009) Homologous Sequence in Lumican and Fibromodulin Leucine-rich Repeat 5–7 Competes for Collagen Binding. Journal Of Biological Chemistry 284: 534–539.
67. Niewiarowska J, Brezillon S, Sacewicz-Hofman I, Bednarek R, Maquart FX, et al. (2011) Lumican inhibits angiogenesis by interfering with alpha2beta1 receptor activity and downregulating MMP-14 expression. Thromb Res 128: 452–457.
68. Jian J, Zheng Z, Zhang K, Rackhon TM, Hsu C, et al. (2013) Fibromodulin promoted *in vitro* and *in vivo* angiogenesis. Biochemical and Biophysical Research Communication 436.
69. Martin P (1997) Wound healing – aiming for perfect skin regeneration. Science 276: 75–81.
70. Sjoberg A, Onnerfjord P, Morgelin M, Heinegard D, Blom AM (2005) The extracellular matrix and inflammation – Fibromodulin activates the classical pathway of complement by directly binding C1q. Journal of Biological Chemistry 280: 32301–32308.
71. Bossi F, Rizzi L, Bulla R, Tripodo C, Guarnotta C, et al. (2011) C1q induces in vivo angiogenesis and promotes wound healing. Molecular Immunology 48: 1676–1677.
72. Sinno H, Malholtra M, Lutfy J, Jardin B, Winocour S, et al. (2013) Topical application of complement C3 in collagen formulation increases early wound healing. Journal of Dermatological Treatment 24: 141–147.
73. Roberts AB, Sporn MB (1996) Transforming growth factor-beta. In: Clark RAF, editor. The Molecular and Cellular Biology of Wound Repair. New York: Plenum Press. pp. 275–308.
74. Ikushima H, Miyazono K (2012) TGF-beta signal transduction spreading to a wider field: a broad variety of mechanisms for context-dependent effects of TGF-beta. Cell Tissue Res 347: 37–49.
75. Leask A, Abraham DJ (2004) TGF-beta signaling and the fibrotic response. Faseb Journal 18: 816–827.
76. Massague J (2012) TGFbeta signalling in context. Nat Rev Mol Cell Biol 13: 616–630.
77. Beanes SR, Dang C, Soo C, Ting K (2003) Skin repair and scar formation: the central role of TGF-beta. Expert Rev Mol Med 5: 1–22.
78. Levine JH, Moses HL, Gold LI, Nanney LB (1993) Spatial and Temporal Patterns of Immunoreactive Transforming Growth-Factor-Beta-1, Beta-2, and Beta-3 during Excisional Wound Repair. American Journal of Pathology 143: 368–380.
79. Frank S, Madlener M, Werner S (1996) Transforming growth factors beta 1, beta 2, and beta 3 and their receptors are differentially regulated during normal and impaired wound healing. Journal of Biological Chemistry 271: 10188–10193.
80. Goldberg M, Septier D, Oldberg A, Young MF, Ameye LG (2006) Fibromodulin-deficient mice display impaired collagen fibrillogenesis in predentin as well as altered dentin mineralization and enamel formation. Journal of Histochemistry & Cytochemistry 54: 525–537.
81. Ranjzad P, Salem HK, Kingston PA (2009) Adenovirus-mediated gene transfer of fibromodulin inhibits neointimal hyperplasia in an organ culture model of human saphenous vein graft disease. Gene Ther 16: 1154–1162.
82. Oldberg A, Kalamajski S, Salnikov AV, Stuhr L, Morgelin M, et al. (2007) Collagen-binding proteoglycan fibromodulin can determine stroma matrix structure and fluid balance in experimental carcinoma. Proc Natl Acad Sci U S A 104: 13966–13971.
83. Mayr C, Bund D, Schlee M, Moosmann A, Kofler DM, et al. (2005) Fibromodulin as a novel tumor-associated antigen (TAA) in chronic lymphocytic leukemia (CLL), which allows expansion of specific CD8(+) autologous T lymphocytes. Blood 105: 1566–1573.
84. Mikaelsson E, Danesh-Manesh AH, Luppert A, Jeddi-Tehrani M, Rezvany MR, et al. (2005) Fibromodulin, an extracellular matrix protein: characterization of its unique gene and protein expression in B-cell chronic lymphocytic leukemia and mantle cell lymphoma. Blood 105: 4828–4835.
85. Levens E, Luo XP, Ding L, Williams RS, Chegini N (2005) Fibromodulin is expressed in leiomyoma and myometrium and regulated by gonadotropin-releasing hormone analogue therapy and TGF-beta through Smad and MAPK-mediated signalling. Molecular Human Reproduction 11: 489–494.
86. Qian H, Xiao Y, Bartold PM (2004) Immunohistochemical localization and expression of fibromodulin in adult rat periodontium and inflamed human gingiva. Oral Diseases 10: 233–239.

Methylation State of the *EDA* Gene Promoter in Chinese X-Linked Hypohidrotic Ectodermal Dysplasia Carriers

Wei Yin[1,2], Xiaoqian Ye[1], Huali Fan[3], Zhuan Bian[1]*

1 The State Key Laboratory Breeding Base of Basic Science of Stomatology (Hubei-MOST) and Key Laboratory of Oral Biomedicine Ministry of Education, School and Hospital of Stomatology, Wuhan University, Wuhan, Hubei, China, **2** Department of Endodontics and Periodontics, College of Stomatology, Dalian Medical University, Dalian, Liaoning, China, **3** The Second General Department, Hangzhou Stomatology Hospital, Hangzhou, Zhejiang, China

Abstract

Introduction: Hypodontia, hypohidrosis, sparse hair and characteristic faces are the main characters of X-linked hypohidrotic ectodermal dysplasia (XLHED) which is caused by genetic ectodysplasin A (*EDA*) deficiency. Heterozygous female carriers tend to have mild to moderate XLHED phenotype, even though 30% of them present no obvious symptom.

Methods: A large Chinese XLHED family was reported and the entire coding region and exon–intron boundaries of *EDA* gene were sequenced. To elucidate the mechanism for carriers' tempered phenotype, we analyzed the methylation level on four sites of the promoter of *EDA* by the pyrosequencing system.

Results: A known frameshift mutation (c.573–574 insT) was found in this pedigree. Combined with the pedigrees we reported before, 120 samples comprised of 23 carrier females from 11 families and 97 healthy females were analyzed for the methylation state of *EDA* promoter. Within 95% confidence interval (CI), 18 (78.26%) carriers were hypermethylated at these 4 sites.

Conclusion: Chinese XLHED carriers often have a hypermethylated EDA promoter.

Editor: Francesc Palau, Instituto de Ciencia de Materiales de Madrid - Instituto de Biomedicina de Valencia, Spain

Funding: This work was supported by grants from the National Natural Scientific Foundation of China (30500562, 30772417, 30930099 (Monumental Projects) and 81120108010 (International cooperation and exchange projects)), the Chenguang Plan for Distinguished Youth of Wuhan, China (200850731374), the Open Research Fund Program of Hubei-MOST KLOS & KLOBME (201103), the Foundation for the Author of National Excellent Doctoral Dissertation (2007B69) and the Program for New Century Excellent Talents in University, Ministry of Education, China. The funders had no role in study design, data collection and analysis, decision to publish, or preparation of the manuscript.

Competing Interests: The authors have declared that no competing interests exist.

* E-mail: bz@whuss.com

These authors contributed equally to this work.

Introduction

Mutations in *EDA* gene can lead to X-linked hypohidrotic ectodermal dysplasia (XLHED), the most common form of ectodermal dysplasias (EDs). The incidence is less than one in per 100'000 [1]. Mutant *EDA* affects cell signaling transduction or cell migration during the epithelial-mesenchymal inductive process. The structures of ectodermal origin are affected. Patients with XLHED have prominent clinical features: sparse hair, eyelashes and eyebrows, small, misshapen or missing teeth, diminished sweating with a history of high fevers in hot weather, decreased salivary secretions, and a characteristic special facial appearance. Facial features include prominent forehead, narrow and short maxillary regions, small palatal depth, small cranial length, and depressed nasal root and bridge of the nose. However most heterozygous carriers only show minor to moderate degrees of these abnormalities [2].

DNA methylation refers to the biological process that a methyl group added to cytosine that stands directly before a guanine molecule by DNA methyltransferases after DNA duplication. In living cells, methylation has been reported as one of the most common covalent modifications of DNA. It has both epigenetic and mutagenic effects on specific gene expression, cell differentiation, chromatin inactivation, embryo growth, and cancer.

EDA contains a large CpG island in its promoter. CpG islands located in gene promoters represent a major target for DNA hypermethylation, which impairs transcription upon regional or specific methylation events. It has been confirmed that promoter CpG island hypermethylation contributed to gene silencing by inhibiting the binding of certain transcription factors to their recognition sequence, attracting methylated DNA-binding proteins, and/or through chromatin remodeling [3–11]. However, whether aberrant methylation is related to XLHED carriers' phenotype has been controversial.

In the present study, we report a causative *EDA* mutation (c. 573–574 insT) in a Chinese XLHED family. We investigated the methylation of *EDA* promoter of this family' carrier as well as other 22 carriers we reported before [12,13] to study correlations between the phenotype of carriers and the methylation state of the promoter. *EDA* gene in eighteen (78.26%) of the carriers were hypermethylated, and this result demonstrated that there was a

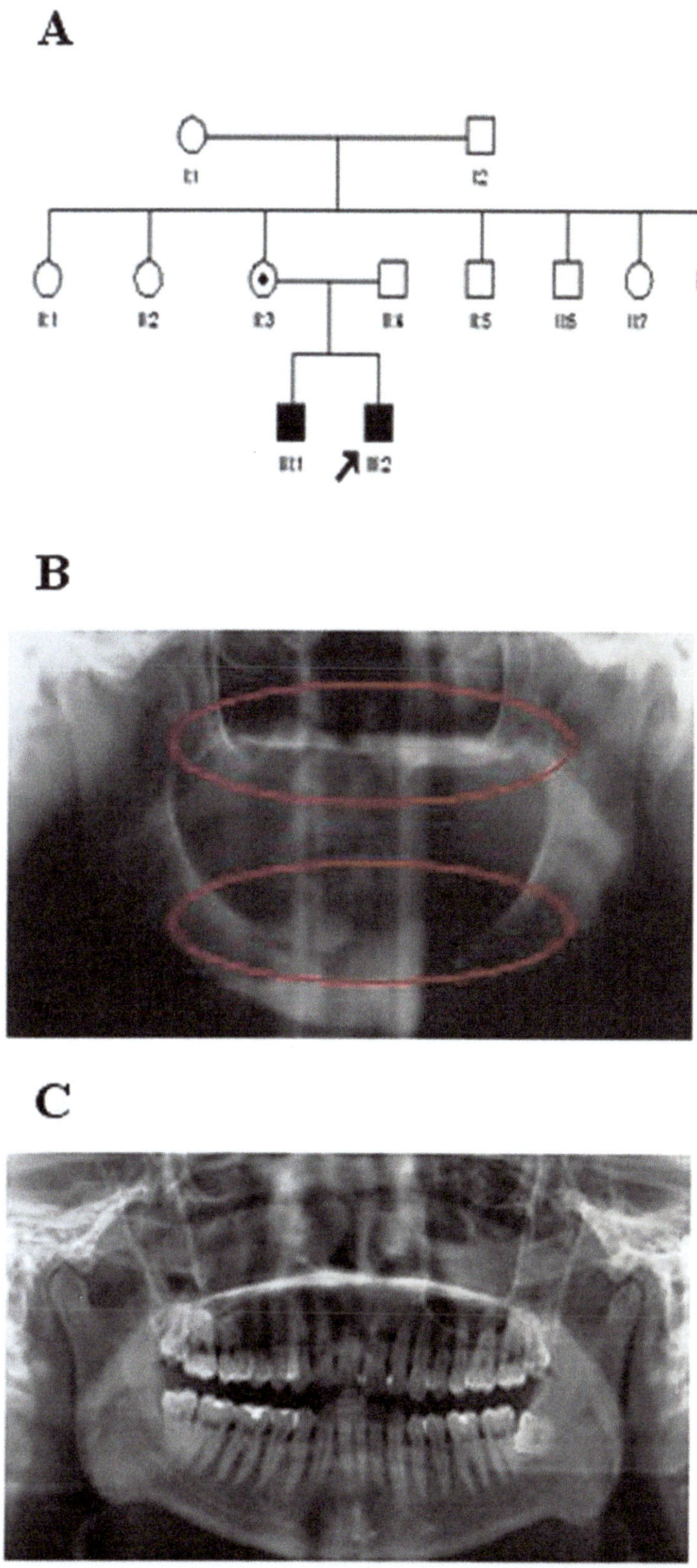

Figure 1. Pedigree and tooth development features of the Chinese family. (A) Males are indicated by squares, females by circles. Affected individuals are indicated by filled symbols and unaffected individuals by white symbols. Circle containing a dot refers to carrier. An arrow indicates the proband. (B) The panoramic radiographs of the proband confirmed there was no tooth germ in the alveolar bone (red circle) which was the severest symptom of tooth dysplasia. (C) The panoramic radiographs of a healthy control with normal tooth development.

Table 1. Clinical phenotypes of family members in the Chinese pedigree.

Family ID	Person ID	Gender	Affection status	Age (years)	Skin		Sparse hair	Hypohidrosis	Facial features	Eczema	Tooth existing (Hypodontia)	Nail dysplasia	Sweat glands dysplasia	Other Manifestations
					Hypoplastic	Thin & wrinkled								
I	II3	F	C	50	-	-	+	-	-	-	NM	-	-	
I	III1	M	A	25	++	++	++	+	+	+	13, 23	+	++	
I	III2	M	A	23	++	++	++	++	+	+	anodontia	+	++	

A: affected; C: carrier; F: female; M: male; NM: no missing; +: positive; number of '+' symbols reflects the degree of these clinical features; -: negative; 13: Right maxillary canine; 23: Left maxillary canine.

correlation between being a XLHED carrier and the hypermethylation status of the *EDA* promoter.

Materials and Methods

Ethical Approval

This study was approved by the Institutional Review Board (IRB) of Hospital and School of Stomatology, Wuhan University. Written informed consents were obtained from all participants or their guardians.

Nomenclature

Gene mutation nomenclature used in this study follows the recommendations of den Dunnen and Antonarakis Gene symbols used in this article follow the protocol created by the HUGO gene nomenclature committee [15].

DNA Sample Collection

All probands were outpatient cases of School and Hospital of Stomatology, Wuhan University. Two professional dentists examined the patients respectively according to the classical diagnosis criteria. Comprehensive physical examinations and panoramic radiograph films were taken thoroughly. Pilocarpine iontophoresis sweat test was used to evaluate the function of sweat gland. – to ++ was scored for normal to absolutely no sweat. After a definite diagnosis was obtained, patients' family members were interviewed and examined. 5–10 ml blood samples were collected with EDTA $2Na^+$ and heparin as anticoagulant. DNA was isolated from leukocytes using the standard sodium dodecyl sulphate–proteinase K–phenol/chloroform method After quality accessing, DNA was frozen at −20°C.

Polymerase Chain Reaction (PCR) and Mutation Screening

The entire *EDA* coding region and exon–intron boundaries of patients and their relatives were amplified using the same primers used in the previous report Amplified fragments were purified with a PCR purification kit (Omega, USA) according to the manufacturer's protocol. DNA sequences were obtained from both strands with an ABI PRISM 3730 genetic analyzer. Sequence analysis was performed by the CHROMAS program and BLAST program of the National Center for Biotechnology Information (NCBI). After identifying nucleotide variants in the *EDA* gene, 200 unrelated controls were examined respectively.

Quantification of *EDA* Promoter's Methylation State by Pyrosequencing

Bisulfite modification of the genome was processed with the CpGenome DNA Modification Kit (Intergen Company, Purchase, NY). The potential methylation sites analyzed in this study were "CGgctgaggcagaCGcagCGgctccCG" located in *EDA* promoter. Specific amplification and sequencing primers were designed by PSQ Assay Design 1.0. One of the PCR primers was labeled with biotin. Blank sample was used as negative control. 97 clinically healthy subjects who had similar ages as carriers were recruited as normal controls.

Pyrosequencing analysis was conducted with PYRO MARK ID (BIOTAGE). The figures and data were analyzed by PSQ96MA 2.1 software. Peak value in the sequencing picture means allele frequency of the DNA sample. The percentage of residual C (Cm) showed how much of each site has been methylated. To insure the reliability of the results, all of the samples underwent pyrosequencing twice.

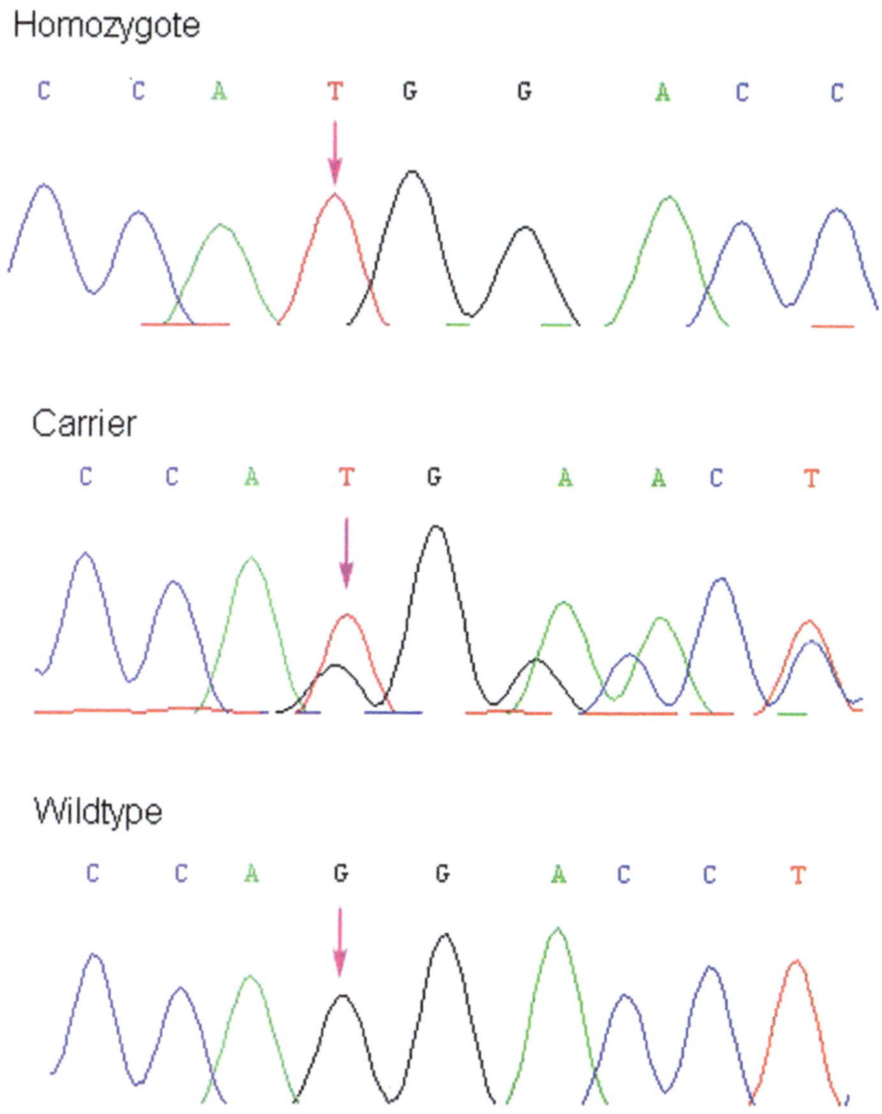

Figure 2. Identification of the causative mutation in *EDA* gene. Arrows indicate the mutation site. The affected male patient and his mother harbored a frameshift mutation c.573–574insT.

Statistical Analysis

Taking advantage of parameter estimation, 95% confidence interval (CI) was employed to do statistical analysis. Within CI, carriers were divided into 3 groups, hypermethylation, normal and hypomethylation groups.

Results

Clinical Data

The clinical features of this Chinese family are listed in Table 1. The 2 patients experienced the classic XLHED symptoms, hypodontia, sparse hair, thin and dry skin and specific facial features (Fig. 1). Both of them were born by a normal delivery, and had normal psychomotor and intellectual development.

The carrier (II3) had no clinical abnormity except for sparse hair. The other 22 carriers we reported before had a similar trait. The most common features were sparse hair and aberrant tooth shape. All of them were Han people which account for 90.56% of the population in China and lived in the middle of China, ranging from teens to 60s in age. They harbored 8 missense mutations, 1 frameshift mutation, 1 splicing site mutation and 2 exon deletions.

Identification of the Causative *EDA* Mutation

Direct sequencing was used to analyze all the coding exons and intron-exon boundaries from both directions. The proband had a nucleotide insertion in exon 5, c.573–574 insT (Fig. 2). His mother (II3) and elder brother (III1) also had the same mutation. The insertion induced a frameshift from amino acid 192 and caused the transcription to stop at amino acid 239. 200 healthy controls did not have this change.

Features of *EDA* Promoter Methylation

The 95% CI for methylation of each site is shown in Fig. 3B. Compared with it, 78.26% (n = 18) carriers were in hypermethylated state while 14.29% (n = 3) were hypomethylated. The other 2 samples were in normal state. The methylation state had no correlation with carriers' mutation type and site (Table 2).

Table 2. The mutations and some selected clinical findings of twenty-three carriers.

Family number	Exon/ intron	Mutation type	Nucleotide changes	Amino acid change	Domain[a]	Sparse hair	Number of tooth missing	Conical shape tooth	Nail dysplasia	Sweat glands dysplasia	Methylation state[b] (Cm value)
II1[12]	1	Missense	c.200A>T	E67V	E	–	1	0	–	–	Hyper
III1[12]	3	Missense	c.463C>T	R155C	F	+	5	0	+	NE[c]	Hyper
III2[12]	3	Missense	c.463C>T	R155C	F	–	NE[c]	NE[c]	–	–	Hyper
IV1[13]	3	Missense	c.467G>A	R156H	F	–	0	0	–	–	Hyper
V1[12]	3	Missense	c.491A>C	E164A	E	+	0	0	-	–	Normal
V2[12]	3	Missense	c.491A>C	E164A	E	+	0	0	+	–	Normal
VI1*	3	Deletion	–	–	E	+	7	0	+	NE[c]	Hyper
VI2*	3	Deletion	–	–	E	+	7	1	–	–	Hyper
VI3*	3	Deletion	–	–	E	–	0	0	–	–	Hyper
VI4*	3	Deletion	–	–	E	–	0	2	–	–	Hyper
VII1*	3	Deletion	–	–	E	–	0	0	–	–	Hyper
VII2*	3	Deletion	–	–	E	–	0	0	–	–	Hyper
VII3*	3	Deletion	–	–	E	–	0	4	–	–	Hyper
VII4*	3	Deletion	–	–	E	–	0	4	–	–	Hyper
VII5*	3	Deletion	–	–	E	–	0	2	–	–	Hyper
VII6*	3	Deletion	–	–	E	–	0	2	–	–	Hyper
I1	5	Frameshift	573insT	FS at 192 Term	C	–	0	0	–	–	Hyper
VIII1[12]	5	Splice donor site	IVS5+1 g>a	Altered splicing	C	–	0	0	–	–	Hypo
VIII2[12]	5	Splice donor site	IVS5+1 g>a	Altered splicing	C	–	0	0	–	–	Hypo
IX1[12]	7	Missense	c.758T>C	L253P	T	+	9	0	+	–	Hyper
X1[12]	9	Missense	c.926T>G	V309G	T	+	3	0	–	–	Hypo
XI1[13]	9	Missense	c.1045G>A	A349T	T	+	6	0	–	–	Hyper
XI2[13]	9	Missense	c.1045G>A	A349T	T	–	0	0	–	–	Hyper

[a]E: Extracellular domain; F: Furin domain; C: Collagen domain; T: TNF homology domain.
[b]Hyper: hypermethylation; Hypo: hypomethylation.
[c]not examined.
*unpublished data.

A

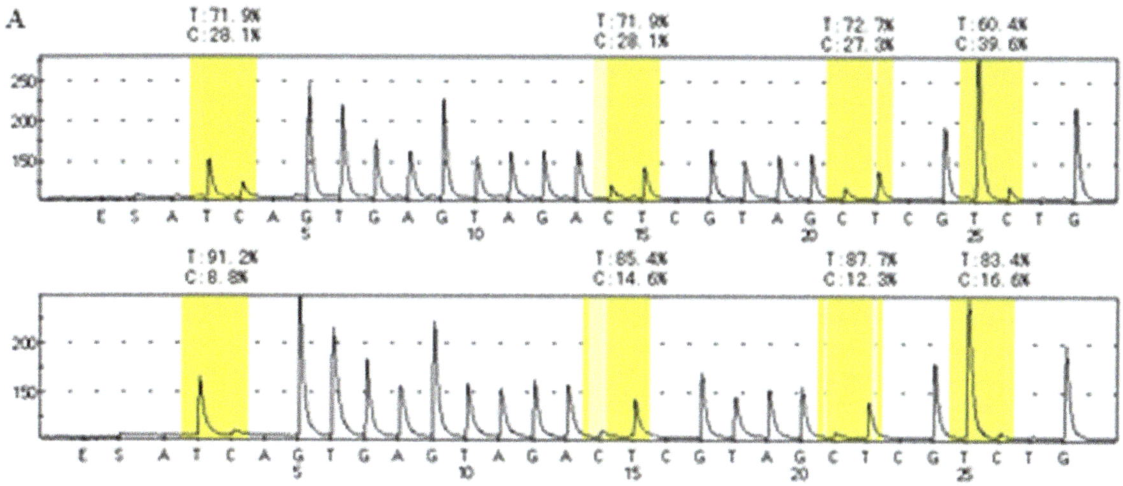

B

Site	I	II	III	IV
95%CI	21.46-26.79	22.01-25.57	19.47-23.25	27.12-31.79

C

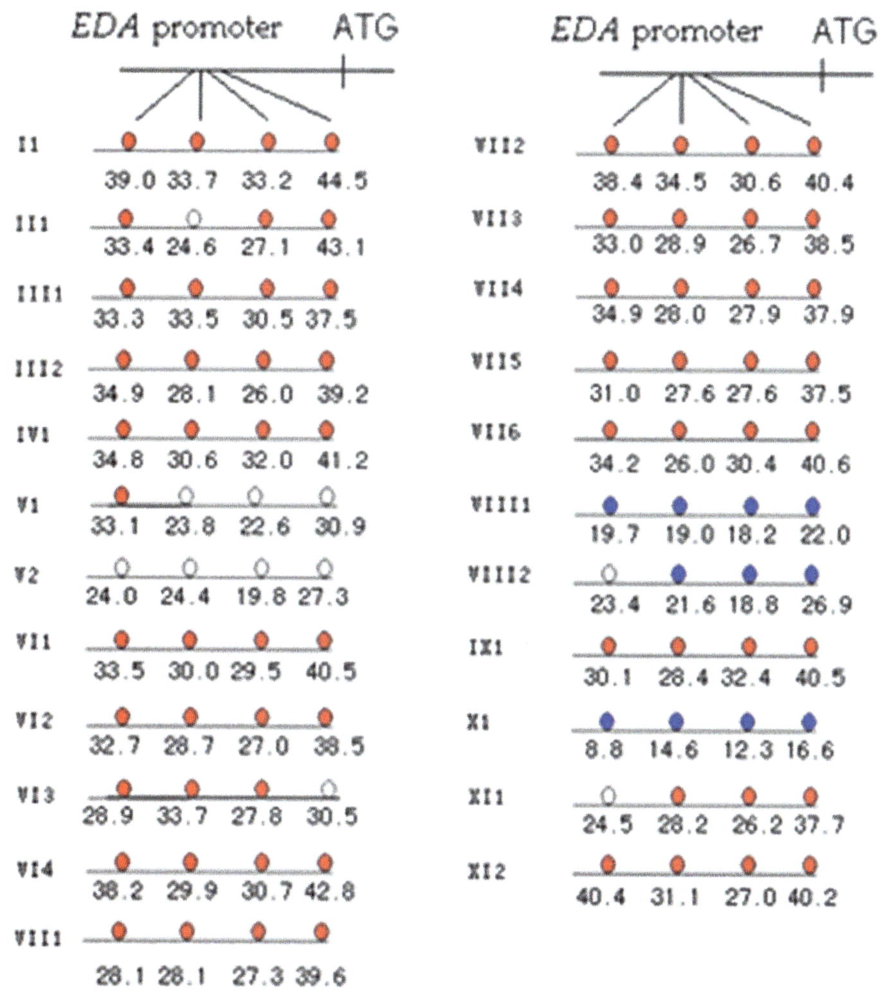

Figure 3. *EDA* promoter's methylation analysis of 23 carriers. (A) Pyrosequencing graphs of 2 samples, a hypermethylation carrier and a hypomethylation carrier. Peak heights are proportional to the number of identical residues incorporated. Percentage in pictures means allele frequency of each site. (B) The 95% CI for the 4 sites. The figures which refer to methyl-cytosine percent at that site are calculated as described in the text. (C) The methylation state of each carriers in the 4 sites. Red, white and blue refer to hypermethylation, normal and hypomethylation respectively.

Similarly, methylation state and phenotype also had no correlation. However, hypermethylated group was inclined to have more defects in nails and tooth shape when compared to hypomethylated carriers (Fig. 4).

Discussion

EDA is a trimeric type II membrane protein that co-localizes with cytoskeletal structures at the lateral and apical surfaces of cells The protein includes intracellular domain, transmembrane domain, furin subdomain, collagen subdomain and TNF homology subdomain As a member of the TNF-related ligand family, EDA is involved in the early epithelial-mesenchymal interaction So far hundreds of mutations have been identified. About 80% of them are small intragenic changes, including point mutations, small deletions and insertions, and more than half of them are found in exons 1, 3 and 5. Large deletions, including entire exon loss and complete gene deletion, have also been reported But the type of mutations, the phenotype and disease severity showed no obvious correlation especially for heterozygous carriers. About 30% of them do not even have obvious symptoms, rendering accurate diagnosis of carrier status difficult [2].

In this study, we reported a known frameshift mutation in the *EDA* gene. The frameshift mutation, c.573–574insT, caused aberrant transcription from codon192 and a premature stop at 239. So far, at least 14 frameshift mutations have been reported in exon 5, but only 3 were insertions. Mutant *EDA* missed partial collagen subdomain and the whole TNF homology subdomain. The TNF homology domain consisted of 10 predicted antiparallel b-sheets linked by variable loops, in common with other members of the TNF family, which was necessary for the homotrimerization of ligands and the binding of *EDA* to its receptor Therefore the mutant *EDA* was predicted not to bind *EDAR* at all.

In the post-genomic era, it is becoming increasingly evident that epigenetic controlling of gene expression plays an important role in determining the phenotype. Histone modifications and DNA methylation-demethylation events are central to the epigenetic regulations of development XLHED female carriers are mosaics of functionally normal and abnormal cells. The carriers' clinical features are likely to depend on the percentage of abnormal cells having participated to the process of ectodermal appendage formation. But it is presently unclear whether EDA promoter methylation contributes at all to the phenotype of carriers.

To obtain more precise hints, we chose the quantitative method, pyrosequencing system [22,23], to analyze the methylation level of *EDA* promoter. Besides the carrier of this family, we additionally recruited 22 other carriers that we reported before. Most of them showed mild symptoms of tooth and hair impairments. All of the causative mutations were distributed in the extracellular domain. 18 of the carriers displayed hypermethylation of the *EDA* promoter. Some of them were even 50% higher in methylation level than normal controls. Although hypermethylated carriers were inclined to have more conical shaped tooth and nail dysplasia than that of hypomethylated group, no regular pattern seemed to

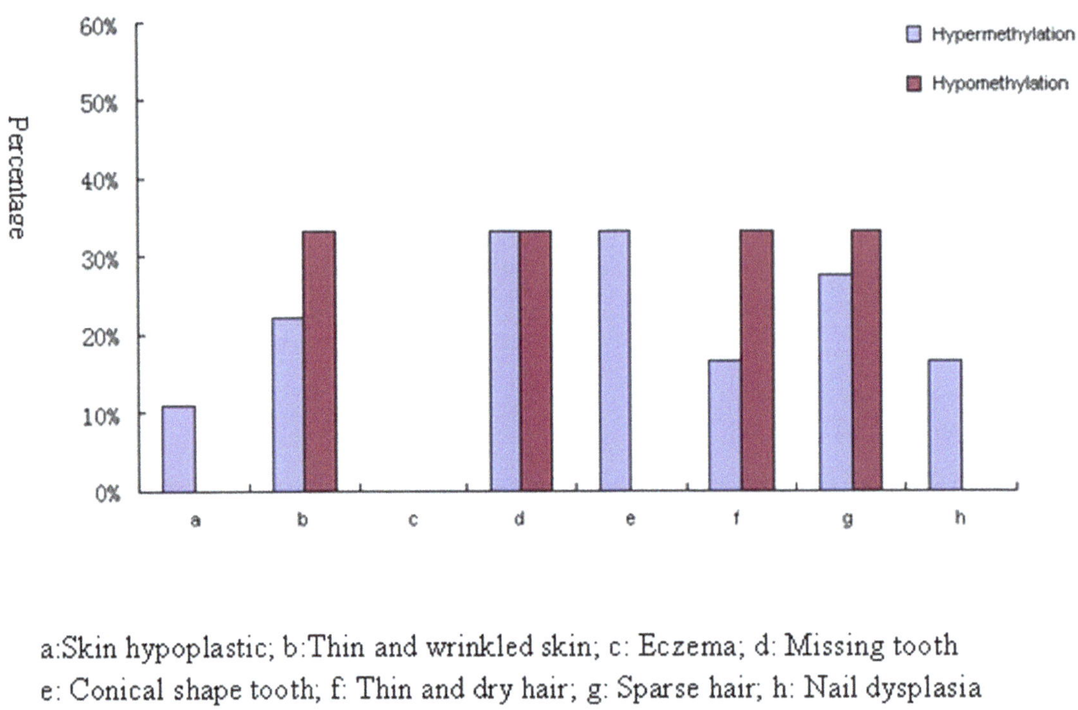

Figure 4. Relationship between methylated state and phenotype of XLHED carriers. Hypermethylated carriers are inclined to have more conical shaped tooth and nail dysplasia than hypomethylated group.

exist among methylation state, mutation type, mutation site and clinical features. Some hypermethylated carriers appeared clinically normal, but some even had as many as 7 missing teeth, conical tooth and sparse hair. The 3 hypomethylated carriers came from 2 families. The 2 carriers who had a mutation in splice donor site were totally normal. The other carrier had sparse hair and missing tooth. Her missense mutation was located at the end of the transcript. The phenotypic changes may be due to the modulation of selection at another X chromosome locus or polymorphism at a locus controlling inactivation. The 2 methylation normal individuals came from the same family. They exhibited mild sparse hair. The mutation occurred between the furin cleavage site and the collagen-like domain.

In addition, the measure of promotor's methylation by pyrosequencing is for both WT and mutated allele on both active and inactive X chromosomes, further studies are needed to explain whether this effect is specific to the *EDA* promoter or is generalized to the entire X chromosome.

In conclusion, a recurrent *EDA* missense mutation, c.573–574 insT in a Chinese patient was reported. We also performed the first study to elucidate the variation of DNA methylation patterns in *EDA* promoters on Chinese XLHED carriers. The results suggest most of these Chinese XLHED carriers' have hypermethylated EDA promoter.

Acknowledgments

We appreciate the patients and their families for participating in this study.

Author Contributions

Conceived and designed the experiments: WY XQY HF ZB. Performed the experiments: WY XQY HF. Analyzed the data: WY XQY ZB. Contributed reagents/materials/analysis tools: ZB. Wrote the paper: WY XQY HF ZB.

References

1. Chassaing N, Bourthoumieu S, Cossee M, Calvas P, Vincent MC (2006) Mutations in EDAR account for one-quarter of non-ED1-related hypohidrotic ectodermal dysplasia. Hum Mutat 27: 255–259.
2. Vincent MC, Biancalana V, Ginisty D, Mandel JL, Calvas P (2001) Mutational spectrum of the ED1 gene in X-linked hypohidrotic ectodermal dysplasia. Eur J Hum Genet 9: 355–63.
3. Rivenbark AG, Jones WD, Coleman WB (2006) DNA methylation-dependent silencing of CST6 in human breast cancer cell lines. Lab Invest 86: 1233–42.
4. Douglas DB, Akiyama Y, Carraway H, Belinsky SA, Esteller M, et al. (2004) Hypermethylation of a small CpGuanine-rich region correlates with loss of activator protein-2alpha expression during progression of breast cancer. Cancer Res 64: 1611–1620.
5. Prendergast GC, Ziff EB (1991) Methylation-sensitive sequence-specific DNA binding by the c-Myc basic region. Science 251: 186–189.
6. Deng G, Song GA, Pong E, Sleisenger M, Kim YS (2004) Promoter methylation inhibits APC gene expression by causing changes in chromatin conformation and interfering with the binding of transcription factor CCAAT-binding factor. Cancer Res 64: 2692–2698.
7. Meehan RR, Lewis JD, McKay S, Kleiner EL, Bird AP (1989) Identification of a mammalian protein that binds specifically to DNA containing methylated CpGs. Cell 58: 499–507.
8. Lewis JD, Meehan RR, Henzel WJ, Maurer-Fogy I, Jeppesen P, et al. (1992) Purification, sequence, and cellular localization of a novel chromosomal protein that binds to methylated DNA. Cell 69: 905–914.
9. Hendrich B, Bird A. (1998) Identification and characterization of a family of mammalian methyl-CpG binding proteins. Mol Cell Biol 18: 6538–6547.
10. Nan X, Tate P, Li E, Bird A (1996) DNA methylation specifies chromosomal localization of MeCP2. Mol Cell Biol 16: 414–421.
11. Lux W, Klobeck HG, Daniel PB, Costa M, Medcalf RL, et al. (2005) In vivo and in vitro analysis of the human tissue-type plasminogen activator gene promoter in neuroblastomal cell lines: evidence for a functional upstream kappaB element. J Thromb Haemost 3: 1009–1017.
12. Fan H, Ye X, Shi L, Yin W, Hua B, et al. (2008) Mutations in the EDA gene are responsible for X-linked hypohidrotic ectodermal dysplasia and hypodontia in Chinese kindreds. Eur J Oral Sci 116: 412–7.
13. Fan HL, Ye XQ, Shi B, Zhang YL, Bian Z (2007) Mutations in the ED1 gene in families with X-linked hypohidrotic ectodermal dysplasia. Zhonghua Kou Qiang Yi Xue Za Zhi 42: 272–5.
14. den Dunnen JT, Antonarakis SE (2001) Nomenclature for the description of human sequence variations. Hum Genet 109: 121–4.
15. Povey S, Lovering R, Bruford E, Wright M, Lush M, et al. (2001) The HUGO gene nomenclature committee (HGNC). Hum Genet 109: 678–80.
16. Yin W, Ye X, Shi L, Wang QK, J Huixi, et al. (2010) *TP63* Gene Mutations in Chinese P63 Syndrome Patients. J DENT RES 89: 813–817.
17. Monreal AW, Zonana J, Ferguson B (1998) Identification of a new splice form of the EDA1 gene permits detection of nearly all X-linked hypohidrotic ectodermal dysplasia mutations. Am J Hum Genet 63: 380–9.
18. Ezer S, Bayés M, Elomaa O, Schlessinger D, Kere J (1999) Ectodysplasin is a collagenous trimeric type II membrane protein with a tumor necrosis factor-like domain and co-localizes with cytoskeletal structures at lateral and apical surfaces of cells. Hum Mol Genet 8: 2079–86.
19. Schneider P, Street SL, Gaide O, Hertig S, Tardivel A, et al. (2001) Mutations leading to X-linked hypohidrotic ectodermal dysplasia affect three major functional domains in the tumor necrosis factor family member ectodysplasin-A. J Biol Chem 276: 18819–27.
20. Pääkkönen K, Cambiaghi S, Novelli G, Ouzts LV, Penttinen M, et al. (2001) The mutation spectrum of the EDA gene in X-linked anhidrotic ectodermal dysplasia. Hum Mutat 17: 349.
21. Laurikkala J, Kassai Y, Pakkasjärvi L, Thesleff I, Itoh N (2003) Identification of a secreted BMP antagonist, ectodin, integrating BMP, FGF, and SHH signals from the tooth enamel knot. Dev Biol 264: 91–105.
22. Tao R, Jin B, Guo SZ, Qing W, Feng GY, et al. (2006) A novel missense mutation of the EDA gene in a Mongolian family with congenital hypodontia. J Hum Genet 51: 498–502.
23. Castaldo I, Pinelli M, Monticelli A, Acquaviva F, Giacchetti M, et al. (2008) DNA methylation in intron 1 of the frataxin gene is related to GAA repeat length and age of onset in Friedreich ataxia patients. J Med Genet 45: 808–12.

4

Targeting Cx43 and N-Cadherin, Which Are Abnormally Upregulated in Venous Leg Ulcers, Influences Migration, Adhesion and Activation of Rho GTPases

Ariadna Mendoza-Naranjo[1]*, Peter Cormie[1], Antonio E. Serrano[1], Rebecca Hu[2], Shay O'Neill[2], Chiuhui Mary Wang[1], Christopher Thrasivoulou[1], Kieran T. Power[1], Alexis White[2], Thomas Serena[3], Anthony R. J. Phillips[2], David L. Becker[1]*

1 Department of Cell and Developmental Biology, University College London, London, United Kingdom, **2** CoDa Therapeutics, Auckland, New Zealand, **3** Newbridge Medical Research Corp, Warren, Pennsylvania, United States of America

Abstract

Background: Venous leg ulcers can be very hard to heal and represent a significant medical need with no effective therapeutic treatment currently available.

Principal Findings: In wound edge biopsies from human venous leg ulcers we found a striking upregulation of dermal N-cadherin, Zonula Occludens-1 and the gap junction protein Connexin43 (Cx43) compared to intact skin, and in stark contrast to the down-regulation of Cx43 expression seen in acute, healing wounds. We targeted the expression of these proteins in 3T3 fibroblasts to evaluate their role in venous leg ulcers healing. Knockdown of Cx43 and N-cadherin, but not Zonula Occludens-1, accelerated cell migration in a scratch wound-healing assay. Reducing Cx43 increased Golgi reorientation, whilst decreasing cell adhesion and proliferation. Furthermore, Connexin43 and N-cadherin knockdown led to profound effects on fibroblast cytoskeletal dynamics after scratch-wounding. The cells exhibited longer lamelipodial protrusions lacking the F-actin belt seen at the leading edge in wounded control cells. This phenotype was accompanied by augmented activation of Rac-1 and RhoA GTPases, as revealed by Förster Resonance Energy Transfer and pull down experiments.

Conclusions: Cx43 and N-cadherin are potential therapeutic targets in the promotion of healing of venous leg ulcers, by acting at least in part through distinct contributions of cell adhesion, migration, proliferation and cytoskeletal dynamics.

Editor: Johanna M. Brandner, University Hospital Hamburg-Eppendorf, Germany

Funding: This work was supported in part by Action Medical Research, and the Henry Smith Charity. The funders had no role in study design, data collection and analysis, decision to publish, or preparation of the manuscript.

Competing Interests: The authors have read the journal's policy and have the following conflicts: The patented antisense technology targeting Cx43 is being developed by CoDa Therapeutics Inc which is currently in phase2B clinical trial treating venous leg ulcers. Patent: DL Becker and CR Green PCT No. WO 00/44409 USA No. PCT/GB00/00238 Formulations comprising antisense nucleotides to connexins. New Zealand patent 513154 awarded, Australia 21193, USA09/890363, Canada 2361251, Europe 901236 and Japan 00/595711. DLB holds shares in CoDa and RH, SO, AW and ARJP are employed by CoDa.

* E-mail: d.becker@ucl.ac.uk (DLB); a.mendoza@ucl.ac.uk (AMN)

Introduction

Chronic wounds, such as diabetic foot ulcers, pressure ulcers, and venous leg ulcers (VLU) are an increasing problem worldwide, with estimates that 1–2% of the population in Western countries will develop a chronic wound over the course of their lifetime [1]. Chronic wounds represent a major economic burden on healthcare services with an estimated annual USA expenditure of $25 billion [2,3]. With the growing numbers of elderly and diabetics in the population this expenditure figure is expected to rise in coming years. Unfortunately there is little in the way of effective therapeutic options for these debilitating wounds and there remains a significant need for effective new treatments.

Cx43 is the most ubiquitous connexin in the skin, expressed in keratinocytes and fibroblasts, endothelial cells and dermal appendages [4,5]. We have reported that topical application of a Cx43-specific antisense containing gel to acute wounds in rodent models significantly accelerates the healing process whilst reducing inflammation and scar size [6,7].

In the normal healing process Cx43 protein becomes down-regulated in keratinocytes in the first 24–48 hours as they become migratory and crawl forward to close the wound [8,9,10,11,12]. Following experiments in Cx43 conditional knockout mice it was later reported that downregulation of Cx43 appears to be a pre-requisite for the coordinated proliferation and mobilization of keratinocytes during wound healing [13,14]. In contrast, we showed that in STZ diabetic rats, a model for chronic wounds, Cx43 is upregulated in wound edge keratinocytes instead of being down-regulated, and that migration is delayed until downregulation occurs [15]. Application of a Cx43 antisense to STZ diabetic rat wounds prevented the abnormal upregulation of Cx43 and restored wound closure to normal rates or better [15]. Over-expression of Cx43 was also shown to inhibit corneal endothelial wound healing in an *in vivo* rat corneal scrape injury model, while knockdown with Cx43 antisense sped it up [16]. Cx43 was also reported to be detected in the cells at the wound margins of the majority of biopsies taken from nine mixed and two diabetic leg ulcers [11].

One of the key impediments to the healing of chronic wounds is the failure of fibroblasts to migrate, proliferate and generate granulation tissue. Most previous reports have concentrated on epidermal Cx43 in wound healing and little attention has been paid to Cx43 in dermal fibroblasts. In the present work, we used a combination of *in vivo* and *in vitro* models to analyze the implications of elevated Cx43 expression, which we have discovered to be detrimentally upregulated in the dermis of human chronic VLU, and to correlate with reduced rates of migration of scratch-wounded fibroblasts over-expressing Cx43. In addition to Cx43, we also discovered that ZO-1 and N-cadherin, which interact with Cx43 and each other [17], are abnormally overexpressed in the dermis of human chronic VLU. Targeting Cx43 reduced the expression levels of ZO-1 and N-cadherin both *in vitro* and *in vivo*. Knock down of Cx43 and N-cadherin, but not ZO-1, accelerated cell migration in a scratch wound-healing assay. Reduction of Cx43 or N-cadherin also increased Golgi polarization whilst reducing proliferation and cell adhesion in fibroblasts. Targeting of Cx43 or N-cadherin, furthermore, was accompanied by cytoskeletal changes, increased lamellipodia protrusion, and activation of Rho GTPases. These findings support the idea that Cx43 and N-cadherin are therapeutic targets for improvement of wound repair through a mechanism involving remodeling of cell contacts and adhesion-dependent cytoskeletal modifications in fibroblasts.

Results

Cx43, N-cadherin and ZO-1 are dramatically upregulated in the dermis of human VLU

Skin punch biopsies, 2 mm, from healthy human volunteers (Figure 1A), and chronic wound edge biopsy samples, 4 mm, from 6 human VLU (Figure 1D and E), together with corresponding intact skin samples from the same patients (Figure 1E), were used to analyze Cx43 protein levels in the dermis of chronic vs. acute wounds. In acute wounds, downregulation of Cx43 was seen at dermal wound margins 4 hours after excisional wounding (Figure 1A), similar to that observed in the wound-edge dermis in a murine model after an excisional wounding (Figure S1, A) while Cx43 has been reported to persist at the wound edge epidermis of a majority of mixed diabetic leg ulcers [11]. Human and murine skin punch biopsies analysis showed that Cx43 was significantly reduced at the wound edge, with levels increasing towards normal with progressive distance from the injury site (Figure 1, A, B and C; $p<0.01$; and Figure S1, A, arrowheads; $p<0.005$). In sharp contrast, biopsies from the wound edge of VLU had not only failed to downregulate Cx43, but also showed significantly elevated expression of Cx43 throughout the dermis of the whole 4 mm biopsy (Figure 1, E and F; $p<0.005$).

Cx43 can interact with adherens junction proteins such as N-cadherin [17,18], and with the tight junction associated protein ZO-1 [19] which also interact with each other. We investigated the expression and distribution of these proteins in the dermis of chronic VLU biopsies and matched non-wounded skin (Figure 2, A and B). ZO-1 and N-cadherin levels were significantly higher in chronic VLU samples than in matched non-wounded control dermis (Figure 2, C and D; $p<0.01$ and $p<0.005$, respectively). Taken together, these data indicate that human chronic VLUs not only fail to downregulate Cx43 in the dermal wound margins, but also that N-cadherin and ZO-1 are abnormally upregulated compared to their levels in intact skin.

Cx43 expression is tightly linked to N-cadherin and ZO-1 expression in fibroblasts

We have previously shown that Cx43 downregulation significantly accelerates the skin healing process [6,7]. Here we investigated the effects of Cx43 knockdown on ZO-1 and N-cadherin protein expression *in vivo*. To this end we used a mouse model of wound healing where full thickness skin excision wounds were treated with Cx43 antisense, or sense oligodeoxynucleotide control (Cx43asODN and Cx43sODN, respectively).

Immunohistochemical analysis revealed positive ZO-1 staining in dermal sense-treated wounds, where ZO-1 was frequently co-localized with Cx43 (Figure S1, B). Treatments with Cx43asODN, on the other hand, induced a significant decline not only of Cx43, but also of ZO-1 in the dermal wound margins (Figure S1, B; Figure 3A, $p<0.05$). Analysis of N-cadherin expression revealed a preferential distribution in the dermis in sense-treated wounds, and significant protein downregulation after treatment with the Cx43asODN (Figure S1, C; Figure 3B, $p<0.01$). These data demonstrate that Cx43 expression is tightly linked to ZO-1 and N-cadherin expression in the dermis, and that targeting Cx43 can reduce ZO-1 and N-cadherin expression *in vivo*.

In order to better understand the effects of Cx43, N-cadherin and ZO-1 on fibroblast migration in response to a wounding stimulus we turned to the 3T3 fibroblast cell line. This can be easily transfected or transduced with shRNA constructs and avoids the variability of primary human fibroblasts derived from different patients. ZO-1 and N-cadherin expression was evaluated in fibroblasts transduced with a Cx43 short-hairpin RNA (Cx43shRNA) that suppresses Cx43 expression [20], or a p.Sup control plasmid. Cx43 protein expression and gap junction-mediated intercellular communication (GJIC) were effectively prevented in the Cx43shRNA cells, in contrast to p.Sup control cells (Figure 3C; Figure S2, G and I). With regard to ZO-1 expression, ZO-1 protein levels were downregulated in Cx43shRNA-transduced cells (Figure 3D). ZO-1 distribution was also analyzed in fibroblast scratch wound assays generated with Cx43shRNA and control cells. The Cx43shRNA-transduced cells showed a reduction of ZO-1 located at cell contacts at both the leading edge (LE) and in regions more internal to the wound (IA), accompanied by a loss of ZO-1 from the leading edge lamellipodia (Figure 3E, arrowheads). In p.Sup-transduced fibroblasts, however, ZO-1 was predominantly restricted to the contact margins between cells, often co-localizing with Cx43 (Figure 3E). With regard to N-cadherin, protein levels were significantly reduced in Cx43shRNA-transduced fibroblasts (Figure 3F; $p<0.01$) and N-cadherin was found located predominantly in the cytosol (Figure 3G, arrows) rather than the preferential plasma membrane localization found in p.Sup-transduced control fibroblasts (Figure 3G, arrowheads).

We also studied α- and β-catenin expression and distribution in p.Sup and Cx43shRNA-transduced cells. Whereas total β-catenin protein levels did not change significantly after Cx43 knockdown (Figure S3B), its cellular distribution was altered. In p.Sup-transduced cells, β-catenin was mainly localized to the plasma membrane at sites of cell-cell contact (Figure S3A), but relocation to the cytosol was additionally found in Cx43shRNA-transduced fibroblasts (Figure S3A, arrows), with evidence for some nuclear localization (Figure S3A, arrowhead). Alpha-catenin was seen localized in both the plasma membrane and the cytosol in p.Sup and Cx43shRNA-transduced cells (Figure S3C), and expression levels and location did not change with Cx43 knockdown (Figure S3D).

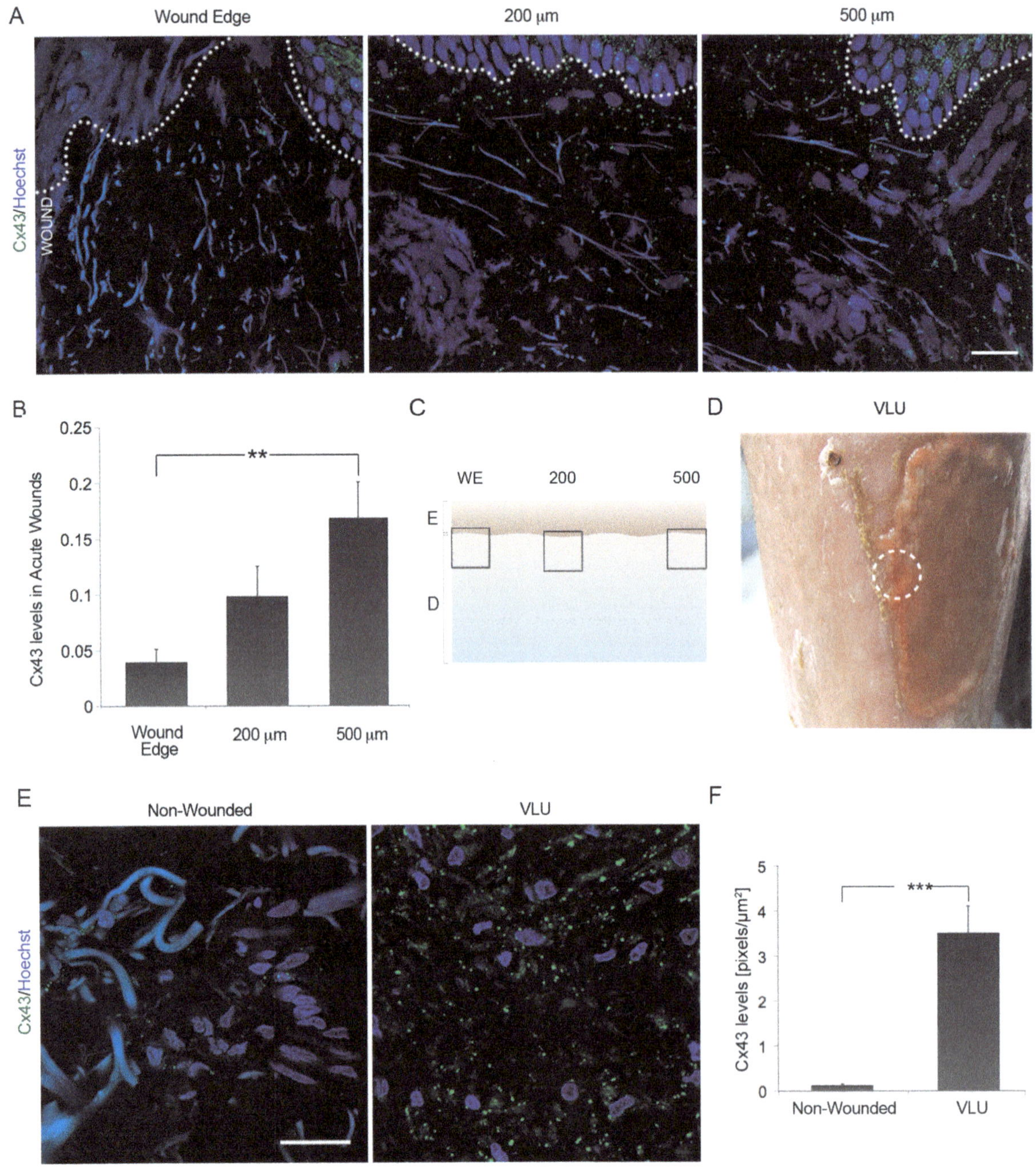

Figure 1. Dermal Cx43 is greatly upregulated in human chronic VLU. (A) Cx43 expression levels are reduced at the dermal wound margins 4 hours after leg punch biopsy of the skin of healthy volunteers. Scale bar = 25 μm. Blue signal is Hoechst staining of nuclei and collagen bundle autofluorescence. The dotted white line shows the border between the epidermis and the dermis (B) Cx43 levels increased with progressive distance from the injury site (C). Values represent mean ± SD (n = 3; ** $p<0.01$). (D) A representative picture of a chronic VLU in the lower leg of a patient, from which a wound edge punch biopsy has been taken – white dotted circle. (E) Dermal Cx43 expression levels were significantly upregulated in chronic VLU in comparison to matched non-wounded samples (n = 6; *** $p<0.005$). (F) Graph depicting Cx43 levels in VLU vs. non-wounded skin. Values were expressed as mean ± SEM. Scale bar = 25 μm.

Cx43 and N-cadherin, but not ZO-1 knockdown accelerate the rate of fibroblast migration

Targeting Cx43 for knockdown accelerates the rate of wound closure *in vivo* [6]. However, the underlying mechanism remains unknown. We investigated whether the increase in cell migration following a reduction in Cx43 expression was associated with reduction of ZO-1 protein levels or decreased cell adhesion (ZO-1 or N-cadherin down-regulation, respectively).

We first evaluated the migration rate of fibroblasts transduced with Cx43shRNA or p.Sup vectors, or cells treated with Cx43asODN or control Cx43sODN. Similar to Cx43shRNA cells, fibroblasts treated with Cx43asODN showed greatly reduced Cx43 protein levels and GJIC compared to Cx43sODN, or

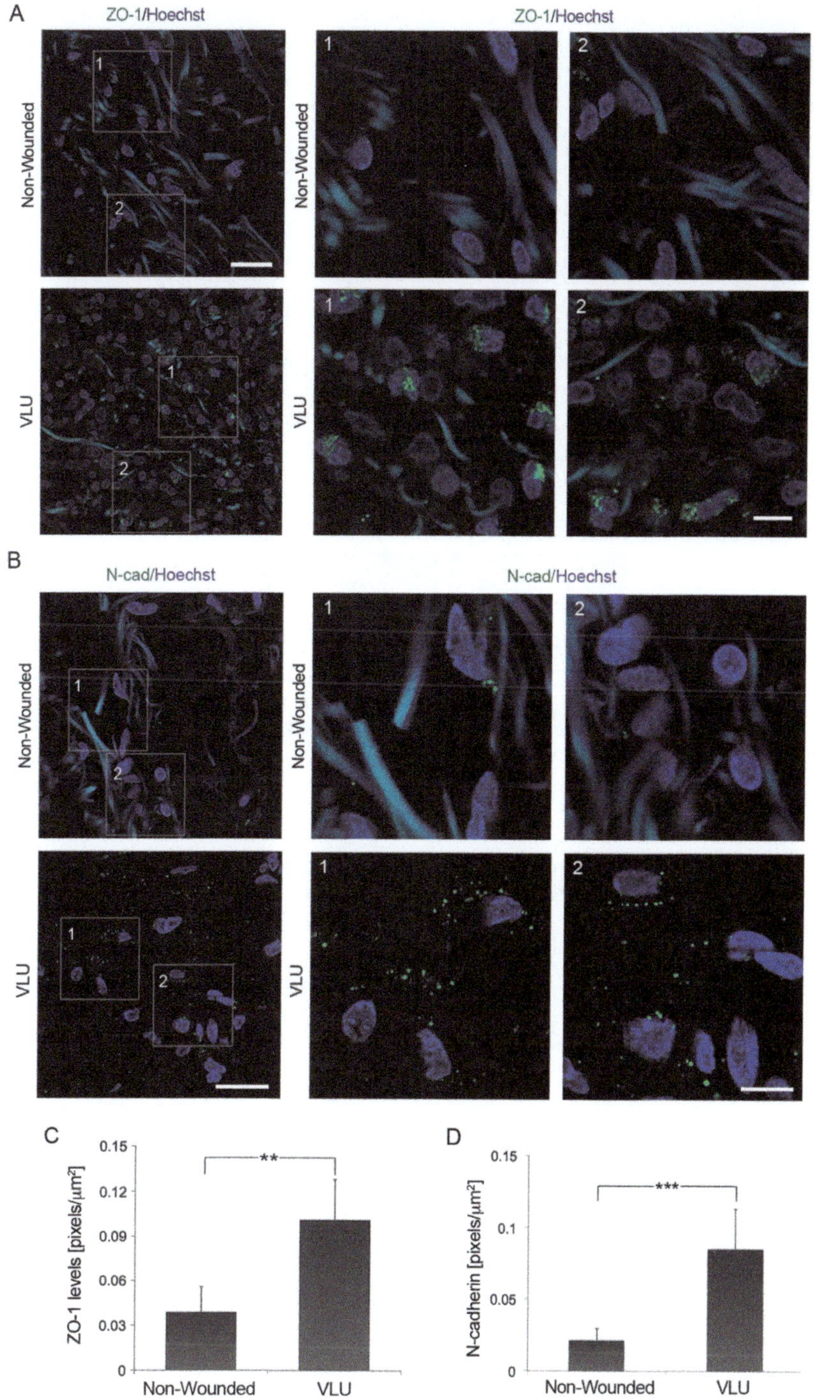

Figure 2. Increased expression of N-cadherin and ZO-1 in the dermis of human chronic VLU (A) ZO-1 expression levels are elevated in the dermis of chronic VLU compared to matched non-wounded controls (n = 6). Scale bar = 25 μm. Higher magnifications of VLU and intact skin (boxed regions 1 and 2) stained for ZO-1 (green) and Hoechst (blue) are shown. Scale bar = 10 μm. (B) N-cadherin is significantly upregulated in chronic VLU compared to matched non-wounded samples (n = 6). Scale bar = 25 μm. The boxed regions 1 and 2 show high magnifications of VLU and non-wounded skin samples stained for N-cadherin (green) and Hoechst (blue). Scale bar = 10 μm. Values represent mean ± SD. (C and D) Graphs show ZO-1 and N-cadherin expression levels in VLU vs. non-wounded skin. Values for ZO-1 and N-cadherin were expressed as mean ± SD; $^{**}p<0.01$ and $p<0.005$, respectively.

untreated cells (Figure S2, A and B, respectively; $p<0.05$ and $p<0.01$). We also transiently transfected fibroblasts with a bicistronic pIRES-GFP empty vector (pGFP) or with a matching vector encoding GFP and either wild-type Cx43 (Cx43-WT), or a dominant negative Cx43 construct (Cx43-DN) that interferes with the traffic of endogenous Cx43 protein to the plasma membrane, thereby blocking GJIC [21].

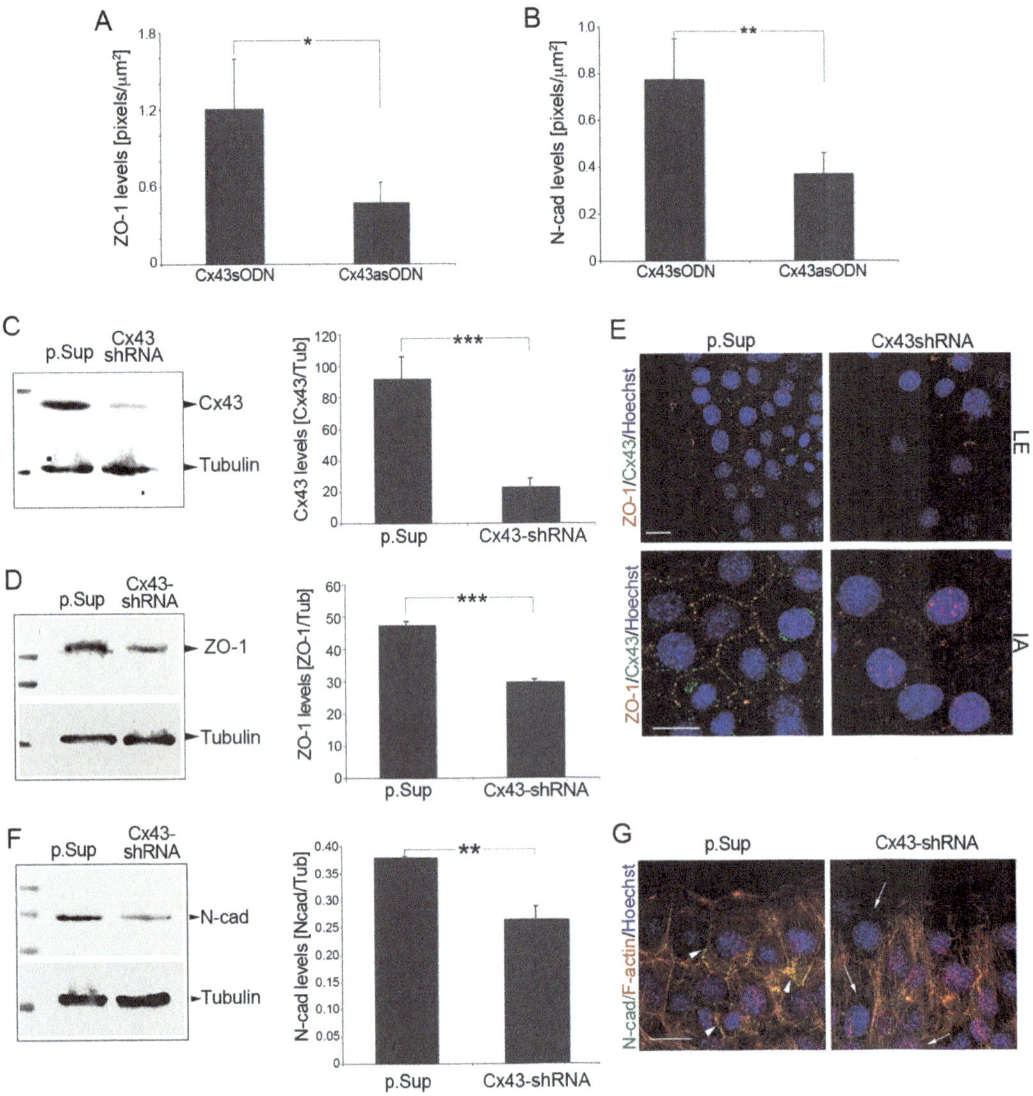

Figure 3. Targeting Cx43 reduces N-cadherin and ZO-1 expression in fibroblasts. (A) ZO-1 or (B) N-cadherin expression levels were examined in mouse skin wounds treated *in vivo* with Cx43sODN or Cx43asODN (n = 6). Downregulation of ZO-1 and N-cadherin was found in the dermis of mice after Cx43 knockdown. Graphs represent mean ± SD; * $p<0.05$ and ** $p<0.01$. (C–D) ZO-1 and Cx43 levels were analyzed by Western blot in Cx43shRNA and p.Sup-transduced fibroblasts. Tubulin was included as loading control. Quantification shows that knockdown of Cx43 reduced the expression of ZO-1 (*** $p<0.005$; n = 3). (E) ZO-1 (red) and Cx43 (green) expression and distribution in leading edge (LE) and internal areas (IA) were analyzed by confocal microscopy in wounded Cx43shRNA or p.Sup-transduced cells (n = 4). Cells were also counterstained with Hoechst (blue). Scale bar = 20 μm. (F) N-cadherin expression levels were significantly reduced after targeting Cx43 (** $p<0.01$; n = 3). (G) N-cadherin (green) redistribution from membrane (arrowheads) to cytosolic compartments (arrows) was analyzed along with F-Actin (red) in p.Sup and Cx43shRNA fibroblasts 3 h after scratch wounding of confluent 3T3 monolayers (n = 3). Scale bar = 20 μm.

The velocity of migration of Cx43shRNA and Cx43asODN cells was significantly faster than p.Sup or Cx43sODN control cells, respectively (Figure 4, C and D, $p<0.005$; Movie S1; Figure S2, C and D; Movie S2). Cx43 knockdown cells also displayed much more extensive lamellipodia than control cells (Figure 4C, Movie S1). Similarly, Cx43-DN-transfected fibroblasts migrated faster than their untransfected neighbors or pGFP control cells, and also extended larger than usual lamellipodia at the leading edge (Figure S2, E and F; Movie S3). Conversely, fibroblasts overexpressing Cx43 (Cx43-WT) migrated significantly slower than either pGFP or Cx43-DN constructs (Figure S2, E and F; $p<0.05$ and $p<0.01$ respectively; Movie S3). These data provide further evidence for an inverse correlation between Cx43 protein levels and the rate of fibroblast migration after scratch wounding. However, there have also been reports that siRNA reduction of Cx43 can slow cell migration in 3T3 cell scratch wound assays that have been serum starved for 2 days [22]. We repeated these experiments in serum starved conditions and in the presence of normal amounts of cell culture serum. We found that in serum-starved conditions reducing Cx43 protein levels slowed migration whilst in more normal media conditions with serum, reducing Cx43 significantly sped migration (Figure S2 J).

We then analyzed the velocity of migration of fibroblasts transduced with N-cadherin or Mock shRNA constructs (N-cadshRNA and Mock, respectively). The N-cadshRNA construct effectively suppressed N-cadherin expression in NIH3T3 fibro-

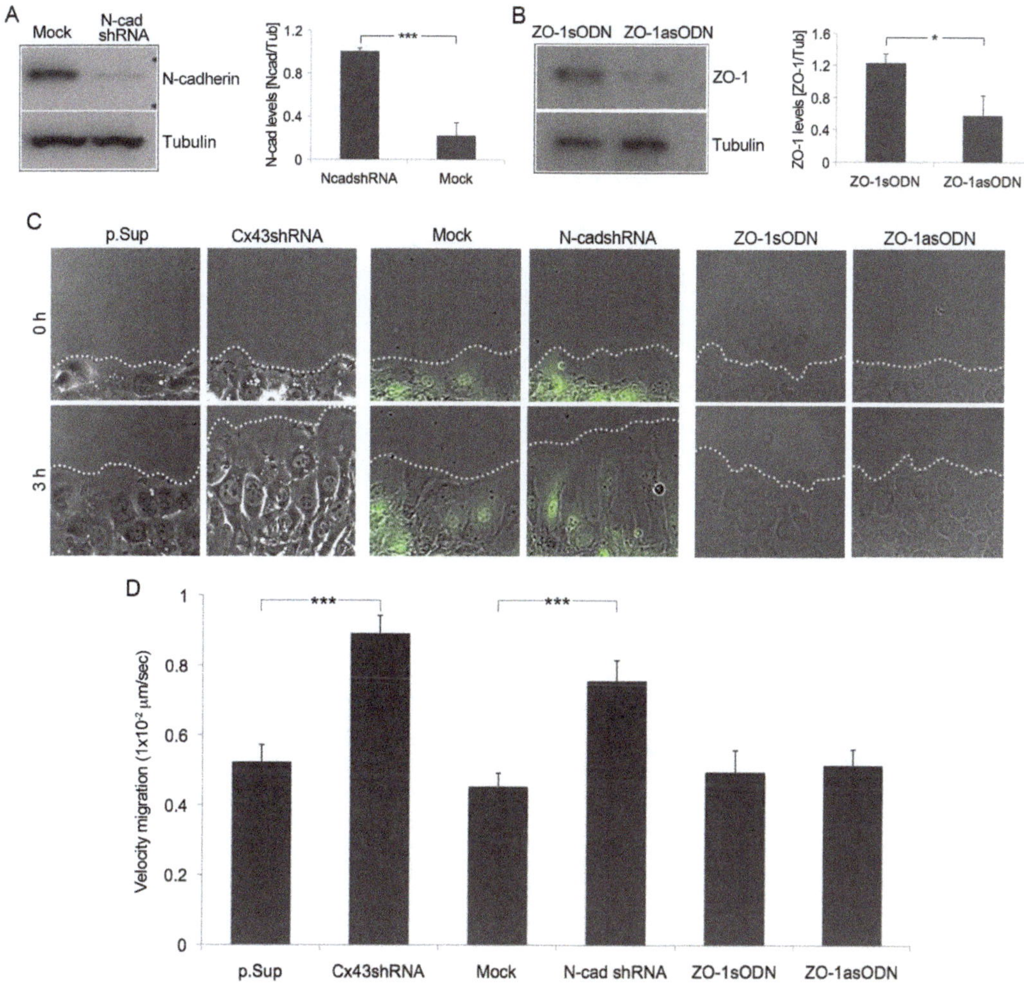

Figure 4. Cx43 and N-cadherin knockdown accelerates the rate of fibroblast migration. (A and B) N-cadherin and ZO-1 expression was evaluated by Western blot in Mock or N-cadshRNA-transduced cells, and in ZO-1asODN or sense-treated (ZO 1sODN) cells, respectively. Values represent mean ± SD (n = 3, ***$p<0.005$; n = 3, *$p<0.05$). (C) Cx43shRNA and p.Sup cells, Mock and N-cadshRNA cells, or fibroblasts treated with ZO-1sODN and ZO-1asODN were allowed to migrate into a wound for 3 h. Pictures of cells at the beginning of the migration recording (0 h) and at the end (3 h) are shown. (D) The graph shows the velocity of migration for all the aforementioned conditions. Values represent mean ± SEM (***$p<0.005$).

blasts (Figure 4A), as previously described [23], which accelerated cell migration in scratch wound assays almost to the same extent as in Cx43shRNA transduced cells (Figure 4, C and D). To reduce ZO-1 expression in fibroblasts, cells were treated with ZO-1 sense and antisense oligodeoxynucleotide (ZO-1sODN and ZO-1asODN), previously described as able to effectively reduce ZO-1 expression [24]. Contrary to Cx43 and N-cadherin, ZO-1 down-regulation (Figure 4B) did not have any effect on the rate of fibroblast migration or wound closure (Figure 4, C and D). These results indicate that targeting Cx43 may additionally contribute to cell migration by reducing N-cadherin, but not ZO-1 protein levels in fibroblasts.

Cx43 and N-cadherin regulate cell adhesion, polarization and proliferation in fibroblasts

Downregulation of the machinery of cell-cell adhesion is one of the ways in which different cell types, including skin cells, reactivate themselves to acquire a migratory phenotype [25]. Hanging drop assays have previously been used to characterize the strength of intercellular adhesion [26,27]. We used this strategy to compare cell-cell adhesion properties by measuring the size of cell clusters that formed in suspended drops, and which resisted trituration with a micropipette tip [27]. Clusters were evaluated by morphometric image analysis and classified into three size groups according to their area [26]. Cx43shRNA and N-cadshRNA-transduced cells formed fewer trituration-resistant clusters (area $>2.5\times10^3$ μm^2) and smaller clusters (area $<7.5\times10^2$ μm^2) characteristic of reduced cell-cell adhesion (Figure 5, A and B; $p<0.005$).

The redistribution of the Golgi apparatus is an important event in the polarization and migration of many types of cells, including fibroblasts [28]. To examine the role of Cx43 and N-cadherin in cell polarity during cell migration, we analyzed the localization of the Golgi protein GM130 in fibroblasts transduced with Cx43shRNA, N-cadshRNA, or their respective controls. Increased GM130 polarization towards the wound was observed in Cx43shRNA and N-cadshRNA cells compared to p.Sup and Mock controls, 3 h after wounding (Figure 5, C and D; $p<0.05$).

Cell proliferation was also investigated using an IncuCyte^{TM} live-cell imaging system. A clear reduction of cell growth was

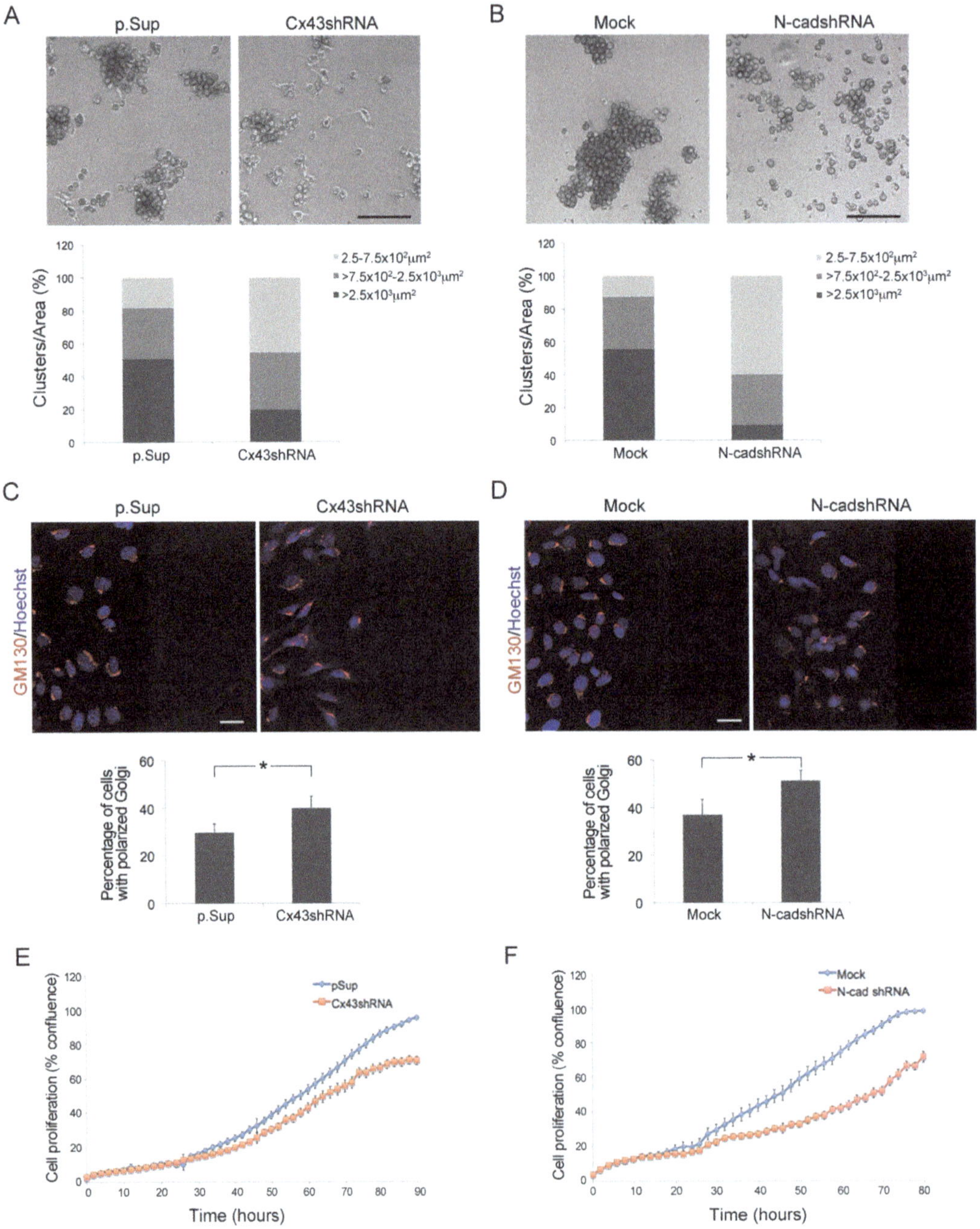

Figure 5. Cx43 and N-cadherin contribute to cell polarization, adhesion, and proliferation in fibroblasts. (A–B) Cell–cell adhesion upon suspension in hanging drops was assessed for Cx43shRNA and p.Sup, and for Mock and N-cadshRNA cells. The areas of cell clusters in six random fields taken from six different hanging drops were determined for each condition. Graphs represent the average number of clusters falling into each of three size ranges for each condition. Scale bar = 300 μm. (C–D) Cx43shRNA and p.Sup, and Mock and N-cadshRNA cells were wounded, allowed to migrate for 3 h, and then fixed and immunostained with anti-GM130 (red) and Hoechst (blue). Scale bar = 25 μm. The percentage of cells with Golgi located in the 120° arc facing the wound were scored as positive. Between 66–106 cells were evaluated in n = 3 independent experiments. Data represent the mean ± SEM (*$P<0.05$). Growth curves showing cell proliferation of fibroblasts transduced with (E) p.Sup and Cx43shRNA, and (F) Mock and N-cadshRNA constructs are shown. Data represent mean ± SD of three independent experiments, performed in duplicate.

observed in Cx43shRNA and N-cadshRNA transduced cells, compared to p.Sup and Mock control cells (Figure 5, E and F), indicating a direct correlation between Cx43 and N-cadherin expression, and cell proliferation in fibroblasts.

Altogether these data confirm the important contribution of Cx43 and N-cadherin to the regulation of cell polarization, adhesion and proliferation processes in fibroblasts during wound repair.

Targeting Cx43 induces cytoskeletal changes in leading-edge fibroblasts

Using scratch wound assays we observed that polarized Cx43 knockdown cells in the wound edge extended larger than usual lamellipodial protrusions (Movies S1 and S2). Directional cell locomotion requires complex interactions between actin filaments (F-actin) and microtubules, and we analyzed the distribution of F-actin, and tyrosinated and acetylated tubulin in wounded monolayers after targeting Cx43 expression in fibroblasts. Front-row control Cx43sODN, pGFP-transfected and p.Sup fibroblasts displayed the F-actin belt typical of polarized migratory cells (Figures 6A and 7A arrowhead; Figure S4A), which is regulated by adherens junctions [29]. In contrast, Cx43asODN, Cx43-DN and Cx43shRNA wound-edge cells developed rich lamelipodial protrusions oriented in the direction of movement, and lacked the F-actin belt found in control cells (Figures 6A and 7B arrowhead; Figure S4A). Under control conditions, tyrosinated and acetylated microtubules (TyrTub and AcetTub, respectively) were arranged very much as previously described in wounded fibroblast monolayer experiments [30], fanning out from the perinuclear region towards the wound margin. In Cx43asODN, Cx43shRNA, and Cx43-DN cells, which tended to be more extended, tyrosinated microtubules were predominantly oriented perpendicularly to the wound edge (Figures 6A and 7B arrowhead; Figure S4A). Cells over-expressing Cx43 (Cx43-WT) showed microtubules and lamellipodia that were less extensive than pGFP-transfected control cells (Figure 7C).

Lamellipodial dynamics were analyzed in more detail by transfecting fibroblasts with a red fluorescent protein (RFP)-actin construct. Sixteen hours after RFP-actin transfection a confluent monolayer was scratch-wounded and imaged for 1.5 hours by confocal microscopy. The p.Sup cells showed active, actin-rich lamellipodia and filopodia (Movie S4) and actin remodeling, characterized by dynamic formation and collapse of filopodia and actin ruffles in front-row cells. Cx43shRNA transduced fibroblasts displayed considerably more extensive actin-rich membrane protrusions at the front of the leading-edge cells (Movie 4). We quantified the extent of the cell protrusion and found that Cx43asODN, Cx43-DN and Cx43shRNA cells displayed almost twice the average protrusion length exhibited by Cx43sODN, pGFP and p.Sup control cells (Figures 6B and 7D; Figure S4B).

Following demonstration that Cx43 knockdown reduced N-cadherin expression, which also contributes to accelerate cell migration in fibroblasts (Figure 4D), we analyzed the distribution of polymerized actin in N-cadshRNA and Mock transduced cells 3 h after wound-scratch experiments. Similar to Cx43 knockdown fibroblasts, wound edge N-cadherin-targeted cells extended rich lamellipodial protrusions oriented towards the direction of cell migration (Figure S5A), and quantification showed more extensive lamellipodia protrusions compared to Mock control cells (Figure S5B).

Targeting Cx43 and N-cadherin increases Rac1 and Rho-A GTPase activities in fibroblasts

Rho GTPases are key regulators of actin and microtubule dynamics and have an essential role in controlling different actin-based structures critical for cell motility and chemotactic responses [31]. We examined the effect of Cx43 and N-cadherin knockdown on Rho family GTPase activation in fibroblasts, using pull-down assays with specific GST fusion protein-binding domains for activated Rac1, Cdc42 and RhoA (GTP-bound forms). Quantitative analysis showed enhanced Rac1 and RhoA activity in Cx43shRNA and N-cadshRNA cells compared to p.Sup and Mock controls, respectively (Figure 8, A and B). In contrast, no differences in Cdc42 GTPase activity were detected.

To examine the activation of Rho GTPases in more detail, biosensors for Rac1, RhoA and Cdc42 [32,33] were transfected into either p.Sup or Cx43shRNA-transduced cells and FRET was used to examine the activity of these GTPases in leading edge fibroblasts 3 hours after scratch-induced migration. Targeting Cx43 with Cx43shRNA induced a two-fold increase in Rac1 and RhoA activity over the p.Sup control (Figure 8, C and E; $p<0.05$), but had no effect on the activity of Cdc42 (Figure 8E). These findings support a direct role for Cx43 in the regulation of cytoskeletal dynamics in fibroblasts during cell migration.

Discussion

Chronic wounds are a significant and growing global problem and place a great burden on both patients and healthcare system resources. While chronic wounds can occur anywhere on the body, most fall within the categories of VLUs, diabetic foot ulcers and pressure ulcers, which fail to progress through an organized, orderly and timely sequence of wound repair. Acceleration or even stimulation of wound closure is important for these chronic wounds, which are often infected and inflamed, making them painful and debilitating for the growing numbers of elderly and diabetic patients, and putting them at risk of lower limb amputation. Here we show that Cx43 is markedly upregulated in the dermis of human chronic VLU, similar to what was found in the wound edge epidermis of STZ diabetic rats, a feature that underlies impaired migration and healing [15]. We do not have ethical approval to biopsy and treat human VLU with Cx43 antisense and then resample these hard to heal wounds with additional biopsies. We therefore utilised a fibroblast cell line where we could reliably manipulate Cx43 protein expression and explore the effects on the dynamics of cell migration in a scratch wound healing assay. Whilst this is not as authoratative as in vivo human studies, they are useful for exploring the effect of Cx43 modulation on fibroblast behaviour. In these cell-culture experiments, fibroblast migration was impaired when Cx43 protein levels and GJIC were elevated after transfection with a Cx43-WT construct. These findings support a conclusion that the impaired healing observed in human chronic VLU wounds might be a consequence of the reduced rate of fibroblast migration caused by elevated levels of Cx43 protein.

However, elevated levels of Cx43 may not be the only factor that compromises healing in VLU. Cx43 reportedly forms a multiprotein complex or 'nexus' with ZO-1, α- and β-catenin, and N-cadherin [17,18,34], proteins that are likely to influence both cell adhesion and migration in wound healing. In fact, when compared to intact skin, we found that both ZO-1 and N-cadherin were significantly upregulated in the dermis of human chronic VLU, along with Cx43 upregulation. Clinically relevant is the observation that silencing Cx43 accelerated the velocity of fibroblast migration, supporting the idea that this process can be therapeutically controlled. Using *in vitro* models it was recently reported that connexin mimetic peptides also improve the migration rates of dermal fibroblasts [35], as well as keratinocyte and fibroblast migration in organotypic models and 2D cultures [36], which further reinforce our observations. These studies reported that levels of Cx43 protein were not changed by the peptide but phosphorylation of Cx43 was increased and cell adhesion decreased [35,36]. We found that directly targeting Cx43 protein production additionally reduced N-cadherin and ZO-1 protein levels *in vivo*, with redistribution of both proteins from the plasma membrane to the cytosol. In the case of ZO-1, the protein was noticeably lost from the leading edge lamellipodia, which is normally a feature of fibroblast migration in scratch assay wound healing [37] and this may bring about changes in the distribution of the cytoskeletal components to which it binds.

The cytoplasmic tail of Cx43 is able to interact with the PDZ2 domain on ZO-1 but this interaction can be competed out by the addition of a mimetic peptide (ACT-1) to the last 9 amino acids of the Cx43 tail [38]. This peptide has been reported to stabilize

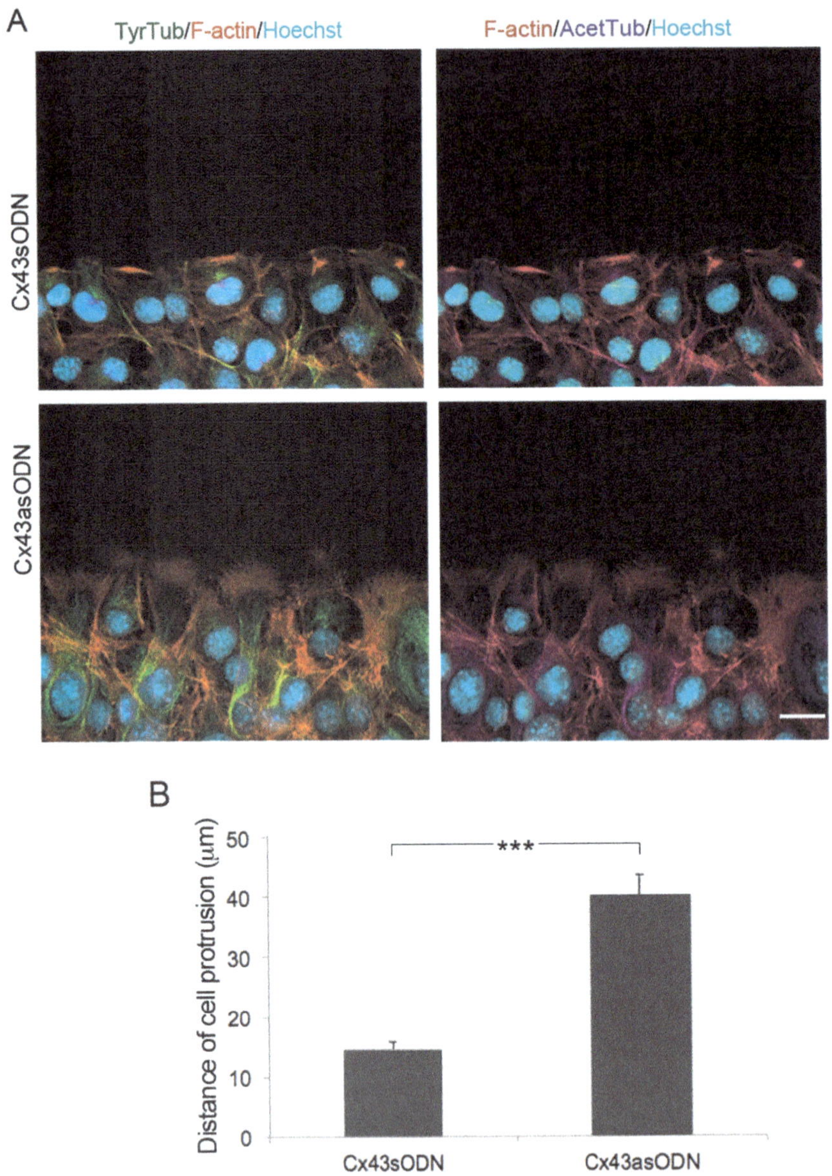

Figure 6. Targeting Cx43 induces cytoskeletal changes in leading-edge fibroblasts. (A) Representative images showing the distribution of F-actin (red), and tyrosinated (green) and acetylated (blue) tubulin (TyrTub and AcetTub, respectively) in leading edge Cx43sODN and C43asODN fibroblasts, 3 h after wounding. Cells were also counterstained with the nuclear marker Hoechst. Scale bar = 20 µm. (B) The graph shows the length of the protrusions of wound edge cells. Data represent the distance (mean ± SEM) from the nucleus to the leading edge in n = 3 experiments (***$P<0.005$).

Cx43 in the cell membrane forming larger gap junction plaques [38]. Applied to acute skin lesions this peptide is reported to accelerate wound healing whilst reducing scar formation, actions that are similar to those of the Cx43 antisense [39,40,41]. The mechanism behind the reported action of the peptide on wound healing is not at all clear at present. Interestingly, while knockdown of Cx43 and N-cadherin accelerated cell migration in a scratch wound-healing assay, targeting of ZO-1 failed to speed up fibroblast migration, indicating that ZO-1 down-regulation does not account for the faster migration that occurs when Cx43 is downregulated. It would be interesting in future studies to see if the ACT-1 peptide is able to accelerate fibroblast migration.

The literature regarding GJ communication and cell migration contains conflicting reports. Elevated connexin expression has been associated with reduced migration [42,43], while other authors have reported the opposite effect [44,45]. Using a different approach, *in vitro* studies performed on NIH 3T3 cells showed that the dynamic spreading movement, over an hour, of individual isolated and non-wounded cells appeared to be reduced when Cx43 was downregulated with siRNAs [17]. This discrepancy may reflect the different cell states (wounded vs. non-wounded) and different models used (cell migration into a scratch-wound vs. the spreading of non-wounded cells in sparse cultures). More recently the same group reported that Cx43 KO mouse embryonic fibroblasts migrated more slowly in scratch wound assays than those with Cx43 [22]. The reasons for these divergent observations are not clear but may be related to their serum starving of the cells for 48 hours prior to performing the scratch wound assay. We

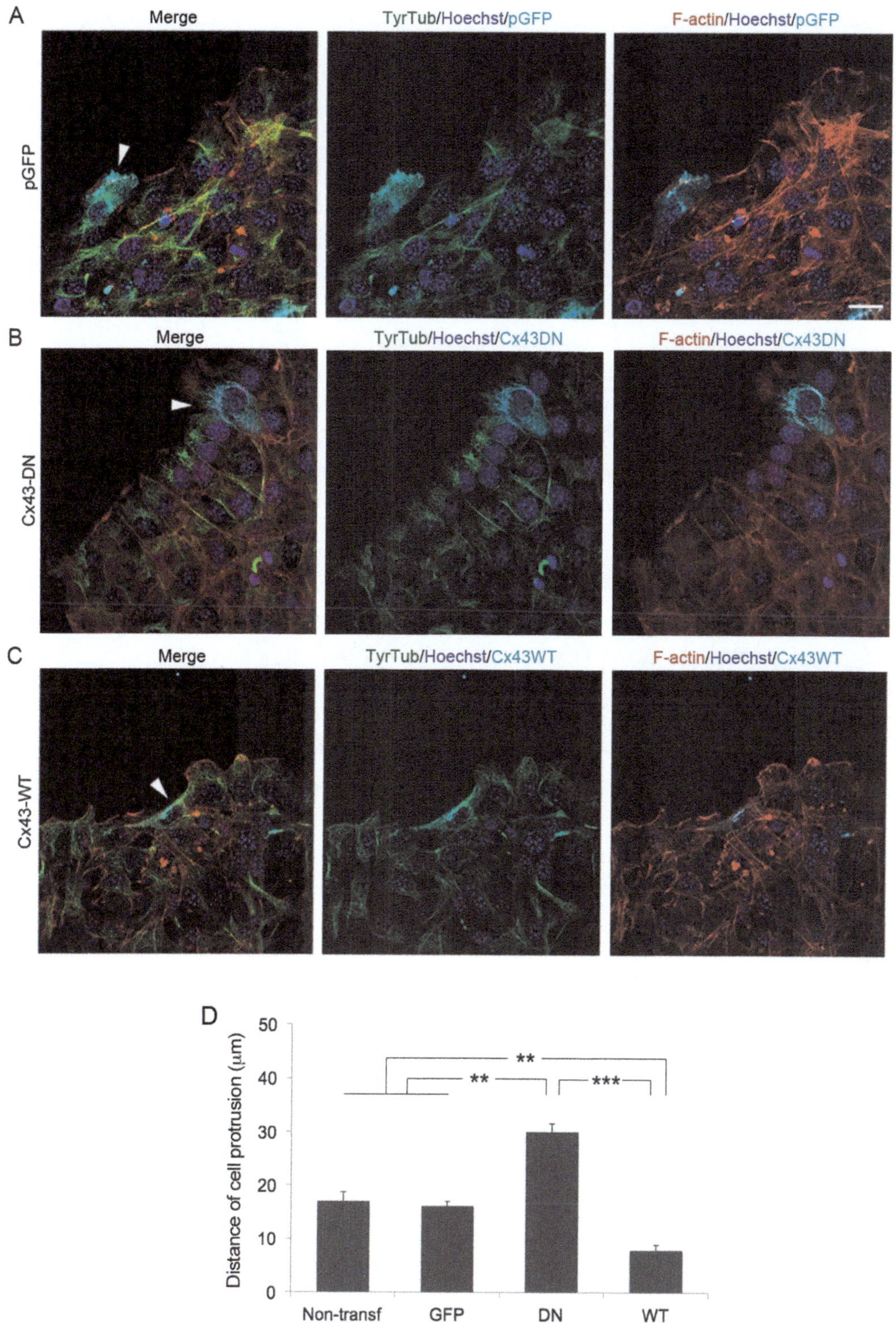

Figure 7. Modulation of Cx43 levels influence wound-edge cytoskeletal architecture in fibroblasts. Representative images of leading-edge cells transfected (arrowhead) with (A) a control pGFP construct (B) Cx43-DN, or (C) Cx43-WT, stained for TyrTub, F-actin and Hoechst. Scale bar = 20 μm. (D) Graph depicting the length of lamelipodial protrusions of fibroblasts transfected with the different constructs is shown (**$p<0.01$; ***$P<0.005$; n = 3).

repeated the migration experiments with control 3T3 cells and 3T3 cells transduced with Cx43shRNA to reduce Cx43 expression. One batch was serum starved for 2 days, whilst the other was not. Cultures were then scratch wounded and imaged for 4 hours. We found that serum starved cells with reduced Cx43 migrated more slowly whereas reducing Cx43 in the absence of serum starvation speeded migration. As serum starvation would not be expected to match the conditions found in an acute wound in vivo,

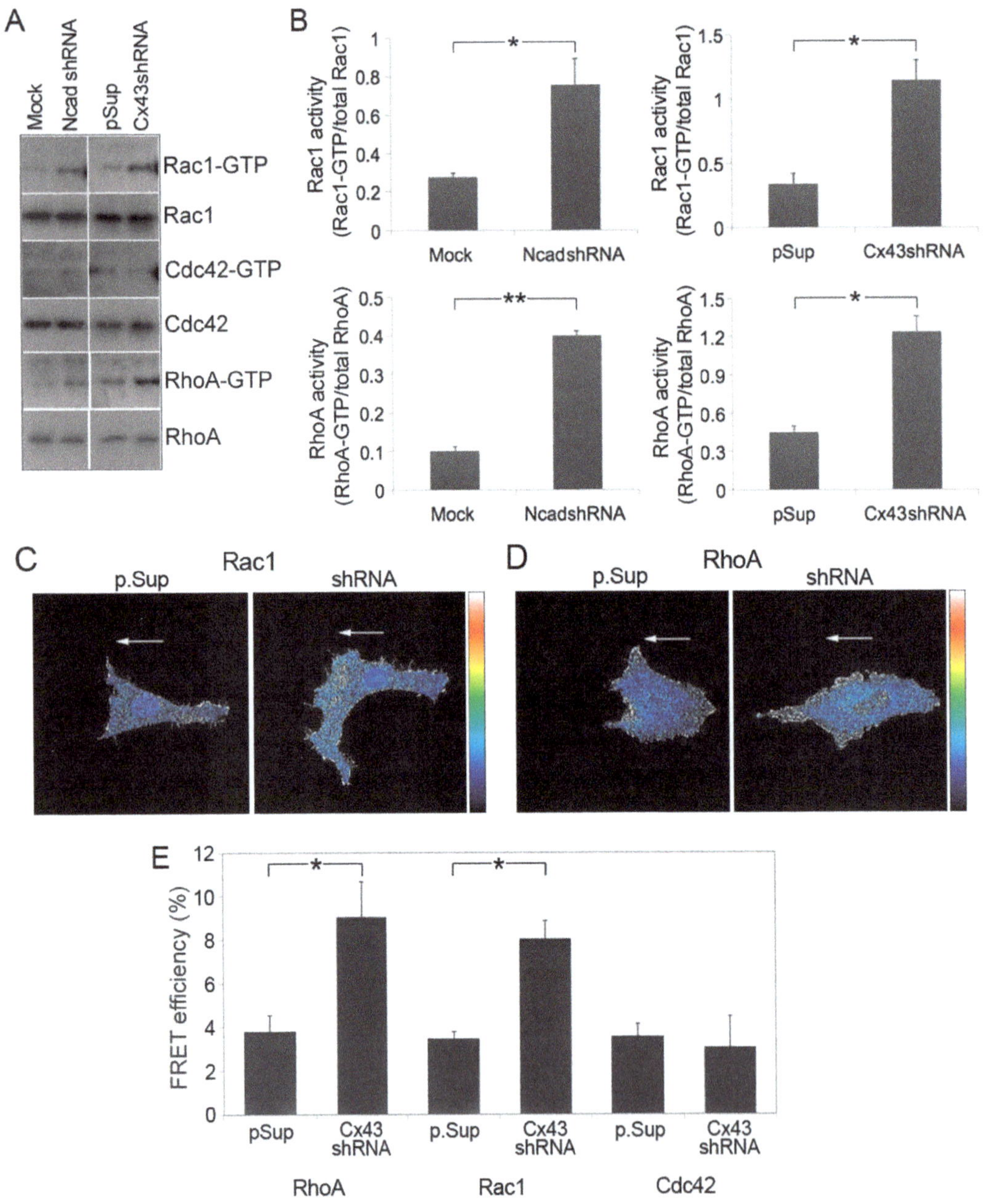

Figure 8. Cx43 and N-cadherin knockdown increases Rac1 and RhoA GTPase activity in fibroblasts. (A) Rho GTPase (GTP) activities in wounded fibroblasts were measured by pull-down assays using the PBD domain of PAK (Rac1 and Cdc42), or the RBD domain of Rhotekin (RhoA), followed by immunoblotting with the respective antibodies. Additionally, Rac1, Cdc42 and RhoA from total lysates were used as loading controls. (B) Graphs show active Rac1 and RhoA GTPase activity (GTP levels/total levels; mean ± SEM, $^*P<0.05$); n = 3 independent experiments. Representative images of leading edge Cx43shRNA and p.Sup transduced cells showing (C) Rac1, and (D) RhoA GTPase activities, 3 h after wounding of confluent monolayers. Scale bar = 10 μm. Arrows indicate the direction of migration. (E) FRET efficiency analysis show a two-fold increase in Rac1 and RhoA activities in Cx43shRNA vs. p.Sup-transduced cells, while no differences were observed for Cdc42. Data is representative of n = 3 experiments per condition; $^*p<0.05$.

where we and others have shown that down regulating Cx43 speeds migration of fibroblasts and keratinocytes, we can only assume that it is the abnormal conditions of serum starvation that is triggering the anomalous response.

Cadherin-mediated cell–cell adhesion is reported to coordinate junction development with cell movement and cell polarization, and to maintain junction integrity by forming links with actin filaments [46]. Disruption of N-cadherin has been reported to increase the rate of Schwann cell migration on astrocytes by enhancing both the number of migrating cells, and the maximum migration distance [47]. Here we demonstrated that targeting Cx43, which consistently reduced N-cadherin expression, significantly diminished cell-cell adhesion, while increasing cell polarization in fibroblasts. This was further demonstrated by targeting N-cadherin, which provided similar results. It is also possible that decreased cell-cell adhesion is contributed to by a direct loss of Cx43–Cx43 connexon docking in Cx43-targeted fibroblasts. This was previously confirmed in cadherin null human squamous carcinoma cells [48], and also in other models in which expression of Cx43 increased cell adhesitivity [49,50]. In the same way, interfering with Cx43 in individual cells of the 8–16 cell mouse embryo has previously been shown to reduce adhesion and produce decompaction of the targeted cell [51], whereas ZO-1 has recently been described to be essential for the compaction step [52]. Based on the findings described here we conclude that Cx43 down-regulation may prevent maturation of stable cell–cell adhesions by reducing N-cadherin expression and/or docking of connexons themselves.

We found that sustained reduction of the expression of either Cx43 or N-cadherin in 3T3 cells, by transduction with shRNA resulted in reduced cell proliferation. At first this observation does not seem to fit with previous reports from our group and others relating to Cx43 and cell proliferation. We have found that applying Cx43 antisense to an excisional wound on a mouse results in increased proliferation of fibroblasts and nascent keratinocytes but this was 1, 2 & 7 days after the treatment by which time the antisense was no longer preventing Cx43 protein production [7]. Pollock et al., 2011 [36] reported that the mimetic peptide GAP27 could in some cases enhance cell proliferation at the leading edge of a scratch wound assay of keratinocytes or fibroblasts. This effect was brought about without apparently reducing Cx43 protein levels and so the differences observed when Cx43 protein is significantly reduced may reflect the direct effect of the presence of the Cx43 protein on cell proliferation rather than the effect of Cx43 based gap junctional communication.

Trafficking of Cx43 hemichannels to cell–cell junctions takes place through a pathway that is dependent on microtubules [18], and it is well known that the cytoplasmic tail of Cx43 is able to interact with various components of the cytoskeleton, including microtubules and actin [18,53,54,55,56]. Here we show that front-row migrating fibroblasts lacking N-cadherin or Cx43 adopt an elongated phenotype with lamellipodia extended into the wound bed in the direction of migration. In contrast, actin organization in control-wounded fibroblasts was characterized by the F-actin belt typical of polarized migratory cells, known to be regulated by adherens junctions [29]. We also identified enhanced Rac1 and RhoA activities in Cx43 and N-cadherin-targeted fibroblasts, yet the molecular mechanism by which these proteins regulate Rho GTPase activation remains to be elucidated. However, these findings correlate with a reported role for RhoA in regulating fibroblast protrusion as an initiator of actin polymerization at the onset of the protrusion-retraction cycle [57]. Rac1, on the other hand, can influence the reinforcement and stabilization of newly expanded protrusions [57], which may help to explain the faster migration and more extensive lamellipodia observed in Cx43-targeted fibroblasts. The organization of the microtubule cytoskeleton was also investigated and found to be altered after reducing Cx43 levels, indicating that Cx43 not only interacts directly with microtubules, but may also affect microtubule dynamics during fibroblast migration. A finding that is in agreement with recent observations by Francis et al 2011showing altered microtubule dynamics in Cx43 KO mouse embryonic fibroblasts [22].

Overall, this study provides insight into why chronic VLUs that we have found to overexpress Cx43 in the dermis are slow to heal, and the cellular mechanisms as to how reducing Cx43 and N-cadherin expression accelerates fibroblast migration, pointing to a potential therapeutic solution to this debilitating problem. Our findings support the concept that the role of Cx43 is not simply to form GJ channels, but also to stabilize a nexus or multiprotein complex comprising N-cadherin, amongst others, that is required for cell-cell adhesion and adhesion-dependent actin dynamics, and must be broken down to facilitate efficient fibroblast migration. A large Phase 2 clinical trial is now underway using the Cx43asODN to reduce Cx43 expression in subjects with VLUs after an initial clinical trial showed significant improvement in complete healing.

Materials and Methods

Human chronic VLU and matched intact skin samples

Collection of wound edge punch biopsies from chronic venous ulcer leg wounds and normal arm biopsies was approved by the Western Institutional Review Board, Olympia, Washington State, USA. Punch biopsies from the thigh of healthy volunteers were under approval by the Northern X Regional Ethics Committee, Auckland, New Zealand. All biopsies were taken after written informed consent was obtained and the clinical research executed in accordance with the principles of the Declaration of Helsinki. Briefly for the VLUs a single 4 mm punch biopsy was taken from the wound edge under local anaesthesia in patients with clinically confirmed venous ulceration. A second 4 mm punch biopsy was taken from normal skin on the forearm in the same subjects. In all, biopsies from 6 subjects with clinically confirmed VLU (3 male and 3 female; range 38–79 years) were taken: median ulcer duration 6 months (range 1.5–36 months), and median size 10 cm^2 (range 2–113 cm^2). The VLU biopsies were initially fixed overnight with 4% paraformaldehyde (PFA), then transferred to 25% sucrose, and stored at 4°C until processing. For immunohistochemistry, tissue biopsies were embedded in OCT (BDH, UK). Samples were cryo-sectioned (10 μm) for immunohistochemistry analysis. For the normal (acute) wound biopsies an initial 6 mm punch biopsy was performed under local anesthetic on the anterolateral thigh of 3 healthy male volunteers (range 20–36 years) and then 4 hours later the punched wound site was excised with a larger 10 mm punch, and the resulting wound sutured closed. The 2 mm wide donut shaped biopsy was immediately imbedded in OCT snap frozen in liquid nitrogen and then stored at −80°C until being cryosectioned before analysis.

Mouse and rat cutaneous wound-healing model and ODNs application

Male, 8-week-old ICR mice or Sprague-Dawley rats from UCL's Biological Services Unit were maintained according to UK Home Office animal regulations. Excisional lesions were performed as previously described [7]. Single topical applications of 10 μM unmodified Cx43asODN and control Cx43sODN (Sigma-Genosys) were delivered to each of two independent wounds in 30% Pluronic F-127 gel (Sigma). Two days after wounding, animals were humanely sacrificed and the wound tissue was harvested.

Cell cultures and ODNs treatment

3T3 fibroblasts were grown in DMEM-GlutaMAX^{TM}-1 (Gibco, Invitrogen) supplemented with 10% FBS (Gibco, Invitrogen) in 5% CO_2 at 37°C. For ODN treatments fibroblasts were washed with PBS to eliminate any traces of serum, and were incubated in serum free media for 2 hours with 20 μM Cx43asODN or Cx43sODN [6] (Sigma-Genosys); or with 10 μM ZO-1asODN or ZO-1sODNs [24] (Sigma-Genosys). Following this incubation, the medium with the ODNs was removed and replaced by 10% FBS in DMEM.

Transfection; retroviral and lentiviral constructs and transduction

A retroviral pSuper vector containing the Cx43-specific shRNA target sequence GGTGTGGCTGTCAGTGCTC [20], kindly donated by W.H. Moolenaar and here designated Cx43shRNA, was used to establish a stable knockdown of Cx43 in 3T3 fibroblasts. A pSuppressor (p.Sup) retroviral vector (Imgenex Co) was used as control. The packaging cell line GP2–293 (Clontech) was transfected with the p.Sup and Cx43shRNA constructs as previously described [58]. Mock and N-cad shRNA constructs [23], kindly provided by S Arai and T Suda, were transfected into HEK 293T cells according to [59]. 3T3 fibroblasts were transduced with retrovirus or lentivirus for 2 days, and Cx43shRNA and N-cadshRNA and Mock-transduced cells were selected on the basis of resistance to 2 μg/ml puromycin or 500 μg/ml of geneticin (for p.Sup).

Fugene HD (Roche) was used to transfect 70% confluent fibroblasts with 1 μg/ml pGFP, Cx43-DN or Cx43-WT constructs ([21]) according to manufacturer's recommendation. Media was changed the following morning and 24 h later cells were used on different set of experiments.

Immunohistochemistry of murine and human skin samples

Immunostaining was carried out on 6-μm cryostat sections of wounded rat and mouse skin, or 10-μm human chronic VLU or matched non-wounded skin, fixed in acetone at 4°C for 5 minutes. Primary antibodies (Abs) for Cx43 (diluted 1:2000; Sigma, 6219), N-cadherin (diluted 1:100; Abcam, ab18203) and ZO-1 (diluted 1:100; Zymed Laboratories, 61–7300) were incubated for 1 hour at room temperature. Sections were washed with PBS and then incubated with the respective secondary Abs: swine anti-rabbit FITC-conjugated (DAKO) and goat anti-mouse Cy3-conjugated (Pierce). Secondary Abs incubation in the absence of primary Abs was used as negative control. Sections were then counterstained for 10 minutes with 5 μg/ml of the nuclear dye Hoechst 33342 (Sigma) and single optical sections were acquired on a Leica SP2 confocal microscope (Leica Microsystems, UK). All parameters during image acquisition were kept constant throughout each experiment to allow direct comparison of all of the 8 bit digital images. Immunostaining levels were quantified per unit area using a well-established pixel-counting method [15] using ImageJ software (NIH). Images were converted to binary images using an identical threshold. Objects greater than 2 pixels were counted in order to generate a readout of the number of positive pixels per unit area for comparison between conditions.

Immunostaining

Confluent fibroblast monolayers were wounded and fixed 3 h later with 4% PFA for 10 minutes and permeabilized with 0.1% Triton X-100. Primary Abs for Cx43 (diluted 1:2000; Sigma), ZO-1 (diluted 1:100; Zymed Laboratories), N-cadherin (diluted 1:100; Abcam), β-catenin (diluted 1:200; ab6302 Abcam), α-catenin (diluted 1:200; C2081 Sigma), tyrosinated tubulin (diluted 1:400; YL1/2; Ab6160 Abcam) and acetylated tubulin (diluted 1:200; T7451 Sigma) were used according to the manufacturer's recommendations. Incubation with the appropriate secondary Abs (Alexa 488 or 633; Molecular Probes) was followed by 10 minutes application of 5 μg/ml of the nuclear dye Hoechst 33342 (Sigma). Secondary Ab incubation in the absence of primary Ab was used as negative control. TRITC-phalloidin (Sigma) was included in some experiments for visualization of F-actin. Cells were imaged using a 63×, 1.25 NA objective on a Leica SP2 confocal microscope (Leica Microsystems, UK). At least three images, from 3–5 independent experiments were acquired. All acquisition parameters were kept constant throughout each experiment and staining was quantified based on pixel counts [15].

Golgi reorientation measurements

Measurement of Golgi reorientation was performed as described previously [60]. Confluent fibroblasts were scratched and incubated for 3 h. After this time, cells were fixed with 4% PFA and stained with anti-GM130 (BD Biosciences) and Hoechst 33342 nuclear stain (Sigma). One hundred cells in ten randomly selected fields were evaluated for Golgi orientation.

Cell proliferation

3T3 fibroblasts (1×10^4 cells) transduced with pSup, Cx43shRNA, Mock and N-cadshRNA constructs were plated into 96-well plates and cell growth was monitored in real-time using the IncuCyte™ live-cell imaging system (Essen Instruments, Ann Arbor, MI). Experiments were performed at least three times in duplicate and data was expressed as percentage of confluence.

Measurement of protrusion length

Confluent fibroblasts transduced with Cx43shRNA, p.Sup, N-cadshRNA and Mock constructs, or transfected with pGFP, Cx43-DN or Cx43-WT were wounded and fixed with 4% PFA 3 h later. The cells were then stained with Hoechst 33342 nuclear stain (Sigma). To quantify the protrusions' length, the distance from the nuclei to the leading edge of wound edge cells was measured. In each of three independent experiments, 3–5 transfected cells, or 30 transduced cells in randomly selected fields were analyzed to calculate the average length of these protrusions.

Western blot

Cell pellets from harvested fibroblasts (Cx43shRNA- or p.Sup-transduced) were suspended at 4°C in ice-cold RIPA buffer plus protease inhibitors. Equal amounts of protein were resuspended in Laemmli 4× sample buffer, separated by 10% SDS-PAGE and visualized with primary Abs to Cx43 (diluted 1:2000; Sigma), ZO-1 (diluted 1:500; Zymed Laboratories), α-catenin (diluted 1:200; Sigma), β-catenin β-catenin (diluted 1:1000; Abcam) or N-cadherin (diluted 1:500; Abcam). Abs against α-tubulin or actin (both from Sigma) were used as loading controls. Secondary antibodies were HRP-conjugated, and protein levels were visualized using an enhanced chemiluminescence (ECL) system (Amersham). The ratio protein/tubulin or/actin was determined by scanning and quantifying the bands, using ImageJ software (NIH).

Dye-transfer assay

Dye-injection was carried out according to the method described previously [61]. Cells were impaled under visual control and filled with dye by iontophoresis. Communication was assessed 1 minute after cessation of iontophoresis. At least 10 injections were performed for each set of experimental conditions. The coupling was tested in cells: a) treated with Cx43sODN, Cx43asODN, or control untreated cells; b) transiently transfected with Cx43-DN, Cx43-WT or pGFP; and c) Cx43shRNA or p.Sup-transduced cells. Images of microinjected cells were acquired with a 40×0.8 NA objective on a Leica DMLFS microscope (Leica Microsystems, UK) using Volocity acquisition software (Improvision/Perkin Elmer).

Cell migration assay

Confluent cultures of Cx43sODN, Cx43asODN, ZO-1asODN and ZO-1sODN-treated fibroblasts; or Cx43shRNA, p.Sup, N-cadshRNA and Mock-transduced cells; as well as Cx43-WT, Cx43-DN and pGFP-transfected fibroblasts were subjected to a mechanical scratch-wound. In some experiments, Cx43shRNA and p.Sup fibroblasts were serum starved (SS) or incubated in the presence of serum (FBS) for 48 h as described [22]. After this period of time, cells were wounded and incubated in DMEM supplemented with serum. Time-lapse images were taken soon after wounding at intervals of 5 minutes for 3–4 hours, and were acquired on an inverted Zeiss LSM AxioPlan 400 fluorescence microscope (Zeiss, UK), equipped with a Orca CCD camera (Hamamatsu, UK), using a 40×1.2NA objective with an incubation chamber at 37° and 5% CO_2. Time-lapse images were captured using OpenLab image acquisition software (Improvision/Perkin Elmer, UK). The migration velocities of individual fibroblasts were quantified using Volocity4 analysis software (Improvision/Perkin Elmer) by measuring the distance between the initial and final positions of leading edge cells 3 hours after wounding. For each experimental condition, velocities were presented as mean ± SD (μm/sec).

Rho GTPase activition assays

Fresh lysates were used for Rac1/Cdc42 and RhoA-pulldown assays, using the Rac/Cdc42-binding domain (p21-binding domain, PBD) of PAK, as previously described [62], or GST-Rhotekin (kind gift of P Rodriguez-Viciana) to detect relative amounts of RhoA-GTP. Bound protein (GTP-bound Rac1, Cdc42 or RhoA) levels were detected by western blot. Total Rac1, Cdc42 and RhoA from total cell lysates were also analyzed as loading controls.

Förster resonance energy transfer (FRET)

Plasmids encoding FRET probes [Raichu-Rac1, Raichu-Cdc42 [32] and RhoA biosensor [33] were transfected into Cx43shRNA or p.Sup-transduced fibroblasts using Fugene HD (Roche). The FRET efficiency of the cells expressing the EYFP-ECFP fusion construct was measured using confocal fluorescence microscopy and acceptor photobleaching. Leading-edge transfected cells were imaged using an Olympus FluoView 1000 laser scanning confocal microscope and a 60×1.4NA oil objective (Olympus Microscopes, UK). The CFP and YFP channels were excited using the 440 nm and 515 nm lasers, respectively. The two emission channels were 460–510 nm for CFP and 520–620 nm for YFP. The gain for each channel was set to approximately 75% of dynamic range (12-bit, 4096 grey levels) and offsets set such that backgrounds were zero. Pre- and post-bleach CFP and YFP images were acquired and the FRET mode was used to collect images for each channel after acceptor bleaching with 10–12 scans of the 515 nm argon laser line at maximum power (to bleach YFP). The Olympus FluoView 1000 software was used to analyze donor and acceptor intensity values before (pre) and after (post) bleaching and values were then extracted from pixels falling inside the cell of interest, as well as an equal-sized bleached region outside the cell, and the mean ratio was determined for each region. The FRET efficiency ratio over the whole cell was calculated using the following formula: FRET efficiency = $[ID_{(post)} - ID_{(pre)}]/ID_{(post)}$, where ID_{pre} and ID_{post} refer to the intensity of the donor (CFP) before (pre) and after (post) photobleaching of the acceptor (YFP).

Hanging drop assay

Approximately 20,000 single cells were suspended in 35 μl drops of 10% FBS in DMEM from the lids of 24-well dishes for 4 hours. Water was placed at the bottom of each well to maintain humidity. The drops were pipetted five times up and down with 200 μl yellow tips, fixed with 4% paraformaldehyde, and aliquots were spread on coverslips. Images of six random fields from six individual samples for each condition studied (p.Sup and Cx43shRNA-transduced cells) were taken with a 4×0.1 NA objective on an inverted Axiovert Zeiss LSM microscope. An area of approximately 2.5×10^2–7.5×10^2 μm^2 corresponds to a cluster of 1–3 cells and 2.5×10^3 μm^2 corresponds to about 10 cells. The area of each cell cluster was determined using a custom-written plug-in for ImageJ software (NIH). The area occupied by single cells was measured in parallel to estimate the amount of cells per unit area.

Statistical analysis

Statistical differences were determined using Wilcoxon Matched-Pairs Signed-Ranks Test for paired data, or one-way analysis of variance (ANOVA) for data sets of multiple comparisons. A two-tailed Chi-squared test was used for the analysis of cell cluster sizes in the hanging drop assay of adhesion. All data are presented as the mean ± SD except where stated. Criterion levels for the individual tests are given in the Results.

Supporting Information

Figure S1 Cx43 is downregulated in fibroblasts after wounding. (A) The expression and distribution of Cx43 in mouse's skin dermis was examined by immunohistochemistry 2 d after excisional wounding. Wound-edge Cx43 was reduced in dermal fibroblasts after such wounds. Arrowheads show how Cx43 becomes more prevalent with increasing distance from the wound edge. Scale bar = 25 μm. Cx43 levels were quantified along the wound site and were significantly lower at the wound edge; $p<0.005$. Values are expressed as mean ± SD. (B) ZO-1 (green) and Cx43 (red) were examined in mouse skin wounds treated *in vivo* with Cx43sODN or Cx43asODN (n = 6). Cells were also counterstained with Hoechst (blue). A clear downregulation of ZO-1 was found in the dermis of mice treated with the Cx43asODN. Scale bar = 100 μm. (B) Excisional wounds treated with Cx43asODN or control Cx43sODN were used to evaluate the distribution of N-cadherin (green) by immunohistochemistry. Scale bar = 100 μm.

Figure S2 Knockdown of Cx43 induces cytoskeletal changes. (A) Cx43 expression levels and (B) cell-cell communication were evaluated in Cx43asODN or LiCl-treated 3T3 fibroblasts, and in untreated or sense-treated (Cx43-sODN) controls. Values are expressed as mean ± SD (*$p<0.05$; **$p<0.01$ and ***$p<0.005$; n = 4). (C) Confluent monolayers treated with Cx43sODN, Cx43asODN or LiCl were wounded and allowed to migrate for 3 hours. Pictures of cells at the beginning of the migration recording (0 hours) and at the end (3 hours) are shown. Scale bar = 25 μm. (D) The graph shows the velocity of migration, which was inversely correlated with both dye coupling and Cx43 expression. Values represent mean ± SEM (*$p<0.01$; ***$p<0.05$; n = 6). (E) Cells transfected with Cx43-DN, Cx43-WT or pGFP constructs (n = 3), as well as Cx43shRNA or p.Sup-infected cells (n = 6), were allowed to migrate into a wound for 3 hours. Images were taken at the beginning of the migration recording (0 hours; arrows pointing to Cx43-DN, Cx43-WT, or pGFP-transfected cells) and 3 hours later (arrowheads pointing to Cx43-DN, Cx43-WT or pGFP). Cx43shRNA and Cx43-DN cells accelerated migration, while Cx43-WT slowed it. Scale bar = 25 μm. (F) The graph shows the velocity of migration for each treatment and confirms that either silencing of Cx43 or transfection with Cx43-DN induce a significant increase in the rate of migration relative to the other conditions analyzed. Data are expressed as mean ± SD (*$p<0.05$; **$p<0.01$; n = 4). (G) Cx43 levels and dye coupling after LY microinjection were assessed in

Cx43shRNA or p.Sup-infected 3T3 fibroblasts. Cx43shRNA was effective in downregulating Cx43 and eliminating communication with neighbouring cells. Values represent mean ± SEM for Cx43 levels, and mean ± SD for cell coupling (***$p<0.005$; n = 4). (J) Cx43shRNA and p.Sup cells were grown in the presence (FBS) or absence (SS) of serum and allowed to migrate into a wound for 4 h. The graph shows the velocity of migration; values represent mean ± SEM of n = 3 independent experiments (***$p<0.005$).

Figure S3 Analysis of α- and β-catenin expression and distribution after targeting Cx43. (A and C) Protein distribution of α- and β-catenin was analyzed in p.Sup and Cx43shRNA-infected fibroblasts 3 h after wound scratch of confluent 3T3 monolayers. Arrows in (A) indicate cytoplasmic relocation of β-catenin from the plasma membrane to the cytosol in Cx43shRNA-infected cells. The single arrowhead indicates a site of putative nuclear localization of β-catenin in Cx43shRNA-infected fibroblasts. Scale bar = 25 μm. (B and D) The expression levels of these proteins were also evaluated by Western blot and values were normalized with respect to actin or tubulin (Tub).

Figure S4 Knockdown of Cx43 induces cytoskeletal changes. The distribution of TyrTub, AcetTub, and F-actin was studied 3 h after wounding confluent monolayers of Cx43shRNA and p.Sup transduced fibroblasts. Scale bar = 25 μm. The graph shows the length of the protrusions of wound edge cells and data represent the distance from the nucleus to the leading edge (mean ± SEM; n = 3 experiments; ***$P<0.005$).

Figure S5 Knockdown of N-cadherin increases lamellipodial protrusions. (A) The distribution of F-actin was studied 3 h after wounding confluent monolayers of Cx43shRNA and p.Sup transduced fibroblasts. Targeting N-cadherin induces cytoskeletal changes in wound edge cells. Scale bar = 25 μm. (B) The graph shows the length of the protrusions of control (Mock) and NcadshRNA wound edge cells. Data represent the distance from the nucleus to the leading edge (mean ± SEM; n = 3 experiments; ***$P<0.005$).

Movie S1 Cx43 expression influences the velocity of migration scratch wounded fibroblasts. Time-lapse recordings of cells treated with Cx43sODN, Cx43asODN or LiCl were performed at intervals of 5 min for a period of 3 h. Cx43asODN-treated cells migrated almost twice as fast as Cx43sODN treated cells and displayed an extensive lamellipodial protrusion at the leading edge. Incubation with LiCl significantly reduced the rate of migration.

Movie S2 Knockdown of Cx43 accelerates the rate of fibroblasts migration. Fibroblasts stably transfected with Cx43shRNA or p.Sup were monitored for 3 h and time-lapse images were taken at 5 min intervals. Cells transfected with the Cx43shRNA migrated faster than their respective controls, further confirming the close relationship between Cx43 expression levels and the rate of migration in fibroblasts. Cx43shRNA-transfected cells also displayed the same phenotype observed in Cx43asODN treated fibroblasts, characterized by the formation of extensive lamellipodia during migration.

Movie S3 Cx43-DN transfected cells migrate faster than Cx43-WT or eGFP-transfected cells after wounding. Fibroblasts were transiently transfected with bicistronic pIRES-GFP expression vectors encoding Cx43-WT, Cx43-DN or eGFP alone. The migration rates were monitored for 3 h and time-lapse images were taken at 5 min intervals. Cells transfected with the Cx43-DN migrated faster than their respective controls, and also extended a large lamellipodial membrane protrusion at the leading edge in the direction of the migration.

Movie S4 Actin dynamics is affected after silencing Cx43. The effect of silencing of Cx43 on actin cytoskeleton dynamics was analyzed after sequentially transfecting p.Sup or Cx43shRNA-stable transfected fibroblasts with an RFP-actin construct. Confocal time-lapse images were taken at intervals of 2 min for 1 ½ h after a scratch wounding confluent cultures.

Acknowledgments

We are grateful to Prof WH Moolenaar for the gift of the Cx43shRNA; Dr S Arai and Dr T Suda for the gift of the N-cadshRNA and Mock constructs; Prof M Matsuda for the gift of Rac1 and Cdc42 FRET probes; Prof KM Hahn for the gift of the RhoA FRET probe; and Dr P Rodriguez-Viciana for the gift of the GST-Rhotekin-RBD and the GST-PBD. We would also like to thank Dr Silvia Purro and Dr Jeremy Cook for helpful discussions; and Daniel Ciantar for the Image J plug-in.

Author Contributions

Conceived and designed the experiments: AMN ARJP DLB. Performed the experiments: AMN PC AES RH SO CMW CT KTP TS DLB. Analyzed the data: AMN AES RH CT DLB. Contributed reagents/materials/analysis tools: TS AW ARJP. Wrote the paper: AMN ARJP DLB. Obtained ethics for human tissue: TS AW.

References

1. Gottrup F (2004) A specialized wound-healing center concept: importance of a multidisciplinary department structure and surgical treatment facilities in the treatment of chronic wounds. Am J Surg 187: 38S–43S.
2. Sen CK, Gordillo GM, Roy S, Kirsner R, Lambert L, et al. (2009) Human skin wounds: a major and snowballing threat to public health and the economy. Wound Repair Regen 17: 763–771.
3. Walmsley S (2002) Advances in wound management: executive summary. London: PJB Publications, Ltd.
4. Coutinho P, Qiu C, Frank S, Tamber K, Becker D (2003) Dynamic changes in connexin expression correlate with key events in the wound healing process. Cell Biol Int 27: 525–541.
5. Guo H, Acevedo P, Parsa FD, Bertram JS (1992) Gap-junctional protein connexin 43 is expressed in dermis and epidermis of human skin: differential modulation by retinoids. J Invest Dermatol 99: 460–467.
6. Qiu C, Coutinho P, Frank S, Franke S, Law LY, et al. (2003) Targeting connexin43 expression accelerates the rate of wound repair. Curr Biol 13: 1697–1703.
7. Mori R, Power KT, Wang CM, Martin P, Becker DL (2006) Acute downregulation of connexin43 at wound sites leads to a reduced inflammatory response, enhanced keratinocyte proliferation and wound fibroblast migration. J Cell Sci 119: 5193–5203.
8. Goliger JA, Paul DL (1995) Wounding alters epidermal connexin expression and gap junction-mediated intercellular communication. Mol Biol Cell 6: 1491–1501.
9. Saitoh M, Oyamada M, Oyamada Y, Kaku T, Mori M (1997) Changes in the expression of gap junction proteins (connexins) in hamster tongue epithelium during wound healing and carcinogenesis. Carcinogenesis 18: 1319–1328.
10. Richards TS, Dunn CA, Carter WG, Usui ML, Olerud JE, et al. (2004) Protein kinase C spatially and temporally regulates gap junctional communication during human wound repair via phosphorylation of connexin43 on serine368. J Cell Biol 167: 555–562.
11. Brandner JM, Houdek P, Husing B, Kaiser C, Moll I (2004) Connexins 26, 30, and 43: differences among spontaneous, chronic, and accelerated human wound healing. J Invest Dermatol 122: 1310–1320.

12. Coutinho P, Qiu C, Frank S, Wang CM, Brown T, et al. (2005) Limiting burn extension by transient inhibition of Connexin43 expression at the site of injury. Br J Plast Surg 58: 658–667.
13. Kretz M, Euwens C, Hombach S, Eckardt D, Teubner B, et al. (2003) Altered connexin expression and wound healing in the epidermis of connexin-deficient mice. J Cell Sci 116: 3443–3452.
14. Kretz M, Maass K, Willecke K (2004) Expression and function of connexins in the epidermis, analyzed with transgenic mouse mutants. Eur J Cell Biol 83: 647–654.
15. Wang CM, Lincoln J, Cook JE, Becker DL (2007) Abnormal connexin expression underlies delayed wound healing in diabetic skin. Diabetes 56: 2809–2817.
16. Nakano Y, Oyamada M, Dai P, Nakagami T, Kinoshita S, et al. (2008) Connexin43 knockdown accelerates wound healing but inhibits mesenchymal transition after corneal endothelial injury in vivo. Invest Ophthalmol Vis Sci 49: 93–104.
17. Wei CJ, Francis R, Xu X, Lo CW (2005) Connexin43 associated with an N-cadherin-containing multiprotein complex is required for gap junction formation in NIH3T3 cells. J Biol Chem 280: 19925–19936.
18. Shaw RM, Fay AJ, Puthenveedu MA, von Zastrow M, Jan YN, et al. (2007) Microtubule plus-end-tracking proteins target gap junctions directly from the cell interior to adherens junctions. Cell 128: 547–560.
19. Giepmans BN, Moolenaar WH (1998) The gap junction protein connexin43 interacts with the second PDZ domain of the zona occludens-1 protein. Curr Biol 8: 931–934.
20. van Zeijl L, Ponsioen B, Giepmans BN, Ariaens A, Postma FR, et al. (2007) Regulation of connexin43 gap junctional communication by phosphatidylinositol 4,5-bisphosphate. J Cell Biol 177: 881–891.
21. Becker D, Ciantar D, Catsicas M, Pearson R, Mobbs P (2001) Use of pIRES vectors to express EGFP and connexin constructs in studies of the role of gap junctional communication in the early development of the chick retina and brain. Cell Commun Adhes 8: 355–359.
22. Francis R, Xu X, Park H, Wei CJ, Chang S, et al. (2011) Connexin43 modulates cell polarity and directional cell migration by regulating microtubule dynamics. PloS one 6: e26379.
23. Hosokawa K, Arai F, Yoshihara H, Iwasaki H, Nakamura Y, et al. (2010) Knockdown of N-cadherin suppresses the long-term engraftment of hematopoietic stem cells. Blood 116: 554–563.
24. Underwood JL, Murphy CG, Chen J, Franse-Carman L, Wood I, et al. (1999) Glucocorticoids regulate transendothelial fluid flow resistance and formation of intercellular junctions. Am J Physiol 277: C330–342.
25. Alt-Holland A, Shamis Y, Riley KN, DesRochers TM, Fusenig NE, et al. (2008) E-cadherin suppression directs cytoskeletal rearrangement and intraepithelial tumor cell migration in 3D human skin equivalents. J Invest Dermatol 128: 2498–2507.
26. Elbert M, Cohen D, Musch A (2006) PAR1b promotes cell-cell adhesion and inhibits dishevelled-mediated transformation of Madin-Darby canine kidney cells. Mol Biol Cell 17: 3345–3355.
27. Redfield A, Nieman MT, Knudsen KA (1997) Cadherins promote skeletal muscle differentiation in three-dimensional cultures. J Cell Biol 130: 1323–1331.
28. Magdalena J, Millard TH, Etienne-Manneville S, Launay S, Warwick HK, et al. (2003) Involvement of the Arp2/3 complex and Scar2 in Golgi polarity in scratch wound models. Mol Biol Cell 14: 670–684.
29. Yonemura S, Itoh M, Nagafuchi A, Tsukita S (1995) Cell-to-cell adherens junction formation and actin filament organization: similarities and differences between non-polarized fibroblasts and polarized epithelial cells. J Cell Sci 108 (Pt 1): 127–142.
30. Gundersen GG, Bulinski JC (1988) Selective stabilization of microtubules oriented toward the direction of cell migration. Proc Natl Acad Sci U S A 85: 5946–5950.
31. Jaffe AB, Hall A (2005) Rho GTPases: biochemistry and biology. Annu Rev Cell Dev Biol 21: 247–269.
32. Itoh RE, Kurokawa K, Ohba Y, Yoshizaki H, Mochizuki N, et al. (2002) Activation of rac and cdc42 video imaged by fluorescent resonance energy transfer-based single-molecule probes in the membrane of living cells. Mol Cell Biol 22: 6582–6591.
33. Pertz O, Hodgson L, Klemke RL, Hahn KM (2006) Spatiotemporal dynamics of RhoA activity in migrating cells. Nature 440: 1069–1072.
34. Wei CJ, Xu X, Lo CW (2004) Connexins and cell signaling in development and disease. Annu Rev Cell Dev Biol 20: 811–838.
35. Wright CS, van Steensel MA, Hodgins MB, Martin PE (2009) Connexin mimetic peptides improve cell migration rates of human epidermal keratinocytes and dermal fibroblasts in vitro. Wound Repair Regen 17: 240–249.
36. Pollok S, Pfeiffer AC, Lobmann R, Wright CS, Moll I, et al. (2010) Connexin 43 mimetic peptide Gap27 reveals potential differences in the role of Cx43 in wound repair between diabetic and non-diabetic cells. J Cell Mol Med.
37. Taliana L, Benezra M, Greenberg RS, Masur SK, Bernstein AM (2005) ZO-1: lamellipodial localization in a corneal fibroblast wound model. Invest Ophthalmol Vis Sci 46: 96–103.
38. Hunter AW, Barker RJ, Zhu C, Gourdie RG (2005) Zonula occludens-1 alters connexin43 gap junction size and organization by influencing channel accretion. Mol Biol Cell 16: 5686–5698.
39. Gourdie RG, Ghatnekar GS, O'Quinn M, Rhett MJ, Barker RJ, et al. (2006) The unstoppable connexin43 carboxyl-terminus: new roles in gap junction organization and wound healing. Annals of the New York Academy of Sciences 1080: 49–62.
40. Ghatnekar GS, O'Quinn MP, Jourdan LJ, Gurjarpadhye AA, Draughn RL, et al. (2009) Connexin43 carboxyl-terminal peptides reduce scar progenitor and promote regenerative healing following skin wounding. Regenerative medicine 4: 205–223.
41. Rhett JM, Ghatnekar GS, Palatinus JA, O'Quinn M, Yost MJ, et al. (2008) Novel therapies for scar reduction and regenerative healing of skin wounds. Trends in biotechnology 26: 173–180.
42. McDonough WS, Johansson A, Joffee H, Giese A, Berens ME (1999) Gap junction intercellular communication in gliomas is inversely related to cell motility. Int J Dev Neurosci 17: 601–611.
43. Batten BE, Haar JL (1979) Fine structural differentiation of germ layers in the mouse at the time of mesoderm formation. Anat Rec 194: 125–141.
44. Xu X, Francis R, Wei CJ, Linask KL, Lo CW (2006) Connexin 43-mediated modulation of polarized cell movement and the directional migration of cardiac neural crest cells. Development 133: 3629–3639.
45. Huang GY, Cooper ES, Waldo K, Kirby ML, Gilula NB, et al. (1998) Gap junction-mediated cell-cell communication modulates mouse neural crest migration. J Cell Biol 143: 1725–1734.
46. Pokutta S, Weis WI (2002) The cytoplasmic face of cell contact sites. Curr Opin Struct Biol 12: 255–262.
47. Wilby MJ, Muir EM, Fok-Seang J, Gour BJ, Blaschuk OW, et al. (1999) N-Cadherin inhibits Schwann cell migration on astrocytes. Mol Cell Neurosci 14: 66–84.
48. Chakraborty S, Mitra S, Falk MM, Caplan SH, Wheelock MJ, et al. (2010) E-cadherin differentially regulates the assembly of Connexin43 and Connexin32 into gap junctions in human squamous carcinoma cells. J Biol Chem 285: 10761–10776.
49. Lin JH, Takano T, Cotrina ML, Arcuino G, Kang J, et al. (2002) Connexin 43 enhances the adhesivity and mediates the invasion of malignant glioma cells. J Neurosci 22: 4302–4311.
50. Cotrina ML, Lin JH, Nedergaard M (2008) Adhesive properties of connexin hemichannels. Glia 56: 1791–1798.
51. Becker DL, Davies CS (1995) Role of gap junctions in the development of the preimplantation mouse embryo. Microsc Res Tech 31: 364–374.
52. Wang H, Ding T, Brown N, Yamamoto Y, Prince LS, et al. (2008) Zonula occludens-1 (ZO-1) is involved in morula to blastocyst transformation in the mouse. Dev Biol 318: 112–125.
53. Li W, Hertzberg EL, Spray DC (2005) Regulation of connexin43-protein binding in astrocytes in response to chemical ischemia/hypoxia. J Biol Chem 280: 7941–7948.
54. Butkevich E, Hulsmann S, Wenzel D, Shirao T, Duden R, et al. (2004) Drebrin is a novel connexin-43 binding partner that links gap junctions to the submembrane cytoskeleton. Curr Biol 14: 650–658.
55. Giepmans BN, Verlaan I, Hengeveld T, Janssen H, Calafat J, et al. (2001) Gap junction protein connexin-43 interacts directly with microtubules. Curr Biol 11: 1364–1368.
56. Theiss C, Meller K (2002) Microinjected anti-actin antibodies decrease gap junctional intercellular commmunication in cultured astrocytes. Exp Cell Res 281: 197–204.
57. Machacek M, Hodgson L, Welch C, Elliott H, Pertz O, et al. (2009) Coordination of Rho GTPase activities during cell protrusion. Nature 461: 99–103.
58. Carr AJ, Whitmore D (2005) Imaging of single light-responsive clock cells reveals fluctuating free-running periods. Nat Cell Biol 7: 319–321.
59. Demaison C, Parsley K, Brouns G, Scherr M, Battmer K, et al. (2002) High-level transduction and gene expression in hematopoietic repopulating cells using a human immunodeficiency [correction of imunodeficiency] virus type 1-based lentiviral vector containing an internal spleen focus forming virus promoter. Hum Gene Ther 13: 803–813.
60. Magdalena J, Millard TH, Machesky LM (2003) Microtubule involvement in NIH 3T3 Golgi and MTOC polarity establishment. J Cell Sci 116: 743–756.
61. Becker DL, Evans WH, Green CR, Warner A (1995) Functional analysis of amino acid sequences in connexin43 involved in intercellular communication through gap junctions. J Cell Sci 108 (Pt 4): 1455–1467.
62. Mendoza-Naranjo A, Gonzalez-Billault C, Maccioni RB (2007) Abeta1-42 stimulates actin polymerization in hippocampal neurons through Rac1 and Cdc42 Rho GTPases. J Cell Sci 120: 279–288.

5

Dysregulation of Suppressor of Cytokine Signaling 3 in Keratinocytes Causes Skin Inflammation Mediated by Interleukin-20 Receptor-Related Cytokines

Ayako Uto-Konomi[1,2], Kosuke Miyauchi[1], Naoko Ozaki[2], Yasutaka Motomura[1], Yoshie Suzuki[1], Akihiko Yoshimura[3], Shinobu Suzuki[2], Daniel Cua[4], Masato Kubo[1,5]*

1 Laboratory for Signal Network, Research Center for Allergy and Immunology, RIKEN Yokohama Institute, Yokohama, Kanagawa, Japan, **2** Department of Molecular and Cellular Biology, Kobe Pharma Research Institute, Nippon Boehringer Ingelheim Co., Ltd., Kobe, Hyogo, Japan, **3** Department of Microbiology and Immunology, Keio University School of Medicine, Tokyo, Japan, **4** Schering-Plough Biopharma, Palo Alto, California, United States, **5** Division of Molecular Pathology, Research Institute for Biological Science, Tokyo University of Science, Noda, Chiba, Japan

Abstract

Homeostatic regulation of epidermal keratinocytes is controlled by the local cytokine milieu. However, a role for suppressor of cytokine signaling (SOCS), a negative feedback regulator of cytokine networks, in skin homeostasis remains unclear. Keratinocyte specific deletion of *Socs3* (*Socs3* cKO) caused severe skin inflammation with hyper-production of IgE, epidermal hyperplasia, and S100A8/9 expression, although *Socs1* deletion caused no inflammation. The inflamed skin showed constitutive STAT3 activation and up-regulation of IL-6 and IL-20 receptor (IL-20R) related cytokines, IL-19, IL-20 and IL-24. Disease development was rescued by deletion of the *Il6* gene, but not by the deletion of *Il23*, *Il4r*, or *Rag1* genes. The expression of IL-6 in *Socs3* cKO keratinocytes increased expression of IL-20R-related cytokines that further facilitated STAT3 hyperactivation, epidermal hyperplasia and neutrophilia. These results demonstrate that skin homeostasis is strictly regulated by the IL-6-STAT3-SOCS3 axis. Moreover, the SOCS3-mediated negative feedback loop in keratinocytes has a critical mechanistic role in the prevention of skin inflammation caused by hyperactivation of STAT3.

Editor: Christianne Bandeira de Melo, Instituto de Biofisica Carlos Chagas Filho, Universidade Federal do Rio de Janeiro, Brazil

Funding: This work was supported by a grant from Grant in Aid for Scientific Research (B) and Grant in Aid for Scientific Research on Priority Areas of the Ministry of Education, Culture, Sports, Science, and Technology (Japan) and the Program for Promotion of Fundamental Studies in Health Sciences of the National Institute of Biomedical Innovation (NIBIO). The funders had no role in study design, data collection and analysis, decision to publish, or preparation of the manuscript.

Competing Interests: Ayako Uto-Konomi, Naoko Ozaki and Shinobu Suzuki are employed by Nippon Boehringer Ingelheim Co., Ltd., and Daniel Cua is employed by Schering-Plough Biopharma. There are no patents, products in development or marketed products to declare. Other authors have declared that no competing interests exist.

* E-mail: raysolfc@rcai.riken.jp

Introduction

The suppressor of cytokine signaling (SOCS) family of proteins plays a role in the negative regulation of cytokine-JAK-STAT signaling by inhibiting JAK tyrosine kinase activity. There are eight proteins in this family, each of which has a central SH2 domain and a C-terminal 40-amino-acid conserved domain called the SOCS box. SOCS1 inhibits STAT1 activation in the IFN-γ signaling cascade, while SOCS3 is a major negative regulator of IL-6-STAT3 signaling [1,2]. Additionally, SOCS3 negatively regulates skin wound healing through inhibition of the gp130-STAT3 pathway [3], suggesting a pivotal role for SOCS proteins in skin inflammatory responses. However, the regulatory role of SOCSs in the maintenance of skin homeostasis remains unclear.

The skin consists of two major layers, the epidermis and the dermis. The epidermis consists of keratinocytes, which proliferate in the basal layer and differentiate into cells that migrate towards the outer layer to form the stratified epithelium that provides the skin barrier. The epidermis is in a continuous equilibrium of growth and differentiation and has the remarkable capacity for complete self-renewal, relying on its rich reservoir of stem cells. The dermis contains mainly fibroblasts and a large population of immune cells, along with structures important for skin function including blood vessels, nerves, hair follicles, and glands. The dermis also provides the epidermis with mechanical support and nutrients [4],[5]. Epidermal homeostasis is dependent on proper repair after injury and on maintenance of a tight junction with the underlying basement membrane, both of which are precisely regulated by various cytokines. Keratinocytes are now proposed to play important roles in the regulation of skin homeostasis by producing a variety of cytokines [5]. TNF-α, IL-1 and IL-6 have been shown to have regulatory roles in skin wound healing, and also in skin permeability [6,7,8]. For example, IL-6 deficiency caused delayed skin repair, and topical application of IL-6 to barrier-disrupted skin enhanced repair of the skin barrier [8].

STAT3 is one of the key components for IL-6 receptor signaling, and it is thought to be an important transcription factor in skin homeostasis [8,9]. Activated (phosphorylated) STAT3 expression is enhanced at sites of injured epidermis compared with the normal epidermis, and STAT3 related signaling also affects the survival of keratinocyte stem cells, which are important for keratinocyte renewal and wound healing. Besides IL-6, other cytokines/growth factors also stimulate the phosphorylation of STAT3 and the subsequent STAT3 mediated nuclear signaling.

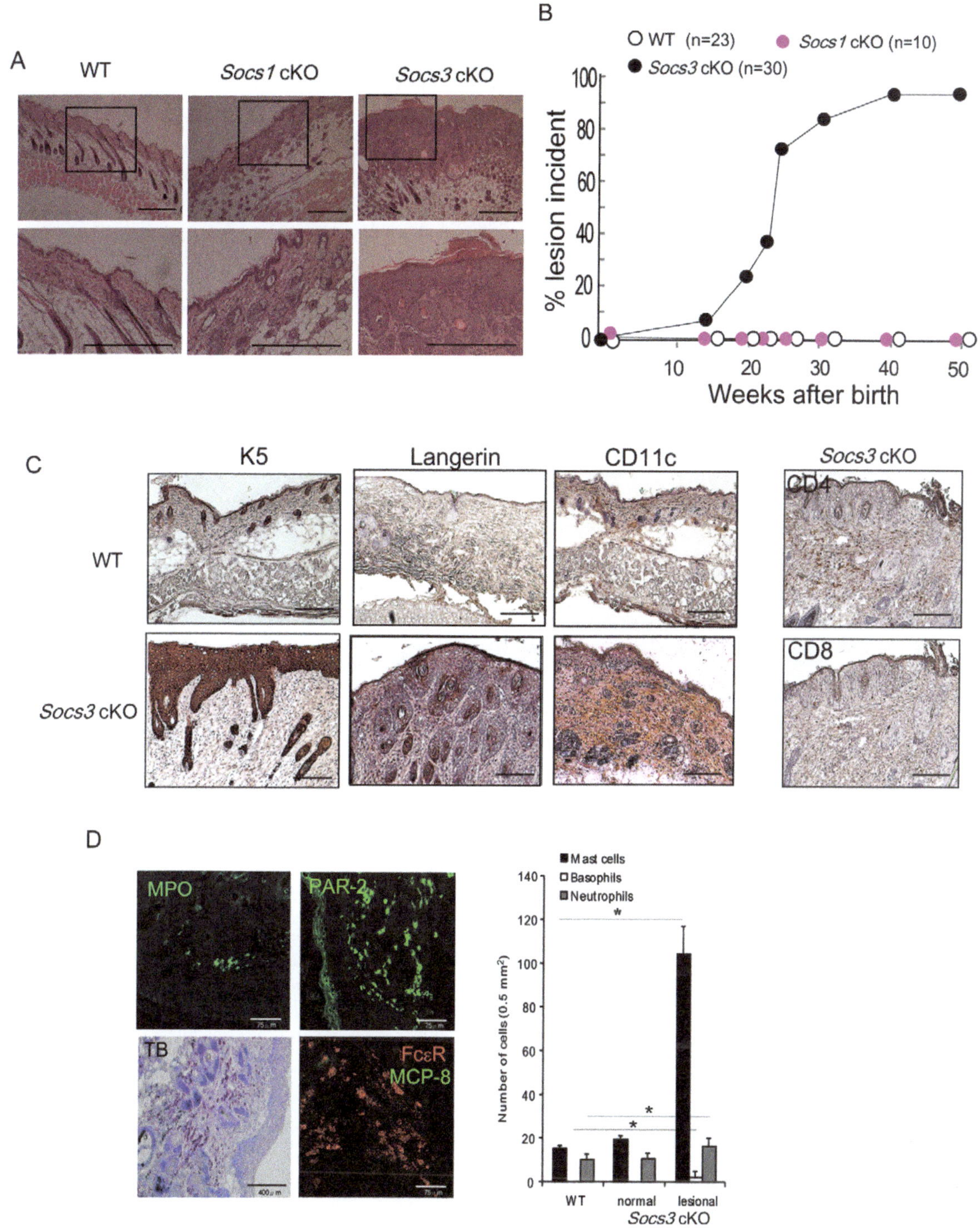

Figure 1. Socs3 cKO spontaneously developed epidermal hyperplasia and skin inflammation. A) Upper and bottom panels show histopathological analysis of K5-Cre (WT) (left), *Socs1* cKO (center) and *Socs3* cKO (right) mice skin with hematoxylin and eosin staining. Magnification of upper and lower panels are x40 and x100, respectively. Scale bar in each section indicates 750 υm. B) Percentage of mice showing skin lesion incidences in wild type (WT) (open circle), *Socs1* cKO (closed purple circle) and *Socs3* cKO (closed-black circle) mice. Disease incidence was monitored weekly up to 50 weeks after birth. Percentage of mice showing incidence of disease is shown on the Y axis at each time point. The number of mice used in each group is indicated in the figure. C) Localization of keratinocytes (K5), Langerhans cells (Langerin), and CD11c^{+} dendritic cells (CD11c) in epidermis and dermis of the diseased *Socs3* cKO skin was assessed by immunohistlogical staining (x40) (left panel). Wild type (WT) mice skin was stained as a control. CD4 and CD8 positive T cells were also identified in epidermis and dermis of the diseased *Socs3* cKO skin (right panel). Scale bar in each section indicates 750 υm. D) Neutrophil number was confirmed by counting MPO positive cells in epidermis and dermis of the diseased *Socs3* cKO skin by immunohistlogical staining (x400) (upper left panel). PAR-2, TB staining, FceR and MCP-8 positive cells in epidermis and dermis of the diseased *Socs3* cKO skin are shown (upper right, lower left, and lower right panel, respectively). Scale bar in each section indicates 75 υm. Number of neutrophils, mast cells and basophils in epidermis and dermis are shown in the right bar graphs. *$P<0.01$. Data are the mean from three independent experiments. Error bars are SD.

Thus a sophisticated cytokine network is required for the homeostatic events in the proliferation and differentiation of keratinocytes. Disruption of this homeostasis has pathological consequences. For example, the overexpression of active-*Stat3* resulted in impaired wound healing and increased keloid pathogenesis [9] and augmented the development of spontaneous psoriatic skin disease [10]. Therefore, dysregulation of STAT3 activation results in the breakdown of keratinocyte homeostasis, sometimes leading the development of skin carcinogenesis [11].

Phosphorylation of STAT3 is regulated by IL-6, IL-10, EGF and many other cytokines, including the interleukin-20 receptor (IL-20R) related cytokines, IL-19, IL-20, and as well as IL-24 [12]. The IL-20RI is composed of two chains, IL-20RA and IL-20RB, and its ligands are IL-19, IL-20 and IL-24, which are highly expressed in keratinocytes [13]. These cytokines are important in the manifestation of psoriatic lesions [14] and, recently, an association of polymorphisms of IL-20 with psoriasis has been described [15]. IL-19, IL-20 and IL-24 are reported to induce epidermal hyperplasia and STAT3 activation in the reconstituted human epidermis [16], and are highly expressed in psoriatic inflammatory sites [17].

In the present study, we investigated the role of SOCS3 in keratinocyte function using keratinocyte-specific SOCS3 gene deficient mice, and found that these mice spontaneously developed a severe form of skin inflammation. Here we identified a critical role for SOCS3 as a negative regulator of STAT3 hyperactivation in keratinocytes that restored skin homeostasis. Moreover, in the absence of SOCS3, excessive IL-6 signaling resulted in skin lesions that were also strongly correlated with increased IL-19/IL-24 cytokines and the expression levels of anti-microbial peptides, β-defensin and S100A8/A9.

Results

Loss of SOCS3 in keratinocytes resulted in skin inflammation

To examine the role of SOCS proteins in the epidermis, we generated keratin 5-specific *Socs1* and *Socs3* conditional knockout mice (*Socs1* cKO and *Socs3* cKO respectively; See Materials and Methods). At age 40 weeks or older, mice lacking SOCS3 in keratinocytes spontaneously developed a severe form of skin inflammation, with a disease incidence of >90% (**Fig. 1A&B**). Histopathological analysis revealed epidermal hyperplasia and massive leukocyte infiltration in the skin of the *Socs3* cKO mice, whereas the deletion of *Socs1* did not cause such inflammation. These findings suggested that SOCS3 expression in keratinocytes is required for the maintenance of normal skin. Additionally, we analyzed the cell types in the skin lesions (**Fig. 1C&D**). Keratin 5 (K5) staining showed a thickened epithelium in *Socs3* cKO mice as a result of an extensive expansion of keratinocytes. Compared to the control K5-Cre mice (with a wild type *Socs3* locus), *Socs3* cKO mice displayed an increased infiltration of Langerin$^+$ Langerhans cells and CD11c$^+$ dendritic cells (DCs). We also identified an increased number of CD4$^+$ but not CD8$^+$ T cells in the dermis of *Socs3* cKO mice (**Fig. 1C, right panel**). In addition, we performed an immunohistochemical staining of neutrophils, connective tissue type mast cells and basophils in the epidermis and dermis of *Socs3* cKO mice, using toluidine blue or antibodies for myeloperoxidase (MPO), PAR-2, FcεR and MCP-8 (**Fig. 1D**). Compared to the wild type littermates, elevated numbers of mast cells were identified in both the epidermis and dermis of *Socs3* cKO mice, and there was also an increased infiltration of neutrophils and basophils. These findings indicated that the loss of SOCS3 rendered the mice prone to spontaneous skin inflammation.

The skin inflammation in Socs3 cKO mice is T and B cell independent

We examined whether this skin inflammation was due to an atopic type Th2 response and, interestingly, we found that total serum levels of the prototypical Th2-type immunoglobulin, IgE, were markedly increased in the diseased *Socs3* cKO mice, but not in pre-disease *Socs3* cKO mice. Moreover, we observed that there was a positive correlation between the IgE levels and the severity of inflammation in the diseased *Socs3* cKO mice (**Fig. 2A**). Therefore, in order to understand if any atopic response associates with this skin pathology, the *Socs3* cKO mice were crossed with *Il4 receptor (Il4r)* KO mice and monitored for the spontaneous development of skin inflammation over time. We found that *Il4r* KO mice still developed skin lesions similar to those observed in *Il4r*$^{+/-}$ mice, even with complete attenuation of the increased serum IgE levels (**Fig. 2B**). This further demonstrates that the skin inflammation observed in *Socs3* cKO mice completely segregated from the IgE-mediated as well as the IL-4/IL-13-mediated responses.

As shown in Fig. 1D, we found massive infiltration of CD4$^+$ cells but not CD8$^+$ T cells in the dermis of the diseased skin. We therefore asked whether T cells were involved in the actual development of skin lesions, or were only needed for maintenance of the disease situation in an ongoing inflammation. To answer the question, we crossed *Socs3* cKO mice onto a *Rag1* KO background, in which T and B cells were completely absent. Interestingly, spontaneous skin lesions still occurred in these mice (**Fig. 2C**). Our results indicate that the development of skin lesion in *Socs3* cKO mice was independent of CD4 T cells, and that CD4 T cells in the lesions might accumulate locally as a result of the inflammation.

Cytokine profile in the lesional skin of Socs3 cKO mice

To understand the mechanism underlying the development of skin inflammation in *Socs3* cKO mice, we examined the cytokine profiles. Cytokines, cytokine receptors, and anti-microbial peptide gene panels, that are known to play a role in skin homeostasis or diseases, were analyzed by quantitative real-time PCR in normal skin from controls and *Socs1* cKO mice, as well as in the inflamed skin of *Socs3* cKO mice. We found clear induction of IL-1β, IL-4, IL-6, IL-19, IL-20 and IL-24 expression in *Socs3* cKO derived skin (**Fig. 3A&B**). It has been reported that the cytokines IL-19, IL-20 and IL-24 are highly expressed in the inflammatory sites of psoriasis, and may thus mediate the progression of psoriasis [13,17]. Only STAT3, but no other STAT family member (STAT1, STAT5, or STAT6), is highly phosphorylated in the skin of *Socs3* cKO mice (**Fig. 3C, Fig. S1**). Immunohistochemical analysis revealed that IL-6, IL-19 and IL-24 protein levels are also elevated in *Socs3* cKO mouse skin (**Fig. 3D**). However, the inflamed skin had no expression of IL-23, IL-17A, IL-17F, IL-22, and RORγt (**Fig. 3A&B Fig. S2**), which are known to be expressed by Th17 cells, a critical helper T cell population in various inflammatory conditions including psoriasis [18]. On the other hand, the inflamed skin expressed significantly high levels of the anti-microbial peptides; S100A8, S100A9, and β-defensin (**Fig. 3A&B**)

IL-6 plays a regulatory role in skin wound healing through its effect on skin barrier homeostasis [8]. This indicates that IL-6 might be a key cytokine to enhance the hyperactivation of STAT3 in the skin of *Socs3* cKO mice. IL-23 is also well known to be an important STAT3 cytokine related to skin disorders such as

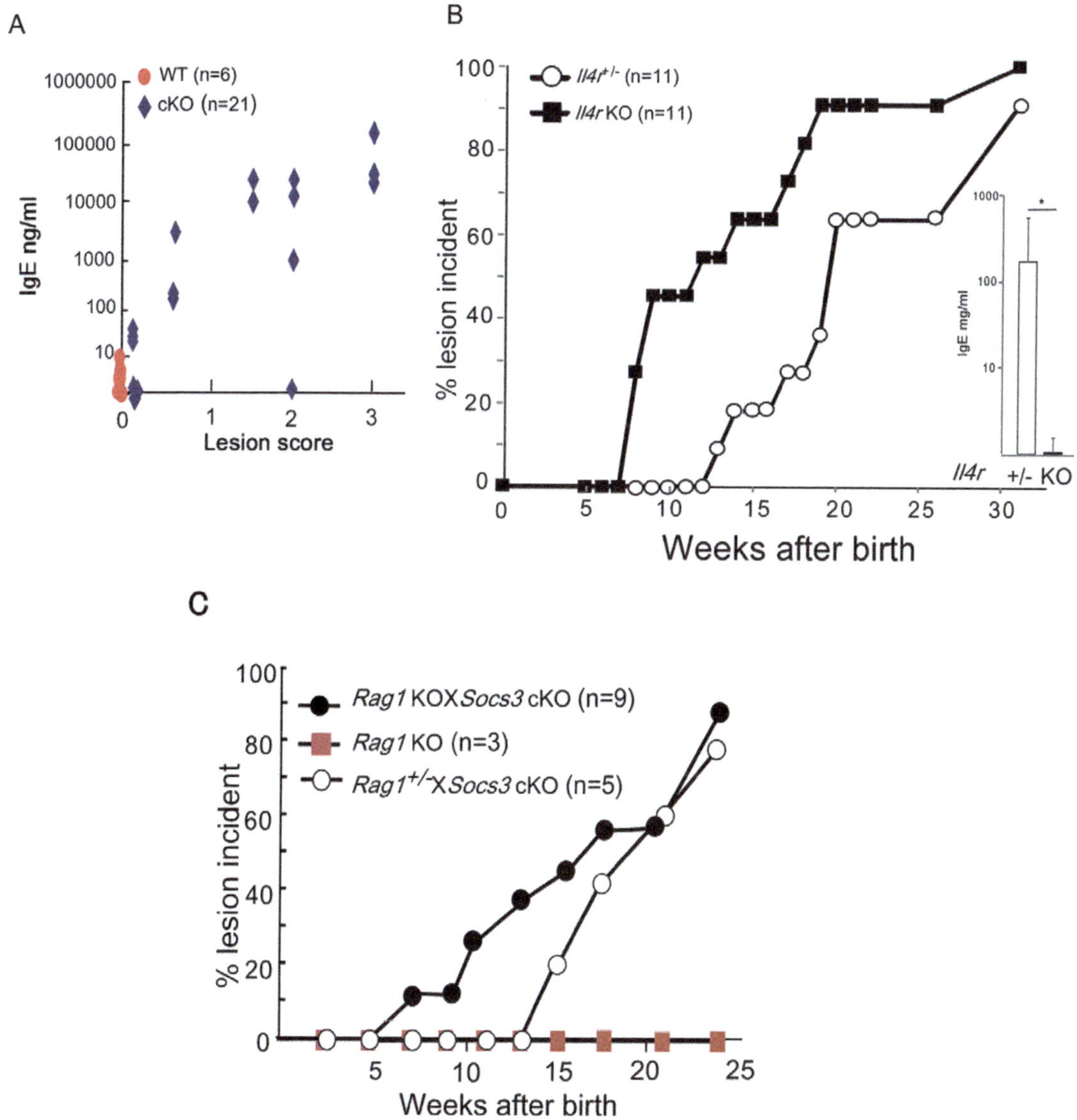

Figure 2. T cell responses are not required for initiation of the skin disease in Socs3cKOmice. A) Serum level of IgE was measured in wild type (WT) and *Socs3* cKO mice and is shown on the Y axis. X axis indicates skin disease severity (Lesion score). Red symbols indicate WT mice (n = 6) and blue symbols indicate *Socs3* cKO with or without skin lesions (n = 21). B) Lesion incidence was examined in *Socs3* cKO with *Il4r*$^{+/-}$ (shown as *Il4r*$^{+/-}$ in the figure, open circle, n = 11) and *Il4r* null *Socs3* cKO (shown as *Il4* KO in the figure, closed circle, n = 11). Serum IgE in individual *Socs3* cKO with *Il4r*$^{+/-}$ (+/−) and *Socs3* cKO with *Il4r* KO mice (KO) was measured at 30 weeks of age and the mean +/− SD is shown (right). C) Role of T-B cells in the development of the skin lesions in *Socs3* cKO mice. Lesion incidence was examined in *Rag1* KO (red-square, n = 3), *Socs3* cKO with *Rag1* KO (Rag1 KOX*Socs3* cKO, closed circles, n = 9), and *Socs3* cKO with *Rag1*$^{+/-}$ (*Rag1*$^{+/-}$X*Socs3* cKO, open circles, n = 5) mice. Each mouse strain was monitored until 24 weeks after birth (X axis). The percentage of mice with lesions is shown on the Y axis at each time point after birth.

psoriasis [19,20,21]. Therefore, we tested *Socs3* cKO mice crossed with either *Il6* KO or *Il23* KO mice to identify which cytokine is more important for disease development. We found that crossing *Socs3* cKO mice with *Il6* KO mice markedly restored the skin condition (**Fig. 4A**). By contrast, skin from *Socs3* cKO mice crossed with *Il23* KO mice did not show any improvement in disease development (**Fig. 4B**). These results demonstrate that IL-6 is a key cytokine for the regulation of homeostasis in keratinocytes, and that STAT3 activation and aberrant expression of IL-19 and IL-24 may promote development of skin inflammation.

IL-6 induces IL-20-RI related cytokines in Socs3 KO keratinocytes

As shown in Fig. 3C, the STAT3 pathway is highly active in *Socs3* deficient skin. To confirm the prolonged activation of STAT3 in the SOCS3 deficient condition, keratinocytes were isolated from wild type and pre-diseased *Socs3* cKO mice and cultured with IL-6 before analyzing their STAT3 phosphorylation status. Ten minute stimulation of KO keratinocytes induced similar levels of STAT3 phosphorylation to that of wild type keratinocytes. However, after 60 min, there was a significant reduction in STAT3 phosphorylation in control keratinocytes, whereas the phosphorylation levels in KO keratinocytes was markedly sustained (**Fig. 5A**).

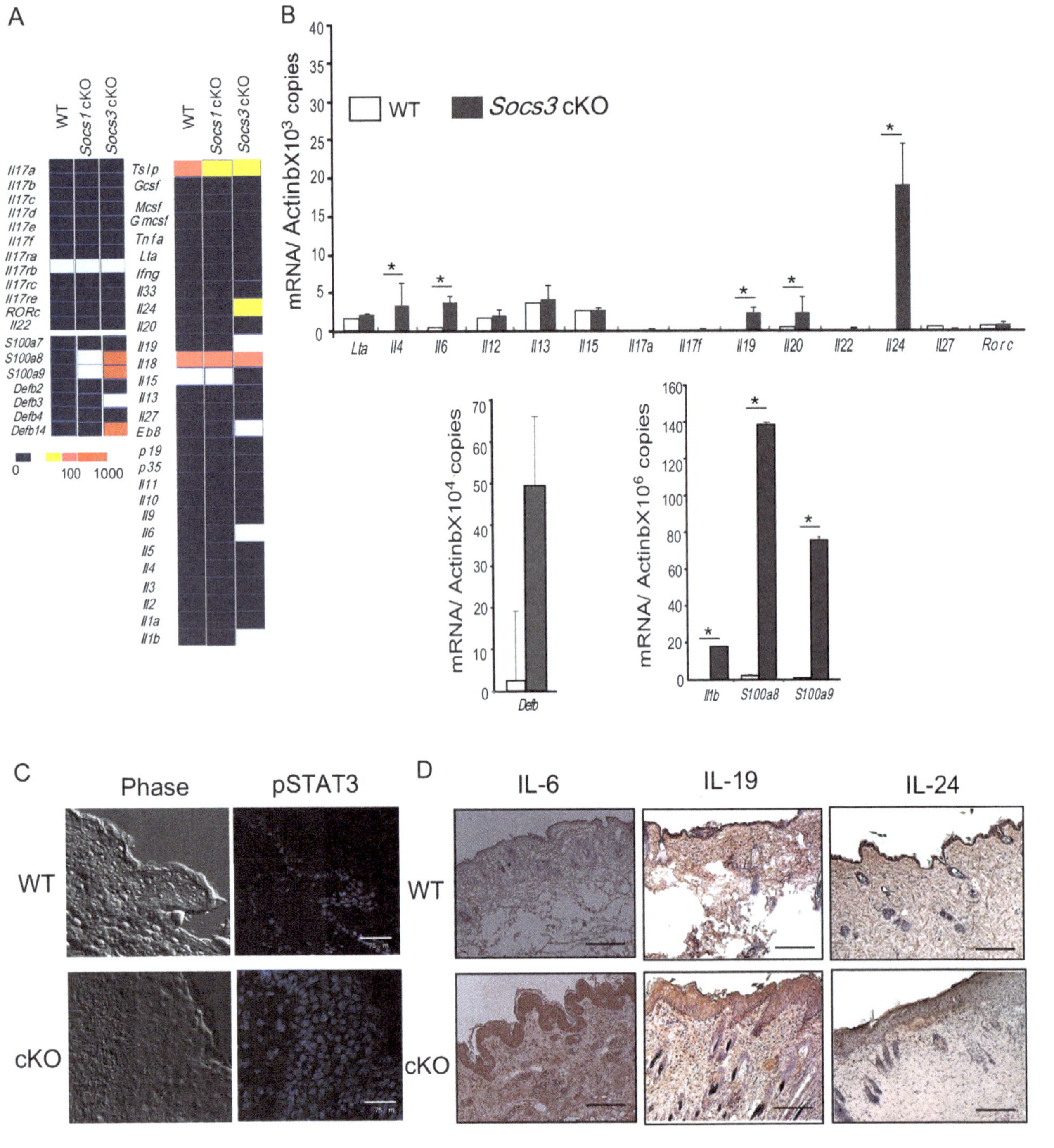

Figure 3. Cytokine expression in the diseased skin. A) Expression profiles. RNA was prepared from skin of K5-Cre (WT), *Socs1* cKO, and the diseased *Socs3* cKO mice, and analyzed using a TAQMAN™ real-time quantitative PCR system. Copy numbers are depicted by the color indicators shown on the lower left. B) Quantitative RT-PCR analysis of the cytokine and *Rorc* panel (upper), *Defb* (lower left) and *S100a8* and *S100a9* (lower right) expression. Skin from K5-Cre (WT, open column) and *Socs3* cKO (closed column) mice was analyzed by SYBR green real-time qPCR. Data are normalized to β-actin mRNA copy number and the mean and SEM (n = 5) are indicated. Statistical significance was determined using the Student's t-test. * $p<0.05$. C) Skin sections from K5-Cre control (WT) and the diseased *Socs3* cKO mice (cKO) were stained with Alexa 488 labeled anti-pSTAT3. Left panels represent phase contrast of skin section, and right panels represent pSTAT3 (green) in the skin section (x400). Scale bar in each section indicates 75 υm. D) Protein expression of IL-6, IL-19, and IL-24 in the frozen skin sections from K5-Cre (WT) and the diseased *Socs3* cKO mice were analyzed by immunohistochemical staining (x40). Scale bar in each section indicates 750 υm.

We further examined the effect of IL-6 on *Socs3* deficient keratinocytes in the induction of expression of IL-20R related cytokine genes, *Il19*, *Il20* and *Il24*. Socs3 deficient keratinocytes showed much higher IL-20RI related cytokine mRNA levels than the control keratinocytes (**Fig. 5B**). Our results revealed a prolonged STAT3 activation in response to IL-6 in the *Socs3* deficient keratinocytes, eventually leading to the expression of IL-19, IL-20 and IL-24 by keratinocytes. Furthermore, we found

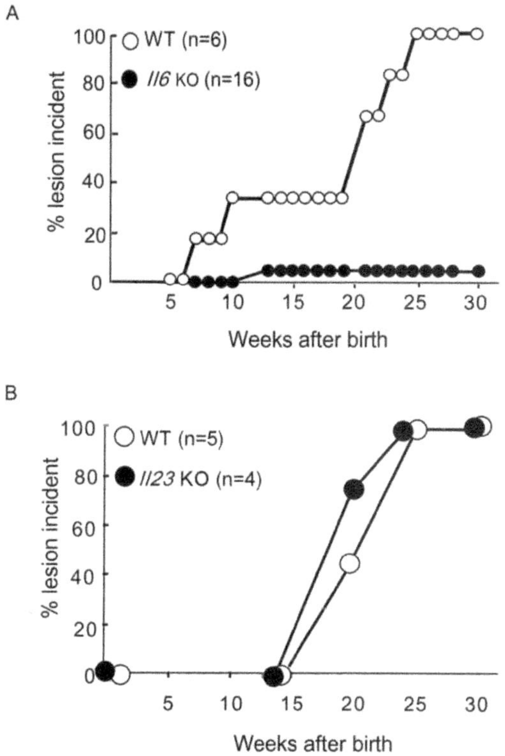

Figure 4. Lesion incidences in Socs3 cKO mice and in combined Il6$^{-/-}$- or Il23$^{-/-}$-Socs3 cKO mice. A) Lesion incidences were examined in K5-Cre mice (WT, open circle, n = 6) and *Il6*$^{-/-}$ *Socs3* cKO (*Il6* KO, closed circle, n = 16) mice. Each mouse strain was monitored up to 30 weeks after birth. The percentage of the mice showing disease incidence is shown on the Y axis in all examined mice at each time point. B) Lesion incidences were examined in K5-Cre mice (WT, open circle, n = 5) and *Il23*$^{-/-}$ *Socs3* cKO (*Il23* KO, closed circle, n = 4) mice. Each mouse strain was monitored for up to 30 weeks after birth. The percentage of the mice showing disease incidence is shown on the Y axis in all examined mice at each time point.

enhanced expression of IL-20R2, the receptor for IL-19, IL-20, and IL-24, on the keratinocytes of the diseased Socs3 cKO mice (**Fig. 5C**).

IL-20R related cytokines induce epidermal hyperplasia in Socs3 cKO skin

Up-regulation of IL-20R related cytokines, IL-19, IL-20 and IL-24, has often been reported in several skin diseases [22]. We therefore examined the effect of IL-20R related cytokines on skin pathology using the air pouch system. Recombinant IL-19 was injected into the air space generated in the skin of control and *Socs3* cKO mice. Interestingly, treatment with IL-19 in the pouches of *Socs3* cKO skin induced KC and MCP-1 production, but not IL-12p40 production (**Fig. 6A**). We further injected small amounts of IL-6 and IL-19 (10 ng/mouse) intradermally into *Socs3* deficient skin, and pathological signatures were assessed by histological analysis with K5 and MPO staining 14 days after the injection (**Fig. 6B**). This amount of IL-6 and IL-19 is not sufficient to induce skin diseases in wild type mice. However, in *Socs3* cKO mice, both IL-6 and IL-19 independently caused epidermal hyperplasia and massive neutrophil migration, while control treatment (PBS) showed no pathological changes (**Fig. 6B**); an indication that IL-19 expression in the keratin layer led to the skin inflammation through the attraction of neutrophils.

We further investigated whether IL-20R related cytokines are required for the IL-6 induced epidermal hyperplasia. We first tested the inhibitory properties of two independent reagents, IL-20Rβ-Fc fusion protein and anti-IL-20Rα antibody. The inhibitory activity was assessed by IL-6 production from IL-19 activated keratinocytes, and the inhibition was observed with the IL-20Rβ-Fc fusion protein (**Fig. S3**). Next, *Socs3* deficient mice were injected intradermally with IL-6 (20 ng/mouse) along with either control Ig or the IL-20Rβ-Fc fusion protein, and pathological signatures were assessed as epidermal hyperplasia at fourteen days after treatments. Treatment with the IL-20Rβ-Fc fusion protein completely abrogated the IL-6 induced epidermal hyperplasia (**Fig. 6C**). The same inhibition also observed in the mice treated with anti-IL-20 antibody (**Fig. S4**). These results demonstrated that IL-6-induced pathogenesis in the skin disease occurs though the induction of expression of IL-20R related cytokines.

Physical stimuli induced expression of IL-20R related cytokines and hyperplasia in Socs3 cKO mice

Skin lesions of *Socs3* cKO mice were consistently observed on the head and face, where mice were able to scratch by themselves, suggesting that physical stimulation by scratching might be a key event responsible for the disrupted skin barrier. To examine this possibility, artificial stimulation was provided by shaving hair on the dorsal skin where mice are unable to directly scratch. Five days after shaving, *Socs3* cKO mice, but not control mice, exhibited scaly skin and scabs at the shaved site, and the level of IL-19, IL-20 and IL-24 expression was comparably increased (**Fig. 7A**). *Socs3* KO skin showed signs of epidermal hyperplasia on day 4 (**Fig. 7B&C**), and this symptom completely resolved by day 14. Therefore, in the absence of SOCS3, shaving is sufficient for the induction of hyperplasia. The hyperplasia was only partially resolved in *Socs3* KO mice crossed with *Il6*$^{+/-}$ mice, but was completely resolved in *Socs3* KO mice crossed with *Il6* KO mice. *Il6* KO skin exhibited very weak expression of IL-19 in the shaved area (**Fig. 7B**). These results clearly demonstrated that IL-6 is a critical cytokine in the initiation of the epidermal hyperplasia induced by physical stimulation.

The shaving-induced epidermal thickening was inhibited by Tetracyclic Pyridone 6 (P6), a pan-JAK inhibitor that has a higher sensitivity in the JAK1-STAT3 activation pathway [23]. A low dose of P6 (1 mg) showed no effect, while high dose (2 mg) treatment almost totally inhibited the shaving-induced epidermal thickening (**Fig. 7D**). These results indicate that the epidermal hyperplasia induced by physical stimulation is exacerbated through hyperactivation of the JAK-STAT pathway.

Discussion

Recently, accumulating evidence has pointed to a crucial role for cytokines in chronic skin inflammation. The present study proposed that negative regulator for cytokine signaling SOCS3 plays a crucial role to maintain the keratinocyte homeostasis, and showed that defective SOCS3 expression causes inflammatory skin disease. We also found that the disruption of SOCS3 leads to excess activation of the IL-6-STAT3-IL-20R related cytokine signaling pathway. It is suggested that the balance among IL-6, STAT3 and SOCS3 controls normal skin homeostasis and maintains normal keratinocyte growth and proliferation. Imbalance of this skin homeostasis caused increased expression of IL-20R-related cytokines, eventually leading to the psoriatic inflammation in skin. Keratinocyte-specific Socs3 deficient mice provided us with a quite useful window on the disease process explained by the combined initiation of STAT3 activation and the

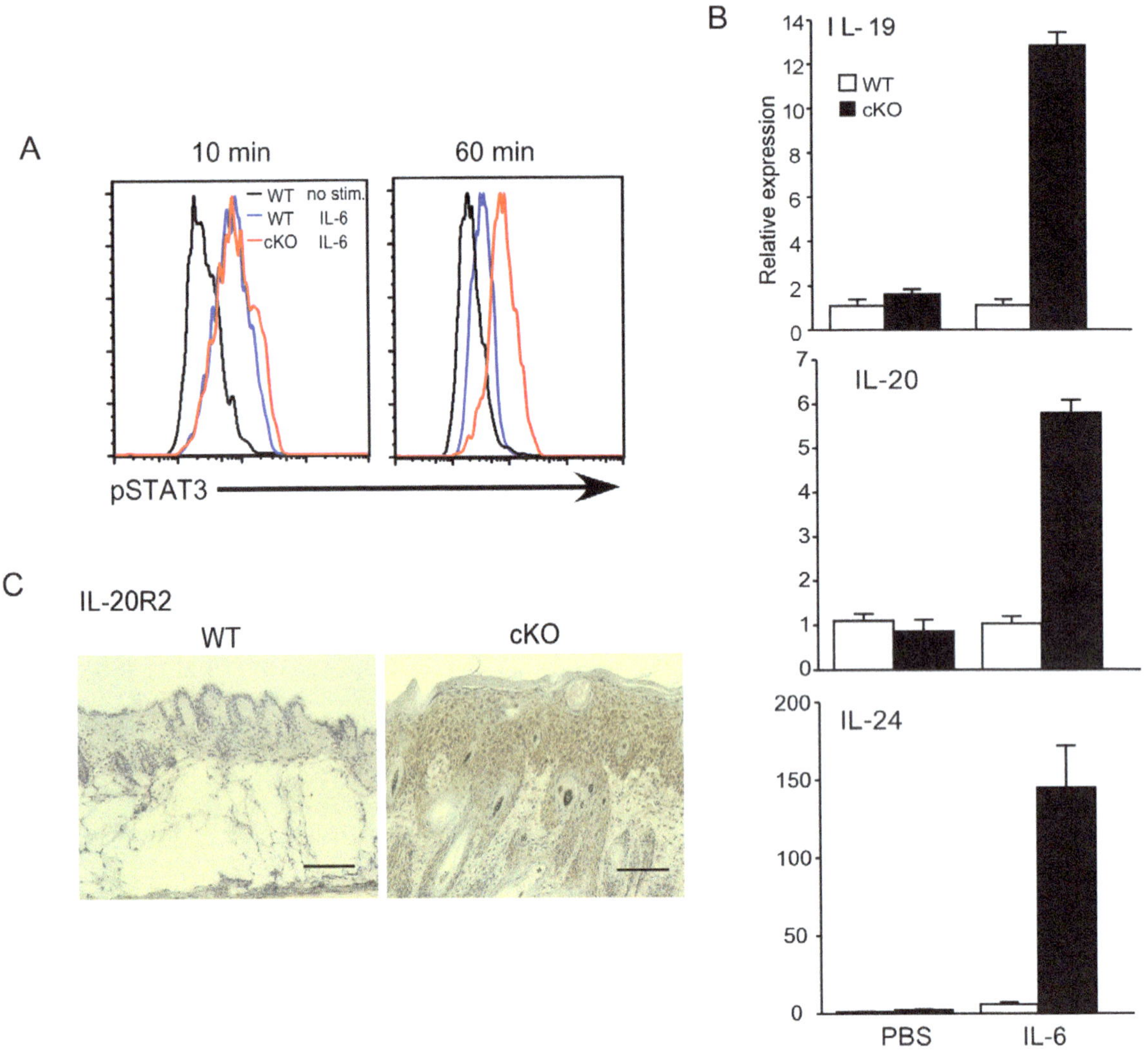

Figure 5. The effect of IL-6 on primary keratinocytes derived from Socs3 cKO mice. A) Mouse primary keratinocytes were stimulated with 10 ng/ml of IL-6 for 10 or 60 min and pSTAT3 was analyzed by flow cytometry. Black lines show the PBS control, blue lines show the keratinocytes from normal C57BL/6 mice, and red lines show the keratinocytes from *Socs3* cKO mice. Data are representative of 3 separate experiments. B) mRNA expression of IL-20R related cytokines in the keratinoyctes. Mouse primary keratinocytes were stimulated with or without IL-6 for 24 hrs and the expression of IL-19, IL-20 and IL-24 mRNA was investigated by quantitative RT-PCR. Open bars show the keratinocytes from C57BL/6 mice (WT), and closed bars show those of *Socs3* cKO mice. Data are relative expression to PBS-treated C57BL/6 keratinocytes. Data are mean ± SEM, n = 3. C) Increased expression of IL-20R2 protein in the diseased skin of *Socs3* cKO mice. Protein levels of IL-20R2 in the frozen skin sections from K5-Cre (WT) and the diseased *Socs3* cKO mice were analyzed by immunohistochemical staining (x200). Scale bar in each section indicates 150 um.

IL-20R-related cytokine mediated psoriatic skin inflammation, and the understanding of the entire disease process.

Many skin diseases such as seborrheic dermatitis, atopic dermatitis and psoriasis involve inflammation, and in these skin disorders, T cells or T cell-derived cytokines are thought to associate with disease development and aggravation. However, our observations revealed that the dysregulation of cytokine signaling only in the keratinocytes is enough to induce severe inflammation. In *Socs3* cKO mice, the serum IgE level is up-regulated but this seems not to play a critical role in the disease development, suggesting that the up-regulation of IgE may be a secondary event in this skin disease.

In our study, IL-6 seems to be a trigger for the spiral of inflammation in *Socs3* KO skin. Regarding the source of IL-6 in the skin, neuropeptides are possible triggers. Several substances, including Substance P (SP) and vasoactive intestinal peptide (VIP) which is released from dermal nerve endings, are known to stimulate keratinocytes to produce cytokines including IL-6 [24]. These neuropeptides like VIP can be induced under various stressful conditions including mental stress, alcohol consumption, and smoking. Bacterial infection could be another case for IL-6 induction, because we found plaque of streptococcus in the inflamed skin area of some, but not all, *Socs3* cKO mice (data not shown). Bacterial infections cause an acute form of inflammatory response leading to elevation of IL-6 production in the skin.

In the diseased *Socs3* cKO mouse skin, STAT3 is highly activated but other STAT family members are not (data not shown), indicating that SOCS3 in keratinocytes specifically regulates STAT3 activity. Furthermore, improvement of the skin disease by treatment with the P6 pan-JAK inhibitor confirmed that key cytokine signaling here utilizes the JAK/STAT pathway. SOCS3 specifically inhibits IL-6-induced STAT3 activation by

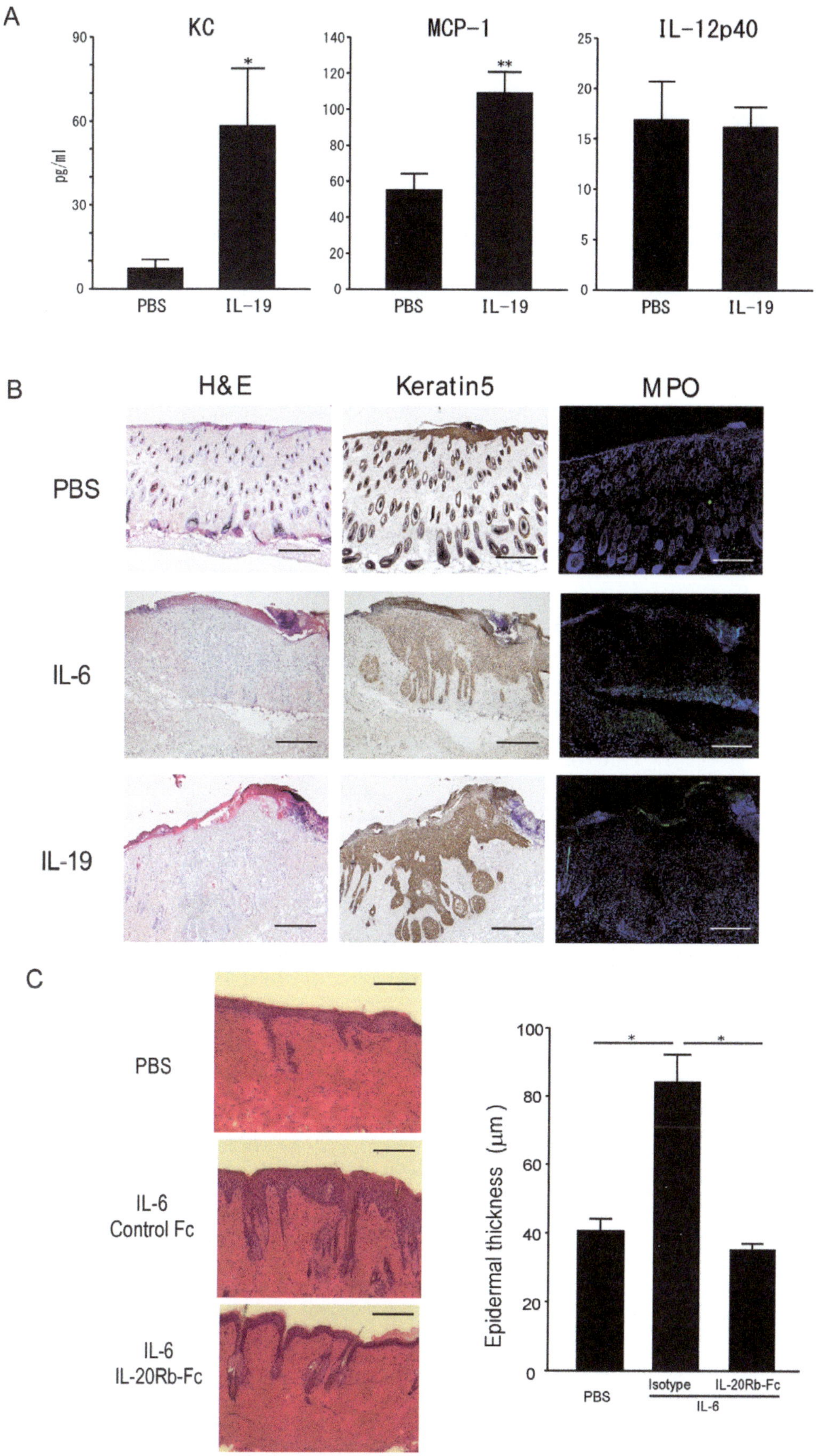
A
KC
MCP-1
IL-12p40
pg/ml
PBS
IL-19
B
H&E
Keratin5
MPO
PBS
IL-6
IL-19
C
PBS
IL-6
Control Fc
IL-6
IL-20Rb-Fc
Epidermal thickness (μm)
PBS
Isotype
IL-20Rb-Fc
IL-6

Figure 6. Effect of IL-19 on skin inflammation in the Socs3 cKO mice. A) Amounts of KC, MCP-1 and IL12p40 in the air pouches after IL-19 injection into C57BL/6 mice. IL-19 or PBS was injected into mouse air pouches, and chemokine concentration in the pouch lavage was measured after 5 hrs. Data are mean ± SEM, n = 5–6. B) IL-6 and IL-19 induced skin inflammation in the *Socs3* cKO mice. *Socs3* cKO mice were injected with PBS (upper rows), 10 ng of IL-6 (middle rows) or 10 ng of IL-19 (bottom rows) was injected intradermally and skin sections were obtained two weeks later. Left panels show the H&E staining, middle panels show K5 immunostaining, and right panels show MPO^+ neutrophils (x40). Scale bar in each section indicates 750 υm. C) *Socs3* cKO mice were injected with PBS (upper rows) or 20 ng of IL-6 (middle and bottom rows) intradermally with 5 υg of control Fc or IL-20Rβ fusion Fc (IL-20Rβ-Fc). After two weeks, skin sections were stained with H&E and epidermal thickness was measured at the injection site (x200). Scale bar in each section indicates 150 υm. Bar graph (right panel) indicates the mean and SEM (n = 3) of epidermal thickness (υm).

binding to the STAT3 docking site (Tyr759) in one of the components of the IL-6 receptor, gp130 [25,26]. This pivotal role for SOCS3 in skin inflammation is supported by recent reports showing that a specific microRNA, miR203, is highly expressed in human psoriatic skin and inhibits the expression of SOCS3 [27]. IL-20R-related cytokines, IL-19, IL-20 and IL-24, transmit their signal through IL-20Rα/IL-20Rβ receptor complex. These cytokines have been reported to play important roles in the skin, and are often thought to be pro-inflammatory cytokines [28]. Here we report that IL-6 induced higher levels of IL-19, IL-20 and IL-24 mRNA in SOCS3 deficient keratinocytes than in the WT keratinocytes, consistent with IL-6 mediated IL-20 induction in human keratinocytes [29]. Together, these findings indicate that in the healthy condition, SOCS3 is required for inhibition of the IL-6 induced increases in pro-inflammatory IL-20R-related cytokines. The up-regulation of these cytokines leads to neutrophil accumulation directly or indirectly through the induction of neutrophil chemoattractants, S100A8/S100A9.

In conclusion, we have demonstrated that skin homeostasis is maintained by a balance among IL-6, STAT3 and SOCS3 in keratinocytes. Furthermore, when this balance is broken and STAT3 activation is out of control, inflammatory skin disease is induced without any abnormalities in the immune cells. This SOCS3 mediated homeostatic function plays a key role in negatively regulating STAT3 activity. The relation among IL-6, STAT3, and SOCS3 provides a useful tool for understanding the mechanism of chronic skin inflammation in humans.

Materials and Methods

Reagents

Polylactide-glycoside (PLGA) nanospheres have been reported as useful pulmonary drug delivery carriers for improving the pharmacological effect of drugs [30]. The pan-JAK inhibitor Tetracyclic Pyridone 2-tert- butyl- 9-fliro- 3,6-dihydro- 7H-benz[h]-imidaz[4,5-f]isoquinoline-7-one (P6) [23] was packaged with PLGA nanospheres by Hosokawa Powder Technology Research Institute (Osaka). P6 was dissolved in PBS when applied onto the skin of mice. The dorsal skin area of *Socs3*cKO was shaved with depilatory cream, and P6 (1 mg or 2 mg) or PBS was injected intradermally into the shaved area. Five days after shaving, skin samples were prepared and frozen for sectioning and H&E staining.

Mice

K5 Cre Tg [31], $Socs1^{f/f}$ [32], $Socs3^{f/f}$ [33], $Il23^{-/-}$ [34], $Il4r^{-/-}$ [35], $Rag1^{-/-}$ [36] and $Il6^{-/-}$ [37] mice are described elsewhere. All mice used in this study except $Il4r^{-/-}$ were backcrossed into C57BL/6 mice, and $Il4r^{-/-}$ mice were maintained on a BALB/c background. C57BL/6 and BALB/c mice were purchased from CLEA Japan, Inc. (Tokyo, Japan). All mice were maintained in SPF conditions.

Monitoring disease incidences

The clinical scoring was assessed with the incidence number of regions: 0, no lesion; 1, lesion in ear; 2, lesion in half of face; 3, lesion in whole face. The scoring was done until week 50.

Antibodies and Cytokines

Immunohistochemistry was carried out with the following antibodies. Biotinylated rat anti-mouse CD4 (H129.19), biotinylated mouse anti-ClassII ($I-A^b$) (KH74), rat-anti-IL-17A (TC11-18H10)-PE, mouse anti-pSTAT3 (4/P-STAT3)-Alexa 488 and rat anti-IFNγ (XMG1.2)-PE antibodies were purchased from BD Biosciences (San Diego, CA). Biotinylated rat anti-CD8 (53–6.7), biotinylated hamster anti-CD11c (N418), rat-anti-Langerin (eBioL31), biotinylated rat anti-FcεRIα (MAR-1) and rat anti-IL-20R2 (20RNTC) were purchased from e-Biosciences (San Diego, CA). Goat anti-IL-6 (AF-406-NA), rat anti-IL-19 (350105), recombinant murine IL-23R Fc chimera (1686-MR), rat anti-IL-24 (303308), rat anti-IL-20 (380605) antibodies and recombinant murine IL-20Rβ Fc chimera (4388-MR) were purchased from R&D Systems, Inc. (Minneapolis, MN). Rabbit anti-pSTAT1 (9171), anti-pSTAT5 (9351) and anti-pSTAT6 (9361) were purchased from Cell Signaling Technology (Massachusetts, MA). Rabbit anti-K5 (PRB-160P) was obtained from Covance Research Products Inc. (Denver, PA). Goat anti-PAR2 (sc-8205) was purchased from Santa Cruz Biotechnology, Inc. (Santa Cruz, CA). Rabbit MPO polyclonal antibody (PA1-28215) was obtained from Pierce Biotechnology (Rockford, IL). Rat anti-MCP-8 (TUG8) was purchased from BioLegend (San Diego, CA). Rabbit anti-IL-20Rα antibody (ab25922) was obtained from abcam (Cambridge, UK). Murine anti-rat and goat antibodies (Histofine MAX-PO), Histo-fine streptavidin, anti-rat IgG Alexa Fluor 488 and streptavidin Alexa Fluor 546 (Invitrogen), anti-human IgG HRP (Jackson immune research, Pennsylvania, PA) were used for 2nd antibodies for Immunohistochemistry. Recombinant murine IL-6 and IL-19 were purchased from Peprotech Inc. and R&D Systems, Inc., respectively.

In vitro keratinocyte culture

Primary keratinocytes were obtained from epidermis isolated from mouse ears. The epidermis was separated from the dermis following 1 hour incubation at 37°C in 0.25% trypsin/EDTA (Nacalai Tesque, Kyoto Japan) followed by filtration through 70 υm nylon mesh cell strainers (BD). Keratinocytes were suspended in the keratinocyte growth media (KGM-2, Lonza, Basel, Switzerland) containing 4 ng/ml mouse epidermal growth factor (EGF) and seeded at 5×10^5 cells/ml. Before cytokine stimulation, keratinocytes were deprived of growth factors for 4 hours, then stimulated with recombinant IL-6 (10 ng/ml). After 10 or 60 min stimulation, cells were harvested and intracellular staining of pSTAT3 was performed. The flow cytometric analysis was done with a FACS Calibur (BD). For the detection of mRNA expression, after 24 hours stimulation, cells were harvested and

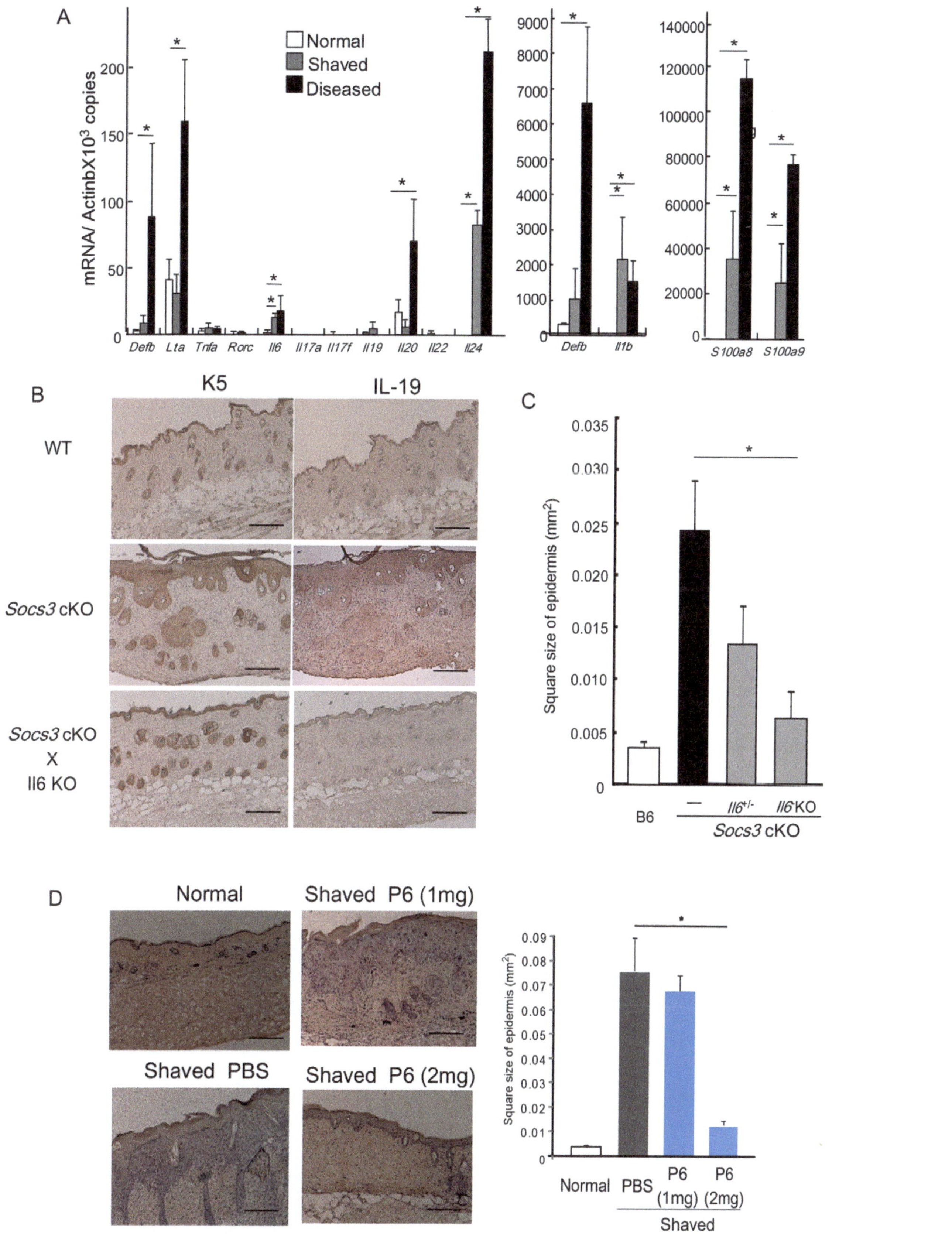

Figure 7. Physical stimulation initiates epidermal hyperplasia. A) mRNA was prepared from the skin of healthy K5-Cre (Normal), the shaved *Socs3* cKO mice (Shaved) and the diseased *Socs3* cKO mice (Diseased), and analyzed for the expression of the indicated genes by SYBR green real-time qPCR analysis. B) Immunohistochemical staining of keratinocytes (K5, left panels) and IL-19 positive cells (IL-19, left panels) in epidermis and dermis of

K5-Cre (WT), *Socs3* cKO mice and *Socs3* cKO mice crossed with *Il6* KO mice (*Socs3* cKO X *Il6* KO) (x40). Scale bar in each section indicates 750 υm. C) The role of IL-6 on the development of epidermal hyperplasia in *Socs3* cKO mice. B6, *Socs3* cKO mice, *Socs3* cKO mice crossed with $Il6^{+/-}$ or *Il6* KO mice were studied. The square area of epidermis (0.25 mm^2) in the section was measured at day 5 after shaving and is indicated on the Y-axis. Data are mean of the square size and error bars indicate SEM (n = 3). D) Effect of PLGA-P6 on physical stimulation-induced epidermal hyperplasia in *Socs3* cKO mice. Left; The dorsal skin area of *Socs3* cKO was shaved with depilatory cream and PLGA-P6 (1 mg or 2 mg) or PBS was injected intradermally into the shaved area. The shaved area (Shaved) was then compared to the non-treated area (Normal). At day 5 after shaving, skin sections were examined by H&E staining to assess the appearance of hyperplasia. The images are representative of three independent experiments (x40). Scale bar in each section indicates 750 υm. Right; the square size of the epidermis (0.25 mm^2) in the sections shown in the left image was measured at day 5 after shaving and is indicated on the Y-axis. Data are mean of the square size and error bars indicate SEM (n = 3).

RNA was extracted with RNAeasy mini kit (Qiagen). RT-PCR was done with SYBR green real-time quantitative PCR assay.

Histology and immunohistochemistry

The frozen skin sections were fixed with acetone and then stained with H&E. After blocking the sections with 3% BSA/PBS for 30 min, they were treated with primary abs in 1% BSA/PBS and were incubated for 30 min at room temperature. When the secondly abs were labeled with HRP, sections were then visualized by using DAB for 5 to 15 minutes. After washing the sections with water for 10 mins, sections were treated with EtOH and xylene and observed under light microscopy. When the secondly antibodies were fluorescently labeled, the sections were washed with PBS(−)−0.05% Tween20 after secondly antibody treatment. After washing the sections with water for 10 mins they were mounted with VECTA SHIELD/Prolong Gold reagent and imaged using an LSM 510 confocal microscopy system (Carl Zeiss, Germany). For the quantification of mast cells, basophils and neutrophils, toluidine blue, MCP-8 and MPO were used as cell markers respectively. We randomly picked four fields on the sections from each mouse for analysis.

Gene expression analysis

For gene expression analysis, total RNA was isolated using RNA STAT-60 (Tel-Test, Friendswood, TX, USA). Total RNA (5 υg) was subjected to treatment with DNase (Roche). DNase-treated total RNA was reverse-transcribed using Superscript II (Gibco/ BRL). Primers were designed using Primer Express (PE Biosystems), or obtained commercially from Applied Biosystems. Real-time quantitative PCR on 10 ng of cDNA from each sample was performed using either of two methods. In the first method, two gene-specific unlabelled primers were utilized at 400 nM in a Perkin Elmer SYBR green real-time quantitative PCR assay utilizing an ABI 5700 instrument. In the second method, two unlabelled primers at 900 nM each were used with 250 nM of FAM-labeled probe (Applied Biosystems) in a TAQMAN™ real-time quantitative PCR reaction on an ABI 7700 sequence detection system. The absence of genomic DNA contamination was confirmed using primers that recognize the genomic region of the CD4 promoter – samples with detectable DNA contamination by real-time PCR were excluded from the study. Ubiquitin levels were measured in a separate reaction and used to normalize the data by the $\Delta - \Delta$ Ct method, using the mean cycle threshold (Ct) value for ubiquitin and the gene of interests for each sample; the equation 1.8 e (Ct ubiquitin – Ct gene of interest) x 10^4 was used to obtain the normalized values.

Air pouch

C57BL/6 mice (8–9 wks) were injected with 5 ml of sterile air into the subcutaneous tissue of the back, followed by a second injection of 3 ml of sterile air into the pouch 3 days later. IL-19 (1 mg) in 1 ml of sterile PBS, or sterile PBS as a control were injected into the pouch 7 days after the first injection of air. After 5 hrs, mice were killed and pouch fluids were harvested by injecting 0.5 ml of PBS. After centrifugation, the supernatant were analyzed for cytokines/chemokines concentrations with Bioplex Cytokine assay kit (Bio-Rad Laboratories, Hercules, CA, USA) according to the manufacturer's protocol.

Supporting Information

Figure S1 Skin sections from the diseased Socs3 cKO mice were stained with anti-pSTAT1, anti-pSTAT5, or anti-pSTAT6, and the sections were further probed with HRP labeled secondary antibody. Control indicates secondary antibody alone.

Figure S2 Expression of IL-17A and IL-23 protein in frozen sections of K5-Cre control (WT) and the diseased skin from Socs3 cKO (cKO) mice was analyzed by immunohistochemical staining. The images are representative of five independent experiments (x40).

Figure S3 Isolated keratinocytes were cultured with IL-19 in the presence of IL-20Rβ-Fc fusion protein or anti-IL-20Rα antibody. After 6 hrs, IL-6 production in culture supernatant was measured by ELISA. Data are mean and SEM of three independent cultures.

Figure S4 Socs3 deficient mice were injected intradermally with IL-6 (10 ng/mouse) with either control Ig (isotype) or anti-IL-20 antibody (100 υg). After two weeks, skin sections were stained with H&E and epidermal thickness was measured at the injection site (x200). Scale bar in each section indicates 150 υm. Bar graph (right panel) indicates the mean and SEM (n = 3) of epidermal thickness (υm).

Acknowledgments

The authors thank Dr. Shigetoshi Sano, Dr. Hiromitsu Hara, Dr. Douglas Osei-Hyiaman and Dr. Peter Barrows, for critical review and comments on the manuscript and Y. Sato, H. Dohi, Uno, T., Natsume, M., Miura, E., Ohmori, A., and Hayashi, E., for technical assistance.

Author Contributions

Conceived and designed the experiments: AU SS MK. Performed the experiments: AU KM NO YM YS DC. Analyzed the data: AU KM SS DC MK. Contributed reagents/materials/analysis tools: AY DC. Wrote the paper: AU KM SS MK.

Reference

1. Kubo M, Hanada T, Yoshimura A (2003) Suppressors of cytokine signaling and immunity. Nat Immunol 4: 1169–1176.
2. Yoshimura A, Naka T, Kubo M (2007) SOCS proteins, cytokine signalling and immune regulation. Nat Rev Immunol 7: 454–465.
3. Zhu BM, Ishida Y, Robinson GW, Pacher-Zavisin M, Yoshimura A, et al. (2008) SOCS3 negatively regulates the gp130-STAT3 pathway in mouse skin wound healing. J Invest Dermatol 128: 1821–1829.
4. Margadant C, Charafeddine RA, Sonnenberg A (2010) Unique and redundant functions of integrins in the epidermis. FASEB J 24: 4133–4152.
5. Wullaert A, Bonnet MC, Pasparakis M (2011) NF-kappaB in the regulation of epithelial homeostasis and inflammation. Cell Res 21: 146–158.
6. Jensen JM, Schutze S, Forl M, Kronke M, Proksch E (1999) Roles for tumor necrosis factor receptor p55 and sphingomyelinase in repairing the cutaneous permeability barrier. J Clin Invest 104: 1761–1770.
7. Shornick LP, De Togni P, Mariathasan S, Goellner J, Strauss-Schoenberger J, et al. (1996) Mice deficient in IL-1beta manifest impaired contact hypersensitivity to trinitrochlorobenzone. J Exp Med 183: 1427–1436.
8. Wang XP, Schunck M, Kallen KJ, Neumann C, Trautwein C, et al. (2004) The interleukin-6 cytokine system regulates epidermal permeability barrier homeostasis. J Invest Dermatol 123: 124–131.
9. Sano S, Chan KS, DiGiovanni J (2008) Impact of Stat3 activation upon skin biology: a dichotomy of its role between homeostasis and diseases. J Dermatol Sci 50: 1–14.
10. Sano S, Chan KS, Carbajal S, Clifford J, Peavey M, et al. (2005) Stat3 links activated keratinocytes and immunocytes required for development of psoriasis in a novel transgenic mouse model. Nat Med 11: 43–49.
11. Kataoka K, Kim DJ, Carbajal S, Clifford JL, DiGiovanni J (2008) Stage-specific disruption of Stat3 demonstrates a direct requirement during both the initiation and promotion stages of mouse skin tumorigenesis. Carcinogenesis 29: 1108–1114.
12. Pestka S, Krause CD, Sarkar D, Walter MR, Shi Y, et al. (2004) Interleukin-10 and related cytokines and receptors. Annu Rev Immunol 22: 929–979.
13. Kunz S, Wolk K, Witte E, Witte K, Doecke WD, et al. (2006) Interleukin (IL)-19, IL-20 and IL-24 are produced by and act on keratinocytes and are distinct from classical ILs. Exp Dermatol 15: 991–1004.
14. Stenderup K, Rosada C, Worsaae A, Clausen JT, Norman Dam T (2007) Interleukin-20 as a target in psoriasis treatment. Ann N Y Acad Sci 1110: 368–381.
15. Kingo K, Koks S, Nikopensius T, Silm H, Vasar E (2004) Polymorphisms in the interleukin-20 gene: relationships to plaque-type psoriasis. Genes Immun 5: 117–121.
16. Sa SM, Valdez PA, Wu J, Jung K, Zhong F, et al. (2007) The effects of IL-20 subfamily cytokines on reconstituted human epidermis suggest potential roles in cutaneous innate defense and pathogenic adaptive immunity in psoriasis. J Immunol 178: 2229–2240.
17. Leng RX, Pan HF, Tao JH, Ye DQ IL-19, IL-20 and IL-24: potential therapeutic targets for autoimmune diseases. Expert Opin Ther Targets 15: 119–126.
18. Sabat R, Philipp S, Hoflich C, Kreutzer S, Wallace E, et al. (2007) Immunopathogenesis of psoriasis. Exp Dermatol 16: 779–798.
19. Chan JR, Blumenschein W, Murphy E, Diveu C, Wiekowski M, et al. (2006) IL-23 stimulates epidermal hyperplasia via TNF and IL-20R2-dependent mechanisms with implications for psoriasis pathogenesis. J Exp Med 203: 2577–2587.
20. Lee E, Trepicchio WL, Oestreicher JL, Pittman D, Wang F, et al. (2004) Increased expression of interleukin 23 p19 and p40 in lesional skin of patients with psoriasis vulgaris. J Exp Med 199: 125–130.
21. Nair RP, Duffin KC, Helms C, Ding J, Stuart PE, et al. (2009) Genome-wide scan reveals association of psoriasis with IL-23 and NF-kappaB pathways. Nat Genet 41: 199–204.
22. Ouyang W, Rutz S, Crellin NK, Valdez PA, Hymowitz SG (2011) Regulation and functions of the IL-10 family of cytokines in inflammation and disease. Annu Rev Immunol 29: 71–109.
23. Pedranzini L, Dechow T, Berishaj M, Comenzo R, Zhou P, et al. (2006) Pyridone 6, a pan-Janus-activated kinase inhibitor, induces growth inhibition of multiple myeloma cells. Cancer Res 66: 9714–9721.
24. Park YM, Kim CW (1999) The effects of substance P and vasoactive intestinal peptide on interleukin-6 synthesis in cultured human keratinocytes. J Dermatol Sci 22: 17–23.
25. Schmitz J, Weissenbach M, Haan S, Heinrich PC, Schaper F (2000) SOCS3 exerts its inhibitory function on interleukin-6 signal transduction through the SHP2 recruitment site of gp130. J Biol Chem 275: 12848–12856.
26. Lehmann U, Schmitz J, Weissenbach M, Sobota RM, Hortner M, et al. (2003) SHP2 and SOCS3 contribute to Tyr-759-dependent attenuation of interleukin-6 signaling through gp130. J Biol Chem 278: 661–671.
27. Bostjancic E, Glavac D (2008) Importance of microRNAs in skin morphogenesis and diseases. Acta Dermatovenerol Alp Panonica Adriat 17: 95–102.
28. Boniface K, Lecron JC, Bernard FX, Dagregorio G, Guillet G, et al. (2005) Keratinocytes as targets for interleukin-10-related cytokines: a putative role in the pathogenesis of psoriasis. Eur Cytokine Netw 16: 309–319.
29. Otkjaer K, Kragballe K, Johansen C, Funding AT, Just H, et al. (2007) IL-20 gene expression is induced by IL-1beta through mitogen-activated protein kinase and NF-kappaB-dependent mechanisms. J Invest Dermatol 127: 1326–1336.
30. Hara K, Tsujimoto H, Tsukada Y, Huang CC, Kawashima Y, et al. (2008) Histological examination of PLGA nanospheres for intratracheal drug administration. Int J Pharm 356: 267–273.
31. Tarutani M, Itami S, Okabe M, Ikawa M, Tezuka T, et al. (1997) Tissue-specific knockout of the mouse *Pig-a* gene reveals important roles for GPI-anchored proteins in skin development. Proc Natl Acad Sci U S A 94: 7400–7405.
32. Tanaka K, Ichiyama K, Hashimoto M, Yoshida H, Takimoto T, et al. (2008) Loss of suppressor of cytokine signaling 1 in helper T cells leads to defective Th17 differentiation by enhancing antagonistic effects of IFN-gamma on STAT3 and Smads. J Immunol 180: 3746–3756.
33. Yasukawa H, Ohishi M, Mori H, Murakami M, Chinen T, et al. (2003) IL-6 induces an anti-inflammatory response in the absence of SOCS3 in macrophages. Nat Immunol 4: 551–556.
34. Cua DJ, Sherlock J, Chen Y, Murphy CA, Joyce B, et al. (2003) Interleukin-23 rather than interleukin-12 is the critical cytokine for autoimmune inflammation of the brain. Nature 421: 744–748.
35. Mohrs M, Ledermann B, Kohler G, Dorfmuller A, Gessner A, et al. (1999) Differences between IL-4- and IL-4 receptor alpha-deficient mice in chronic leishmaniasis reveal a protective role for IL-13 receptor signaling. J Immunol 162: 7302–7308.
36. Mombaerts P, Iacomini J, Johnson R, Herrup K, Tonegawa S, et al. (1992) RAG-1-deficient mice have no mature B and T lymphocytes. Cell 68: 869–877.
37. Kopf M, Baumann H, Freer G, Freudenberg M, Lamers M, et al. (1994) Impaired immune and acute-phase responses in interleukin-6-deficient mice. Nature 368: 339–342.

6

Subcutaneous Fascial Bands—A Qualitative and Morphometric Analysis

Weihui Li[1]*, Andrew C. Ahn[1,2]

1 Martinos Center for Biomedical Imaging, Massachusetts General Hospital, Charlestown, Massachusetts, United States of America, 2 Division of General Medicine and Primary Care, Beth Israel Deaconess Medical Center, Boston, Massachusetts, United States of America

Abstract

Background: Although fascial bands within the subcutaneous (SQ) layer are commonly seen in ultrasound images, little is known about their functional role, much less their structural characteristics. This study's objective is to describe the morphological features of SQ fascial bands and to systematically evaluate the bands using image analyses tools and morphometric measures.

Methods: In 28 healthy volunteers, ultrasound images were obtained at three body locations: the lateral aspect of the upper arm, medial aspect of the thigh and posterior aspect of lower leg. Using image analytical techniques, the total SQ band area, fascial band number, fascial band thickness, and SQ zone (layer) thickness were determined. In addition, the SQ spatial coherence was calculated based on the eigenvalues associated with the largest and smallest eigenvectors of the images.

Results: Fascial bands at these sites were contiguous with the dermis and the epimysium forming an interconnected network within the subcutaneous tissue. Subcutaneous blood vessels were also frequently encased by these fascial bands. The total SQ fascial band area was greater at the thigh and calf compared to the arm and was unrelated to SQ layer (zone) thickness. The thigh was associated with highest average number of fascial bands while calf was associated with the greatest average fascial band thickness. Across body regions, greater SQ zone thickness was associated with thinner fascial bands. SQ coherence was significantly associated with SQ zone thickness and body location (calf with statistically greater coherence compared to arm).

Conclusion: Fascial bands are structural bridges that mechanically link the skin, subcutaneous layer, and deeper muscle layers. This cohesive network also encases subcutaneous vessels and may indirectly mediate blood flow. The quantity and morphological characteristics of the SQ fascial band may reflect the composite mechanical forces experienced by the body part.

Editor: Bradley Steven Launikonis, University of Queensland, Australia

Funding: This research was supported by grant number K23-AT003238, P30AT005895, and K24-AT004095 of the National Center for Complementary Alternative Medicine (NCCAM) and supported in part by a gift from The Bernard Osher Foundation. The project described was supported by Clinical Translational Science Award UL1RR025758 to Harvard University and Beth Israel Deaconess Medical Center from the National Center for Research Resources. The content is solely the responsibility of the authors and does not necessarily represent the official views of the National Center for Complementary Alternative Medicine or the National Center for Research Resources or the National Institutes of Health. The funders had no role in study design, data collection and analysis, decision to publish, or preparation of the manuscript.

Competing Interests: The authors have declared that no competing interests exist.

* E-mail: weihuil@gmail.com

Introduction

Subcutaneous (SQ) tissue is an adipose rich loose connective tissue layer lying underneath the dermal layer of the skin. It links the skin to the deeper muscular layers and bones [1]. It also acts as a storage depot for metabolic fuel and as a protective cushion for the deeper tissues and organs. For the past century, the main focus of the SQ region has been the adipocytes and traversing structures such as superficial nerves and vessels. The extracellular macromolecules such as collagenous and elastin fibers have garnered considerably less attention in the field of anatomy - partly due to the lack of clarity regarding their functional significance and partly due to difficulties in isolating them from the muscular fascia during dissections of an embalmed cadaver. With the increased availability and widespread use of ultrasonography, however, the existence of lateral band-like structures distinct from muscle, vessels or nerves is readily apparent within the subcutaneous layers. These bands appear as white, echogenic linear structures that span the width of the ultrasound image and have been matched to immune-histological staining of large collagenous fibers [2]. Anatomists and histologists have variably termed these extracellular fibers as "textus connectives compactus", "Fascia superficialis", "membrane layers", and "Straffes Bindegewebe" [3]. For the purpose of clarity and uniformity, these collagenous bands will be termed "SQ fascial bands" in this manuscript.

Past studies have qualitatively assessed the characteristics of these SQ fascial bands and have described variability in both the number of bands and band thickness across body sites and across individuals [3]. To our knowledge, however, no study has quantitatively evaluated the morphological characteristics of these SQ fascial bands and identified factors associated with them. This study's objective is to systematically evaluate the morphological features of SQ fascial bands in healthy volunteers by analyzing ultrasound images obtained at three separate extremity sites – the upper arm, thigh, and calf. Image analytical techniques were used to quantify various aspects of SQ fascial bands - including the number of bands, band thickness, and total fascial band area – while also determining SQ zone thickness. We additionally evaluated the spatial anisotropy of the SQ zone with the use of a spatial coherence measure. The detailed description of the bands' morphology and their quantitative assessments may create the initial foundation for better understanding the physiological significance of these fascial bands.

Methods

Ethics Statement

This study was reviewed and approved by the institutional review board at the Beth Israel Deaconess Medical Center. Each study participant read and signed an informed consent form.

Human Subject Recruitment

We recruited 28 subjects (19 females 9 males) in the study via flyers throughout Boston campus areas near Beth Israel Deaconess Medical Center and via postings in Craigslist (www.Craigslist.org). Subjects were excluded if they were under 18 years old or pregnant, used anticoagulation medications, had history of bleeding disorder, had an implanted ventricular defibrillator, had a chronic skin condition (such as eczema, psoriasis), or had a collagen disorder (scleroderma, mixed connective tissue disorder, Marfan's). Subjects' age was 28.6±7.9 (mean ± SD) years of BMI 23.5±3.6. Demographic representation was 23 non-Hispanic White, 1 Hispanic, and 4 Asian. Each subject was compensated for participation. The testing was performed in the General Clinical Research Center at the Beth Israel Deaconess Medical Center.

Ultrasound Image Data Acquisition and Processing

A GE Logiq Book XP scanner (GE, Waukesha, Wisconsin) with a 38 mm linear array transducer (10MHz, 8L-RS) was used to image the subcutaneous region. Imaging depth was set at 40 mm and the focal depth was kept at 12.5 mm. Ultrasound transducer was placed in the direction longitudinal to the long axis of the extremities and swept anteriorly or posteriorly at a velocity of 1 cm/sec for a total of 6 seconds, as in Figure 1A. To standardize the measurements, transducer was held perpendicular to the skin. Minimal amounts of compression were applied on the skin to avoid deformation of the skin during ultrasound image acquisition. Recording mode was set to a cine loop setting – a 301 frame video loop was obtained for each sweep.

The videos were obtained at three different segments on the skin surface: the lateral aspect of the upper arm, medial aspect of the thigh and posterior aspect of lower leg, as previously reported [4] and shown in Figure 1B. These sites were predefined and localized according to adjacent body landmarks to reduce inter-subject measurement variability. Each video was then segmented to individual images (Figure 1C as an example) with Avidemux, a multi-platform video editor by Free Software Foundation Inc. (Boston, MA, USA). The segmented images were in jpeg format. Of the 301 images of each video, we evenly selected 6 images for imaging analysis. In cases where the imaging quality was in question (due to shadows or other imaging artifacts), the closest neighboring image without quality problems was chosen. We averaged the measurements from the 6 images and used this average for statistical analyses. In total, seventy five data sets from 450 images, 25 subjects, and 3 body sites (16 female and 9 male, 3 subjects' data were not analyzed due to poor image quality) were analyzed.

We used ImageJ software (National Institute of Health, USA) for imaging analysis. Images were first converted to 8-bit images with pixel intensity ranging from 0 to 255 (0 is no echogenicity and 255 is maximal echogenicity). The SQ layer was then marked out manually in the images to delineate the regions of interest (ROI), as shown in Figure 1D shaded with yellow. The

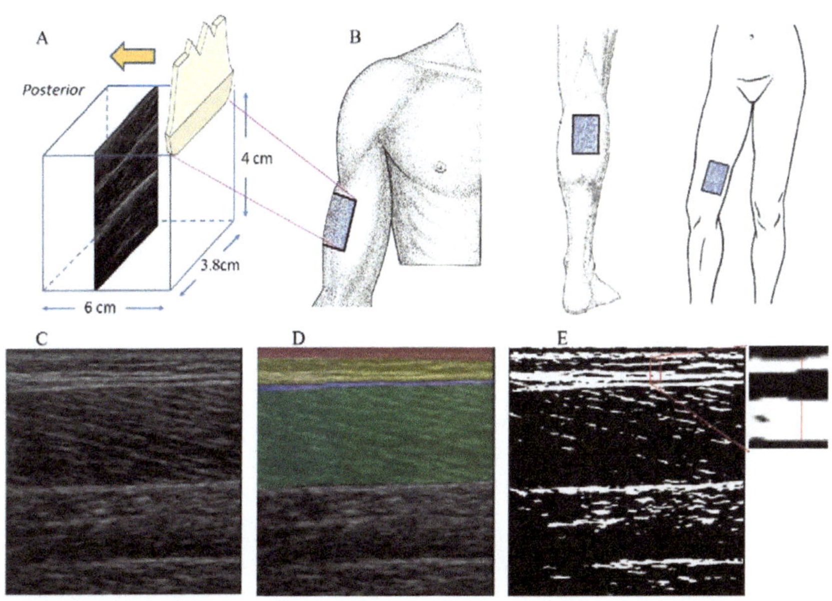

Figure 1. Three test segments with ultrasound image samples. (A) Illustration of ultrasound scanning longitudinal to the long axis of the extremities; (B) The locations where images were obtained: arm (left), calf (middle) and thigh (right); (C). Sample of ultrasound image; (D). Zones demarcated by color: dermal zone (red), SQ zone (yellow), epimysium zone (blue) and muscular zone (green); (E). Binary image with a pixel intensity threshold of 90.

red, blue and green zones in the figure were dermal, epimysial (dense connective tissue ensheathing the entire muscle) and muscular zones respectively, that were not included in the ROI. The depth and location of the SQ zone was confirmed by visualizing adjacent images within the video loop where the distinction between muscle and SQ zone was clear. Total pixel number in SQ was counted as the *total SQ zone area. SQ zone thickness* was calculated out by dividing total SQ zone area by the width of the SQ tissue.

We converted the images to binary images with a pixel intensity of 90 set as threshold. Pixels with intensity between 90 and 255 were regarded as echogenic. To eliminate the contribution of small, echogenic speckles to the total band area, high-intensity pixels with an aggregate area smaller than 20 pixels were categorized as non-echogenic. Figure 1E shows a sample of binary image. The threshold was determined by principal components analysis in JMP program (SAS institute Inc), as described below.

In the binary image, the total number of echogenic pixels in SQ zone was referred to as *total fascial band area. Fascial band* was defined as a continuous, transverse line composed of high-intensity pixels. *Fascial band number* was the average number of fascial bands within the SQ zone and was determined by totaling the number of fascial band segments across all the pixel columns and dividing by the total number of columns. The inset of Figure 2F shows two sample fascial band segments, each marked with a red line. *Fascial band thickness* was estimated by dividing the total fascial band area by the fascial band number. *Fascial band density* was computed by dividing total fascial band area by total SQ zone area. In the image analyses, one-pixel was considered a unit. Each ultrasound image had dimensions of 390×412 pixels. With a linear array transducer width of 38 mm and imaging depth of 40 mm, we converted the pixel dimensions into metric units: 1 pixel = 0.00956 mm^2 in area and 1 pixel = 0.097 mm in length.

We also calculated the coherence (Coh) for the SQ tissue with formula shown below:

$$Coh = \begin{cases} \left(\frac{\lambda 1 - \lambda 2}{\lambda 1 + \lambda 2}\right)^2 & if \ (\lambda 1 + \lambda 2) > 0 \\ 0 & otherwise \end{cases}$$

$\lambda 1$ and $\lambda 2$ are the first and second eigenvalues corresponding to the largest and smallest eigenvectors. Coherence is an indication of whether the local area is anisotropic. Coh is 1 when the local structure has one dominant orientation. The Coh is 0 when the local area is isotropic [5].

Principal Components Analysis

Principal components analysis is a method that works with high-dimensional data and determines the vectors with greatest variances. By doing so, it reduces the dimensionality of the data and thus helps retrieve hidden patterns.

In this study, pixel intensities ranged from 0 to 221. No pixels in any of the ultrasound images had intensities above 221. The pixels were categorized into decades forming 22 variables. Each decade variable contained the number of pixels whose intensities fit within a specific range (e.g. 0–9 for the first decade variable) for each ultrasound image. These variables were used for the principal components analysis.

Our aim was to objectively categorize the images into high echogenicity (fascial band) and low echogenicity areas (non-band tissue). This implied the existence of two principal components. Figure 2A displays the loading plot from JMP and shows the eigenvector coordinates of each decade variable on the two-principal-components axes. To identify the most appropriate intensity threshold for differentiating echogenic and non-echogenic tissue, each decade variable was systematically used to divide all the variables into two groups. A summed vector was computed for each group, represented by the two thick black lines as shown in Figure 2A as an example (in this case, the summed vectors represent the first four vectors in one group and the remaining 18 vectors in the other group). These two vectors formed an angel α. Figure 2B showed the cosine values of the angle α for each decade variable, and the decade variable associated with the smallest magnitude of $\cos(\alpha)$ was considered the optimal intensity threshold (α nearing 90 degrees indicates independence between the two vectors). In Figure 2B, $\cos(\alpha)$ crosses the x-axis between pixel intensity variable 90 and 100. For this reason, pixel intensity threshold of 90 was chosen: pixels with intensity below 90 were treated non-echogenic and pixels with intensity above 90 were considered echogenic tissue.

Statistical analysis

The study includes repeated measurements at three different locations on each subject for total 28 volunteers. With location as the dependent variable within each subject, different variables were analyzed to explore their location dependence with least-

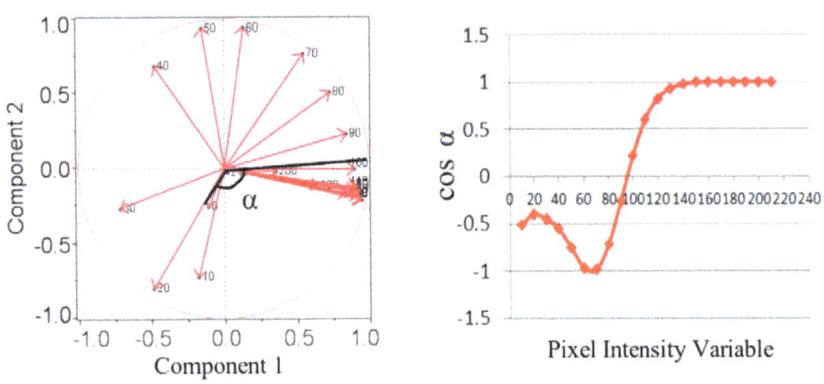

Figure 2. Determination of pixel intensity threshold by principal component analysis. (A). Eigenvectors of 22 decade variables plotted with respect to two principal components; (B). Value of cos(α) with respect to decade variables: α represents the angle formed between vector 1 (vector sum of all decade variables below designated decade variable) and vector 2 (vector sum of all decade variables above designated decade variable). (see text for detail).

square means method. Pairwise comparison was also performed and adjusted with SCHEFFE algorithm [6]. To demonstrate the relationships between SQ zone variables, we conducted a bivariate linear fit. We used multilevel mixed model in determining the effect of location, SQ collagen band thickness, SQ collagen band number and SQ zone thickness on SQ coherence. The p value of 0.05 was set as the significant level.

Results

Structural morphologies of SQ collagen band

Figure 3A shows sample ultrasound images from calf (panel C1, C2, C3), arm (panel A1, A2, A3) and thigh (panel T1, T2, T3) from different subjects. "M" and "SQ" in the figure labels the muscular layer and SQ layer respectively. Vertical blue lines are visual representation of the average SQ zone thickness. The layer above the top of the blue line is the dermal layer; the echogenic layer directly below the SQ zone is the epimysium layer.

SQ zone thickness (the length of the blue lines) greatly varied across individuals. For example, in the calf images, the SQ zone in C1 was approximately 2 mm while it was approximately 10 mm in panel C3. Similarly, in the arm and thigh images, SQ zone in panel A1 (about 3 mm) and T1 (about 5 mm) were thinner when compared to SQ zones in A3 (about 10 mm) and T3 (about 35 mm).

The morphology of fascial bands also differed across subjects. Fascial bands in panel A1 and T1 were generally linear and coherent whereas the bands in panel T3 were fragmented and curved. In general, individuals with decreased SQ zone thickness had more linear and less fragmented fascial bands compared to individuals with thicker SQ zones. The fascial band number also varied across individuals. More than two distinct echogenic bands are seen in panel T2 and only one relatively dimmer and less contiguous band is present in panel A1. In many cases, the SQ fascial bands are found aggregated close to the epimysium and less frequently near the dermis (C3, T1, T3 as examples). Among these

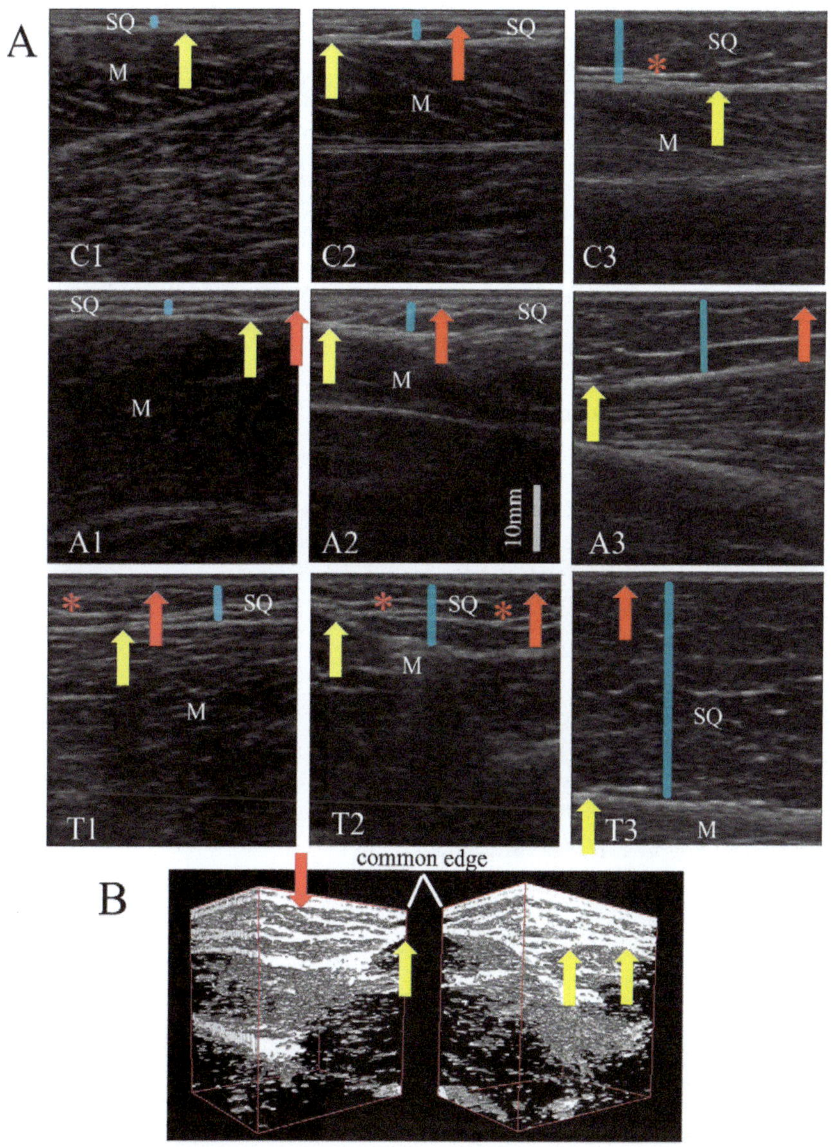

Figure 3. Ultrasound images showing the morphological characteristics of fascial bands. (A). Ultrasound images from calf, arm and thigh; (B). Three dimensional reconstruction of a video sweep, visualized from two different perspective angles.

images, some fascial bands are branched (below the red stars) while others are not.

The SQ fascial bands are, in many cases, contiguous with the epimysium and dermis, as demonstrated in Figure 3A. Red arrows indicate the site where SQ fascia plane extends towards the dermis, and the yellow arrows point to sites where epimysium and SQ fascial bands are fused. Figure 3B shows a three-dimensional reconstruction of serial binary images obtained from a video sweep and visualized from two different perspective angles. Again, the yellow and red arrows point to sites where the SQ fascial bands attach to the epimysium and dermis, respectively.

Multiple images revealed that subcutaneous veins are often encased by the fascial bands – either between SQ fascial bands or between the SQ fascial bands and epimysium. Figure 4A, 4B, 4C show sample images from the thigh, calf and arm. Figure 4D shows a cubic tissue reconstructed from the video sweep associated with Figure 4A. These two panels were viewed from two opposite direction with vein revealed as a black tunnel (also see "Video S1"). Within a span of only 6 cm, the fascial band's structural relationship with the vein can vary. As seen in the right panel of Figure 4D, the vein is located between two parallel, coherent fascial bands while, in the left panel, the fascial bands appears not to be as cohesive.

Quantitative analysis of SQ fascial bands

Table 1 lists the mean and standard deviations for the variables of fascial band number, fascial band thickness, total fascial band area, SQ zone thickness, and fascial band density regardless of locations. Their dependence on body site is presented in Figure 5 with pairwise comparison p values.

The thigh was associated with statistically greater number of SQ fascial bands when compared to the calf and arm (Figure 5A); SQ fascial band thickness was significantly greater at the calf compared to that of the arm and thigh (Figure 5B); the thigh had the greatest amount of total fascial band area while the arm had the least (Figure 5C).

Figure 5D shows the mean thickness of the SQ zone at different body sites. SQ zone was thickest at the thigh and thinnest at the calf. The thigh was associated with a statistically greater SQ zone thickness compared to the arm and calf. Body site dependence of fascial band density is presented in Figure 5E. Only the pairwise comparison between the calf and thigh was statistically significant.

Figure 6 shows the bivariate linear fit between the various fascial band variables in the SQ zone. Data from arm, thigh and calf were color coded as shown in the figure. There was a significant direct relationship between fascial band thickness and fascial band number ($p = 0.0375$). Fascial band number was not significantly associated with SQ zone thickness ($p = 0.2543$). There was significant correlations between fascial band thickness and SQ zone thickness ($p < 0.0001$). The association between total total fascial band area and SQ zone thickness was also not statistically significant ($p = 0.3879$).

The bivariate relationship between SQ coherence and various SQ variables - including fascial band number, fascial band thickness, total fascial band area, SQ zone thickness and fascial band density are presented in Figure 7. SQ coherence was not significantly associated with fascial band number ($p = 0.8978$) or total fascial band area ($p = 0.2969$), but was positively associated with fascial band thickness ($p = 0.0051$), fascial band density ($p = 0.0229$) and negatively correlated with SQ zone thickness ($p < 0.0001$).

When SQ coherence was modeled in a multilevel mixed model with location, fascial band number, fascial band thickness and SQ zone thickness as independent variables, body site ($p < 0.0001$) and SQ zone thickness ($p < 0.0001$) were statistically significant factors (Table 2) while fascial band number and fascial band thickness were not ($p = 0.6906$ and 0.225 respectively). SQ coherence was greatest on the calf and least on the arm (Table 3). SQ coherence on the thigh was 0.711, significantly greater than on the arm ($p = 0.0155$) and comparatively reduced than on the calf ($p = 0.3116$).

Discussion

This study highlights the interconnectedness of the fascial bands. These bands not only intertwined and connected with other fascial bands at different depths, but they also merged with the epimysium immediately beneath the subcutaneous layer and

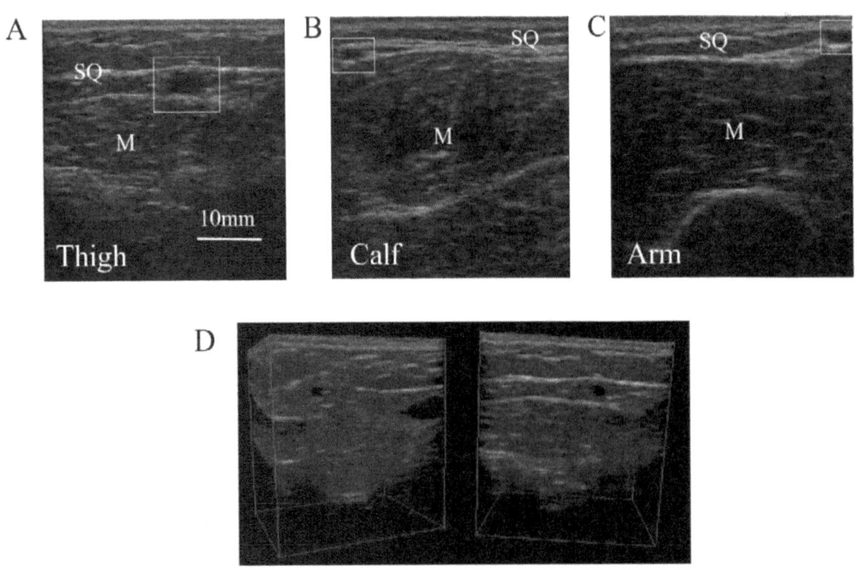

Figure 4. Ultrasound images showing the subcutaneous blood vessels encapsulated by fascial bands. (A). From the site of thigh; (B). From the site of calf ; (C) From the site of arm; (D). Three-dimensional reconstruction of a site with a vessel.

Table 1. Means and standard deviations of ultrasound-image derived variables.

Variables	Mean	Std Dev
Fascial Band Number	2.44	0.7
Fascial Band Thickness (mm)	0.51	0.08
Total Fascial Band Area (mm^2)	48.12	17.06
SQ Zone Thickness (mm)	9.3	5.7
Fascial Band Density	0.21	0.17

ascended superficially to intersect with the skin's dermis. As confirmed by multiple 2D images and 3D reconstructed renditions, the SQ fascial bands formed a coherent network of fibers that ensured various layers of the skin structurally and mechanically linked. These finding corroborates what others have reported in the literature. In a cadaveric study of the extremities, trunk, anterior chest wall, and neck, Abu-Hijleh MF [3] observed interconnecting and merging fascial membranes within the subcutaneous layer at all locations studied. Johnson D [7] and Nash [8] also observed fascial bands radiating toward the skin from deeper subcutaneous/epimysial layers to form adherent junctions with the dermis. These junctions termed "skin ligaments" were identified in the abdomen and the extremities far more frequently than what is commonly perceived as limited to certain locations (i.e. Zygomatic ligament in the cheek and Coopers ligament in the breast) [7]. This ubiquitous fascial network likely serves to maintain structural cohesiveness between the skin and the underlying muscle and bones. Without the tensile resilience afforded by the collagen fibers and without the structural junctions to serve as anchors, skin would otherwise be prone to disengaging and completely detaching from the body. Importantly, this structural arrangement also ensures that the skin and its structural components are not mechanically isolated. Substantial muscular movement or large skin displacements would generate mechanical strain along the fascial bands that can theoretically span well beyond a focal location and thus affect fibroblast mechanotransduction and even nerve activity at a large spatial scale. Within this framework, the fascial network may conceivably form a body-wide network that not only helps mediate mechanical forces but also cellular and nervous activities as well [9].

Subcutaneous blood vessels were also extensively integrated in this fascial network. In our ultrasound images at all three locations, SQ fascial bands were found to compartmentalize and encase the blood vessels (Figure 4). At the spatial resolution of our ultrasound, the vessel wall appeared inseparable from the fascial bands, particularly at the most superficial and deep aspect of the vessel. Past authors have equated this structural arrangement with the "Egyptian eye" and reported such morphologies at both the saphenous vein [10] and the cephalic vein [11]. For both these veins, the blood vessels were bounded by subcutaneous fascial bands superficially and by perimuscular fascia at a deeper level. Our images have identified similar arrangements, although

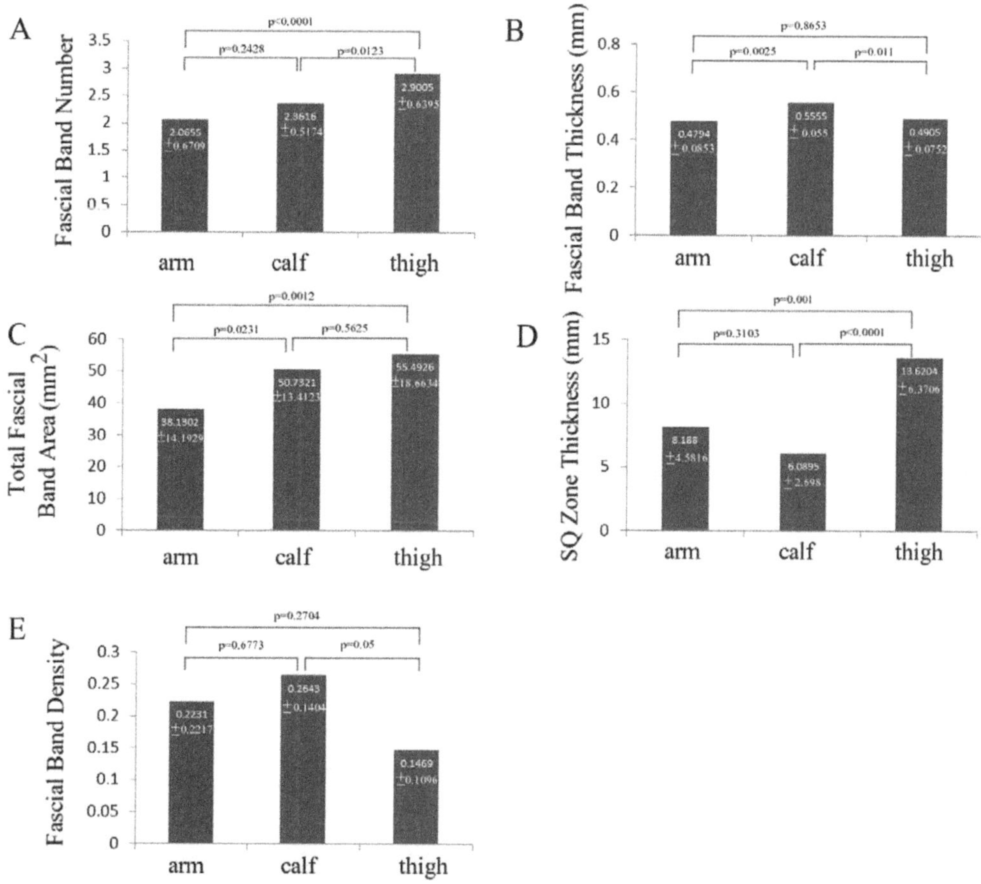

Figure 5. Body-location dependence of SQ zone variables with pairwise comparisons.

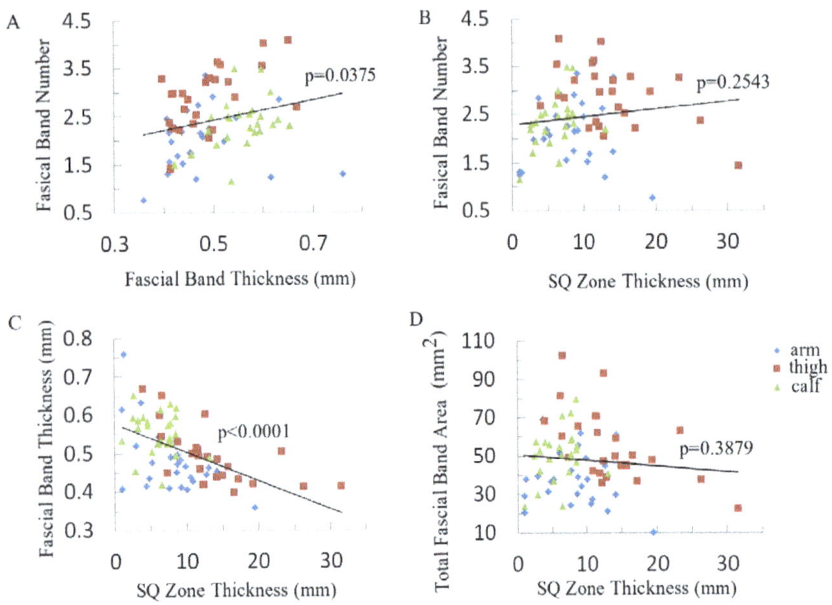

Figure 6. Bivariate linear fit between SQ zone variables.

subcutaneous vessels were at times bound by subcutaneous fascial bands on the deeper aspect of the vessel as well. From a clinical perspective, these fascial bands help prevent excessive dilatation of the veins and account for why veins constrained by fascia are less prone to develop varicosities relative to tributary veins without fascia sheathing [12]. Given the fact that fascial bands are contiguous with both skin and muscles, they may transmit mechanical forces arising from muscle contraction or from skin shear movement to the vessel wall and thus help modify blood flow in a manner that is beneficial to the affected limb. Moreover, the variable structural arrangements between the vein and fascial bands seen in Figure 4D may be strategically formed in such a way that only specific segments of the vein are affected by mechanical stresses.

Quantitative analyses of the ultrasound images revealed that the total SQ fascial band area was greatest at the calf and thigh and smallest at the arm. This difference may be attributed to the greater mechanical forces typically generated at the lower extremities. Daily ambulation and the need to chronically sustain the weight of the body are two conditions that likely facilitate a sustained increase in fascial band content. Future studies may consider evaluating how daily activities or weight training would affect the total fascial content in the subcutaneous layer, and whether greater total fascial band area would be identified in more active and possibly heavier individuals.

According to our quantitative analysis, the total fascial band area in the calf was statistically similar to that of the thigh, despite the thigh's thicker SQ zones (greater SQ fat layer). This decreased fascial band densities at the thigh was manifested by a comparatively greater number of fascial bands but an overall reduced fascial band thickness and was revealed by the fragmented and curved appearance of echogenic bands in Figure 3 panel T3 in contrast to fewer yet thicker bands seen in the calf images (Figure 3, Panel C1–C3). This inverse relationship between the average SQ fascial band thickness and SQ zone thickness was observed across body sites (including the arm) and across individuals as well ($p<0.0001$, Figure 6C). Interestingly, a statistically significant correlation between band number and SQ zone thickness was not observed when comparisons were made across individuals ($p = 0.2543$, Figure 6B). Why these patterns exist remains unclear, but one may speculate that thinner SQ layers would sustain greater amounts of mechanical (both shear and lateral) forces per volume and thus require thicker and more cohesive fascial bands. A thicker SQ layer, on the other hand, should dissipate such forces over its full depth and thus may not require the thicker, cohesive collagenous bands. The fact that band thickness was significantly correlated with SQ zone thickness and not total band number suggests that the SQ tissue preferentially alters the band's *thickness* rather than to change the *number* of bands to respond to these hypothetical mechanical forces. This, however, cannot be conclusively established without more microscopic imaging techniques, larger sample size, or more prospective data (e.g. temporal response to changes in mechanical force).

Paradoxically, in our study, increased average fascial band number was associated with an increase in fascial band thickness (Figure 6A). A reasonable functional explanation for this finding cannot be given, although it may reflect regional differences. The thigh, in particular, appears to have increased band thickness as the band number is increased while the other two regions did not.

To investigate the possible functional significance of the SQ fascial bands, we investigated the anisotropy of the SQ zone using a spatial coherence measure. In material science, anisotropy typically indicates a directional preference and implies the ability of a material to handle mechanical forces along a specific axis. In biological tissue, anisotropy exists either to facilitate a functional role or to adapt to persistent mechanical forces. Muscles, for instance, are characterized by high anisotropy ensuring that it is optimized for generating tensile force along a specific axis; bones are usually able to withstand greater tensile forces along the longitudinal axis compared to the transverse direction. Collagenous fibers, similarly, possess anisotropy and respond to mechanical force by aligning along the primary direction of tension. In a recent in vitro experiment involving collagen and fibroblasts, strong collagen fiber alignment and densification occurred in response to applied strains greater than 5% [13]. Fiber alignment was permanently imprinted when the material was cyclically

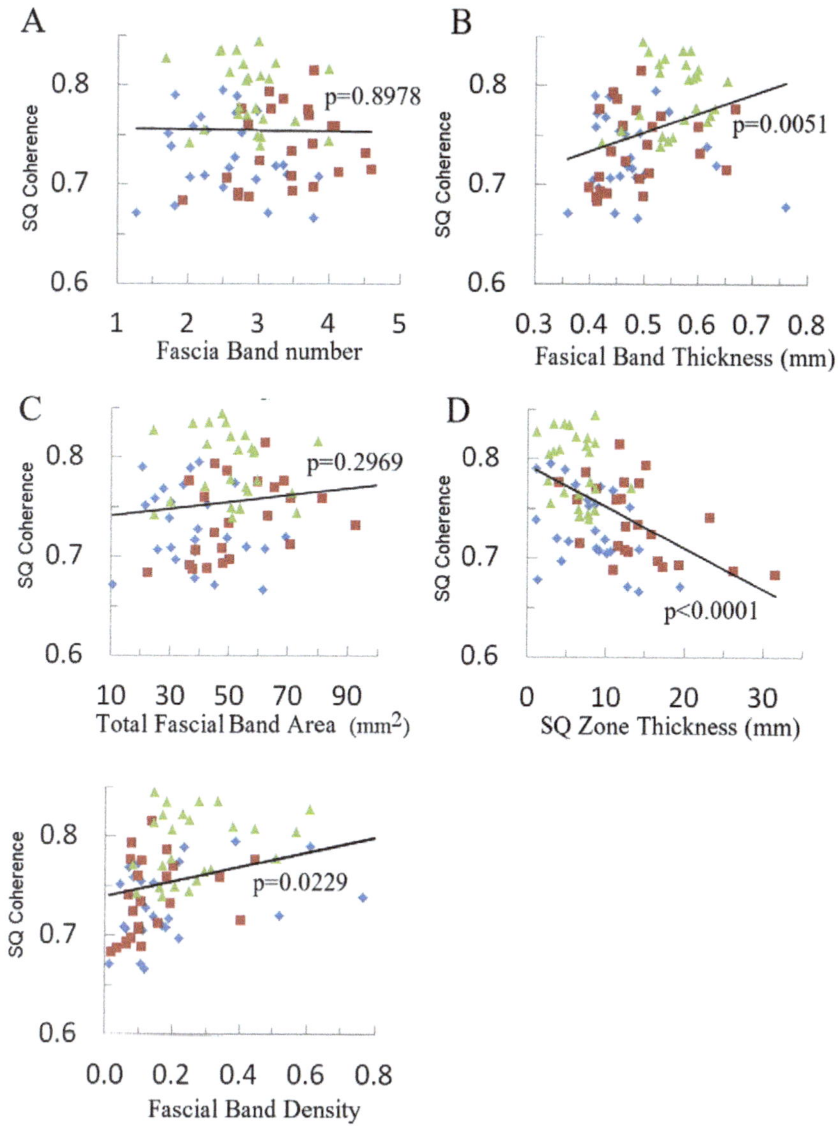

Figure 7. Bivariate linear fit between SQ coherence and various SQ zone variables. Green represents the data from arm, red from thigh and blue from calf.

stretched up to strains of 15%. Our in vivo analysis of SQ zone coherence suggests that, SQ anisotropy is significantly associated with SQ zone thickness and body site. Reduced SQ zone thickness was associated with increased SQ anisotropy and implies that mechanical stress is distributed across the subcutaneous tissue. Thinner subcutaneous tissues are more likely to concentrate the mechanical forces and thus are associated with increased spatial anisotropy. This multivariable analysis also reveals that the calf is associated with greater anisotropies and thus theoretically more

Table 2. Factors associated with SQ coherence: results from a multilevel model with SQ coherence as dependent variable.

Variables	Intercept	Slope	p value
Locaiton			<0.0001
arm	0.76501		
calf	0.82475		
thigh	0.8045		
Fascial Band Number		-0.00291	0.6906
Fascial Band Thickness (mm)		-0.08691	0.225
SQ Zone Thickness (mm)		-0.00453	<0.0001

Table 3. Pair-wise comparisons of SQ coherence between body locations after accounting for other image derived variables.

Location	Means	Pair-Wise Comparison
arm	0.6715	arm vs calf: p<0.0001
calf	0.7313	calf vs thigh: p = 0.3116
thigh	0.711	arm vs thigh: p = 0.0155

likely to experience mechanical stress than the arm or thigh.

This study has a number of limitations. First, it involved a limited number of patients, evaluated three specific body locations, and did not have sufficient power to evaluate the effects of gender, age or ethnicity. Future studies may consider evaluating other body segments and other locations within the extremity of a larger, more diverse study cohort. Second, the study relied on static ultrasound images for characterizing the SQ fascial system. Functional, dynamic measures were not obtained. Third, spatial anisotropy is only a surrogate marker of mechanical force and cannot be interpreted as a direct measure of stress. Finally, the ultrasound device itself has technical limitations. Ultrasonography relies on heterogenic impedance of acoustic waves traveling axially from skin to deeper layers. Vertical structures poorly reflect acoustic waves traveling in an axial (vertical) trajectory and thus are not well characterized on the ultrasound images. This will generate an intrinsic anisotropy within the image that should be considered prior to interpreting the data.

Despite these limitations, this study has a number of advantages that adds to the existing, albeit limited, SQ fascia literature. In vivo ultrasonography was used to quantify and characterize the SQ fascial bands – a method that is more likely to be valid to real-life physiology than cadaveric-dissection studies. In addition, novel techniques incorporating principal component analysis, three dimensional reconstruction, and spatial coherence measures were incorporated in this study to better reveal the morphological features of the SQ fascial bands. These methods and techniques collectively have revealed that SQ Fascia is an interconnected network that likely transmits mechanical forces over large spatial scales and across various tissues. The exact functional significance of this behavior remains unclear and awaits additional study.

Supporting Information

Video S1 An animation of a three-dimensional cubic tissue with 360 degree rotation in the ImageJ software (National Institute of Health, USA); transparency was set at 70. The video shows a vein tunnel enclosed between a SQ fascial sheet and the epimysial sheet.

Author Contributions

Conceived and designed the experiments: ACA. Performed the experiments: ACA. Analyzed the data: WL ACA. Contributed reagents/materials/analysis tools: WL ACA. Wrote the paper: WL ACA.

References

1. Hollinshead WH, Rosse C (1985) Textbook of anatomy. Philadelphia: Harper and Row.
2. Langevin HM, Rizzo DM, Fox JR, Badger GJ, Wu J, et al. (2007) Dynamic morphometric characterization of local connective tissue network structure in humans using ultrasound. BMC Systems Biology 1: 25.
3. Abu-Hijleh MF, Roshier AL, Al-Shboul Q, Dharap AS, Harris PF, et al. (2006) The membranous layer of superficial fascia: evidence for its widespread distribution in the body. Surg Radiol Anat 28(6): 606–19.
4. Ahn AC, Park M, Shaw JR, McManus CA, Kaptchuk TJ, et al. (2010) Electrical impedance of acupuncture meridians: the relevance of subcutaneous collagenous bands. PLoS ONE 5(7): e11907.
5. Jahne B (1993) Spatial-temporal image processing: theory and scientific applications. Berlin: Springer-Verlag.
6. Hsu, C J (1992) The factor analytic approach to simultaneous inference in the general linear model. Journal of Computational and Graphical Statistics 1(2): 151–68.
7. Johnson D, Dixon AK, Abrahams PH (1996) The abdominal subcutaneous tissue: computed tomographic, magnetic resonance, and anatomical observations. Clinical Anatomy 9(1): 19–24.
8. Nash LG, Phillips MN, Nicholson, H, Barnett R, Zhang M (2004) Skin ligaments: regional distribution and variation in morphology. Clinical Anatomy 17(4): 287–93.
9. Langevin HM (2006) Connective tissue: a body-wide signaling network? Medical Hypotheses 66(6): 1074–7.
10. Caggiati A (2001) Fascial relationships of the short saphenous vein. J Vasc Surg 34: 241–6.
11. Lockwood TE (1991) Superficial fascial system (SFS) of the trunk and extremities: a new concept. Plast Reconstr Surg 87(6): 1009–18.
12. Caggiati A (2000) Fascial relations and structure of the tributaries of the saphemous veins. Surg Radiol Anat 22(3-4): 191–6.
13. Vader D, Kabla A, Weitz D, Mahadevan L (2009) Strain-induced alignment in collagen gels. PlosOne 4(6): e5902.

7

Haploinsufficiency of Def Activates p53-Dependent TGFβ Signalling and Causes Scar Formation after Partial Hepatectomy

Zhihui Zhu[1], Jun Chen[2], Jing-Wei Xiong[3], Jinrong Peng[1]*

1 Key Laboratory for Molecular Animal Nutrition, Ministry of Education, College of Animal Sciences, Zhejiang University, Hangzhou, China, **2** College of Life Sciences, Zhejiang University, Hangzhou, China, **3** Institute of Molecular Medicine, Peking University, Beijing, China

Abstract

The metazoan liver exhibits a remarkable capacity to regenerate lost liver mass without leaving a scar following partial hepatectomy (PH). Whilst previous studies have identified components of several different signaling pathways that are essential for activation of hepatocyte proliferation during liver regeneration, the mechanisms that enable such regeneration to occur without accompanying scar formation remain poorly understood. Here we use the adult zebrafish liver, which can regenerate within two weeks following PH, as a new genetic model to address this important question. We focus on the role of Digestive-organ-expansion-factor (Def), a nucleolar protein which has recently been shown to complex with calpain3 (Capn3) to mediate p53 degradation specifically in the nucleolus, in liver regeneration. Firstly, we show that Def expression is up-regulated in the wild-type liver following amputation, and that the $def^{hi429/+}$ heteroozygous mutant ($def^{+/-}$) suffers from haploinsufficiency of Def in the liver. We then show that the expression of pro-inflammatory cytokines is up-regulated in the $def^{+/-}$ liver, which leads to distortion of the migration and the clearance of leukocytes after PH. Transforming growth factor β (TGFβ) signalling is thus activated in the wound epidermis in $def^{+/-}$ due to a prolonged inflammatory response, which leads to fibrosis at the amputation site. Fibrotic scar formation in $def^{+/-}$ is blocked by the over-expression of Def, by the loss-of-function of p53, and by treatment with anti-inflammation drug dexamethasone or TGFβ-signalling inhibitor SB431542. We finally show that the Def- p53 pathway suppresses fibrotic scar formation, at least in part, through the regulation of the expression of the pro-inflammatory factor, high-mobility group box 1. We conclude that the novel Def-p53 nucleolar pathway functions specifically to prevent a scar formation at the amputation site in a normal amputated liver.

Editor: Zhiyuan Gong, National University of Singapore, Singapore

Funding: This work was supported financially by the "973 Program" (2012CB944550) and the National Natural Science Foundation of China (31330050). The funders had no role in study design, data collection and analysis, decision to publish, or preparation of the manuscript.

Competing Interests: The authors have declared that no competing interests exist.

* E-mail: pengjr@zju.edu.cn

Introduction

Liver regeneration refers to the process of regaining liver mass by compensatory growth after partial hepatectomy (PH) or toxic injury [1–3], and previous molecular and genetic studies have revealed the involvement of cytokine- and growth factor-mediated pathways in its regulation. Among these, interleukin (IL)-6 and hepatocyte growth factor (HGF) and their related signalling molecules are two well-studied pathways that have been shown to enable hepatocytes to overcome cell-cycle checkpoint controls [1–3]. Transcription factors, such as c-Jun, c-Fos, c-Myc, NF-κB, STAT3 and C/EBP, are also mobilised during liver regeneration [4]. It is noticed that the healing of the resection site in a normal healthy liver after PH is surprisingly not accompanied with fibrotic scar formation [5]. This contrasts to many other types of wound healing (e.g skin) which often leaves a fibrotic scar at the wounding site. The scarless wound healing serves, in fact, as the key basis for liver operation/transplantation. Scar formation is considered to be a consequence of the prolonged inflammation in the wound epidermis [5]. Interestingly, while the vast majority of previous studies have focused on the initiation, progression and termination of liver regeneration after PH, little work has been carried out on the mechanisms that underlie the scarless repair of the amputation site after PH [5].

In recent years, zebrafish has been used as a model to study the development and regeneration of the liver [6–8], and studies have shown that the amputated livers of wild-type zebrafish regained their mass within 15 days post PH [9,10]. Digestion-organ-expansion-factor (Def) is a novel nucleolar factor that is conserved across species, from yeasts to humans [11–13]. In the zebrafish, the loss of Def function in the $def^{hi429/hi429}$ mutant conferred a phenotype characterised by a smaller liver, a shortened exocrine pancreas and thinner intestines [13]. Our recent studies showed that Def complexes with calpain 3 (Capn3) to mediate p53 degradation in the nucleolus in both human and zebrafish cells [14]. This finding defined a unique novel p53 degradation pathway, the Def-CAPN3-p53 pathway, in the nucleolus, and also explained why p53 protein specifically accumulates in the nucleolus in the $def^{hi429/hi429}$ homozygous mutant. Up-regulated p53 then selectively up-regulates the expression of p53 downstream genes, including *Δ113p53* and *p21* to cause cell-cycle arrest, which results in hypoplasia of the digestive organs in the mutant [13].

In this study, we examined the capacity of *def*$^{+/-}$ heterozygous fish to undergo liver regeneration after PH and found that Def haploinsufficiency in the *def*$^{+/-}$ strain activates a p53-dependent, inflammation-mediated transforming growth factor β (TGFβ) pathway that causes scar formation at the amputation site after PH in zebrafish. This function of the Def- p53 pathway is probably achieved partially through the regulation of the expression of high-mobility group box 1 (HMGB1), a pro-inflammatory pathway.

Results

The *def*$^{+/-}$ Zebrafish Is Defective in Recuperating the Lobe Structure At the Amputation Site after PH

Our previous study showed that Def was expressed in the adult zebrafish liver [13]. Here, we compared the levels of *def* transcripts and Def protein, respectively, in the livers of adult wild-type and *def*$^{+/-}$ zebrafish and found that the levels of *def* transcripts were approximately 4.8-fold (Figure 1A) and those of Def protein approximately four fold (Figure 1B) lower in the *def*$^{+/-}$ mutant, demonstrating that the *def*$^{+/-}$ strain is a typical haploinsufficient mutant. Interestingly, we found that the level of Def was up-regulated in the nucleoli of the livers of both wild-type and *def*$^{+/-}$ adults 2 days after PH, but the staining intensity of Def was apparently much stronger in the wild-type (Figure 1C, Figure S1A). Despite of this, a *def*$^{+/-}$ fish grows to its adulthood normally without showing an overt phenotype (data not shown). Therefore, the *def*$^{+/-}$ fish allowed us to assess the effect of haploinsufficiency of Def on liver regeneration after PH.

An adult zebrafish liver comprises two dorsal lobes and one ventral lobe [9,15]. We surgically removed almost the entire ventral lobe from 5 to 7-month-old wild-type and *def*$^{+/-}$ adults and found that, similar to results reported for wild-type livers [7,9,10], *def*$^{+/-}$ fish regained their liver-to-body ratio at 7 days after PH (Figure 2A–F). In addition, haematoxylin andeosin (H&E) staining revealed no obvious structural changes in the liver parenchyma between wild-type and *def*$^{+/-}$ strains 9 months after PH (Figure 2G). We then compared the gross morphology of the

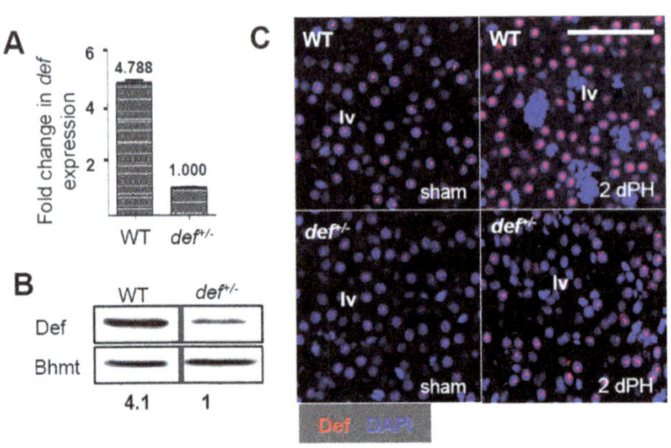

Figure 1. *def*$^{+/-}$ liver suffers from haploinsufficiency of Def. *(A)* qPCR analysis of *def* transcripts in adult wild-type and *def*$^{+/-}$ liver. The expression of *def* was normalised against *elf1a* and is shown as the fold change in expression, with the value from *def*$^{+/-}$ being set at 1. The values plotted represent the means ± standard errors of the mean. *(B)* Western blotting analysis of the Def protein. Bhmt: loading control. Densitometry was performed using Photoshop. The value of Def was obtained by normalising against Bhmt expression. The relative value of Def protein in *def*$^{+/-}$ was set at 1. *(C)* Representative images of immunostaining of Def (red) in wild-type and *def*$^{+/-}$ liver 2 days after PH. lv, liver tissue. Scale bar: 100 μm *(C)*.

liver at the amputation site 3, 7 and 21 days after PH (Figure S2). As expected, the majority of the resected ventral liver lobes (12 out of 15) in the wild-type fish recovered their lobe structure, characterised by a new smooth round lobe tip at the amputation site as early as 7 days after PH (Figure 3A; Figure S2), although the new lobe did not regain its original size up to 60 days after PH (data not shown). In contrast, ~85% (11/13) of *def*$^{+/-}$ fish exhibited an uneven surface and lacked a lobe-like structure at the amputation site 7 days after PH (Figure 3A; Figure S2).

The Wound Epidermis in *def*$^{+/-}$ Fish Failed To Be Remodelled and Finally Formed A Fibrotic Scar At the Amputation Site after PH

The previous result suggested that *def*$^{+/-}$ fish were unable to regenerate the liver structure at the amputation site after PH. The wound healing process can be divided into four sequential phases: haemostasis, inflammation, proliferation and remodelling/maturation [16]. To follow the healing process at the amputation site after PH, we simultaneously assessed cell-cycle entry (by following the nuclear incorporation of 5-ethynyl-2'-deoxyuridine (EdU), a marker for the S-phase) and cell apoptosis (using the terminal deoxynucleotidyl transferase dUTP nick end labeling (TUNEL) assay), together with immunostaining using betaine–homocysteine S-methyltransferase (BhmtHMT) (to mark hepatocytes) [17] antibody at different time points. At 12, 24 and 36 h after PH, we observed no obvious differences in terms of blood clot formation, cell apoptosis or proliferation between the wild-type and *def*$^{+/-}$fish, except that the blood clot was almost detached from the amputation site in the wild-type but was still attached to the liver mass in the *def*$^{+/-}$ fish 36 h after PH (Figure S3).

We then performed immunostaining with the proliferating cell nuclear antigen (PCNA) in the background of the transgenic reporter fish line *Tg(fabp10a::dsRed)*, in which hepatocytes were genetically labelled by red fluorescent protein [18]. Proliferating cells were rarely observed either at the edge of or in the parenchyma in the sham control at 3 days after PH (Figure S4). In contrast, immunostaining with PCNA and Bhmt showed that the number of proliferating cells (PCNA-positive cells, PCNA^{+}) was increased and that they were mainly detected near the amputation site in a similar pattern in both the wild-type and *def*$^{+/-}$ fish at 2 days after PH (Figure 3B). At 3 days after PH, in addition to active proliferating hepatocytes, a new cell mass that was Bhmt-negative (Bhmt^{-}) appeared next to the amputation site in both the wild-type and *def*$^{+/-}$ fish, although fewer such cells were found in the *def*$^{+/-}$ fish (Figure 3C; Figure S1B). The last step of wound healing is the remodelling of the wounded site to restore the tissue structure [19]. Immunostaining with PCNA and Bhmt showed that, by 5.5 days after PH, almost all of the PCNA^{+} cells around the amputation site in the wild-type fish were also Bhmt^{+} (Figure 3D), indicating that the wound epidermis had been successfully remodelled to the liver tissue. In contrast, many PCNA^{+} cells in the *def*$^{+/-}$ livers were still Bhmt^{-} (Figure 3D).

During the wound healing process, fibroblast cells were expected to migrate to the amputation site and then proliferate to form a stratified epithelialised cell mass called the wound epidermis. Following immunostaining with keratin 18, an extracellular matrix marker produced by the epithelial cells [20], we found that the new Bhmt^{-} cells at the amputation site in both wild-type and *def*$^{+/-}$ fish at 3 days after PH (Figure 3C) expressed high levels of keratin 18 (Figure 4A), and that the new cell mass we observed (Figure 3C) therefore actually represented the wound epidermis at the amputation site after PH.

To determine the difference between the wound epidermis of the wild-type and *def*$^{+/-}$ fish, we performed immunostaining with

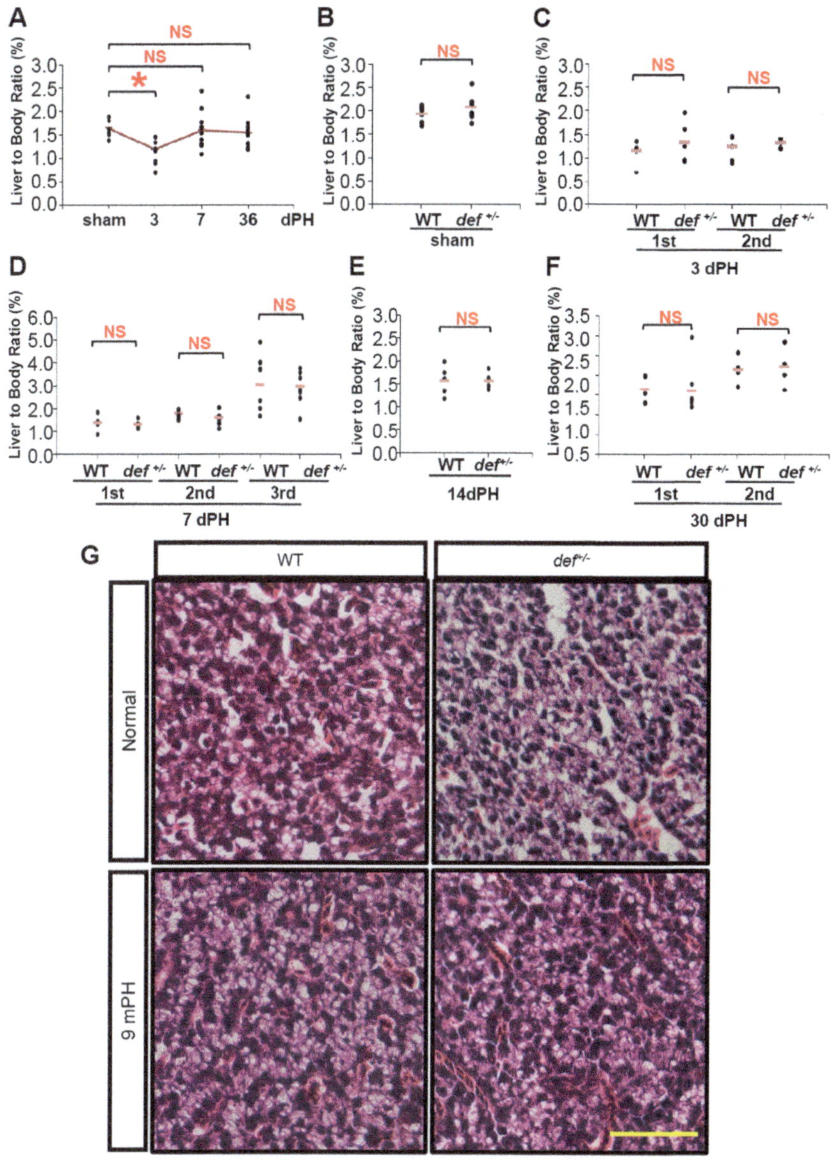

Figure 2. The liver-to-body ratio of the regenerated livers did not differ significantly between the wild-type and *def*$^{+/-}$ mutant fish after PH. (*A*) Liver-to-body ratio of the wild-type sham control and amputated wild-type liver at 3, 7 and 36 days after PH (n≥5). (*B*) Liver-to-body ratios of the sham controls (n≥5) for the wild-type and *def*$^{+/-}$ mutant fish. (*C–F*) Comparison of the liver-to-body ratios of the amputated wild-type and *def*$^{+/-}$ livers 3 days after PH (*C*), 7 days after PH (*D*), 14 days after PH (*E*) and 30 days after PH (*F*) as indicated (n≥5 in each case). NS: not significant; *: $p<0.05$. (*G*) Representative images of haematoxylin-eosin staining of sections across the wild-type or *def*$^{+/-}$ hepatic parenchyma without performing PH or 9 months after PH. Scale bar: 50 μm.

type I collagen (ColI), a marker for fibrotic tissue [21]. The results showed that the wound epidermis (keratin 18$^+$ cells) in the wild-type liver displayed weak ColI expression whereas that in *def*$^{+/-}$ produced large amounts of ColI (Figure 4B; Figure S1C) 3 days after PH, which was further confirmed by Masson staining (the collagen was stained blue) (Figure 5A). By 5.5 days after PH, Masson staining showed that the difference in collagen staining between the amputation site and the liver tissue in the wild-type fish was no longer distinguishable, whereas the wound epidermis in the *def*$^{+/-}$fish was still clearly visible and strongly expressed collagens (Figure 5B). The wound epidermis in the wild-type fish was successfully remodelled to a proper liver structure by 30 days after PH (Figure 5C). In contrast, the wound epidermis in the *def*$^{+/-}$ fish eventually formed a fibrotic scar characterized by the strong staining of collagens at the amputation site (Figure 5C).

Activation of TGFβ Signalling Is Responsible for Collagen Deposition At the Amputation Site after PH in *def*$^{+/-}$ Fish

ColI production is closely related to TGFβ signalling activity [22]. We next examined the status of phosphorylated Smad2 (pSmad2), a hallmark for the activation of TGFβ signalling [23]. At 1.5 and 3 days after PH, the wound epidermis in both the wild-type and *def*$^{+/-}$ fish showed positive pSmad2 staining, with *def*$^{+/-}$ exhibiting a stronger signal intensity (Figure 6A,B). At 5 days after PH, the pSmad2 signal disappeared together with the wound epidermis in the wild-type strain (Figure 6A). Strikingly, in the *def*$^{+/-}$ strain, the wound epidermis failed to be remodelled, with

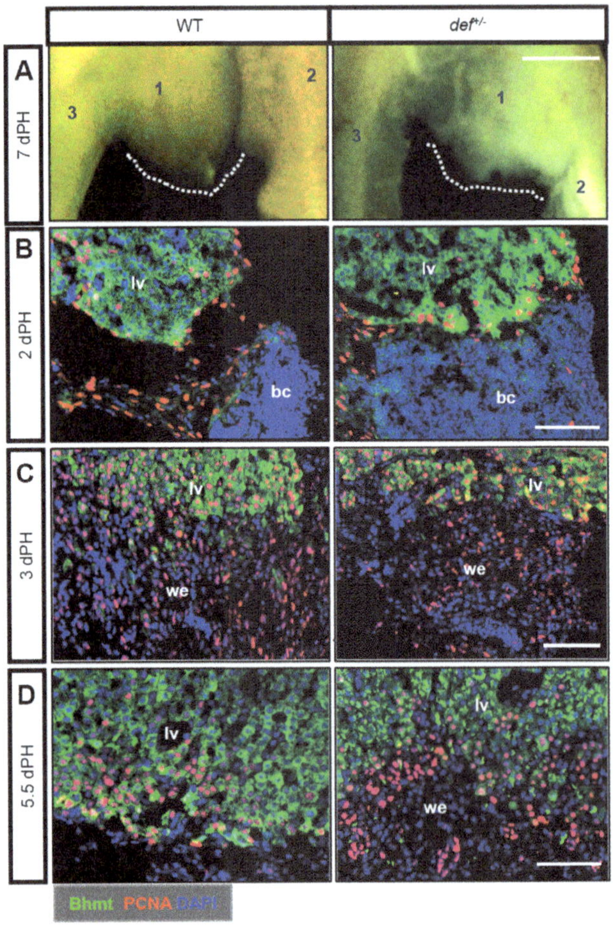

Figure 3. Def haploinsufficiency results in a failure in the remodelling of the wound epidermis to liver tissue. (*A*) Ventral view of the gross morphology of an amputated adult wild-type and *def*$^{+/-}$ liver 7 days after PH. The dotted white line indicates the amputation site. 1: ventral lobe, 2: left dorsal lobe, 3: right dorsal lobe. (*B–D*) Representative images of co-immunostaining of PCNA and Bhmt to compare the process of epithelialisation of the amputation site 2 days after PH (*B*), wound epidermis formation 3 days after PH (*C*), and wound epidermis remodelling 5.5 days after PH (*D*) between the wild-type and the *def*$^{+/-}$ mutant. Nuclei were stained with 4′,6-diamidino-2-phenylindole (DAPI) (blue). In each case or at each time-point, more than 10 sections from at least three wild-type or *def*$^{+/-}$ mutant fish were examined. bc, blood clot; lv, liver tissue; we, wound epidermis. Scale bar: 5 mm (*A*) and 75 μm (*B–D*).

persistent, strong pSmad2 staining at the amputation site (Figure 6B; Figure S5A). To prove that the constitutive activation of TGFβ signalling is responsible for the CollI deposition in *def*$^{+/-}$, we injected SB431542 (Alk5/4-i) intraperitoneally into the amputated fish. SB431542 specifically blocks the TGFβ/activin pathway receptors but does not affect closely related receptors from the bone morphogenetic protein pathway or other signal transduction pathways [24,25]. The results showed that this treatment efficiently down-regulated the expression level of pSmad2 (Figure 6C; Figure S5A) and abolished CollI deposition at the amputation site in the liver of *def*$^{+/-}$fish5 days after PH (Figure 6E and F; Figure S5B).

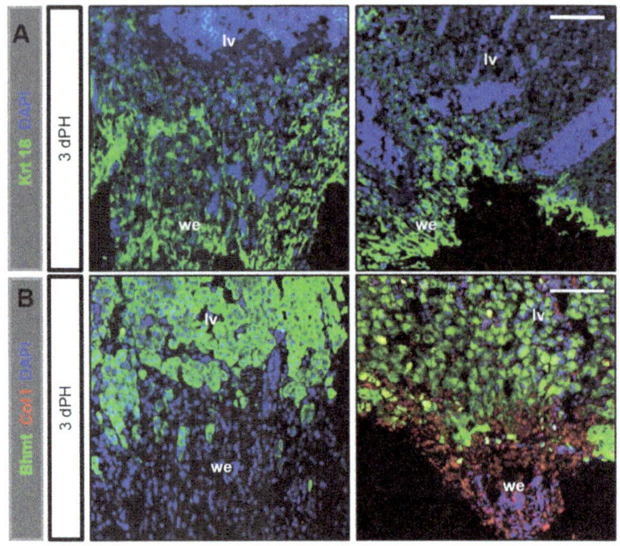

Figure 4. Def haploinsufficiency results in accumulation of CollI at the amputation site after PH. (*A,B*) Representative images of immunostaining of keratin 18 (green) (*A*) and co-immunostaining of CollI (red) and Bhmt (green) (*B*) at the amputation site in wild-type and *def*$^{+/-}$ strains 3 days after PH. Nuclei were stained with DAPI (blue). At each time-point, more than 10 sections from at least three wild-type or *def*$^{+/-}$ mutant fish were examined. lv, liver tissue; we, wound epidermis. Scale bars: 75 μm (*A,B*) and 100 μm (*C*).

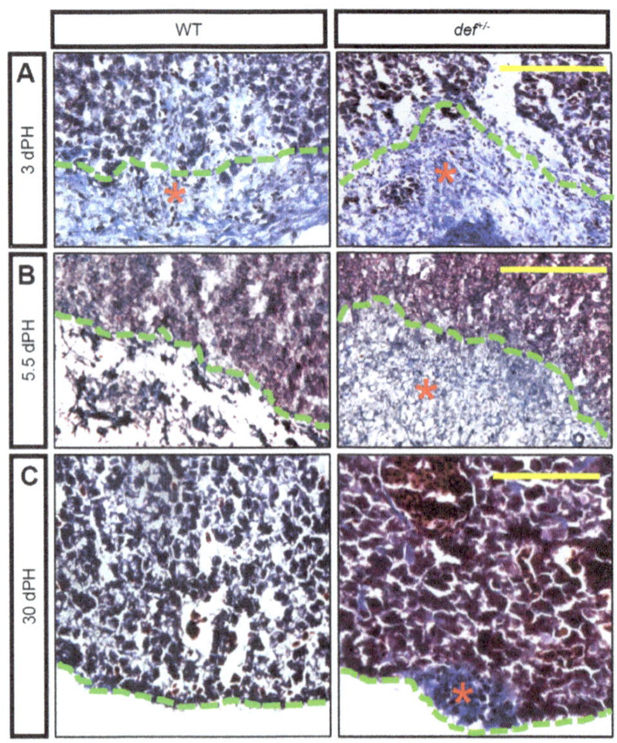

Figure 5. Def haploinsufficiency results in the formation of a fibrotic scar at the amputation site after PH. Masson staining of sections across the amputation site 3 (*A*), 5.5 (*B*) and 30 (*C*) days after PH (dPH), respectively. Fibrotic tissue was stained in blue (highlighted with an asterisk), cytoplasm in light red and nuclei in dark brown. Green, dashed lines outline the amputation site. Scale bar: 100 μm.

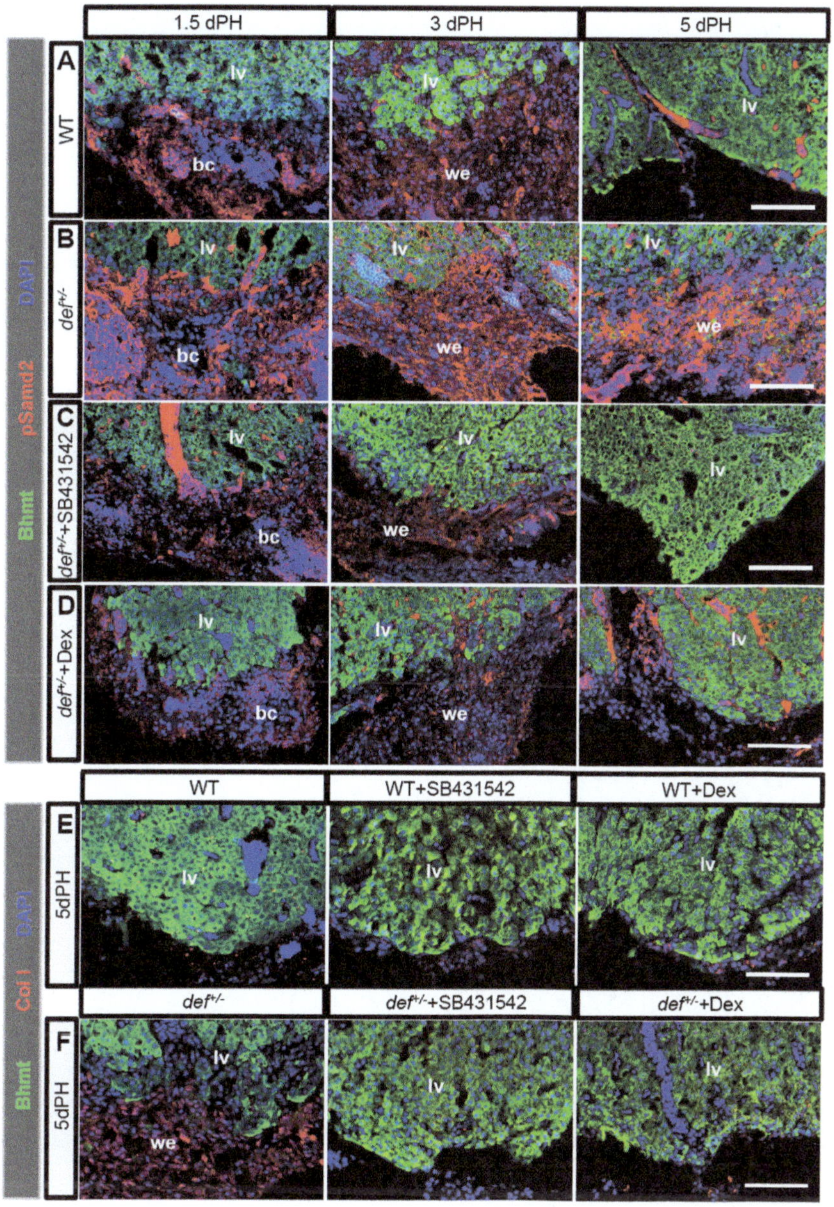

Figure 6. Constitutive activation of TGFβ signalling promotes ColI deposition at the amputation site in *def*$^{+/-}$ fish after PH. (*A–D*) Representative images of immunostaining of pSmad2 (red) and Bhmt (green) in wound epidermis in wild-type (*A*), *def*$^{+/-}$ (*B*), *def*$^{+/-}$ treated with SB431542 (*C*) or *def*$^{+/-}$treated with Dex (*D*) 1.5, 3 and 5 days after PH, respectively. (*E,F*) Representative images of immunostaining of ColI (red) and Bhmt (green) in the wound epidermis in wild-type and *def*$^{+/-}$fish treated or not treated with SB431542 (*E*) or Dex (*F*) 5 days after PH, respectively. Nuclei were stained with DAPI (blue). In each case, more than 10 sections from at least three wild-type or *def*$^{+/-}$ mutant fish were examined. bc, blood clot; lv, liver tissue; we, wound epidermis. Scale bar:75 μm (*A–F*).

An Abnormal Inflammatory Reaction Triggers An Increase in TGFβ Signalling in *def*$^{+/-}$ Fish

We sought the mechanism(s) that activate(s) TGFβ signalling in the wound epidermis. We first treated the fish with two chemicals, diphenyleneiodonium and apocynin (both of which are specific inhibitors of the Duox/Nox enzyme [26]) to down-regulate the production of hydrogen peroxide, which has been shown to be related to the fibrotic scar formation during heart regeneration (Jingwei Xiong, personal communication). We found that neither of these two chemicals induced ColI deposition in the liver of the wild-type fish or inhibited its deposition in the liver of the *def*$^{+/-}$ fish at the amputation site after PH (Figure S6), indicating that the deposition of collagens in this case was independent of the reactive oxygen species signalling pathway. Fibrotic scar formation closely correlates with prolonged local inflammatory reaction. Dexamethasone (Dex) is a potent synthetic member of the glucocorticoid class of steroid drugs that has anti-inflammatory and immunosuppressant properties [27]. Treatment with Dex dramatically down-regulated the expression of pSmad2 in the wound epidermis (Figure 6D; Figure S5A) and efficiently blocked the deposition of ColI at the amputation site in *def*$^{+/-}$fish after PH (Figure 6E and F; Figure S5B).

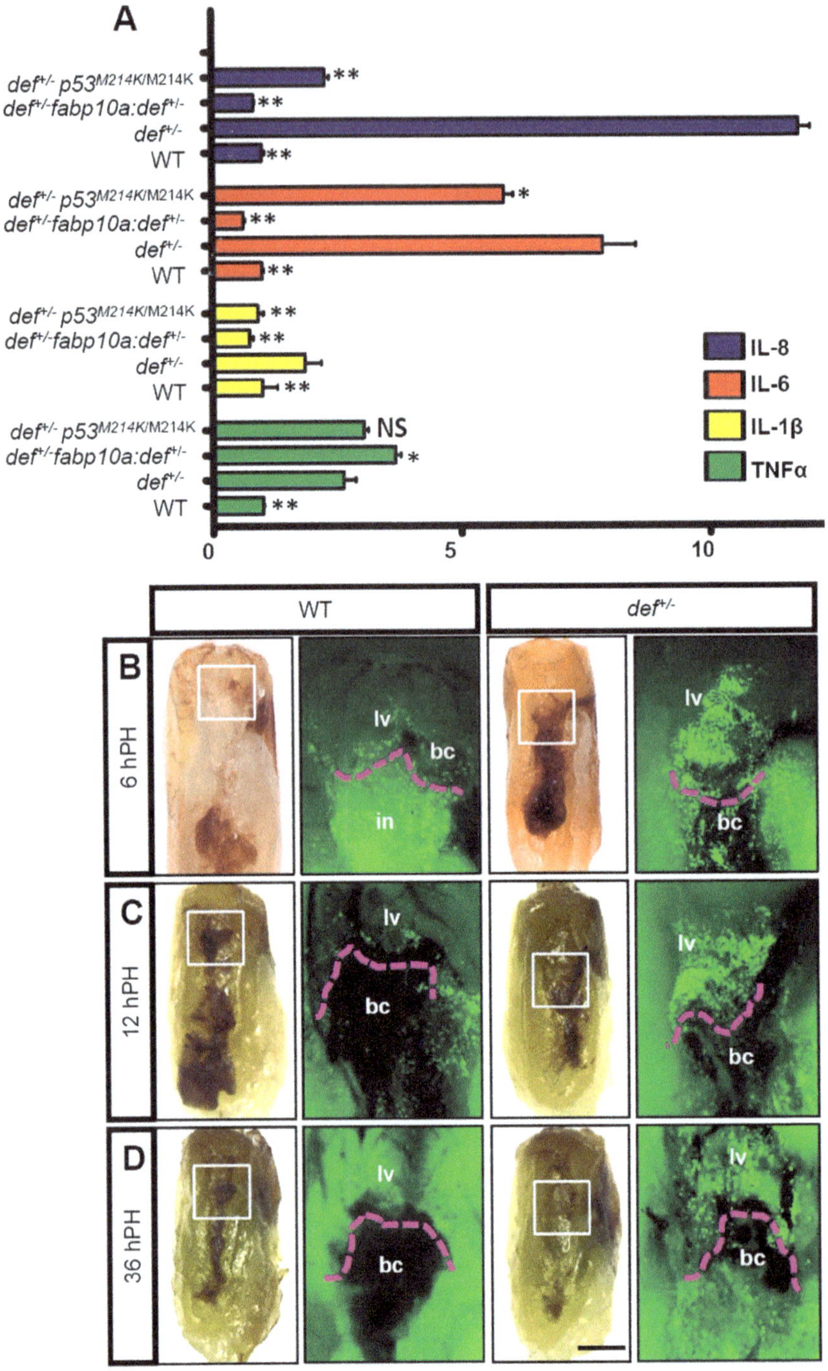

Figure 7. *def*$^{+/-}$ mutant liver exhibited a prolonged inflammatory reaction at the amputation site after PH. (*A*) qPCR analysis of cytokine genes *TNFα*, *IL-1β*, *IL-6* and *IL-8* in adult wild-type, *def*$^{+/-}$, *fabp10a:def*$^{+/-}$ and *def*$^{+/-}$ *p53*$^{M214K/M214K}$ livers prior to the surgical procedure. Gene expression is expressed as the fold change after normalisation against *β-actin*. The value for each gene in the wild-type was set at 1. The *p* value represents the statistical differences between *def*$^{+/-}$ and another corresponding group. *: $p<0.05$, **: $p<0.01$, NS: not significant. (*B–D*) Adult fish of *Tg(zlyz:EGFP)* in a wild-type and *def*$^{+/-}$ background were subjected to PH, and collected 6 h after PH (*B*), 12 h after PH (*C*) and 36 h after PH (*D*) for EGFP fluorescence imaging. Images were taken from the region outlined in white in the corresponding bright field picture shown on the left. The region above the dashed magenta lines is the liver tissue adjacent to the amputation site. Black asterisks highlight the EGFP signal yielded possibly from neutrophils in the intestine. A representative image is shown for each time-point. bc, blood clot; in, intestine; lv, liver tissue. Scale bar: 5 mm (bright field) and 2 mm (GFP field).

Abnormal Expression of Cytokines in the *def*$^{+/-}$ Liver Halted the Timely Migration of Macrophages To the Amputation Site To Clear Neutrophils

The previous result suggested that an abnormal inflammatory response is probably the main mechanism that activates TGFβ signalling and causes scar formation in the *def*$^{+/-}$ liver. To test this hypothesis, we first analysed the expression of pro-inflammatory cytokines, including *tumour necrosis factor α* (*TNFα*), *IL-1β*, *IL-6* and *IL-8* [28–30], in the livers of wild-type and *def*$^{+/-}$ fish prior to surgical operation. We found that *IL-6*, *IL-8* and *TNFα* were expressed at levels several fold higher and *IL-1β* at a significantly higher level in the liver of the *def*$^{+/-}$than in that of the wild-type fish (Figure 7A), which suggested that the innate immune response was probably affected in the *def*$^{+/-}$ fish after acute injury (i.e., after PH).

We then used the *Tg(zlyz:EGFP)* reporter fish to monitor the inflammatory event by observing the dynamics of neutrophils at the amputation site. We noted that the number of neutrophils that accumulated at the amputation site in the *def*$^{+/-}$ fish was much greater than that in the wild-type fish between 6 and 36 h after PH (Figure 7B–D). In addition, while only a few neutrophils remained in the wild-type, a large number of neutrophils still lingered around the amputation site in the *def*$^{+/-}$ fish at 36 hours after PH (Figure 7D), suggesting the amputation site in the *def*$^{+/-}$ fish likely suffered from a prolonged inflammatory reaction due to the delayed clearance of neutrophils by macrophages. This prompted us to examine the behaviour of macrophages using a double-labelled transgenic fish, *Tg(coro1a:eGFP;lyz:dsRed)*. In this reporter fish, both macrophages and neutrophils are genetically labelled by enhanced green fluorescent protein (EGFP) while neutrophils are also labelled by dsRed [31]. We surprisingly found that the number of macrophages at the amputation site was much less in the *def*$^{+/-}$ than that in the wild-type fish at 12 and 36 h after PH. This observation effectively explained why the clearance of neutrophils at the injured site was severely delayed (Figure 8A–D; Figure S7). Treatment with Dex restored the behaviour of the macrophages (Figure 8E,F; Figure S7), demonstrating that the process of wound healing closely correlates with the resolution of inflammation *in situ* in a regenerating liver.

Hepatic Haploinsufficiency of Def Causes Scar Formation in *def*$^{+/-}$ Fish

To determine the role of hepatic Def in the formation of fibrotic scars, we crossed *def*$^{+/-}$ mutants with a transgenic line (*Tg(fabp10:-def)*), in which *def* expression is driven by the promoter of a liver-specific gene *fabp10* [32]. Def expression in the *def*$^{+/-}$*Tg(fabp10a:-def)* progeny was restored to that found in the wild-type fish (Figure 9A). Immunostaining of pSmad2 showed that the aberrantly high level of pSmad2 was almost completely restored to normal in *def*$^{+/-}$ *Tg(fabp10a:def)* progeny at 5 days after PH (Figure 10A; Figure S5A). Immunostaining showed that the amount of ColI deposited at the amputation site in the *def*$^{+/-}$*Tg(fabp10:def)*$^{+/-}$ progeny was down-regulated to a level comparable with that in wild-type fish at 5 days after PH (Figure 10B; Figure S5C). Hepatic over-expression of Def in the *Tg(fabp10a:def)* fish also partially restored the behaviour of macrophages in the *def*$^{+/-}$ strain (Figure 8G–H; Figure S7), which correlated with the down-regulation of *IL-1β*, *IL-6* and *IL-8* in the *def*$^{+/-}$*Tg(fabp10:-def)*$^{+/-}$ fish (Figure 7A). Furthermore, Masson staining showed that the amputation site was successfully remodelled to liver tissue by 14 days after PH (Figure 10C). These results demonstrate that Def haploinsufficiency in hepatocytes is the causative agent of fibrotic scar formation in *def*$^{+/-}$ fish.

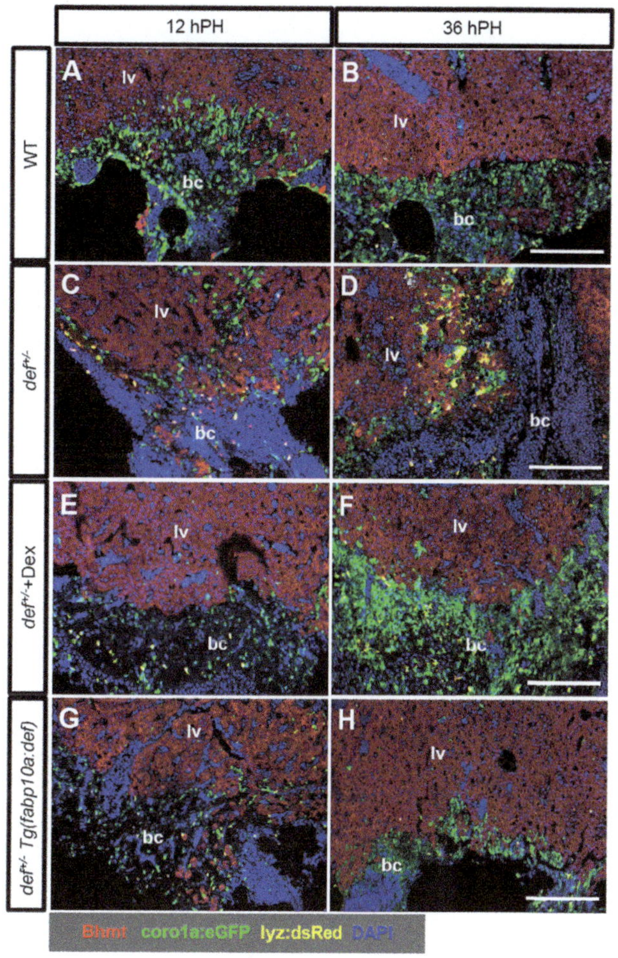

Figure 8. Def haploinsufficiency caused an altered migration behaviour of leukocytes in *def*$^{+/-}$ fish that was rescued by treatment with Dex or ectopic expression of Def in hepatocytes. (*A–H*) Representative images of co-immunostaining of EGFP (green, label macrophage), dsRed (yellow, label neutrophil) and Bhmt (red) in the wound epidermis in wild-type (*A,B*), *def*$^{+/-}$ (*C,D*), *def*$^{+/-}$ treated with Dex (*E,F*) and *def*$^{+/-}$*Tg(fabp10a:def)* progeny (*G,H*) 12 and 36 h after PH, respectively. All are in the background of *Tg(coro1a:eGFP;lyz:dsRED)*. Nuclei were stained with DAPI (blue). In each case, more than 10 sections from at least three wild-type or *def*$^{+/-}$ mutant fish were examined. bc, blood clot; lv, liver tissue. Scale bars: 150 μm (*A–H*).

Loss of Function of p53 Suppresses Scar Formation in *def*$^{+/-}$ Fish after PH

We recently showed that Def complexes with Capn3 to target p53 for degradation in the nucleolus [14]. We first examined the level of p53 and Δ113p53 in *def*$^{+/-}$ fish and found that their expression was up-regulated in the adult *def*$^{+/-}$ liver, and that restoration of the Def protein level in the hepatocytes by *Tg(fabp10a:def)* reduced the p53 and Δ113p53 expression in *def*$^{+/-}$ to a level similar to that exhibited by the wild-type fish (Figure 9B). We then investigated whether constant activation of p53 in the *def*$^{+/-}$ fish promoted inflammation and caused fibrotic scar formation after PH. We crossed the *def*$^{+/-}$ mutant with a *p53*^{M214K} mutant to obtain *def*$^{+/-}$*p53*$^{M214K/M214K}$ progeny for PH. Immunostaining analysis revealed that the loss of function of p53 significantly down-regulated the level of pSmad2 (Figure 10D) and inhibited ColI deposition at the amputation site in the *def*$^{+/-}$ fish

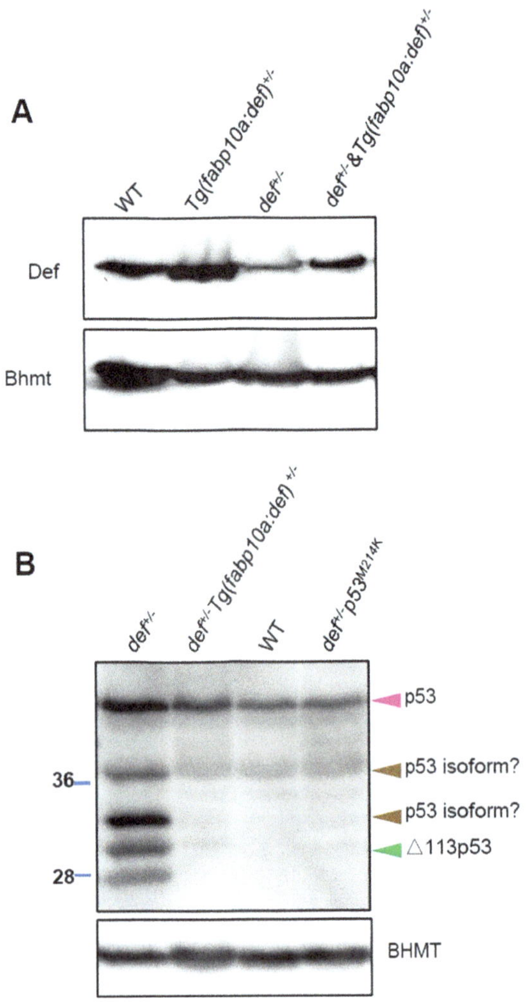

Figure 9. Def expression in the *def*$^{+/-}$ hepatocytes was restored in the *def*$^{+/-}$ *Tg(fabp10a:def)* fish and Def haploinsufficiency up-regulates p53 and Δ113p53 expression in the *def*$^{+/-}$ liver. (*A*) Western blot of Def using an antibody against zebrafish Def to compare its expression levels in the wild-type, *Tg(fabp10a:def)*, *def*$^{+/-}$ and *def*$^{+/-}$ *Tg(fabp10a:def)* adult livers. Bhmt: loading control. (*B*) Western blot of p53 and Δ113p53 in the wild-type, *Tg(fabp10a:def)*, *def*$^{+/-}$ and *def*$^{+/-}$ *p53*$^{M214K/M214K}$ adult livers using an antibody against zebrafish p53. Two uncharacterised p53 isoforms are highlighted by a brown arrow head. Bhmt: loading control.

(Figure 10E; Figure S5C) at 5 days after PH. Moreover, Masson staining also showed that the wound site was completely remodelled without leaving a fibrotic scar at 14 days after PH (Figure 10F). Interestingly, quantitative polymerase chain reaction (qPCR) analysis showed that only the expression of *IL-1β* and *IL-8* but not that of *IL-6* or *TNFα* was down-regulated to a level closer to that found in the wild-type in the *def*$^{+/-}$ *p53*$^{M214K/M214K}$ liver (Figure 7A), suggesting that Def regulates the expression of *IL-6* and *TNFα*, probably through other signalling pathways.

p53 Activation in *def*$^{+/-}$ Fish Up-regulates the Expression of the Pro-inflammatory Factor HMGB1

HMGB1 is a dual function protein that serves either as a nuclear factor that can loosely bind to chromatin or as an extracellular molecule to promote the inflammatory response [33,34]. A recent report showed that p53 activation induces the release of HMGB1 protein to promote inflammation-associated hepatocarcinogenesis [35]. We first compared the expression of HMGB1 in the adult livers from wild-type, *def*$^{+/-}$, *def*$^{+/-}$ *Tg(fabp10a:def)* and *def*$^{+/-}$ *p53*$^{M214K/M214K}$ fish, and found that the level of HMGB1 protein was highly elevated in the *def*$^{+/-}$ fish but was significantly down-regulated to the level found in the wild-type in both the *def*$^{+/-}$ *Tg(fabp:def)* and *def*$^{+/-}$ *p*$^{214K/M214K}$ strains (Figure 11A). We then treated the amputated *def*$^{+/-}$ fish with glycyrrhizic acid ammonium, an inhibitor of HMGB1, and found that it blocked the deposition of ColI at the amputation site(Figure 11B; Figure S5C).

Discussion

Immediately after injury, extravasated blood constituents form a haemostatic plug. Platelets and neutrophils entrapped in the blood clot release a wide variety of factors that serve as chemoattractants to guide the migration of leukocytes, including firstly neutrophils followed by macrophages. Macrophage infiltration into the wound site is responsible for the clearance of neutrophils to resolve local inflammation [36,37]. We found that neutrophil clearance from the amputation site was delayed in *def*$^{+/-}$ fish due to the failure of macrophages to migrate to the injured site in a timely fashion. We believe that this was probably due to disruption of the cytokine gradient because *TNFα*, *IL-1β*, *IL-6* and *IL-8*, four cytokine genes known to modulate leukocyte responses [30], were highly expressed in the *def*$^{+/-}$ liver prior to surgical operation. The prolonged inflammation in the *def*$^{+/-}$ fish consequently activated TGFβ signalling in the wound epidermis that finally resulted in fibrotic scar formation after PH. This conclusion was further confirmed by the fact that treatment with both Dex and SB431542 significantly blocked fibrosis at the amputation site.

Interestingly, we found that the defect (i.e., fibrotic scar formation) in wound healing after PH in the *def*$^{+/-}$ fish was caused by the haploinsufficiency of Def in the hepatocytes, because the restoration of Def expression in the *def*$^{+/-}$ hepatocytes rescued the healing of the amputation site in the *def*$^{+/-}$ fish after PH. We then questioned what role Def, a nucleolar factor, plays in the wound healing process after PH. We recently demonstrated that Def complexes with Capn3 to mediate p53 degradation in the nucleolus and that the level of p53 protein was highly elevated in the *def*$^{-/-}$ homozygous mutant [14]. Here, we show that the loss of function of p53 in the *def*$^{+/-}$ background down-regulated the expression of *IL-1β* and *IL-8* and suppressed fibrotic scar formation after PH. This genetic evidence not only demonstrated unequivocally that the activated p53 pathway contributes to the aberrant expression of cytokines in the *def*$^{+/-}$ liver but also suggested that *IL-1β* and *IL-8* are probably the key players in this process. A recent report showed that constant activation of p53 promotes inflammation by inducing the release of HMGB1 from hepatocytes [35]. Indeed, we found that the expression of HMGB1 was elevated in the *def*$^{+/-}$ liver and that inhibition of the HMGB1 function by the administration of glycyrrhizic acid ammonium blocked the deposition of ColI at the amputation site.

Based on the data available, we propose that the Def-Capn3-p53 pathway negatively affects the inflammatory response in the liver, probably through the regulation of HMGB1 expression. Disruption of this pathway leads to the constant activation of p53 to promote the inflammatory response in the liver that in turn alters the balance between the recruitment and clearance of leukocytes around the amputation site over time after PH, and consequently causes fibrotic scar formation at the amputation site (Figure 11C). However, some key questions remain unanswered. For example, how exactly does p53 regulate the expression of

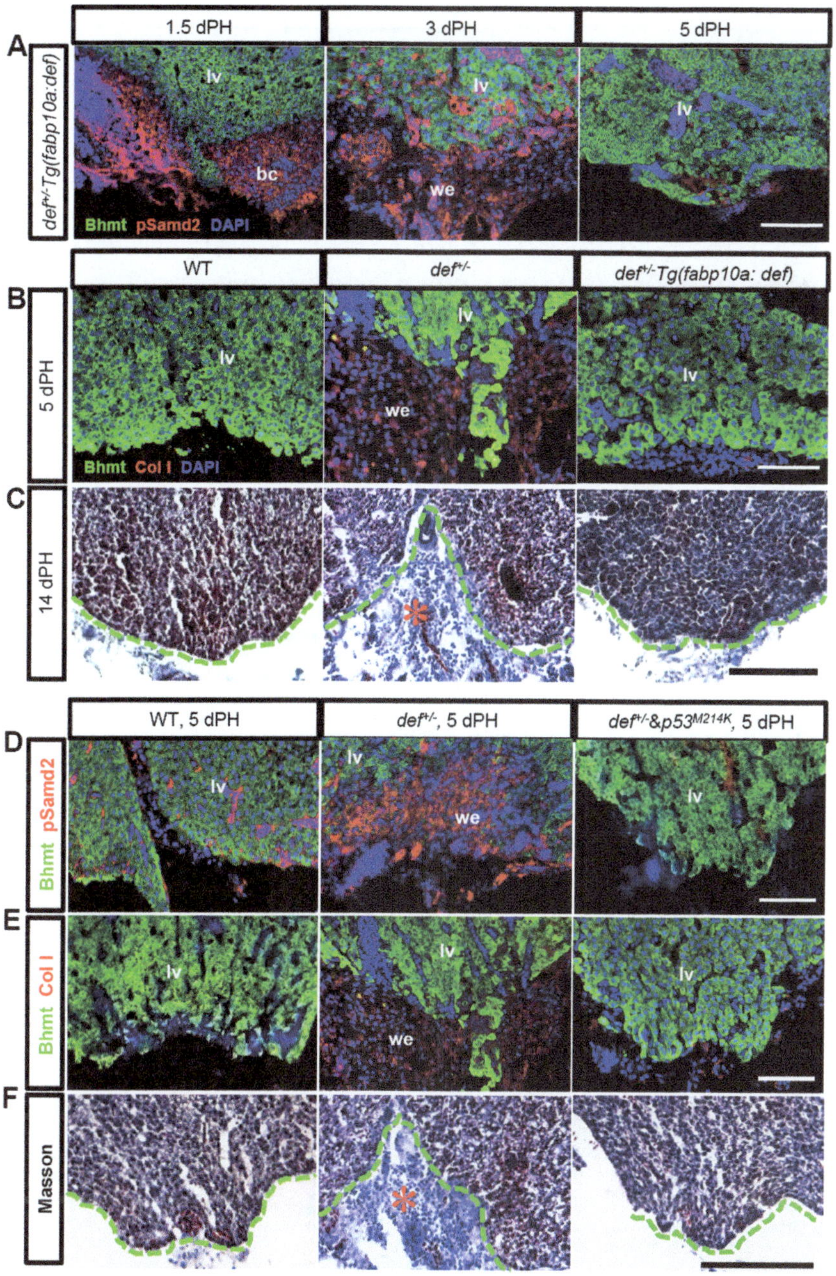

Figure 10. Formation of the fibrotic scar in $def^{+/-}$ fish after PH was mediated by the activation of the p53-pathway. (*A*) Immunostaining of pSmad2 (red) and Bhmt (green) in the wound dermis in $def^{+/-}Tg(fabp10:def)^{+/-}$ progeny 1.5, 3 and 5 days after PH, respectively. (*B*) Immunostaining of ColI (red) and Bhmt (green) in the wild-type, $def^{+/-}$ and $def^{+/-}Tg(fabp10:def)^{+/-}$ progeny 5 days after PH. (*C*) Masson staining of the amputation site (indicated by a green dashed line) in the wild-type, $def^{+/-}$ and $def^{+/-}$ $Tg(fabp10:def)^{+/-}$ progeny 14 days after PH. (*D,E*) Immunostaining of pSmad2 (red) and Bhmt (green) (*D*) and of ColI (red) and Bhmt (green) (*E*) in the wound epidermis in the wild-type, $def^{+/-}$ and $def^{+/-}p53^{M214K/M214K}$ 5 days after PH. (*F*) Masson staining of the amputation site in the wild-type, $def^{+/-}$ and $def^{+/-}p53^{M214K/M214K}$ progeny 14 days after PH. Fibrotic tissue in the $def^{+/-}$ fish is highlighted by a red asterisk. In (*A,B,D,E*), nuclei were stained with DAPI (blue). In each case, more than 10 sections from at least three wild-type or $def^{+/-}$ mutant fish were examined. Representative images are shown here. bc, blood clot; lv, liver tissue; we, wound epidermis. Scale bars: 150 μm (*C,F*) and 75 μm (*A,B,D,E*).

HMGB1? Are other signalling pathways involved in the remodelling of the wound epidermis? The answers to such questions will no doubt help to unravel the mystery of scarless healing of the wound during liver regeneration after PH.

Materials and Methods

Ethics Statement

All animal procedures were performed in full accordance to the requirement by 'Regulation for the Use of Experimental Animals in Zhejiang Province'. This work is specifically approved by the Animal Ethics Committee in the School of Medicine, Zhejiang

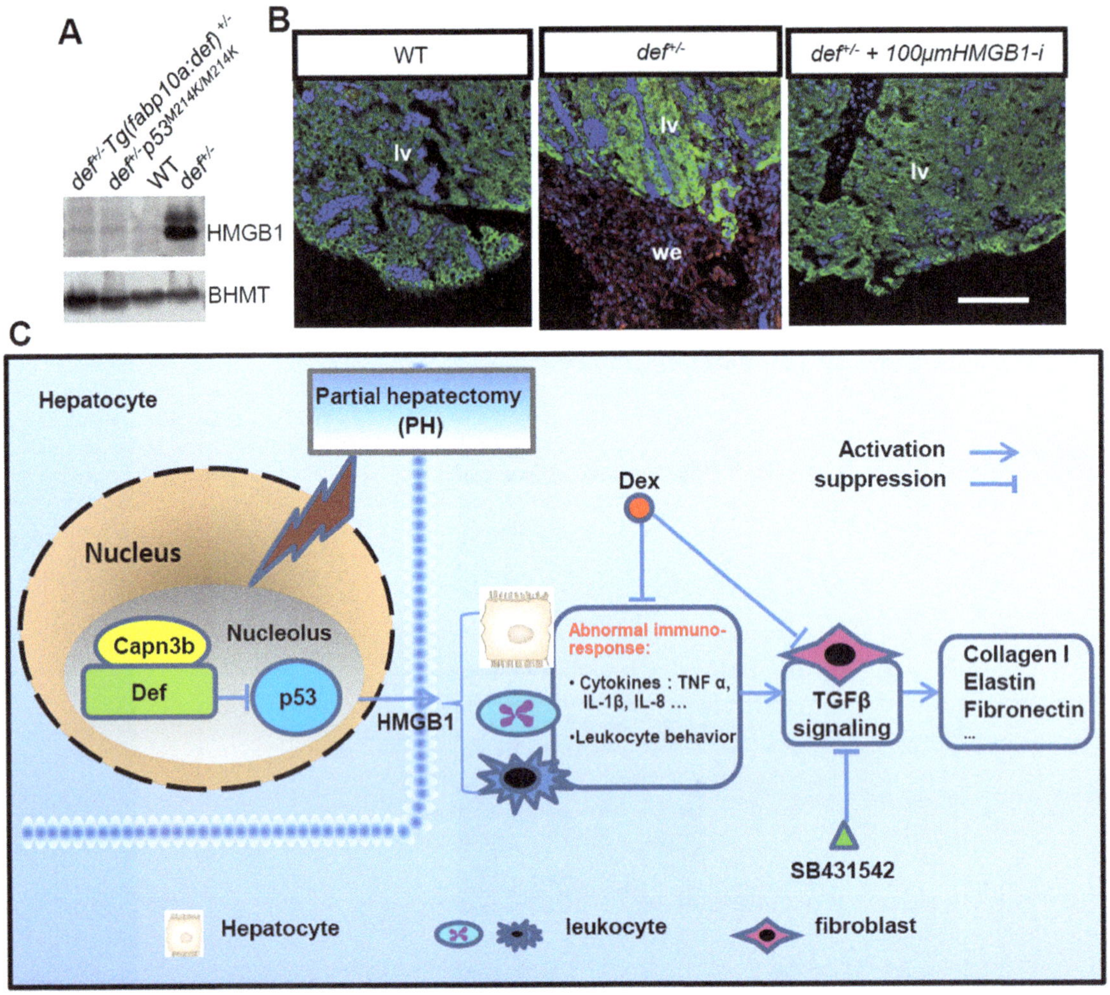

Figure 11. A model to explain how Def haploinsufficiency activates the p53-dependent inflammation-mediated TGFβ signalling and causes fibrotic scar formation in *def*$^{+/-}$ after PH. (*A*) Western blot of HMGB1 in the adult liver from wild-type, *def*$^{+/-}$, *def*$^{+/-}$*Tg(fabp10:def)*$^{+/-}$ and *def*$^{+/-}$*p53*$^{M214K/M214K}$ fish. Loading control: Bhmt. (*B*) Immunostaining of ColI and Bhmt in the wound epidermis in wild-type, *def*$^{+/-}$ and *def*$^{+/-}$fish treated with 100 μM of glycyrrhizic acid ammonium 5 days after PH. lv, liver; we, wound epidermis. (*C*) In a wild-type liver, Def complexes with Capn3 to mediate p53 degradation in the nucleoli to mitigate the inflammatory response after acute injury. In *def*$^{+/-}$ fish, the activity of the Def-Capn3 protein degradation pathway is compromised and p53 protein is thus stabilised, which in turn activates the p53 pathway. Constant activation of the p53 pathway up-regulates the expression of the pro-inflammatory factor HMGB1 that up-regulates the expression of cytokines (e.g., TNFα, IL-1β, IL-6 and IL-8) and other signalling pathways that lead to a prolonged inflammatory response in *def*$^{+/-}$. The prolonged inflammatory response activates TGFβ signalling and causes the over-production of fibrotic molecules (e.g., collagens, elastin and fibronectin) in the wound epidermis that finally forms a fibrotic scar at the amputation site in *def*$^{+/-}$. Fibrotic scar formation in *def*$^{+/-}$ can be blocked by over-expressing Def specifically in the hepatocytes, by the loss of function of p53, and by treatment with Dex (anti-inflammatory drug), SB431542 (inhibitor of TGFβ signalling) or glycyrrhizic acid ammonium (inhibitor of HMGB1 function).

University (ETHICS CODE Permit NO. ZJU2011-1-11-009Y, issued by the Animal Ethics Committee in the School of Medicine, Zhejiang University).

Zebrafish Strains

The two pairs of primers used for genotyping *def*^{hi429} mutants have been described previously [13]. The *Tg(fabp10a:dsRed)* transgenic line was used to label the hepatocytes [38,39], the *Tg(zlyz:EGFP)* transgenic line was used to label the neutrophils [40] and the *Tg(coro1a:eGFP;lyz:dsRed)* transgenic line was used to label macrophages (green) and neutrophils (red), respectively [31]. The *p53*^{M214K} mutant was provided by Prof. Thomas Look [41]. The transgenic and the mutant lines were crossed with a *def*$^{+/-}$ heterozygous mutant.

Zebrafish Manipulation and Measurement of the Liver-versus-Body Ratio

All of the zebrafish used for PH in this study were between 5 and 7 months of age. The PH operation and measurement of the liver-versus-body ratio were performed as described previously [9]. The survival rates of the wild-type and *def*$^{+/-}$ fish after surgery were greater than 95% up to 60 days after PH in all of the experiments described in this work. For drug treatment, 20 μM diphenyleneiodonium (D2926; Sigma) or 200 μM apocynin (W508454; Sigma) was injected into the abdominal cavity daily between days 0 and 2 after PH; 20 mg/L of Dex (D4902; Sigma) was injected immediately after PH; 100 μM of glycyrrhizic acid ammonium salt (50531; Sigma) was injected daily between days 0 and 3 after PH; and 20 µM of SB431542 (ITB1001; Gene Operation) was injected 2 days after PH.

Histological Analysis

Immunohistochemistry was performed as described previously [13]. The antibodies used in this study were mouse anti-PCNA (P8825; Sigma), rabbit anti-red fluorescent protein (ab34771; Abcam), rabbit anti-Collagen I (ab34710; Abcam), rabbit anti-pSmad2 (3101S; Cell Signalling), guinea-pig anti-keratin18 (LS-C22655; Lifespan), chicken anti-GFP (ab13970; Abcam), mouse anti-p53 [14], rabbit anti-Def [13], mouse anti-Bhmt [17] and rabbit anti-HMGB1 (ab18256). The anti-rabbit, -mouse, -guinea, -pig and -chicken secondary antibodies (Invitrogen) were conjugated with Alexa Fluor 647, 568, 633 and 488, respectively. The TUNEL assay was carried out using the In Situ Cell Death Detection Kit, TMR red (Roche). All images were taken under a Leica TCS SP5 microscope or an Olympus FV-ASW confocal microscope.

For the EdU incorporation assay, the fish were anaesthetised in 0.02% Tricaine, and 10 µl of EdU (125 mg/ml in dimethyl sulphoxide solution) was injected into the abdominal cavity immediately after PH followed by another injection 24 h after PH. The fish were then collected and fixed for cryosectioning. EdU staining was performed using an EdU Imaging Kit (Life Technologies). Masson staining was performed according to the protocols described at http://www.ihcworld.com/. All images were taken under a Nikon AZ100 microscope.

Protein and RNA Analysis

Total protein extraction and western blotting were carried out as described previously [42]. The adult zebrafish liver was treated in cell lysis buffer (63 mM of Tris-HCl, 10% glycerol, 5% β-mercaptoethanol, 3.5% sodium dodecyl sulfate) in the presence of a protease inhibitor, Complete (11873580001; Roche). Total RNA extraction and qPCR were performed on a Bio-Rad Real-Time System using the fluorescence-labelled dNTP mix (Bio-Rad) according to the manufacturer's instructions. The experiments were performed in triplicate. The sequences of the primer pairs used for qPCR were as follows: *TNFα* forward primer: GTTTATCAGACAACCGTGGCCA, reverse primer: GATGTTCTCTGTTGGGTTTCTGAC; *il-1β* forward primer: TGGACTTCGCAGCACAAAATG, reverse primer: CACTT-CACGCTCTTGGATGA; *il-6* forward primer:TCAACTTCTC-CAGCGTGATG,reverse primer:TCTTTCCCTCTTTTCCT-CCTG, *il-8* forward primer:GTCGCTGCATTGAAACAGAA, reverse primer:CTTAACCCATGGAGCAGAGG.

Supporting Information

Figure S1 Statistic analysis of the signal intensity of the immunostaining for Def, PCNA and CoII, respectively. (*A*) Comparison of Def signal intensities among WT sham, *def*$^{+/-}$ sham, WT and *def*$^{+/-}$ at 2 dPH as showing in Figure 1C. The relative value of the Def signal intensity in *def*$^{+/-}$ was set at 1. (*B*) Comparison of the index of proliferating cells at the amputation site at 3 dPH as showing Figure 3C. Hepatocytes (Bhmt^{+} cells) and wound epidermal cells (Bhmt^{-} cells) in the same areas at the amputation plane were counted. PCNA+ hepatocytes and wound epidermal cells were also counted. The average ratio of total PCNA^{+} hepatocytes (PH) to total hepatocytes (TH) and total PCNA^{+} epidermal cells (PEC) to total wound epidermal cells (TEC) in WT and *def*$^{+/-}$ were obtained, respectively. The value of PEC/TEC in *def*$^{+/-}$ was set as 1 for the convenience of comparison. Data were collected from three fish for each genotype in each case. (C) Comparison of the CoII signal intensities at the amputation site between WT and *def*$^{+/-}$ at 3dPH as showing in Figure 4B. The relative value of the CoII signal intensity in WT was set as 1. Ten sections from three WT or *def*$^{+/-}$ mutant fish were examined. In (*A–C*), the values plotted represent the means ± standard errors of the mean. The *p*-value was obtained by performing the two-tailed unpaired *t*-test. *** P<0.001; Student's *t* test. Signal intensity in each case was acquired by Photoshop based on the brightness of immunostaining of the targeted protein in a selected region.

Figure S2 The *def*$^{+/-}$ mutant showed defective lobe structure recovery at the amputation site after PH. Lower magnifications of the ventral and lateral views of the gross morphology of the liver 3, 7 and 21 days after PH. The images for 7 days after PH correspond to the closer view of the amputation site shown in Figure 1d. The white, dashed line outlines the amputation site on the ventral tip. The red arrow highlights the ventral lobe in the sham control. VL: ventral lobe; LDL: left dorsal lobe; RDL: right dorsal lobe. Scale bar: 1 cm.

Figure S3 Comparison of the wound healing process between the wild-type and *def*$^{+/-}$ livers after PH. Frontal plane sections of the liver 12, 24 and 36 h after PH were stained for apoptotic cells (in white, using the TUNEL assay), proliferative cells (in red, by EdU incorporation) together with Bhmt (hepatocyte marker) (in green). DAPI was used to stain the nuclei (blue). All images show the part of the hepatic tissue adjacent to the amputation site. Yellow dashed lines outline the amputation site, while regions defined by red brackets represent the blood clot. (*A–D*) The blood clot was clearly formed in both the wild-type (*A*) and *def*$^{+/-}$ mutant (*B*) fish 12 h after PH. Cells in the blood clot underwent massive apoptosis 24 h after PH (*C,D*). (*E,F*) By 36 h after PH, the blood clot was detached from the liver mass in the wild-type fish (*E*), whereas it was still connected to the liver mass in the *def*$^{+/-}$ mutant (*F*). The inset, enlarged view corresponds to the amputation site (*A–F*). bc, blood clot; lv, liver tissue. Scale bar: 250 µm (*A–F*).

Figure S4 Comparison of cell proliferation in the adult liver in the wild-type and *def*$^{+/-}$ sham controls. Representative images of immunostaining of PCNA (in red) in the *Tg(fabp10a:RFP)* background, in which hepatocytes are genetically labelled by expressing the red fluorescent protein (in green), showed that proliferating cells were rarely detected along the epithelial edge of an adult liver in either the wild-type or *def*$^{+/-}$ mutant sham controls. Nuclei were stained with DAPI (blue). lv, liver tissue. Scale bar: 75 µm.

Figure S5 Statistic analysis of the effect of different treatment on the signal intensity of the immunostaining for pSmad2 and CoII at the amputation site, respectively. (*A*). Comparison of the pSmad2 signal intensities in WT, *def*$^{+/-}$, *def*$^{+/-}$ treated with SB431542 or Dex, and *def*$^{+/-}$ *Tg(fabp10a:def)* at 1.5, 3 and 5dPH, respectively, as showing in Figure 6A–D and Figure 10A. Ten sections from three fish for each genotype in each case were examined. (*B*) Comparison of the CoII signal intensities in WT, *def*$^{+/-}$, WT or *def*$^{+/-}$ treated with SB431542 or Dex at 5dPH as showing in Figure 6E and 6F. Ten sections from three fish in each case were examined. (*C*) Comparison of the CoII signal intensities in WT, *def*$^{+/-}$, *def*$^{+/-}$ *Tg(fabp10a:def)*, *def*$^{+/-}$*p53*$^{M214K/M214K}$ or *def*$^{+/-}$ treated with

HMGB1-i at 5dPH as showing in Figure 10B and 10E and Figure 11B. Ten sections from three fish for each genotype in each case were examined. In (*A–C*), the values plotted represent the means ± standard errors of the mean. The *p*-value was obtained by performing the two-tailed unpaired *t*-test. *** P<0.001; NS: non significant. Signal intensity in each case was acquired by Photoshop based on the brightness of immunostaining of the targeted protein in a selected region.

Figure S6 ColI deposition at the amputation site in *def*$^{+/-}$ is not mediated by the reactive oxygen species signalling pathway. Representative images of co-immunostaining of ColI (red) and Bhmt (green) in the wound epidermis in wild-type, *def*$^{+/-}$ and *def*$^{+/-}$ fish treated with diphenyleneiodonium (DPI) or apocynin (APO), two inhibitors of the reactive oxygen species signalling, 5 days after PH. Nuclei were stained with DAPI (blue). lv, liver tissue; we, wound epidermis. Scale bar: 75 μm.

Figure S7 Comparison of the ratio of macrophages to neutrophils at the amputation site. The number of macrophages and neutrophils at the amputation site were counted, respectively, in WT, *def*$^{+/-}$, *def*$^{+/-}$ treated with Dex, and in *def*$^{+/-}$ *Tg(fabp10a:def)* at 12 and 36 hPH as showing Figure 8. Ten sections from three fish in each case were examined and the ratio of macrophages to neutrophils was obtained for each section to minimize the variation caused by sectioning. The values plotted represent the means ± standard errors of the mean. The *p*-value was obtained by performing the two-tailed unpaired *t*-test. * P< 0.05,** P<0.01. Signal intensity in each case was acquired by Photoshop based on the brightness of immunostaining of the targeted protein in a selected region.

Acknowledgments

We thank Drs Ting Tao and Li Jan Lo for helpful discussions and Drs Zilong Wen, Nicolas P. Harberd, Honghui Huang and Li Li for their critical comments on the manuscript.

Author Contributions

Conceived and designed the experiments: JRP JC. Performed the experiments: ZHZ. Analyzed the data: ZHZ JC JRP. Contributed reagents/materials/analysis tools: JWX. Wrote the paper: ZHZ JRP.

References

1. Taub R (2004) Liver regeneration: from myth to mechanism. Nat Rev Mol Cell Biol 5: 836–847.
2. Fausto N, Campbell JS, Riehle KJ (2006) Liver regeneration. Hepatology 43: S45–S53.
3. Michalopoulos GK (2010) Liver regeneration after partial hepatectomy: critical analysis of mechanistic dilemmas. Am J Pathol 176: 2–13.
4. Costa RH, Kalinichenko VV, Holterman AX, Wang X (2003) Transcription factors in liver development, differentiation, and regeneration. Hepatology 38: 1331–1347.
5. Schachtrup C, Le MN, Passino MA, Akassoglou K (2011) Hepatic stellate cells and astrocytes: Stars of scar formation and tissue repair. Cell Cycle 10: 1764–1771.
6. Tao T, Peng J (2009) Liver development in zebrafish (Danio rerio). J Genet Genomics 36: 325–334.
7. Curado S, Stainier DY (2010) deLiver'in regeneration: injury response and development. Semin Liver Dis 30: 288–295.
8. Shin D, Weidinger G, Moon RT, Stainier DY (2012) Intrinsic and extrinsic modifiers of the regulative capacity of the developing liver. Mech Dev 128: 525–535.
9. Kan NG, Junghans D, Izpisua Belmonte JC (2009) Compensatory growth mechanisms regulated by BMP and FGF signaling mediate liver regeneration in zebrafish after partial hepatectomy. FASEB J 23: 3516–3525.
10. Sadler KC, Krahn KN, Gaur NA, Ukomadu C (2007) Liver growth in the embryo and during liver regeneration in zebrafish requires the cell cycle regulator, uhrf1. Proc Natl Acad Sci U S A 104: 1570–1575.
11. Charette JM, Baserga SJ (2010) The DEAD-box RNA helicase-like Utp25 is an SSU processome component. RNA 16: 2156–2169.
12. Harscoet E, Dubreucq B, Palauqui JC, Lepiniec L (2010) NOF1 encodes an Arabidopsis protein involved in the control of rRNA expression. PLoS One 5: e12829.
13. Chen J, Ruan H, Ng SM, Gao C, Soo HM, et al. (2005) Loss of function of def selectively up-regulates Delta113p53 expression to arrest expansion growth of digestive organs in zebrafish. Genes Dev 19: 2900–2911.
14. Tao T, Shi H, Guan Y, Huang D, Chen Y, et al. (2013) Def defines a conserved nucleolar pathway that leads p53 to proteasome-independent degradation. Cell Res 23: 620–634.
15. Korzh S, Pan X, Garcia-Lecea M, Winata CL, Pan X, et al. (2008) Requirement of vasculogenesis and blood circulation in late stages of liver growth in zebrafish. BMC Dev Biol 8: 84.
16. Stadelmann WK, Digenis AG, Tobin GR (1998) Physiology and healing dynamics of chronic cutaneous wounds. Am J Surg 176: 26S–38S.
17. Yang SL, Aw SS, Chang C, Korzh S, Korzh V, et al. (2011) Depletion of Bhmt elevates sonic hedgehog transcript level and increases beta-cell number in zebrafish. Endocrinology 152: 4706–4717.
18. Dong PD, Munson CA, Norton W, Crosnier C, Pan X, et al. (2007) Fgf10 regulates hepatopancreatic ductal system patterning and differentiation. Nat Genet 39: 397–402.
19. Masuzaki R, Zhao SR, Csizmadia E, Yannas I, Karp SJ (2013) Scar formation and lack of regeneration in adult and neonatal liver after stromal injury. Wound Repair Regen 21: 122–130.
20. Moll R, Franke WW, Schiller DL, Geiger B, Krepler R (1982) The catalog of human cytokeratins: patterns of expression in normal epithelia, tumors and cultured cells. Cell 31: 11–24.
21. Bataller R, Gabele E, Parsons CJ, Morris T, Yang L, et al. (2005) Systemic infusion of angiotensin II exacerbates liver fibrosis in bile duct-ligated rats. Hepatology 41: 1046–1055.
22. Chen SJ, Yuan W, Mori Y, Levenson A, Trojanowska M, et al. (1999) Stimulation of type I collagen transcription in human skin fibroblasts by TGF-beta: involvement of Smad 3. J Invest Dermatol 112: 49–57.
23. Gressner AM, Weiskirchen R, Breitkopf K, Dooley S (2002) Roles of TGF-beta in hepatic fibrosis. Front Biosci 7: d793–d807.
24. Inman GJ, Nicolas FJ, Callahan JF, Harling JD, Gaster LM, et al. (2002) SB-431542 is a potent and specific inhibitor of transforming growth factor-beta superfamily type I activin receptor-like kinase (ALK) receptors ALK4, ALK5, and ALK7. Mol Pharmacol 62: 65–74.
25. Ho DM, Chan J, Bayliss P, Whitman M (2006) Inhibitor-resistant type I receptors reveal specific requirements for TGF-beta signaling in vivo. Dev Biol 295: 730–742.
26. Jaquet V, Scapozza L, Clark RA, Krause KH, Lambeth JD (2009) Small-molecule NOX inhibitors: ROS-generating NADPH oxidases as therapeutic targets. Antioxid Redox Signal 11: 2535–2552.
27. Bhattacharyya S, Brown DE, Brewer JA, Vogt SK, Muglia LJ (2007) Macrophage glucocorticoid receptors regulate Toll-like receptor 4-mediated inflammatory responses by selective inhibition of p38 MAP kinase. Blood 109: 4313–4319.
28. Harada A, Sekido N, Akahoshi T, Wada T, Mukaida N, et al. (1994) Essential involvement of interleukin-8 (IL-8) in acute inflammation. J Leukoc Biol 56: 559–564.
29. Lalani I, Bhol K, Ahmed AR (1997) Interleukin-10: biology, role in inflammation and autoimmunity. Ann Allergy Asthma Immunol 79: 469–483.
30. Radtke S, Wuller S, Yang XP, Lippok BE, Mutze B, et al. (2010) Cross-regulation of cytokine signalling: pro-inflammatory cytokines restrict IL-6 signalling through receptor internalisation and degradation. J Cell Sci 123: 947–959.
31. Li L, Yan B, Shi YQ, Zhang WQ, Wen ZL (2012) Live imaging reveals differing roles of macrophages and neutrophils during zebrafish tail fin regeneration. J Biol Chem 287: 25353–25360.
32. Tao T, Shi H, Huang D, Peng J (2013) Def functions as a cell autonomous factor in organogenesis of digestive organs in zebrafish. PLoS One 8: e58858.
33. Tsung A, Sahai R, Tanaka H, Nakao A, Fink MP, et al. (2005) The nuclear factor HMGB1 mediates hepatic injury after murine liver ischemia-reperfusion. J Exp Med 201: 1135–1143.
34. Scaffidi P, Misteli T, Bianchi ME (2002) Release of chromatin protein HMGB1 by necrotic cells triggers inflammation. Nature 418: 191–195.
35. Yan HX, Wu HP, Zhang HL, Ashton C, Tong C, et al. (2013) p53 promotes inflammation-associated hepatocarcinogenesis by inducing HMGB1 release. J Hepatol 59: 762–768.
36. DiPietro LA, Burdick M, Low QE, Kunkel SL, Strieter RM (1998) MIP-1alpha as a critical macrophage chemoattractant in murine wound repair. J Clin Invest 101: 1693–1698.
37. Wetzler C, Kampfer H, Stallmeyer B, Pfeilschifter J, Frank S (2000) Large and sustained induction of chemokines during impaired wound healing in the

genetically diabetic mouse: prolonged persistence of neutrophils and macrophages during the late phase of repair. J Invest Dermatol 115: 245–253.
38. Her GM, Chiang CC, Chen WY, Wu JL (2003) In vivo studies of liver-type fatty acid binding protein (L-FABP) gene expression in liver of transgenic zebrafish (Danio rerio). FEBS Lett 538: 125–133.
39. Wan H, Korzh S, Li Z, Mudumana SP, Korzh V, et al. (2006) Analyses of pancreas development by generation of gfp transgenic zebrafish using an exocrine pancreas-specific elastaseA gene promoter. Exp Cell Res 312: 1526–1539.
40. Zhang Y, Bai XT, Zhu KY, Jin Y, Deng M, et al. (2008) In vivo interstitial migration of primitive macrophages mediated by JNK-matrix metalloproteinase 13 signaling in response to acute injury. J Immunol 181: 2155–2164.
41. Berghmans S, Murphey RD, Wienholds E, Neuberg D, Kutok JL, et al. (2005) tp53 mutant zebrafish develop malignant peripheral nerve sheath tumors. Proc Natl Acad Sci U S A 102: 407–412.
42. Huang H, Ruan H, Aw MY, Hussain A, Guo L, et al. (2008) Mypt1-mediated spatial positioning of Bmp2-producing cells is essential for liver organogenesis. Development 135: 3209–3218.

Neutralization of IL-8 Prevents the Induction of Dermatologic Adverse Events Associated with the Inhibition of Epidermal Growth Factor Receptor

Nannie Bangsgaard[1]*, Mischa Houtkamp[2], Danita H. Schuurhuis[2], Paul W. H. I. Parren[2], Ole Baadsgaard[3], Hans W. M. Niessen[4], Lone Skov[1]

1 Department of Dermato-allergology, Copenhagen University Hospital Gentofte, Hellerup, Denmark, **2** Genmab, Utrecht, The Netherlands, **3** Genmab, Copenhagen, Denmark, **4** Department of Pathology and Cardiac Surgery, VU University Medical Centre, Amsterdam, The Netherlands

Abstract

Epidermal growth factor receptor (EGFR) inhibitors are widely used in the treatment of cancer. EGFR-targeted treatment is known to be associated with a high incidence of dermatological adverse reactions, including papulopustular rash, which can be dose-limiting and may affect compliance to treatment. Currently, the pathways involved in EGFR inhibitor-induced rash are poorly understood and few treatment options for this adverse event are available. Here, we developed a model for induction of papulopustular rash in healthy human volunteers by subcutaneous injection of the anti-EGFR monoclonal antibody zalutumumab. The injection sites and surrounding skin were evaluated by a dermatologist for the presence or absence of papulopustular rash and skin biopsies were taken to confirm the macroscopical findings by immunohistochemistry. Locally injected zalutumumab induced a papulopustular rash, characterized by acute follicular neutrophil-rich hair follicle inflammation, and thus mimicked adverse events induced by systemic administration of EGFR inhibitors. In this model, we tested the hypothesis that neutrophils, attracted by IL-8, play a central role in the observed rash. Indeed, concomitant local repeat dose treatment with HuMab-10F8, a neutralizing human antibody against IL-8, reduced the rash. Inhibition of IL-8 can therefore ameliorate dermatological adverse events induced by treatment with EGFR inhibitors.

Editor: Lucia Gabriele, Istituto Superiore di Sanità, Italy

Funding: The authors have no support or funding to report.

Competing Interests: The authors have read the journal's policy and have the following conflicts: Mischa Houtkamp, Danita Schuurhuis, Paul Parren and Ole Baadsgaard are employees of Genmab. There are no patents, products in development or marketed products to declare.

* E-mail: Nanban01@geh.regionh.dk

Introduction

Cancer therapy is increasingly shifting towards targeting specific pathogenic pathways. Epidermal growth factor receptor (EGFR; ErbB1) controls proliferation and maturation of epithelial cells in skin. In many solid tumors of epithelial origin, EGFR is up-regulated, making it an attractive target for treatment [1,2,3]. Indeed, inhibitors of EGFR, including both small molecules and monoclonal antibodies (mAb), represent a known example of targeted therapy, and are widely used in daily oncologic clinical practice [4]. EGFR inhibitors are less likely than traditional cytotoxic chemotherapeutics to cause myelosuppression, infection, vomiting and nausea. However, several dermatological adverse events accompany the use of EGFR inhibitors. These adverse events affect the patient's well being, may be dose-limiting and influence treatment compliance. A papulopustular (also called acneiform) skin rash is a common toxicity observed with both EGFR-targeting mAb and tyrosine kinase inhibitors (TKI), with a reported incidence of up to 80% in patients treated with EGFR-targeting agents [5,6,7].

The rash induced by EGFR inhibitors typically appears within one to three weeks of treatment and is characterized by inflammatory follicular papules and pustules. The rash is most commonly affecting the face; but is also seen at the upper chest and back and infrequently at other body sites [8]. The rash appears to be dose-related [9,10], and is reversible upon withdrawal of treatment, but may re-appear or worsen once treatment is resumed. Higher response rates and a significant correlation with increased survival have been observed in patients in whoever rash developed [11,12]. To ensure that patients can continue to receive treatment at the optimal dose, effective treatment strategies are required to actively manage rash and aid compliance. As yet, there are no standardized treatments for these skin side-effects [13,14,15]. A greater understanding of the biological mechanisms responsible for the EGFR inhibitor-induced rash would be highly beneficial for the development of rational and more effective treatment management strategies.

The rash may be related to follicular occlusion due to a lack of epithelial differentiation and epithelial inflammation resulting from release of cytokines as direct results from EGFR inhibition. Because the papulopustular rash is characterized by follicular inflammation with an accumulation of neutrophils [16,17,18], we hypothesized that the cytokine IL-8 might play a role in this pathology. Previously, we have shown that treatment of patients with palmoplantar pustulosis (PPP), an inflammatory disease characterized by skin infiltration with neutrophil granulocytes,

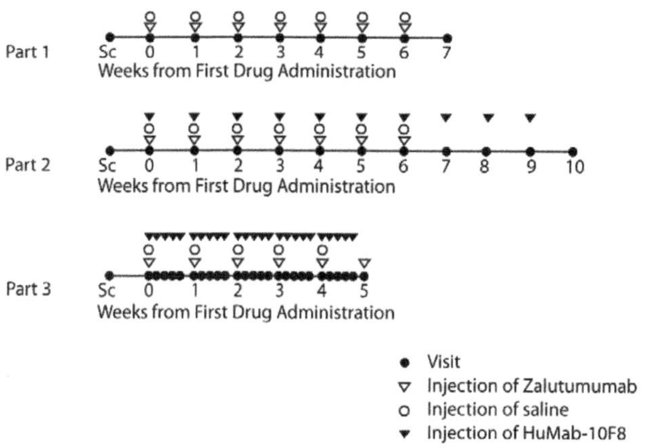

Figure 1. Trial design. Injection schemes for the three different parts of the study are shown. Subjects were injected with different doses of zalutumumab at different sites, as described in Table 1. Sc – screening of patient.

with a neutralizing monoclonal antibody against IL-8, led to a marked improvement in clinical signs concomitant with a reduction in neutrophil infiltration [19].

Here we show, in this proof-of-principle study, that inhibition of IL-8 can ameliorate the dermatological adverse events induced with an EGFR-inhibiting mAb. Further studies addressing the potential of IL-8 inhibition for the prevention of serious dermatological adverse events induced both by small molecule as well as biologic EGFR inhibitors are warranted.

Materials and Methods

An open-label, single-center non-randomized study was performed in healthy volunteers with a single dose escalation set-up. The clinical study was performed at the Department of Dermato-allergology, University Hospital of Copenhagen Gentofte in accordance with the declaration of Helsinki. The study was approved by the local ethics committee (H-KA-20060104) and The Danish Medicines Agency (2006-003253-24). All subjects gave written informed consent prior to enrolment.

A total of nine healthy male volunteers were included in the study. All subjects were Caucasian men and the median age of the group was 24 years (range 22–32 years).

Table 1. Dose escalation schedule for zalutumumab injections.

	Visit						
Injection site	Day 0	Day 7	Day 14	Day 21	Day 28	Day 35	Day 42
1	1 µg	1 µg	1 µg	1 µg			
2		10 µg	10 µg	10 µg	10 µg		
3			100 µg	100 µg	100 µg	100 µg	
4				1 mg	1 mg	1 mg	1 mg

Every injection of zalutumumab was accompanied by a control injection of an identical volume of isotonic saline at a different site. In the third part the dose escalation started at 100 µg.

Injection protocol

The first part of the study was conducted to evaluate whether local subcutaneous (s.c.) injection of zalutumumab could induce a papulopustular rash, similar to that reported in patients treated systemically with EGFR inhibitors. A maximum of four subjects were to be enrolled and attended once weekly for injection of escalating doses of zalutumumab on the upper back. Since there was no experience with s.c. injection of zalutumumab and the local concentration to induce rash was not known, the study was started with a dose-escalation of s.c. zalutumumab (see Table 1 and Figure 1). 1 µg (in 0.2 mL) zalutumumab was injected s.c. on the upper back. The injection site was marked for later identification. One week later, the injection site was inspected macroscopically and scored by a dermatologist for the presence or absence of rash, defined by the appearance of at least one pustule. If there were no signs of pustules, another 1 µg (in 0.2 mL) zalutumumab was injected at the same site. At the same visit, 10 µg (0.2 mL) zalutumumab was injected at another site, marked for later identification. At each visit, a control injection of an identical volume (0.2 mL) of isotonic saline was injected at a different site. The procedure would take place once weekly with a dose-increase of factor 10 each week, over seven weeks or until the subject had a rash considered induced by the zalutumumab treatment. Only one dose level was injected per injection site. Each dose level was applied for a maximum of four weeks or until a rash developed. Part I of the study was performed in a staggered manner (e.g. treatment of subject 2 was only initiated one week after that of subject 1) and this part would be considered completed when at least one volunteer developed a rash.

The second part of the study was conducted to evaluate the effect of the human IL-8 antibody HuMab-10F8 on zalutumumab-induced papulopustular rash. Seven subjects were enrolled. The dose-escalation procedure from the first part was repeated, again starting at 1 µg zalutumumab per dose. Zalutumumab was either injected alone or in combination with 1.25 mg (in 0.25 mL) HuMab-10F8. As a negative control, isotonic saline, in the same volume as the combined zalutumumab/HuMab-10F8 injection (0.45 mL), was injected at a different site at each visit. After the fourth injection of the zalutumumab/HuMab-10F8 combination at one dose level, 1.25 mg HuMab-10F8 was injected alone once weekly for three weeks at the combination injection site (see Figure 1 and Table 1).

In the third and last part of the study, zalutumumab was given in a dose-escalation procedure starting at 100 µg, or 1 mg if the volunteer had received 100 µg earlier in the study. HuMab-10F8 was administered in a repeat dose regimen. Four subjects were enrolled. The procedure was as described for the second part of the study; however, an additional 1.25 mg dose of HuMab-10F8 was administered at four consecutive days after each combined zalutumumab/HuMab-10F8 injection.

Antibodies

The therapeutic antibodies used in this study were zalutumumab (2F8; HuMax-EGFr); a human IgG1, κ mAb specific for EGFR; generated as described in Bleeker et al., by immunizing HuMAb mice with A431 cells and purified EGFR [20]. The clinical batch was produced by Lonza Biologics (Slough, UK) from CHO DG44 cell line DJT33. Zalutumumab binds to domain III on the EGFR and inhibits tumor growth by a dual mechanism of action: blockade of EGFR signaling and induction of Fc-mediated antibody-dependent cell-mediated cytotoxicity (ADCC) [19]. Systemic administration of zalutumumab was shown to induce rash [21]. HuMab-10F8; a human IgG1, κ mAb specific for IL-8

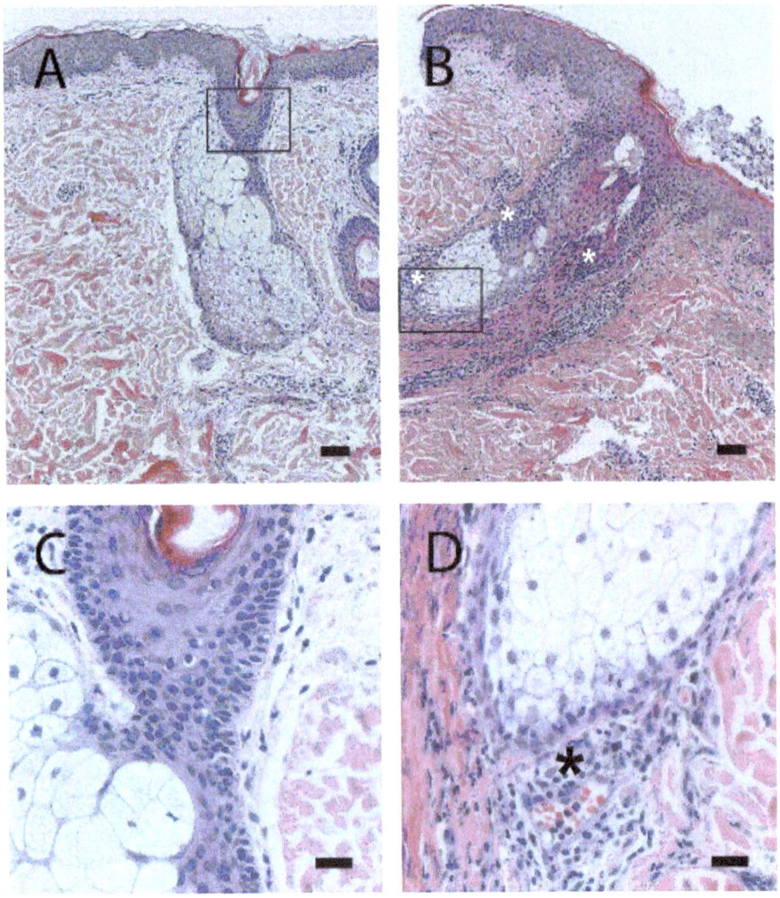

Figure 2. Histology of biopsies from saline- or zalutumumab-injected skin (part I of the study). Representative sections are shown of skin biopsies of one subject for part I of the study (following two injections of 10 μg of zalutumumab). Sections were stained with HE to show nucleated cells and (patho-)histological features. In the saline-injected skin (A, C), inflammatory cells were virtually absent and the hair follicle structure was intact. Note that after zalutumumab injection (B, D), the hair follicle structure was destroyed and extensive influx of inflammatory cells (including neutrophils) in the vicinity of the destroyed hair follicle/glandular structures can be observed (asterisks). Scale bars are 100 μm (A, B) and 20 μm (C, D).

[19]; the clinical batch MDS001 was produced by Medarex Inc. (New Jersey, US).

Clinical Assessment

In each study part, injection sites were evaluated once a week and subjects were instructed to contact the investigator as soon as pustules developed. 4-mm punch skin biopsies were taken from a pustule when a rash was considered to be induced by zalutumumab treatment. At the same time, control biopsies were taken from the isotonic saline injection site and, in part two and three of the study, the positive control site (zalutumumab alone).

The investigator assessed the degree of the rash at the marked injection sites using the following scale from 0 to 3: 0: no rash; +1: mild rash; +2: moderate rash; +3: severe rash. The number of pustules at the injection site was counted and photographic documentation obtained.

Histological and immunohistochemical assessment

Paraffin-embedded skin biopsies were cut at 4 μm thickness, stained with HE and scored as normal or acutely inflamed. Multiple skin sections of each biopsy were examined, to secure that areas with inflammation deeper in the biopsies would not be missed. HE-stained skin biopsies were scored normal when only few diffuse macrophages or lymphocytes were detected in the vicinity of hair follicles (sebaceous glands) and scored acutely inflamed when, in addition to macrophages and lymphocytes, influx of neutrophils was detected (≥50 cells/skin section; semi quantitative score). To confirm the conclusions of the HE staining and identify the inflammatory cells, some skin biopsies were immunostained for EGFR (mouse anti-human EGFR, clone 1F4, cat. # 2239S, specific for the cytoplasmic domain of EGFR; does not compete with zalutumumab for binding to EGFR; Bioke, Leiden, The Netherlands), or with cell type-specific markers identifying neutrophils (mouse anti-human neutrophil elastase, clone NP57, cat. # M0752; Dako, Glostrup, Denmark) and macrophages (mouse anti-human CD68, clone PG-M1; cat. # M0876; Dako). The primary mouse antibodies were detected with a peroxidase-labeled anti-mouse IgG dextran polymer (Envision-PO™ Dako, Glostrup, Denmark; Powervision-PO™, Immunologic, Duiven, The Netherlands) and visualized with AEC (red staining).

Table 2. Histological features of hair follicles in skin biopsies and clinical features of patients treated with zalutumumab, zalutumumab + HuMab-10F8 or saline, based on evaluation of HE staining and clinical observations.

		Saline			Zalutumumab			
Patient ID	**Study Part**	**Histology[a)]**	**#Pustules**	**Degree of reaction**	**Dose/μg**	**Histology**	**#Pustules**	**Degree of reaction**
2	I	Normal	0	None	1	Acute inflammation	10	Mild
1	I	Normal	0	None	1	Acute inflammation	15	Mild
		Zalutumumab			**Zalutumumab + HuMab-10F8**			
Patient ID	**Study Part**	**Histology[a)]**	**#Pustules**	**Degree of reaction**	**Dose/μg**	**Histology**	**#Pustules**	**Degree of reaction**
3	II	Acute inflammation	2	Mild	100	Acute inflammation	0	Mild
4	II	Acute inflammation	3	Mild	1000	Acute inflammation	5	Mild
2	II	Acute inflammation	1	Mild	100	Normal	1	Mild
5	II	Normal	1	Mild	1	Acute inflammation	2	Mild
1	II	Acute inflammation	1	Mild	1000	Acute inflammation	0	Mild
6	II	Acute inflammation	1	Mild	100	Acute inflammation	2	Mild
		Zalutumumab			**Zalutumumab + HuMab-10F8**			
Patient ID	**Study Part**	**Histology[a)]**	**#Pustules**	**Degree of reaction**	**Dose/μg**	**Histology**	**#Pustules**	**Degree of reaction**
6	III	Normal	1	Mild	1000	Normal	0	None
2	III	Acute inflammation	5	Mild	1000	Normal	3	Mild
5	III	Acute inflammation	3	Mild	100	Normal	0	None
1	III	Acute inflammation	6	Mild	1000	Normal	6	Mild

a) semi-quantitative scoring: normal, acute inflammation (based on influx of neutrophils).

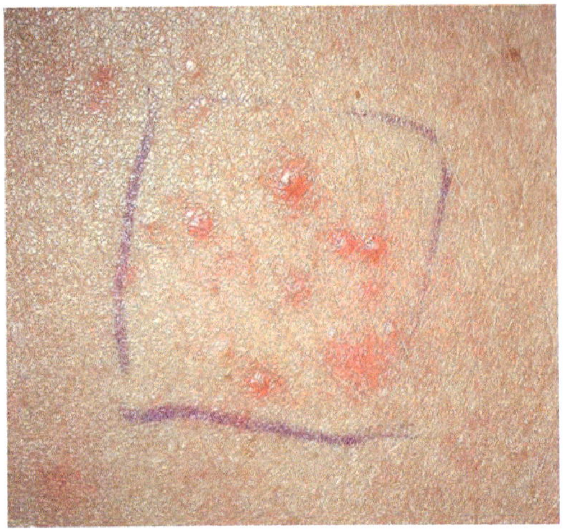

Figure 3. Papulopustular rash was induced by local injection of zalutumumab. The rash observed at the injection site of one subject in part II of the study, following two injections of 100 µg of zalutumumab each, is shown.

Results

Induction of papulopustular rash by local injection of zalutumumab

To set up a human model to study EGFR inhibitor-induced rash, healthy subjects were injected s.c. with the human anti-EGFR antibody zalutumumab. Local injections were used to set up a safe model in human volunteers with limited exposure to the therapeutic antibody.

In part I of the study (Figure 1, Table 1), it was investigated whether s.c. injection of zalutumumab could induce rash. Rash occurred simultaneously in volunteers 1 and 2 on day 14 of the study, which was observed as a mild rash at the 1 µg zalutumumab injection site (i.e. following three 1 µg injections in subject 1 and two injections in subject 2) and a milder rash at 10 µg of zalutumumab (i.e. after two and one 10 µg injections in subjects 1 and 2, respectively). The number of pustules counted is shown in Table 2. Histological examination of skin biopsies from zalutumumab-treated areas showed acute neutrophilic inflammation with follicular localization and signs of disruption of the hair follicles (Table 2, Figure 2B, D), whereas in the saline-treated normal skin, inflammatory cells were virtually absent and the hair follicle structure was intact (Figure 2A, C).

Effect of HuMab-10F8 treatment on zalutumumab-induced papulopustular rash

In part II of the study, it was investigated whether neutralization of IL-8 by a neutralizing antibody, HuMab-10F8, could inhibit the zalutumumab-induced rash. Zalutumumab and HuMab-10F8 were administered concomitantly, once weekly (Figure 1). Seven subjects (including the two subjects from part I) were included in this part of the study. Six of the seven subjects developed pustules following injection of zalutumumab; one at 1 µg, one at 10 µg and four at 100 µg (an example of the rash in shown in Figure 3, the number of pustules counted at the site of biopsy is shown in Table 2). Subject no. 7 was withdrawn due to an adverse reaction (pharyngitis). No clinical or histological differences were observed between the sites with zalutumumab/HuMab-10F8 co-injection compared to sites injected with zalutumumab alone (Table 2). An explanation for these results might be that we did not reach a sufficient local concentration of the IL-8 antibody to achieve a therapeutic effect. Therefore we extended the study with a repeat dose regimen of HuMab-10F8. Four subjects (including the two subjects who completed part I and II of the study and two subjects who completed part II) were included. Zalutumumab was again injected once a week concomitantly with HuMab-10F8 followed by four additional injections of HuMab-10F8 (Figure 1). All four subjects developed pustules following injection of zalutumumab, one at 100 µg and three at 1 mg. Interestingly, an effect of HuMab-10F8 injection on the zalutumumab-induced papulopustular rash was observed in three of four subjects. Clinically, repeat HuMab-10F8 dosing completely suppressed the induction of pustules in two subjects and partially suppressed it in one subject (Table 2). For the zalutumumab positive control alone, induction of pustules was observed in these same subjects (Figure 4). Histological examination supported the clinical findings (Figure 5, Table 2), except in subject no. 6, who had a clinical rash, but normal histology. An extensive influx of inflammatory cells in the vicinity of the hair follicle and signs of folliculitis was observed in the zalutumumab-treated skin (Figure 5 B, D, F, H, J, L). The influx of inflammatory cells consisted predominantly of neutrophils (Figure 5 J, L) and to a lesser extent of macrophages (Figure 5 F, H). In the skin treated with both zalutumumab and repeat doses of HuMab-10F8, the influx of inflammatory cells was virtually absent and sebaceous glands and hair follicles had normal histological features (Fig. 5 A, C, E, G, I, K).

Adverse events

Overall, five subjects experienced at least one adverse event (10 adverse events were experienced in total). Headache (two subjects), influenza (one subject), heamatochezia (one subject) and neutrophil count decrease (one subject) were judged as not related to

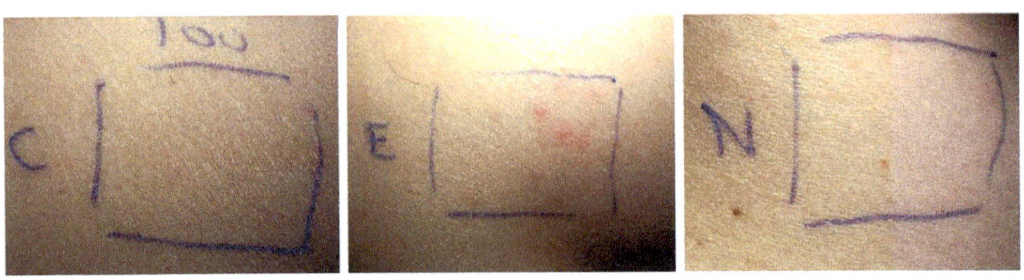

Figure 4. Effect of HuMab-10F8 on zalutumumab-induced pustules. Injection sites of a patient from study part III is shown. Injection of 100 µg zalutumumab alone (E) induced pustules following two injections. Injection of zalutumumab combined with HuMab-10F8, followed by four daily HuMab-10F8 injections (C), suppressed the induction of pustules. The saline control is also shown (N).

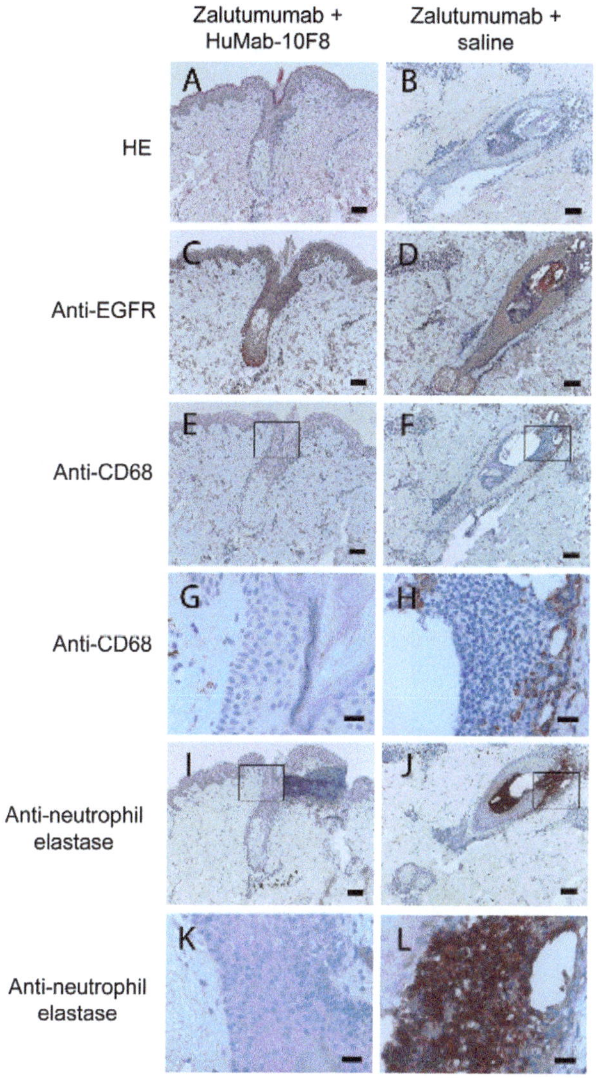

Figure 5. Histology and immunohistochemistry of biopsies from zalutumumab-injected skin treated with HuMab-10F8 or untreated. Data shown are representative sections of skin biopsies of one subject for part III of the study. Biopsies were taken at day 14 after two injections with 100 µg of zalutumumab with [A, C, E, G, I, K] or without HuMab-10F8 [B, D, F, H, J, L]. A, B: HE staining; C, D: staining for EGFR; E–H: staining for macrophages and I–L: staining for neutrophils. Extensive influx of inflammatory cells in the vicinity of the hair follicle with histological signs of folliculitis was observed in zalutumumab-injected skin (right panels), whereas in the zalutumumab-injected skin treated with HuMab-10F8 (left panels) inflammatory cells were virtually absent and sebaceous glands and hair follicles showed normal histological features. Inflammatory infiltrate in the zalutumumab-injected skin was mainly composed of neutrophils (neutrophil elastase positive cells, J, L) and to a lesser extent of macrophages; (CD68 positive cells F, H). Scale bars are 100 µm (A–F, I, J) and 20 µm (G, H, K, L). G, H, K and L are magnifications of the squared areas indicated in E, F, I and J.

zalutumumab treatment; rash distant from the injection site (one subject), fatigue (one subject), pharyngitis (one subject), acne (one subject) and pruritus (one subject) were judged as related to zalutumumab treatment. No serious adverse events were reported.

Discussion

Prevention and management of EGFR inhibitor-induced dermatological toxicities is critical for patients on such treatments. Histologically, the papulopustular skin rash of patients systemically treated with EGFR inhibitors for cancer often presents with neutrophil-rich suppurative folliculitis [16,17,18]. We set up a new model in humans to mimic this adverse event. We here report histological findings, similar to those observed after systemic treatment with EGFR inhibitors, in the skin biopsies from volunteers treated s.c. with zalutumumab. Therefore, this is a model that is very suitable for studying the mechanism behind the development of papulopustular rash and testing potential treatment modalities. Since the model is localized, it is easy to control, and relatively low doses of potential treatments can be studied with minimal risk to the volunteers. We show here that neutralization of IL-8 can ameliorate the symptoms and histological features or EGFR inhibitor-induced papulopustular rash.

Papulopustular rash is reported in up to 80% of patients treated with EGFR inhibitors, both small molecules and mAb [5,6,7]. The papulopustular rash is usually mild and with minimal discomfort [5]; however, serious discomfort and altered quality of life have been reported, resulting in dose reductions or treatment withdrawal [22,23] (out of an 80% overall incidence, grades 1/2 are usually reported at 60%, grades 3/4 at 5–20% [5]). Discontinuation or interruption of cancer therapy may affect clinical outcome. Therefore, effective treatment of these adverse events is required. EGFR inhibitor-induced dermatological toxicities are mainly treated symptomatically, since the mechanisms behind the induction of papulopustular rash by EGFR inhibitors are not well understood. Different agents known to be effective in the treatment of acne such as drying agents, topical antiseptics, topical and systemic antibiotics, topical and systemic retinoids as well as topical and systemic steroids have been used to symptomatically treat the rash, with varying response [5,6].

EGFR is expressed on epidermal keratinocytes, hair follicle epithelium and sebaceous glands [24,25]. Activation of EGFR by its ligands plays a crucial role in keratinocyte proliferation, migration, differentiation and survival, keratinization and development of the hair follicle [26,27,28]. EGFR inhibition in skin induces apoptosis in normal keratinocytes, which increases five-fold between day 4 and 12, and which correlates with median time to rash onset in patients [29]. Furthermore, inhibition of EGFR disrupts growth and differentiation of the hair follicle [16]. Murine studies indicate that complete or partial abrogation of the EGFR gene causes significantly altered and thinned epidermis and abnormal colonic mucosa, which suggests that the down-stream signaling cascade for EGFR is essential for normal development of epithelial tissues [30,31]. Some anti-EGFR mAb, such as RG83852, do not inhibit the tyrosine kinase activity of the receptor. In a phase I study of RG83852, no skin rash was observed at doses that produced a high level of saturation of EGFR *in vivo* [32]. This observation suggests that induction of skin rash requires effective EGFR tyrosine kinase inhibition. However, tyrosine kinase inhibition may be necessary, but not sufficient, for the skin rash to occur.

EGFR blockade has been demonstrated to affect chemokine expression in keratinocytes [33]. Increased chemokine expression after EGFR blockade has been shown to result in enhanced skin inflammation [28]. The induced chemokines could play a role in the inflammation with influx of neutrophils, as observed in the skin biopsies. Several studies have aimed to identify histological and immunohistochemical features of skin in patients treated with EGFR inhibitors [17,18,34]. Thus, the role of tumor necrosis factor-α (TNF-α) and interleukin-1 (IL-1) in the development of EGFR inhibitor-associated skin rash was shown and a possible therapeutic role for anti-TNF agents was suggested [35]. It has previously been described that the EGFR-specific antibody cetuximab induced papulopustular eruptions and induced production of IL-1 and TNF-α [36]. Cetuximab and zalutumumab employ similar mechanisms of action. Both IL-1 and TNF-α can induce IL-8 secretion by fibroblasts [37] and IL-1 can induce IL-8 secretion by keratinocytes [38]. IL-8 attracts and activates neutrophils [37,39,40,41]. It was therefore hypothesized that EGFR inhibition may (indirectly) induce the production of IL-8, which contributes to the induction of EGFR inhibitor-induced rash. However, it was also described that activation of EGFR induced IL-8 production in keratinocytes *in vitro* [42]. This emphasizes the difficulty of extrapolating findings obtained with one cell type *in vitro* to a whole organ *in vivo*, in this case the skin, which contains many different cell types that interact with each other, and may respond distinctly. Our exploratory clinical trial allowed us to test our hypothesis in humans *in vivo*.

Previously, we showed that local injection of HuMab-10F8, a therapeutic human antibody against IL-8, induced a marked reduction of disease activity in PPP patients [19]. In the present study, we tested the hypothesis that local injection of this therapeutic antibody was capable of reducing the papulopustular rash induced by EGFR inhibition. Repeat dose treatment with HuMab-10F8 was shown to reduce papulopustular rash induced by local zalutumumab injections. The effect was not seen when HuMab-10F8 was applied as a single dose once a week. Because of the local nature of the dermatological events, histological data were only used to illustrate that the zalutumumab-induced rash mimicked the adverse events induced by systemic administration of EGFR inhibitors and to examine the composition of the infiltrate.

In addition to a role in inflammation, IL-8 was also demonstrated to play a role in the survival of tumor cells. Blocking IL-8 has been shown to prevent angiogenesis and reduce tumorigenesis of human non-small cell lung cancer in SCID mice [43]. Furthermore, the combination of antibodies targeting IL-8 with those targeting EGFR resulted in increased anti-tumor effects, as compared with anti-EGFR alone, in a metastatic human breast carcinoma model in SCID mice [44]. Thus, anti-IL-8 and anti-EGFR might provide an interesting combination treatment regimen.

In summary, we developed an innovative human model to study dermatological adverse events induced by EGFR inhibitors. Using this model we showed that neutralization of IL-8 by specific mAb is capable of ameliorating these adverse events. Our study provides a proof-of-principle for a role of IL-8-induced neutrophil migration in the biological mechanisms involved in EGFR inhibitor-induced rash.

Author Contributions

Conceived and designed the experiments: LS OB PP. Performed the experiments: NB LS HN. Analyzed the data: NB MH DS PP OB HN LS. Contributed reagents/materials/analysis tools: NB MH DS PP OB HN LS. Wrote the paper: NB MH DS LS.

References

1. Hansen LA, Woodson RL, 2nd, Holbus S, Strain K, Lo YC, et al. (2000) The epidermal growth factor receptor is required to maintain the proliferative population in the basal compartment of epidermal tumors. Cancer Res 60: 3328–3332.
2. Mimeault M, Bonenfant D, Batra SK (2004) New advances on the functions of epidermal growth factor receptor and ceramides in skin cell differentiation, disorders and cancers. Skin Pharmacol Physiol 17: 153–166.
3. Rowinsky EK (2004) The erbB family: targets for therapeutic development against cancer and therapeutic strategies using monoclonal antibodies and tyrosine kinase inhibitors. Annu Rev Med 55: 433–457.
4. Vivanco I, Mellinghoff IK (2010) Epidermal growth factor receptor inhibitors in oncology. Curr Opin Oncol 22: 573–578.
5. Agero AL, Dusza SW, Benvenuto-Andrade C, Busam KJ, Myskowski P, et al. (2006) Dermatologic side effects associated with the epidermal growth factor receptor inhibitors. J Am Acad Dermatol 55: 657–670.
6. Hu JC, Sadeghi P, Pinter-Brown LC, Yashar S, Chiu MW (2007) Cutaneous side effects of epidermal growth factor receptor inhibitors: clinical presentation, pathogenesis, and management. J Am Acad Dermatol 56: 317–326.
7. Lacouture ME (2006) Mechanisms of cutaneous toxicities to EGFR inhibitors. Nat Rev Cancer 6: 803–812.
8. Robert C, Soria JC, Spatz A, Le Cesne A, Malka D, et al. (2005) Cutaneous side-effects of kinase inhibitors and blocking antibodies. Lancet Oncol 6: 491–500.
9. Herbst RS, Giaccone G, Schiller JH, Natale RB, Miller V, et al. (2004) Gefitinib in combination with paclitaxel and carboplatin in advanced non-small-cell lung cancer: a phase III trial–INTACT 2. J Clin Oncol 22: 785–794.
10. Ho C, Sangha R, Beckett L, Tanaka M, Lau DH, et al. (2011) Escalating weekly doses of cetuximab and correlation with skin toxicity: A phase I study. Invest New Drugs 29: 680–687.
11. Cunningham D, Humblet Y, Siena S, Khayat D, Bleiberg H, et al. (2004) Cetuximab monotherapy and cetuximab plus irinotecan in irinotecan-refractory metastatic colorectal cancer. N Engl J Med 351: 337–345.
12. Saltz LB, Meropol NJ, Loehrer PJ, Sr., Needle MN, Kopit J, et al. (2004) Phase II trial of cetuximab in patients with refractory colorectal cancer that expresses the epidermal growth factor receptor. J Clin Oncol 22: 1201–1208.
13. Alexandrescu DT, Vaillant JG, Dasanu CA (2007) Effect of treatment with a colloidal oatmeal lotion on the acneform eruption induced by epidermal growth factor receptor and multiple tyrosine-kinase inhibitors. Clin Exp Dermatol 32: 71–74.
14. Pinto C, Barone CA, Girolomoni G, Russi EG, Merlano MC, et al. (2011) Management of skin toxicity associated with cetuximab treatment in combination with chemotherapy or radiotherapy. Oncologist 16: 228–238.
15. Segaert S, Van Cutsem E (2005) Clinical signs, pathophysiology and management of skin toxicity during therapy with epidermal growth factor receptor inhibitors. Ann Oncol 16: 1425–1433.
16. Busam KJ, Capodieci P, Motzer R, Kiehn T, Phelan D, et al. (2001) Cutaneous side-effects in cancer patients treated with the antiepidermal growth factor receptor antibody C225. Br J Dermatol 144: 1169–1176.
17. Jacot W, Bessis D, Jorda E, Ychou M, Fabbro M, et al. (2004) Acneiform eruption induced by epidermal growth factor receptor inhibitors in patients with solid tumours. Br J Dermatol 151: 238–241.
18. Kimyai-Asadi A, Jih MH (2002) Follicular toxic effects of chimeric anti-epidermal growth factor receptor antibody cetuximab used to treat human solid tumors. Arch Dermatol 138: 129–131.
19. Skov L, Beurskens FJ, Zachariae CO, Reitamo S, Teeling J, et al. (2008) IL-8 as antibody therapeutic target in inflammatory diseases: reduction of clinical activity in palmoplantar pustulosis. J Immunol 181: 669–679.
20. Bleeker WK, Lammerts van Bueren JJ, van Ojik HH, Gerritsen AF, Pluyter M, et al. (2004) Dual mode of action of a human anti-epidermal growth factor receptor monoclonal antibody for cancer therapy. J Immunol 173: 4699–4707.
21. Machiels JP, Subramanian S, Ruzsa A, Repassy G, Lifirenko I, et al. (2011) Zalutumumab plus best supportive care versus best supportive care alone in patients with recurrent or metastatic squamous-cell carcinoma of the head and neck after failure of platinum-based chemotherapy: an open-label, randomised phase 3 trial. Lancet Oncol 12: 333–343.
22. Journagan S, Obadiah J (2006) An acneiform eruption due to erlotinib: prognostic implications and management. J Am Acad Dermatol 54: 358–360.
23. Molinari E, De Quatrebarbes J, Andre T, Aractingi S (2005) Cetuximab-induced acne. Dermatology 211: 330–333.
24. Gusterson B, Cowley G, Smith JA, Ozanne B (1984) Cellular localisation of human epidermal growth factor receptor. Cell Biol Int Rep 8: 649–658.
25. Nanney LB, Stoscheck CM, King LE Jr., Underwood RA, Holbrook KA (1990) Immunolocalization of epidermal growth factor receptors in normal developing human skin. J Invest Dermatol 94: 742–748.
26. Jost M, Kari C, Rodeck U (2000) The EGF receptor – an essential regulator of multiple epidermal functions. Eur J Dermatol 10: 505–510.
27. Nanney LB, Magid M, Stoscheck CM, King LE Jr., (1984) Comparison of epidermal growth factor binding and receptor distribution in normal human epidermis and epidermal appendages. J Invest Dermatol 83: 385–393.
28. Pastore S, Mascia F, Mariotti F, Dattilo C, Mariani V, et al. (2005) ERK1/2 regulates epidermal chemokine expression and skin inflammation. J Immunol 174: 5047–5056.
29. Rodeck U, Jost M, Kari C, Shih DT, Lavker RM, et al. (1997) EGF-R dependent regulation of keratinocyte survival. J Cell Sci 110 (Pt 2): 113–121.

30. Sibilia M, Wagner EF (1995) Strain-dependent epithelial defects in mice lacking the EGF receptor. Science 269: 234–238.
31. Threadgill DW, Dlugosz AA, Hansen LA, Tennenbaum T, Lichti U, et al. (1995) Targeted disruption of mouse EGF receptor: effect of genetic background on mutant phenotype. Science 269: 230–234.
32. Perez-Soler R, Donato NJ, Shin DM, Rosenblum MG, Zhang HZ, et al. (1994) Tumor epidermal growth factor receptor studies in patients with non-small-cell lung cancer or head and neck cancer treated with monoclonal antibody RG 83852. J Clin Oncol 12: 730–739.
33. Mascia F, Mariani V, Girolomoni G, Pastore S (2003) Blockade of the EGF receptor induces a deranged chemokine expression in keratinocytes leading to enhanced skin inflammation. Am J Pathol 163: 303–312.
34. Busam Kea (2001) Cutaneous side-effects in cancer patients treated with the antiepidermal growth factor receptor antibody C225. British Journal of Dermatology 144: 1169–1176.
35. Surguladze D, Deevi D, Claros N, Corcoran E, Wang S, et al. (2009) Tumor necrosis factor-alpha and interleukin-1 antagonists alleviate inflammatory skin changes associated with epidermal growth factor receptor antibody therapy in mice. Cancer Res 69: 5643–5647.
36. Han SS, Lee M, Park GH, Bang SH, Kang YK, et al. (2010) Investigation of papulopustular eruptions caused by cetuximab treatment shows altered differentiation markers and increases in inflammatory cytokines. Br J Dermatol 162: 371–379.
37. Larsen CG, Anderson AO, Oppenheim JJ, Matsushima K (1989) Production of interleukin-8 by human dermal fibroblasts and keratinocytes in response to interleukin-1 or tumour necrosis factor. Immunology 68: 31–36.
38. Takematsu H, Isono N, Kato T, Tagami H (1990) Normal human epidermal keratinocyte-derived neutrophil chemotactic factor. Tohoku J Exp Med 162: 1–13.
39. Hoffmann TK, Schirlau K, Sonkoly E, Brandau S, Lang S, et al. (2009) A novel mechanism for anti-EGFR antibody action involves chemokine-mediated leukocyte infiltration. Int J Cancer 124: 2589–2596.
40. Larsen CG, Anderson AO, Appella E, Oppenheim JJ, Matsushima K (1989) The neutrophil-activating protein (NAP-1) is also chemotactic for T lymphocytes. Science 243: 1464–1466.
41. Schroder JM, Mrowietz U, Morita E, Christophers E (1987) Purification and partial biochemical characterization of a human monocyte-derived, neutrophil-activating peptide that lacks interleukin 1 activity. J Immunol 139: 3474–3483.
42. Pastore S, Mascia F, Mariani V, Girolomoni G (2008) The epidermal growth factor receptor system in skin repair and inflammation. J Invest Dermatol 128: 1365–1374.
43. Arenberg DA, Kunkel SL, Polverini PJ, Glass M, Burdick MD, et al. (1996) Inhibition of interleukin-8 reduces tumorigenesis of human non-small cell lung cancer in SCID mice. J Clin Invest 97: 2792–2802.
44. Salcedo R, Martins-Green M, Gertz B, Oppenheim JJ, Murphy WJ (2002) Combined administration of antibodies to human interleukin 8 and epidermal growth factor receptor results in increased antimetastatic effects on human breast carcinoma xenografts. Clinical Cancer Research 8: 2655–2665.

9

Intestine-Targeted DGAT1 Inhibition Improves Obesity and Insulin Resistance without Skin Aberrations in Mice

Naoto Tsuda[1,2]*, Shin Kumadaki[1], Chika Higashi[1], Makoto Ozawa[1], Mikihiko Shinozaki[1], Yutaka Kato[1], Koutarou Hoshida[1], Satomi Kikuchi[1], Yoshihisa Nakano[1], Yoshihiro Ogawa[2], Shoji Furusako[1]

1 Discovery Research, Mochida Pharmaceutical Company Limited, Shizuoka, Japan, **2** Department of Molecular Endocrinology and Metabolism, Graduate School of Medical and Dental Sciences, Tokyo Medical and Dental University, Tokyo, Japan

Abstract

Objective: Diacylglycerol O-acyltransferase 1 (DGAT1) catalyzes the final committed step in triglyceride biosynthesis. DGAT1 null mice are known to be resistant to diet-induced obesity, and more insulin sensitive relative to the wild-type; however, the mice exhibit abnormalities in the skin. This work determined whether the intestine-targeted DGAT1 inhibitor could improve obesity and insulin resistance without skin aberrations in mice.

Design and Methods: We synthesized 2 DGAT1 inhibitors: Compound A, described in the patent application from the Japan Tobacco, and Compound B (A-922500), reported by Abbott Laboratories. Both compounds were evaluated for inhibitory activities against DGAT1 enzymes and effects on the skin in mice *in vivo*. Compound B was further investigated for effects on obesity and insulin resistance in diet-induced-obese (DIO) mice.

Results: The 2 compounds comparably inhibited the DGAT1 enzyme activity and the cellular triglyceride synthesis *in vitro*, while they showed different distribution patterns in mice *in vivo*. Compound A, which distributed systemically, caused skin aberrations, while Compound B, which preferentially distributed to the intestine, improved obesity and insulin resistance without skin aberrations in DIO mice.

Conclusions: Our results suggest that the intestine is the key tissue in which DGAT1 plays a role in promoting obesity and insulin resistance.

Editor: Yanqiao Zhang, Northeast Ohio Medical University, United States of America

Funding: Mochida Pharmaceutical provided all funds for this work. NT, SK, CH, MO, MS, YK, KH, SK, YN, and SF are current employees of Mochida Pharmaceutical and may own stock or hold stock options in Mochida Pharmaceutical. The funders had no role in study design, data collection and analysis, decision to publish, or preparation of the manuscript.

Competing Interests: Mochida Pharmaceutical provided all funds for this work. NT, SK, CH, MO, MS, YK, KH, SK, YN, and SF are current employees of Mochida Pharmaceutical and may own stock or hold stock options in Mochida Pharmaceutical.

* Email: naoto.tsuda@mochida.co.jp

Introduction

Diacylglycerol O-acyltransferase (DGAT) 1 and DGAT2 catalyze the final committed step in triglyceride biosynthesis [1]. DGAT1 null mice are resistant to diet-induced obesity, and exhibit higher insulin sensitivity compared to the wild-type [2–4]. These results have revealed that DGAT1 plays important roles in the triglyceride synthesis and regulation of energy metabolism. Similarly, DGAT2 also plays a role in mammalian triglyceride synthesis. Although plasma glucose, triglyceride, free fatty acid levels and liver glycogen are decreased in DGAT2 null mice, these mice are lipopenic and die soon after birth due to reduction in substrates for energy metabolism and profound skin aberrations [5]. Thus, the DGAT1 inhibitor is expected to become a novel treatment option for obesity and type-2 diabetes mellitus (T2DM) without the severe adverse events associated with the DGAT2 inhibition. However, DGAT1 null mice exhibit skin aberrations, presumably due to depletion of essential lipids within the skin [3], and thus the DGAT1 inhibitor could induce skin aberrations when systemically administered for the treatment of obesity and diabetes.

Orally taken triglycerides go through hydrolysis and then are rearranged within the enterocyte into triglyceride-rich chylomicrons destined for systemic circulation. Since DGAT1 catalyzes this triglyceride rearrangement, the improvement of metabolic disorders observed in DGAT1 null mice seems to be derived from lack of DGAT1 activity in the intestine. Moreover, the metabolic phenotypes of DGAT1 null mice such as resistance to hepatic steatosis and diet-induced obesity are reported to be lost when DGAT1 is reintroduced into the intestine [6]. Thus the inhibition of the intestinal DGAT1 may be sufficient to improve metabolic disorders, suggesting that the intestine-targeted DGAT1 inhibitor shows beneficial metabolic effects without skin aberrations. Indeed, a previous report [7] aimed for discovery and optimization of intestine-targeted DGAT1 inhibitors. However, detailed comparisons between systemic delivery and intestine-targeted delivery of DGAT1 inhibitors have not been made so far.

In this study, we evaluated the effects of 2 DGAT1 inhibitors with different distribution patterns on skin aberrations in mice. As a result, we have found that the predominantly intestine-targeted DGAT1 inhibitor attenuates metabolic disorders without inducing skin aberrations.

Materials and Methods

Compounds

Compound A (4-[4-(4-amino-2,7,7-trimethyl-7H-pyrimido[4,5-b][1,4]oxazin-6-yl)phenyl]-trans-Cyclohexaneacetic acid, Figure 1A), described in the patent application from the Japan Tobacco [8], has been reported as a potent DGAT1 inhibitor by AstraZeneca [9]. Compound B (A-922500, (1R, 2R)-2-[[4′-[[(Phenylamino)carbonyl]amino][1,1′-biphenyl]-4-yl]carbonyl]cyclopentanecarboxylic acid, Figure 1B) has also been reported as a potent DGAT1 inhibitor by Pfizer and Abbott Laboratories [10,11]. Compound A and B act on the acyl-CoA binding site of DGAT1 and that they compete each other for the binding to DGAT1 [10]. These compounds were synthesized in our laboratory and used for the present study.

Animals

Male C57BL/6J mice were purchased from Charles River Japan. Mice were fed ad libitum with either a standard rodent chow (CE-2; CLEA Japan, Tokyo, Japan) or a high-fat diet (D12492; Research Diets, New Brunswick, NJ). All animals were housed under a 12-h light-dark cycle (lights on from 7:30 am to 7:30 pm) with free access to food and tap water.

All experimental procedures were approved by the Institutional Animal Care and Use Committee of Mochida Pharmaceutical Research Center. Blood sample was withdrawn from venous blood vessels using heparinized syringe. All surgery was performed under isoflurane anesthesia, and all efforts were made to minimize suffering.

Enzyme assays

The effects of the DGAT1 inhibitors were assessed using human (BC015762 from HeLa cell) and mouse DGAT1 (NM_010046 from mouse testis) in Sf9 insect microsomes. To collect the cell S9 fraction, sf9 cells were infected with the recombinant baculovirus containing human DGAT1 coding sequences and harvested after 72 h. The Sf9 cells were homogenized and centrifuged at 600 g for 20 min. Thereafter, the supernatant was centrifuged at 10000 g for 1 h and the precipitate was collected as the S9 fraction.

The reaction was started by adding ^{14}C decanoyl CoA (0.85 kBq; American Radiolabeled Chemicals Inc., Saint Louis, MO) to 5 μg/ml protein of the S9 fraction with Compound A or B, 150 mM $MgCl_2$, 0.01% BSA and 0.15 mM dioleoyl-glycerol in a total volume of 100 μl in 96-well plates. The mixture was incubated at room temperature for 45 min. The reaction was stopped by adding 0.5 M HCl and the incubated mixture was filtered using Multiscreen$_{HTS}$-FB (Millipore, Billerica, MA). The human DGAT1 activity was quantified by counting the radioactivity of synthesized ^{14}C triglycerides by the Microbeta scintillation counter (PerkinElmer, Waltham, MA) in duplicate. The 50% inhibitory concentration (IC_{50}) was calculated using the sigmoidal curve-fitting program (Symyx Assay Explorer 3.1 SP2; Symyx Technologies Inc., Santa Clara, CA). Mouse DGAT1 enzyme assays were carried out in the same way.

Triglyceride synthesis in HT-29 cells and HepG2 cells

The HT-29 cell line (American Type Culture Collection, Manassas, VA) was maintained in the McCoy's 5A medium (Life Technologies, Carlsbad, CA) containing 10% fetal bovine serum. The HepG2 cell line (American Type Culture Collection) was maintained in the Dulbecco's Modified Eagle Medium (Sigma-Aldrich, St. Louis, MO) containing 10% fetal bovine serum. For the experiments, the HT-29 cells were plated in 12-well plates at 3×10^5 cells, the HepG2 cells were plated in 12-well plates at 5×10^5 cells. The cells were cultured in serum-free media for 24 h, and incubated with a compound and oleic acid-albumin (Sigma-Aldrich) solubilized in dimethyl sulfoxide (final 0.1%) for 30 min. The triglyceride synthesis was initiated by the addition of ^{14}C oleic acid (0.2 μCi). The cells were washed in PBS and harvested into the organic phase using hexane:2-propanol (3:2) 30 min after initiation of the triglyceride synthesis. The solvent was evaporated, the extracts were solubilized in chloroform, and lipids were separated via TLC. Incorporation of the radiolabel into the triglyceride fraction was analyzed using BAS2000 in triplicate. The IC_{50} of each compound was calculated using GraphPad Prism.

Compound distribution in mice

Exposure was analyzed using blood, skin, and intestine samples from the C57BL/6J mice orally treated with 30 mg/kg of a compound. At 1, 4, 8, and 24 h after the administration, mice were anesthetized with isoflurane, and blood, skin, and intestine samples were collected. Three mice were used in each group. The blood samples were collected with sodium heparin, subjected to centrifugation, and plasma samples were collected. The skin and the intestine were homogenized and centrifuged to collect samples. The compound concentrations in each tissue sample with values equal to or greater than the lower limit of quantification (LLOQ; 0.005 μg/ml) were used for analyses (HPLC-MS/MS: Shiseido, Tokyo, Japan, Thermofisher Scientific, Waltham, MA).

Effects of Compound A and B on the skin in diet-induced-obese (DIO) mice

After 10 weeks on high-fat diet, mice became obese (36±0.24 g). Mice showed resistance to diet-induced obesity were excluded from the experiment. Fourteen-week-old male DIO mice were orally administered the vehicle (10% Pluronic F-68 for Compound A, 1% Tween 80 for Compound B), 30 mg/kg

A

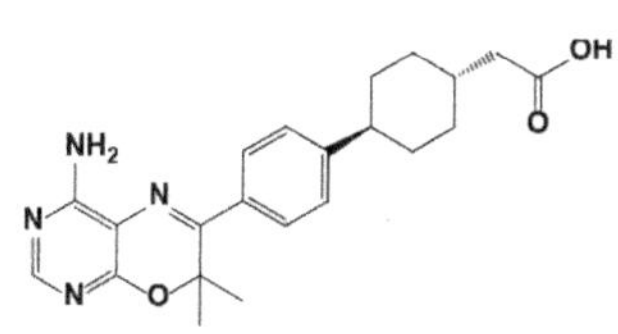

B

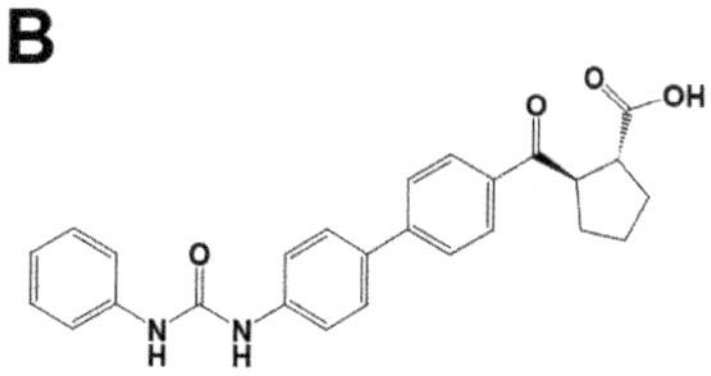

Figure 1. Chemical structures of Compound A (A) and Compound B (B).

Compound A once daily or 30 mg/kg Compound B twice daily. These dosing regimens were decided based on the ratios of concentration at 24 h after the compound administration (C_{24}) in the intestine/the IC50 for mDGAT1 (3.7 for Compound A and 1.2 for Compound B; Table 1) so that both compounds inhibit the intestinal DGAT1 to the same extent at 24 h after their administration. After 4 weeks of the treatment, all the animals were sacrificed. The skin (dorsolateral lesion) was removed and then fixed in 10% neutral buffered formalin, processed, embedded in paraffin, cut into thin sections and stained with Hematoxylin and Eosin. Histopathological examinations were performed. The size of the sebaceous glands were measured using WinROOF (Mitani Corporation, Tokyo, Japan).

Effects of Compound B on postprandial hyperlipidemia in mice

Eight-week-old male C57BL/6J mice were divided into treatment groups, each consisting of 7–8 mice, based on the body weight for the purpose of simplification of dose calculation. Mice were orally administered 1% Tween 80 (vehicle), 0.3, 1, 3, 10, or 30 mg/kg Compound B. Twelve h after administration, mice were orally given 3 ml/kg corn oil. Blood samples were collected 1, 2, and 3 h later, and the plasma triglyceride level was determined by using WAKO TG H (Wako, Osaka, Japan). The area under the curve (AUC) of plasma triglyceride (AUCtriglyceride) was calculated.

Effects of Compound B on glucagon-like peptide-1 (GLP-1) secretion in mice

Mice were divided into treatment groups, each consisting of 6–8 mice, based on the body weight for the purpose of simplification of dose calculation. Mice were orally administered 1% Tween 80 (vehicle), 10, or 30 mg/kg Compound B. Thirty minute after administration, mice were orally given 3 ml/kg corn oil. Blood samples were collected 2 h later, and the plasma GLP-1 level was determined by using Glucagon Like Peptide-1 (Active) ELISA Kit (Linco Research, Inc., St. Charles, MO).

Long-time treatment with Compound B in DIO mice

For evaluation of efficacy of long-time treatment with Compound B, after 10 weeks on high-fat diet, 14-week-old male mice were divided into treatment groups, each consisting of 9–10 animals, based on the body weight and glucose levels. Mice were orally administered 1% Tween 80 (vehicle), 1, 3, 10 or 30 mg/kg Compound B twice daily for 4 weeks. The DIO mice were fed with high-fat diet during the 4-week treatment period. Mice were fasted for 4 hours prior to blood collection. Plasma glucose, insulin, triglyceride, and free fatty acid concentrations were determined by using Glucose CII Test Wako (Wako), ultra sensitive mouse ELISA (Morinaga, Yokohama, Japan), L type WAKO TG H, and HA test WAKO NEFA (Wako), respectively.

Statistical analyses

Data were expressed as means ± SEM or means ± SD. Statistical analyses between the vehicle-treated group and each compound-treated group were performed with the Dunnett's multiple comparison test, and those between the vehicle-treated group and the control group were performed by the t-test, using SAS version 9.1 (SAS Institute Inc, Cary, NC).

Results

Characteristics of the tested compounds *in vitro*

Compound A and B were potent DGAT1 inhibitors for mouse and human DGAT1 (Table 2). These results were consistent with those in the previous reports [9–11].

Inhibition of triglyceride synthesis *in vitro*

In the cellular assay, Compound A was evaluated at concentrations of 0.3 to 3 μM. Compound A inhibited the cellular triglyceride synthesis with the increase in concentrations, and significant inhibition was observed at 1 and 3 μM in HT-29 human colon (Figure 2A) and at all the concentrations tested in HepG2 human liver cells (Figure 2B). Compound B was evaluated at concentrations of 0.1 to 3 μM. Compound B also inhibited the cellular triglyceride synthesis with the increase in concentrations, and significant inhibition was observed at 1 and 3 μM in HT-29 human colon and at all the concentrations tested in HepG2 human liver cells.

Distribution of DGAT1 inhibitors in mice

Figure 3A and 3B show the concentrations of Compound A and B in the plasma, skin, and the intestine of the mice after its oral

Table 1. Pharmacokinetic properties of Compound A and Compound B in mice.

	Compound A	Compound B
T_{max} (h)	1	1
C_{max} in plasma (μM)	240±59	9.1±2.3
plasma/IC_{50}	38±9.2	0.59±0.15
C_{max} in skin (μmol/kg)	14±0.62	1.3±0.51
skin/IC_{50}	2.2±0.097	0.084±0.033
C_{max} in intestine (μmol/kg)	77±37	92±36
intestine/IC_{50}	12±5.8	5.9±2.3
C_{24} in intestine (μmol/kg)	24±1.6	19±3.7
C_{24} in intestine/mDGAT1 IC_{50}	3.7±0.24	1.2±0.24
Intestine/Plasma ratio at T_{max}	0.32±0.090	10±2.8
Intestine/Skin ratio at T_{max}	5.6±2.5	74±8.4

plasma/IC_{50} = C_{max} in plasma/mDGAT1 IC_{50}, skin/IC_{50} = C_{max} in skin/mDGAT1 IC_{50}, intestine/IC_{50} = C_{max} in intestine/mDGAT1 IC_{50}, Three mice were used in each group. Data were expressed as means ± SD.

Table 2. Summary of the effects of Compound A and Compound B.

	Compound A	Compound B
mDGAT1 IC_{50}[a]	6.4 nM	15.5 nM
hDGAT1 IC_{50}[a]	2.6 nM	8.4 nM
Log D	<0.9	<0.9
m plasma protein binding	3.2% free	0.1% free

[a]The 50% inhibitory concentration (IC_{50}) for each compound in the enzymes expressed in insect microsomes.

administration at 30 mg/kg. The time to reach the maximum concentration (Tmax) for Compound A was 1 h, and Compound A exhibited higher concentrations in the plasma and the skin as compared to Compound B (Table 1). The Tmax of Compound B was also 1 h. Compound B exhibited a higher concentration in the intestine in spite of its relatively low concentrations in the plasma and skin. The intestine/plasma and intestine/skin ratios for Compound B (10 and 74) were much higher than those for Compound A (0.32 and 5.6).

Effects of DGAT1 inhibitors on the skin in diet-induced-obese (DIO) mice

The DIO mice treated with Compound A showed skin aberrations derived from atrophy of the sebaceous gland which were characterized by decrease amount and size of sebaceous gland acini (Figure 4A and 4C). All the mice treated with Compound A exhibited skin aberrations, while such aberrations were not observed in the mice treated with the vehicle. Compound A induced no injurious or inflammatory changes, and the skin aberrations recovered 2 weeks after the compound withdrawal. On the other hand, the changes in the skin were not observed in all the DIO mice treated with Compound B, which displayed higher distribution to the intestine over plasma or the skin (Figure 4B and 4C).

Effects of short-time treatment with the intestine-targeted DGAT1 inhibitor on postprandial hyperlipidemia in mice

Compound B was evaluated in a model of postprandial hyperlipidemia by measuring chylomicron-derived triglycerides. Compound B at 0.3, 1, 3, or 10 mg/kg, when orally administered 12 h before the corn oil administration, reduced plasma triglyceride levels with a dose-dependent tendency (Figure 5). The maximum efficacy was achieved at 10 mg/kg. In addition, compound B at 10 and 30 mg/kg also increased plasma glucagon-like peptide-1 (GLP-1) levels after corn oil administration (Figure 5C).

Effects of long-time treatment with the intestine-targeted DGAT1 inhibitor on diet induced obesity in mice

As short-time treatment with Compound B improved postprandial hyperlipidemia, potential anti-obesity effects of Compound B were examined in DIO mice. Following the feeding on high-fat diet for 10 weeks, mice became obese, and exhibited significant increases in the body weight, plasma glucose level, plasma insulin concentration, insulin resistance (HOMA-IR: control vs. DIO = 0.70 vs. 2.0), mesenteric adipose tissue weight, epididymal adipose tissue weight, content of hepatic triglyceride and the content of hepatic total-cholesterol, indicating the development of diet-induced obesity in mice (i.e., DIO mice), as compared to the control mice fed on normal diet. In DIO mice, long-time treatment with Compound B attenuated the body weight gain with the increase in doses (Figure 6A). After the 4-week treatment period, significant attenuation and significant reduction were observed at 10 mg/kg and 30 mg/kg, respectively (Figure 6B). Compound B reduced plasma glucose levels (Figure 6C), and significant reduction was observed at 30 mg/kg. Insulin concentrations tended to decrease in the DIO mice treated with Compound B (Figure 6D). There were also differences in the weight of white adipose tissue (WAT) among the groups.

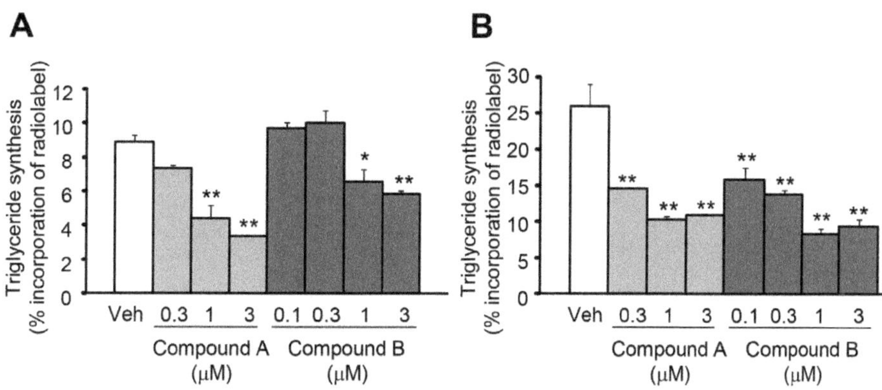

Figure 2. Effects of Compound A and Compound B on the triglyceride synthesis. The effects of Compound A and Compound B on the triglyceride synthesis in HT-29 human colon cells (A) and in HepG2 human liver cells (B). Data are expressed as means + SEM of 3 assays. *$P<0.05$ and **$P<0.01$. Statistical analyses between the vehicle (Veh) group and compound-treated groups were performed by the Dunnett's multiple comparison test.

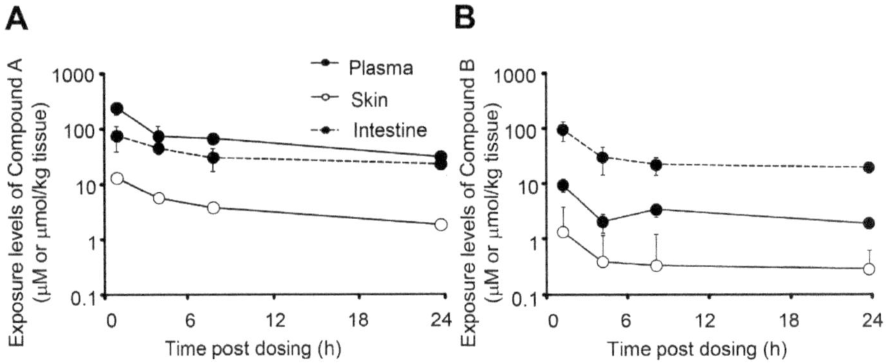

Figure 3. Plasma and tissue concentrations after single oral dosing of Compound A and Compound B. Plasma, skin, and intestine samples were collected from the mice orally administered 30 mg/kg Compound A (A) or B (B). Data are expressed as means ± SD of 3 animals.

Treatment with Compound B reduced the weight of mesenteric (Figure 6E) and epididymal (Figure 6F) fat with the increase in doses and significant reduction was observed at 30 mg/kg. Furthermore, despite lack of differences in the liver weight among the groups (Figure 6G), Compound B reduced concentrations of triglyceride and total-cholesterol in the liver with the increase of doses, and significant reduction was observed at 30 mg/kg (Figure 6H, 6I). Histological analysis also indicated that Compound B attenuated fatty liver (Figure S1).

Discussion

DGAT1 is an endoplasmic membrane bound enzyme which catalyzes the final committed step in triglyceride biosynthesis, distributed in various tissues such as the skeletal muscle, liver, adipose tissue, intestine and the skin. In addition to the metabolic phenotypes of DGAT1 null mice such as resistance to hepatic steatosis and diet-induced obesity, they exhibit skin aberrations owing to lack of DGAT1 in the skin [3]. As the metabolic phenotypes of DGAT1 null mice are lost when DGAT1 is reintroduced into the intestine [6], we raised a hypothesis that the intestine-targeted DGAT1 inhibitor would improve metabolic disorders with minimizing the adverse effect that may be driven by systemic DGAT1 inhibition. In this study, we focused on effects of the 2 DGAT1 inhibitors with different distribution patterns on skin aberrations in mice. Consequently, we found that the predominantly intestine-targeted DGAT1 inhibitor Compound B did not exhibit skin aberrations, while the systemically distributed Compound A caused skin aberrations in DIO mice. We also indicated that the intestine-targeted DGAT1 inhibitor improved metabolic disorders in DIO mice.

The present result showed that Compound A and B similarly inhibited the activities of the mouse and the human DGAT1 enzyme *in vitro* as previously reported [9–11]. Moreover, both compounds inhibited the cellular triglyceride synthesis in HT-29, HepG2, and mouse skin homogenates. In spite of similar profiles *in vitro*, we identified that orally administered Compound A and B exhibited different distribution patterns in mice *in vivo*. The recent publication [12] indicates that distribution of DGAT1 inhibitors to the skin did correlate with its lipophilicity. However lipophilicity (Log D) of Compound A and B were similarly low. Although the precise reason for the difference of distribution has not yet been identified, the intestine-targeted distribution of Compound B may potentially be due to its transporter-mediated efflux from the intestine in the same way as previously discussed with another intestine-targeted DGAT1 inhibitor [7]. It is noteworthy that the intestine/plasma and intestine/skin ratios for Compound B (10 and 74) were much higher than those for Compound A (0.32 and 5.6). Since there is a report that Compound A shows beneficial metabolic effects [10], we focused on whether the predominantly intestine-targeted DGAT1 inhibitor could improve obesity and insulin resistance without skin aberrations in mice in the present study.

In a model of postprandial hyperlipidemia measuring chylomicron-derived triglycerides in mice, single oral administration of Compound B reduced plasma triglyceride levels. This is consistent with the previous observations on the suppression by other DGAT1 inhibitors of postprandial hyperlipidemia [9–11] and the delayed fat absorption in DGAT1 null mice [13–14]. Furthermore, Compound B also increased plasma GLP-1 levels after corn oil administration. The present results support the hypothesis that intestinal DGAT1 might directly regulate the releases of GLP-1 [15]. It might be possible that diacylglycerol accumulated in the intestinal cells following oil administration stimulates the release of GLP-1, since it has been known that the activation of phorbol ester-sensitive protein kinase C leads to GLP-1 release. These results highlighted that pharmacological as well as genetic inhibition of DGAT1 in the intestine would reduce dietary fat absorption and increase plasma GLP-1 levels.

Long-time treatment with Compound B, which selectively inhibits intestinal DGAT1, reduced the body weight gain, weight of white adipose tissues, hepatic triglyceride and the hepatic cholesterol content in DIO mice. In addition, long-time treatment with Compound B reduced plasma glucose levels and tended to reduce insulin concentrations, suggesting that Compound B would improve insulin resistance. In the recent publication [12], the pharmacokinetic/pharmacodynamic relationship of DGAT1 inhibitors between tissue concentration/IC_{50} and its effects was reported. High value (>1) of intestine/IC_{50} of Compound B in spite of its relatively low values of skin/IC_{50} and plasma/IC_{50} supports the consideration that the effects of DGAT1 inhibitors are achieved by the compound in intestine. The beneficial metabolic effects of Compound B may, at least partly, be ascribed to suppressed fat absorption from the intestine via inhibited intestinal DGAT1, as postprandial hyperlipidemia is assumed to promote hepatic steatosis [16] and insulin resistance. In addition to reduction of fat absorption, since it is known that GLP-1 has beneficial metabolic effects such as reduction of body weight gain and improvement of insulin resistance, increased GLP-1 secretion via the inhibition of intestinal DGAT1 would also contribute to the favorable metabolic effects of Compound B.

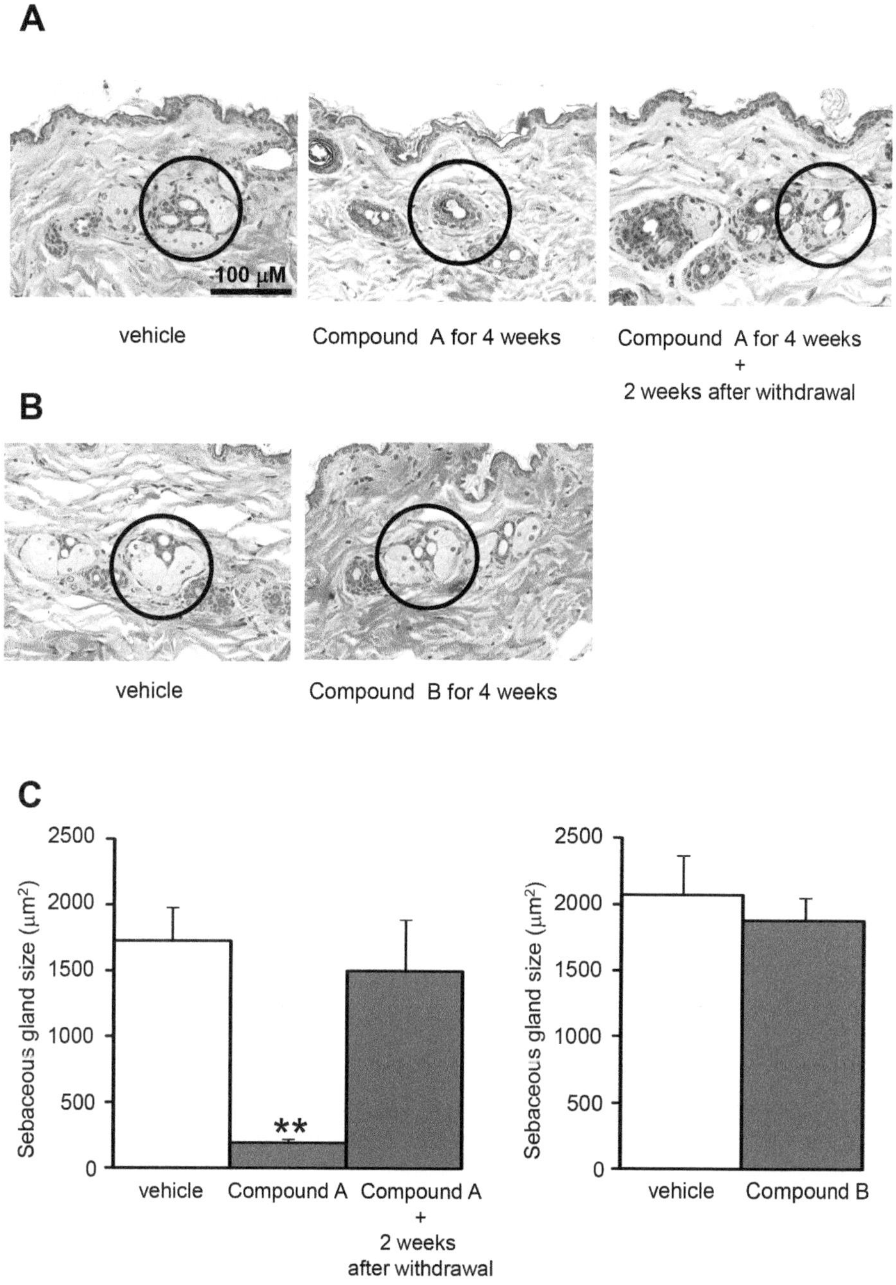

Figure 4. Microphotographs of the skin from the diet-induced-obese (DIO) mice. Microphotographs of the skin from the diet-induced-obese (DIO) mice treated with vehicle (10% Pluronic F-68 for Compound A, 1% Tween 80 for Compound B), 30 mg/kg Compound A once daily (A), or 30 mg/kg Compound B twice daily (B) for 4 weeks. The sebaceous gland is surrounded with a circle. The mice administered Compound A showed moderate skin aberrations derived from atrophy of the sebaceous gland. There were no injurious or inflammatory changes, and the skin aberrations recovered 2 weeks after the Compound A withdrawal. There were no skin aberrations in the mice administered Compound B. The sebaceous gland sizes are plotted (C). Data are expressed as means + SEM (N = 4). ***P*<0.01. Statistical analyses between the vehicle-treated group and Compound-treated groups were performed by the Dunnett's multiple comparison test.

It is well known that obesity, particularly excessive triglyceride deposition in the non-adipose tissues such as the skeletal muscle and the liver, is related to diabetes and insulin resistance [17–21]. DGAT1 inhibition in the whole body may reduce excessive triglyceride deposition in the non-adipose tissues including the skeletal muscle [22], resulting in amelioration of metabolic disorders. In contrast, however, the inhibition of DGAT1 activities in the skeletal muscle or macrophage may cause insulin resistance, leading to aggravation of metabolic disorders, as a result of inhibited conversion of fatty acids substrates which induce insulin resistance into the form of triglyceride [23,24]. Those opposing actions of DGAT1 may explain the reasons why the reintroduction of DGAT1 into the intestine of DGAT1 null mice is sufficient to lose metabolic phenotypes such as resistance to hepatic steatosis and diet-induced obesity, and why long-time treatment with Compound B showed beneficial metabolic effects such as insulin-sensitization and reduction of the body weight gain and hepatic lipids.

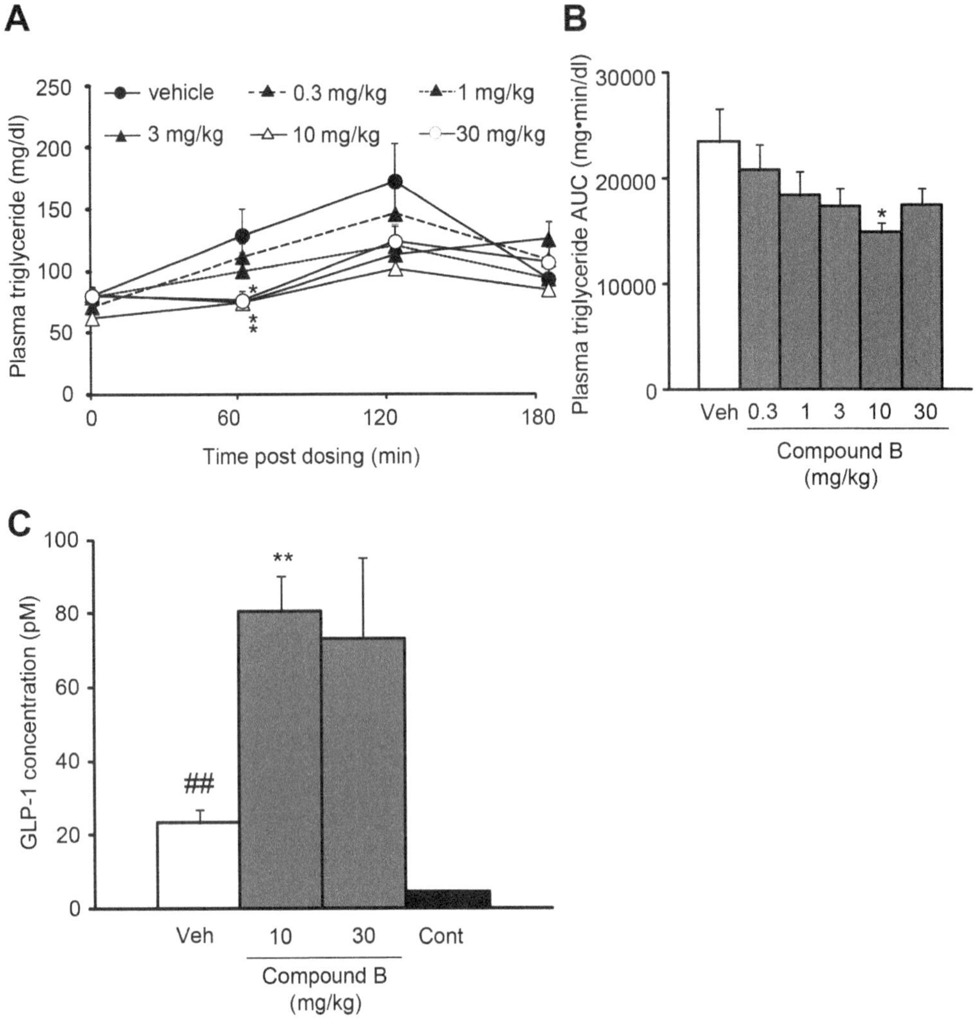

Figure 5. Effects of Compound B on the plasma triglyceride (A, B) and glucagon-like peptide-1 (C) levels. The changes in plasma triglyceride (A) and AUCtriglyceride (−5−180 min) of plasma triglyceride (B), and the plasma GLP-1 levels 2 h following corn oil administration (C) are indicated. The plasma GLP-1 levels of the mice given corn oil are higher than the control mice (Cont). Data are expressed as means + SEM of 6–8 animals. *$P<0.05$ and **$P<0.01$. Statistical analyses between the vehicle (Veh)-treated group and Compound B-treated groups were performed by the Dunnett's multiple comparison test. ##$P<0.01$. Statistical analyses between the vehicle-treated group and the control group were performed by the t-test.

Long-time treatment with Compound B for 4 weeks did not cause any skin aberrations in DIO mice. Long-time treatment with Compound A, in contrast to that with Compound B, caused moderate skin aberrations derived from atrophy of the sebaceous gland which were characterized by decrease amount and size of sebaceous gland acini. The skin aberrations associated with Compound A were not injurious or inflammatory changes, and the aberrations recovered 2 weeks after the compound withdrawal. As these skin aberrations resemble the observations in DGAT1 null mice, depletion of essential lipids due to DGAT1 inhibition is likely to be responsible for the aberrations. The results from the present study and DGAT1 null mice demonstrate that congenital DGAT1 is involved in maintenance and/or development of the sebaceous gland, producing fur essential lipids. As both Compound A and B inhibited the triglyceride synthesis, the lack of skin aberrations in the DIO mice treated with Compound B seems to be due to its minimal distribution to the skin.

Clinical data [25,26] indicate that profound gastrointestinal (GI) adverse events such as nausea, diarrhea, and vomiting appear likely related to DGAT1 inhibition/loss of function in the GI tract. Ideally, a DGAT1 inhibitor as an oral therapeutic agent should overcome those adverse events. In the present study, we cannot deny the possibility that the DGAT1 inhibitor with intestine-restricted distribution may have the same problems in human. Although adverse events would, at least partly, be caused by the inhibition of intestinal DGAT1, their precise mechanisms are unclear. Further clinical studies of intestine-targeted compounds would clarify the therapeutic window of this type of DGAT1 inhibitors.

In conclusion, this study has shown for the first time that the intestine-targeted delivery of the DGAT1 inhibitor improves postprandial hyperlipidemia, body adiposity, hepatic lipid accumulation and insulin resistance without skin aberrations. The presently-observed improvement of metabolic abnormalities is in agreement with other reported results of the studies using DGAT1 inhibitors with different chemical structures [9–11,27–28] or DGAT1 null mice. Collectively, our results provide pharmacological support for the hypothesis that the intestine is the key tissue

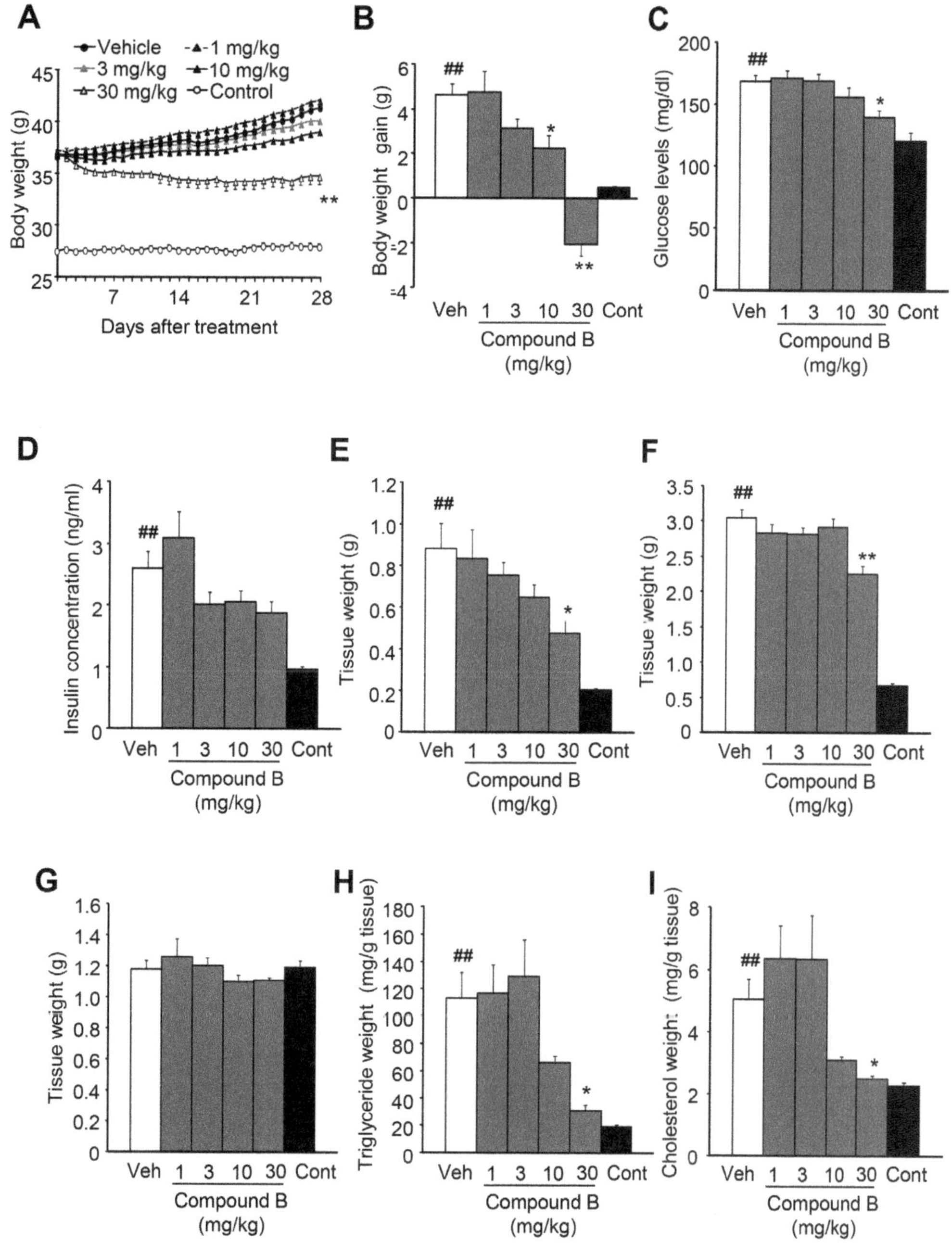

Figure 6. Effects of Compound B in diet-induced-obese (DIO) mice. Mice were orally treated with 1% Tween 80 (vehicle; Veh) or 30 mg/kg Compound B twice daily for 4 weeks. The time-course of body weight changes (A) and the body weight gain at 4 weeks of Compound B treatment (B) are indicated respectively. The body weight of the mice fed a high-fat diet is significantly higher than the control mice (Cont) fed a standard rodent chow during the 4-week treatment period. The plasma glucose level (C), plasma insulin concentration (D), mesenteric adipose tissue weight (E), epididymal adipose tissue weight (F), liver weight (G), content of hepatic triglyceride (H), and the content of hepatic total-cholesterol (I) at 4 weeks of Compound B treatment are indicated respectively. Data are expressed as means ± SEM of 9–10 animals. *$P<0.05$ and **$P<0.01$. Statistical analyses between the vehicle-treated group and Compound B-treated groups were performed by the Dunnett's multiple comparison test. ##$P<0.01$. Statistical analyses between the vehicle-treated group and the control group were performed by the t-test.

in which DGAT1 plays a role in promoting obesity and insulin resistance when exposed to high fat food.

Supporting Information

Figure S1 Effects of Compound B on the hepatic steatosis. Hematoxylin and Eosin staining of liver obtained from the diet-induced-obese (DIO) mice treated with vehicle, 10 or 30 mg/kg Compound B for 4 weeks.

Acknowledgments

We thank the members of the discovery research division of Mochida Pharmaceutical Company Limited, including Akira Karasawa and Junji

Takada for their writing assistant and general support. All authors were involved in writing the paper and have approved the final manuscript.

Author Contributions

Conceived and designed the experiments: NT SK CH MO MS YK KH SK YN YO SF. Performed the experiments: NT SK CH MO MS YK KH SK YN. Analyzed the data: NT SK CH MO KH SK YN. Contributed reagents/materials/analysis tools: NT SK CH MS YK SK YN. Contributed to the writing of the manuscript: NT YK.

References

1. Cases S, Smith SJ, Zheng YW, Myers HM, Lear SR, et al. (1998) Identification of a gene encoding an acyl CoA:diacylglycerol acyltransferase, a key enzyme in triacylglycerol synthesis. Proc. Natl. Acad. Sci. U. S. A. 95: 13018–23.
2. Smith SJ, Cases S, Jensen DR, Chen HC, Sande E, et al. (2000) Obesity resistance and multiple mechanisms of triglyceride synthesis in mice lacking Dgat. Nat Genet. 25: 87–90.
3. Chen HC, Smith SJ, Ladha Z, Jensen DR, Ferreira LD, et al. (2002) Increased insulin and leptin sensitivity in mice lacking acyl CoA:diacylglycerol acyltransferase 1. J. Clin. Invest. 109: 1049–55.
4. Chen HC, Farese RV Jr (2005) Inhibition of triglyceride synthesis as a treatment strategy for obesity: lessons from DGAT1-deficient mice. Arterioscler. Thromb. Vasc. Biol. 25: 482–6.
5. Stone SJ, Myers HM, Watkins SM, Brown BE, Feingold KR, et al. (2004) Lipopenia and skin barrier abnormalities in DGAT2-deficient mice. J. Biol. Chem. 279: 11767–76.
6. Lee B, Fast AM, Zhu J, Cheng JX, Buhman KK (2010) Intestine-specific expression of acyl CoA:diacylglycerol acyltransferase 1 reverses resistance to diet-induced hepatic steatosis and obesity in Dgat1 −/− mice. J. Lipid Res. 51: 1770–80.
7. Michael HSW, Gary MC, Yongjin G, Alan DN, Ricardo C, et al. (2012) Intestinally Targeted Diacylglycerol Acyltransferase 1 (DGAT1) Inhibitors Robustly Suppress Postprandial Triglycerides. ACS Med. Chem. Lett. 3: 411–5.
8. Brian MF, Furukawa N, Hao X, Iio K, Inaba T, et al (2004) Fused bicyclic nitrogen-containing heterocycles. International Patent Application. WO 2004047755 A2.
9. Birch AM, Birtles S, Buckett LK, Kemmitt PD, Smith GJ, et al. (2009) Discovery of a potent, selective, and orally efficacious pyrimidinooxazinyl bicyclooctaneacetic acid diacylglycerol acyltransferase-1 inhibitor. J. Med. Chem. 52: 1558–68.
10. Cao J, Zhou Y, Peng H, Huang X, Stahler S, et al. (2011) Targeting Acyl-CoA:diacylglycerol acyltransferase 1 (DGAT1) with small molecule inhibitors for the treatment of metabolic diseases. J. Biol. Chem. 286: 41838–51.
11. King AJ, Segreti JA, Larson KJ, Souers AJ, Kym PR, et al. (2009) Diacylglycerol acyltransferase 1 inhibition lowers serum triglycerides in the Zucker fatty rat and the hyperlipidemic hamster. J. Pharmacol. Exp. Ther. 330: 526–31.
12. Muise ES, Zhu Y, Verras A, Karanam BV, Gorski J, et al. (2014) Identification and characterization of sebaceous gland atrophy-sparing DGAT1 inhibitors. PLoS One. 18: e88908.
13. Buhman KK, Smith SJ, Stone SJ, Repa JJ, Wong JS, et al. (2002) DGAT1 is not essential for intestinal triacylglycerol absorption or chylomicron synthesis. J. Biol. Chem. 277: 25474–9.
14. Ables GP, Yang KJ, Vogel S, Hernandez-Ono A, Yu S, et al. (2012) Intestinal DGAT1 deficiency reduces postprandial triglyceride and retinyl ester excursions by inhibiting chylomicron secretion and delaying gastric emptying. J. Lipid Res. 53: 2364–79.
15. Okawa M, Fujii K, Ohbuchi K, Okumoto M, Aragane K, et al. (2009) Role of MGAT2 and DGAT1 in the release of gut peptides after triglyceride ingestion. Biochem. Biophys. Res. Commun. 390: 377–81.
16. Musso G, Gambino R, Durazzo M, Biroli G, Carello M, et al. (2005) Adipokines in NASH: postprandial lipid metabolism as a link between adiponectin and liver disease. Hepatology 42: 1175–83.
17. Phillips DI, Caddy S, Ilic V, Fielding BA, Frayn KN, et al. (1996) Intramuscular triglyceride and muscle insulin sensitivity: evidence for a relationship in nondiabetic subjects. Metabolism 45: 947–50.
18. Pan DA, Lillioja S, Kriketos AD, Milner MR, Baur LA, et al. (1997) Skeletal muscle triglyceride levels are inversely related to insulin action. Diabetes 46: 983–8.
19. Ebeling P, Essen-Gustavsson B, Tuominen JA, Koivisto VA. (1998) Intramuscular triglyceride content is increased in IDDM. Diabetologia 41: 111–5.
20. Manco M, Mingrone G, Greco AV, Capristo E, Gniuli D, et al. (2000) Insulin resistance directly correlates with increased saturated fatty acids in skeletal muscle triglycerides. Metabolism 49: 220–4.
21. Virkamaki A, Korsheninnikova E, Seppala-Lindroos A, Vehkavaara S, Goto T, et al. (2001) Intramyocellular lipid is associated with resistance to in vivo insulin actions on glucose uptake, antilipolysis, and early insulin signaling pathways in human skeletal muscle. Diabetes 50: 2337–43.
22. Yamamoto T, Yamaguchi H, Miki H, Kitamura S, Nakada Y, et al. (2011) A novel coenzyme A:diacylglycerol acyltransferase 1 inhibitor stimulates lipid metabolism in muscle and lowers weight in animal models of obesity. Eur. J. Pharmacol. 650: 663–72.
23. Liu L, Zhang Y, Chen N, Shi X, Tsang B, et al. (2007) Upregulation of myocellular DGAT1 augments triglyceride synthesis in skeletal muscle and protects against fat-induced insulin resistance. J. Clin. Invest. 117: 1679–89.
24. Koliwad SK, Streeper RS, Monetti M, Cornelissen I, Chan L, et al. (2010) DGAT1-dependent triacylglycerol storage by macrophages protects mice from diet-induced insulin resistance and inflammation. J. Clin. Invest. 120: 756–67.
25. Haas JT, Winter HS, Lim E, Kirby A, Blumenstiel B, et al. (2012) DGAT1 mutation is linked to a congenital diarrheal disorder. J. Clin. Invest. 122: 4680–8.
26. Denison H, Nilsson C, Löfgren L, Himmelmann A, Mårtensson G, et al. (2014) Diacylglycerol acyltransferase 1 inhibition with AZD7687 alters lipid handling and hormone secretion in the gut with intolerable side effects: a randomized clinical trial. Diabetes Obes. Metab. 16: 334–43.
27. Zhao G, Souers AJ, Voorbach M, Falls HD, Droz B, et al. (2008) Validation of diacyl glycerolacyltransferase I as a novel target for the treatment of obesity and dyslipidemia using a potent and selective small molecule inhibitor. J. Med. Chem. 51: 380–3.
28. Yamamoto T, Yamaguchi H, Miki H, Shimada M, Nakada Y, et al. (2010) Coenzyme A: diacylglycerol acyltransferase 1 inhibitor ameliorates obesity, liver steatosis, and lipid metabolism abnormality in KKAy mice fed high-fat or high-carbohydrate diets. Eur. J. Pharmacol. 640: 243–9.

10

Cutaneous Injury-Related Structural Changes and Their Progression following Topical Nitrogen Mustard Exposure in Hairless and Haired Mice

Neera Tewari-Singh[1]◔, Anil K. Jain[1]◔, David J. Orlicky[2], Carl W. White[3], Rajesh Agarwal[1]*

1 Department of Pharmaceutical Sciences, Skaggs School of Pharmacy and Pharmaceutical Sciences, University of Colorado Denver, Aurora, Colorado, United States of America, **2** Department of Pathology, School of Medicine, University of Colorado Denver, Aurora, Colorado, United States of America, **3** Department of Pediatrics, School of Medicine, University of Colorado Denver, Aurora, Colorado, United States of America

Abstract

To identify effective therapies against sulfur mustard (SM)-induced skin injuries, various animals have been used to assess the cutaneous pathology and related histopathological changes of SM injuries. However, these efforts to establish relevant skin injury endpoints for efficacy studies have been limited mainly due to the restricted assess of SM. Therefore, we employed the SM analog nitrogen mustard (NM), a primary vesicating and bifunctional alkylating agent, to establish relevant endpoints for efficient efficacy studies. Our published studies show that NM (3.2 mg) exposure for 12–120 h in both the hairless SKH-1 and haired C57BL/6 mice caused clinical sequelae of toxicity similar to SM exposure in humans. The NM-induced cutaneous pathology-related structural changes were further analyzed in this study and quantified morphometrically (as percent length or area of epidermis or dermis) of skin sections in mice showing these lesions. H&E stained skin sections of both hairless and haired mice showed that NM (12–120 h) exposure caused epidermal histopathological effects such as increased epidermal thickness, epidermal-dermal separation, necrotic/dead epidermis, epidermal denuding, scab formation, parakeratosis (24–120 h), hyperkeratosis (12–120 h), and acanthosis with hyperplasia (72–120 h). Similar NM exposure in both mice caused dermal changes including necrosis, edema, increase in inflammatory cells, and red blood cell extravasation. These NM-induced cutaneous histopathological features are comparable to the reported lesions from SM exposure in humans and animal models. This study advocates the usefulness of these histopathological parameters observed due to NM exposure in screening and optimization of rescue therapies against NM and SM skin injuries.

Editor: Xiaolin Zi, University of California Irvine, United States of America

Funding: This work was supported by the Countermeasures Against Chemical Threats (CounterACT) Program, Office of the Director National Institutes of Health (OD) and the National Institute of Environmental Health Sciences (NIEHS), [Grant Number U54 ES015678]. The funders had no role in study design, data collection and analysis, decision to publish, or preparation of the manuscript.

* E-mail: Rajesh.Agarwal@ucdenver.edu

◔ These authors contributed equally to this work.

Introduction

Upon cutaneous exposure, only 20% of sulfur mustard (SM) is absorbed, leading to acute and chronic skin lesions [1]. This warfare agent is a weapon of mass destruction, and its toxic skin effects have been observed in the Iranian soldiers and civilians exposed to SM during the Iran-Iraq conflict [2–4]. Depending upon the dose and time of SM exposure, within hours, edema develops and blister formation occurs. This is followed by ulceration, necrosis, desquamation, and pigmentation changes, dry skin after weeks and even years of exposure [5,6]. The histopathology of these human skin lesions show signs of toxicity including pyknotic nuclei and death of some of the basal keratinocytes, and epidermal-dermal separation [7]. Other epidermal changes included parakeratosis, hyperkeratosis, hyperplasia, necrosis, apoptosis, acanthosis and multinucleated giant cells, and pigmentation changes [3,4,8,9]. In addition to epidermal necrosis, dermal necrosis is also observed with infiltration of inflammatory cells, perivascular edema, vascular dilation, and extravasated erythrocytes [4,8]. Animal models showing these toxic lesions by SM are crucial to understand the mechanisms underlying these effects, and to identify and develop effective treatments for SM-induced skin injuries.

Several animal models display many cutaneous lesions and structural changes with SM that are seen in humans [5,8,10–13]. However, there is still a limitation of access to mechanistic examination and routine laboratory efficacy studies in SM models due to its confinement to highly regulated containment facilities. Accordingly, our studies were directed to develop a practical experimental model and establish quantitative endpoints with the easily accessible SM analog of nitrogen mustard (NM). Both SM and NM are vesicating and powerful alkylating agents, and show parallel histopathological and immunohistochemical toxic effects following cutaneous exposure [6,14]. However, comprehensive studies on the histopathological effects of NM skin injury in animal models that parallel SM exposure and can be subjected to useful

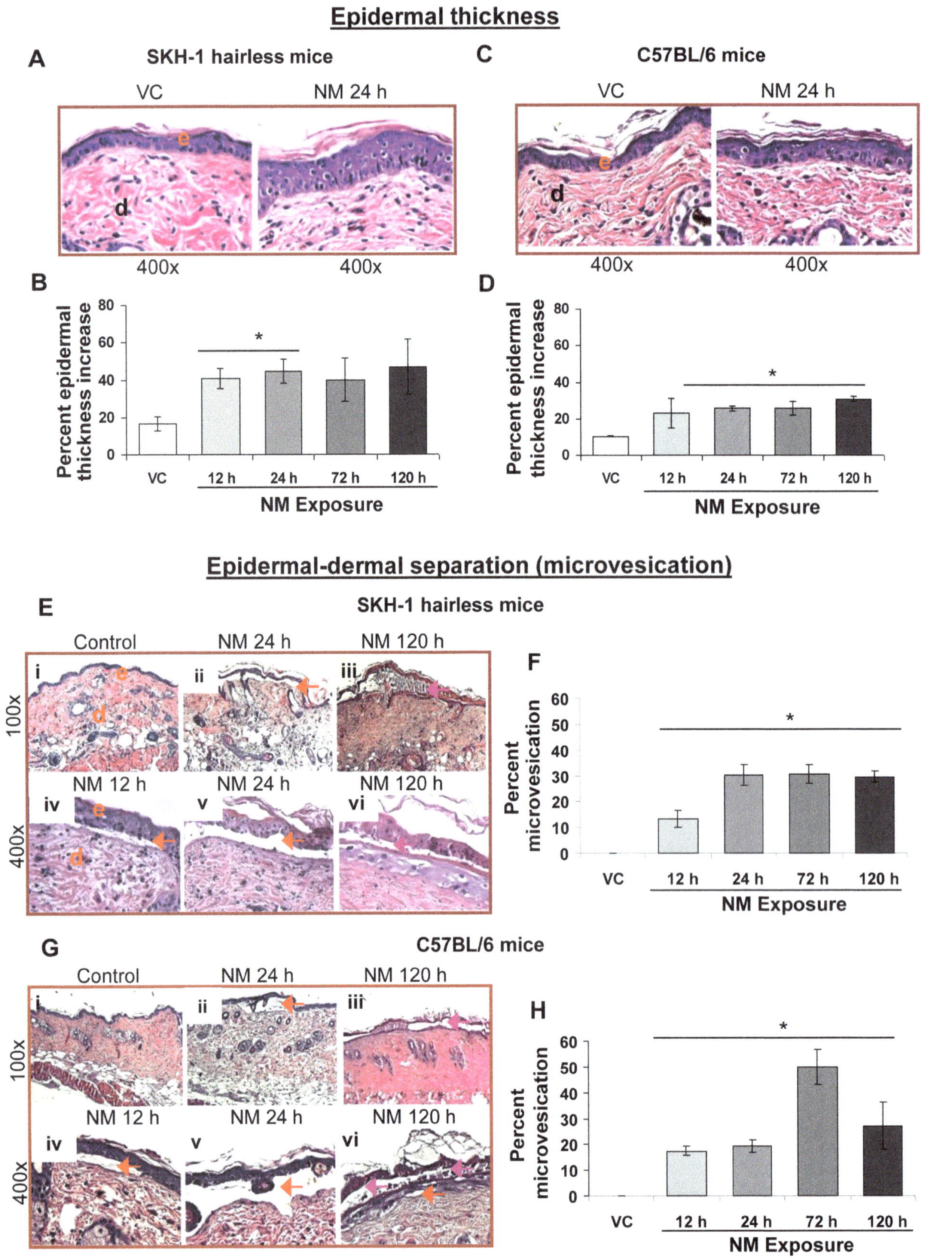

Figure 1. NM exposure causes epidermal thickness and microvesication in the skin of SKH-1 hairless and C57BL/6 mice. Dorsal skin of mice was exposed topically to either 200 μL of acetone or NM (3.2 mg) in 200 μL acetone. After 12, 24, 72 and 120 h of NM exposure, mice were

sacrificed and dorsal skin tissue sections (5 μm) were processed, H&E stained and analyzed as detailed under Materials and Methods. Panels A and C are representative H&E stained skin sections (400× magnification) showing epidermal thickness from vehicle control and 24 h exposed NM exposed skin tissue in SKH-1 and C57BL/6 mice, respectively. Panel E (i–iii) and G (i–iii) are representative H&E stained skin sections (100× magnification), and E (iv–vi) and G (iv–vi) are representative H&E stained skin sections (400× magnification) showing microvesication from vehicle control and 12–120 h NM exposed skin tissue in mice. These NM-related histopathological changes were assessed as detailed under materials and methods, and calculated as percent length of mice skin epidermis showing epidermal thickness (B and D) and microvesication (F and H). Data presented are mean ± SEM of 3–5 animals in each group. *, $p<0.05$ compared to respective vehicle control; VC, vehicle control; NM, nitrogen mustard; e, epidermis; d, dermis; red arrows, microvesication (epidermal and dermal separation); pink arrows, microvesication within the epidermal layer.

efficacy studies are few. Our reported clinical observations with topical NM (3.2 mg) exposure in both SKH-1 hairless and C57BL/6 mice displayed clinical lesions and their progression, which were comparable to those reported in humans and other animal models with SM [15]. Our earlier report also presented clinically-relevant cutaneous injury endpoints that could be useful for efficacy studies to identify therapies against vesicating agents.

In the current study, we sought to further examine the histopathological effects and structural changes responsible for the clinical sequelae of NM-induced toxicity observed in our earlier reported study. Similar to this reported study, both hairless (SKH-1) and haired (C56BL/6) mice were used in this study to analyze the NM-induced histopathological changes. The current assessment will help define any differences in the injury response due to uptake or absorption of NM in the skin of both strains. This study demonstrates that NM cutaneous exposure resulted in epidermal thickness, epidermal-dermal separation, necrolytic/dead epidermis, epidermal denudation and ulceration, scab formation, parakeratosis, hyperkeratosis, and acanthosis associated with hyperplasia in both haired and hairless mice. NM exposure in these mice also caused dermal necrosis and edema, increase in inflammatory cells, and red blood cell extravasation. Overall, NM-induced structural changes in hairless and haired mice evaluated in this study parallel the reported lesions from SM exposure in humans and animal models.

Materials and Methods

Animals and NM Exposure

Both SKH-1 hairless and C57BL/6 (haired) mice (5–6 weeks of age) were purchased from Charles River Labs (Wilmington, MA), and housed under standard conditions and acclimatized before their use in our experimental studies. The Institutional Animal Care and Use Committee (IACUC) of the University of Colorado Denver, CO have specifically approved the studies with mice reported in this article. Mice (n = 5) were either exposed topically to 200 μL acetone alone or to 3.2 mg NM (mechorethamine hydrochloride; Sigma-Aldrich Chemical Co., St. Louis MO) in 200 μL acetone for 12 h, 24 h, 72 h and 120 h. Respective untreated control group was included in the study. C57BL/6 mice were shaved 3 days prior to NM exposure. Following the above mentioned exposures, mice were euthanized, the dorsal skin was collected and either snap frozen in liquid nitrogen or fixed in 10% phosphate buffered formalin as detailed earlier [15–17].

Histopathological Evaluation

The formalin-fixed dorsal skin sample was dehydrated in ascending concentration of ethanol, cleared in xylene, and embedded in PolyFin (Triangle Biomedical Sciences, Durham, NC) as detailed earlier [16,17]. Five-micrometer serial sections were cut and stained with hematoxylin and eosin (H&E), and examined for NM-induced histopathological changes that were scored as follows: a) Percent length or area of mouse skin epidermis or dermis, respectively showing the events listed below and b) incidences of scab formation or outgrowths in skin section.

The histopathological changes were assessed in the three skin sections [(approx.18 mm length per skin tissue section under 400× magnification using Axiovision Rel 4.5 software (Carl Zeiss, Inc. Germany)] from each mouse and an average value was arrived at for each mouse in each exposure group. The infiltration of inflammatory cells was scored as: +, few (less than 100); ++, moderate (100–1000); +++, high (more than 1000) inflammatory cells per skin section (at 400× magnification). The extravasated RBCs were scored as: +, few (less than 10%); ++, moderate (10–30%); +++, high (more than 30%) extravasated RBCs per skin section (at 400× magnification).

Statistical Analysis

Data were analyzed using one-way analysis of variance (one-way ANOVA) to get the statistically significant difference in control versus treated groups, with Tukey or Bonferroni t-test for multiple comparisons (SigmaStat 2.03). Differences were considered significant if the p value was ≤0.05. Data are presented as the mean ± standard error of mean (SEM).

Results

Our published study showed that NM exposure (3.2 mg) for 12–120 h caused edema, erythema, microblister formation, pigmentation changes, dry skin and wounded areas on the skin of SKH-1 hairless and C57BL/6 mice [15]. The skin from these mice was collected, fixed, sectioned and H&E stained to further assess for structural changes associated with these NM-induced lesions.

NM Exposure causes Structural Changes in the Epidermis of the Skin in SKH-1 and C57BL/6 Mice

In the epidermis, death of keratinocytes and epidermal dermal separation, as well as inflammation-related changes with SM exposure were observed [4,18]. Hence, we sought to study these structural changes following NM exposure in hairless and haired mice.

i) Epidermal thickness and microvesication. Our clinical observations in NM (3.2 mg) exposed haired and hairless mice skin revealed increased bi-fold thickness and microblister like appearance [15]. In this study, the histopathology of the skin sections from these NM-exposed mice showed increased epidermal thickness and epidermal-dermal separation (Fig. 1). NM induced more than a two fold increase in areas (percent length of skin section) of epidermal thickness in both SKH-1 and C57BL/6 mice (Fig. 1B and D). In SKH-1 mice, a significant ($p<0.05$) NM-induced increase in thickness of skin sections was observed only at 12 and 24 h after exposure (Fig. 1B). However, in C57BL/6 mice, this NM-induced lesion showed a significant ($p<0.05$) increase after 24, 72 and 120 h of its exposure (Fig. 1D). Our published clinical study showed appearance of small and large areas of yellowish microblisters with swollen skin in both the mouse strains at 12 and 24 h post-NM exposure, respectively. These microblisters covered larger skin area after 72 and 120 h of NM exposure but appeared less swollen and compressed in both these mouse strains [15]. Blister formation on the skin is related to

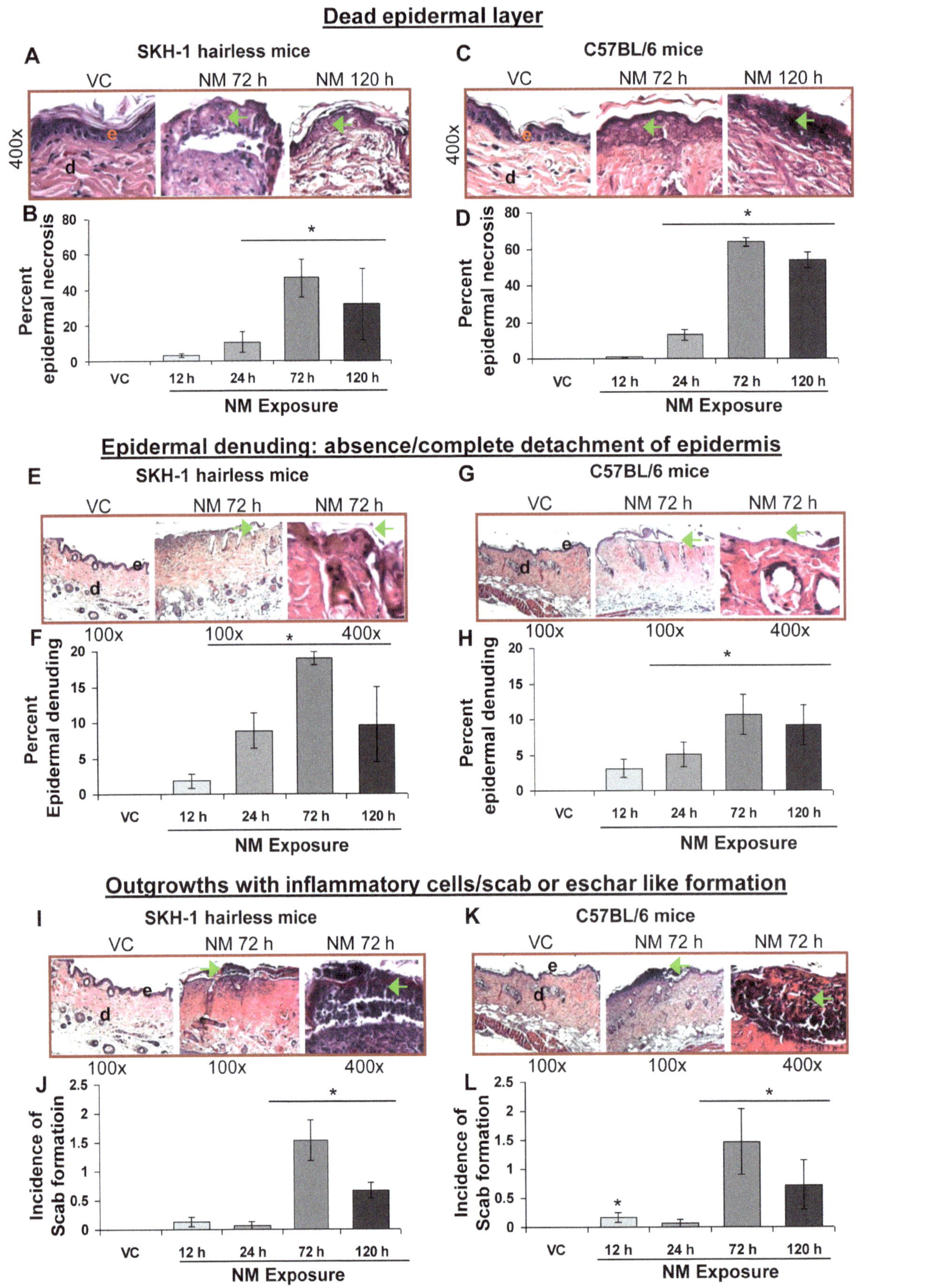
Dead epidermal layer
A
SKH-1 hairless mice
VC
NM 72 h
NM 120 h
400x
e
d
C
C57BL/6 mice
VC
NM 72 h
NM 120 h
400x
e
d
B
Percent epidermal necrosis
80
60
40
20
0
*
VC
12 h
24 h
72 h
120 h
NM Exposure
D
Percent epidermal necrosis
80
60
40
20
0
*
VC
12 h
24 h
72 h
120 h
NM Exposure
Epidermal denuding: absence/complete detachment of epidermis
E
SKH-1 hairless mice
VC
NM 72 h
NM 72 h
e
d
100x
100x
400x
G
C57BL/6 mice
VC
NM 72 h
NM 72 h
e
d
100x
100x
400x
F
Percent Epidermal denuding
20
15
10
5
0
*
VC
12 h
24 h
72 h
120 h
NM Exposure
H
Percent epidermal denuding
20
15
10
5
0
*
VC
12 h
24 h
72 h
120 h
NM Exposure
Outgrowths with inflammatory cells/scab or eschar like formation
I
SKH-1 hairless mice
VC
NM 72 h
NM 72 h
e
d
100x
100x
400x
K
C57BL/6 mice
VC
NM 72 h
NM 72 h
e
d
100x
100x
400x
J
Incidence of Scab formatioin
2.5
2
1.5
1
0.5
0
*
VC
12 h
24 h
72 h
120 h
NM Exposure
L
Incidence of Scab formation
2.5
2
1.5
1
0.5
0
*
*
VC
12 h
24 h
72 h
120 h
NM Exposure

Figure 2. NM exposure causes epidermal cell death, epidermal denuding and ulceration, and scab formation in the skin of SKH-1 and C57BL/6 mice. Dorsal skin of mice was exposed topically to either 200 μL of acetone or NM (3.2 mg) in 200 μL acetone. After 12, 24, 72 and 120 h of NM exposure, mice were sacrificed and dorsal skin tissue sections (5 μM) were processed, H&E stained and analyzed as detailed under Materials and Methods. Panels A and C, E and G and I and K are representative H&E stained skin sections (100 or 400× magnification) showing epidermal cell death, epidermal denuding and scab formation, respectively from vehicle control and 72 or 120 h NM exposed skin tissue in SKH-1 and C57BL/6 mice. These NM-related histopathological changes were assessed as detailed under materials and methods, and calculated as percent length of mice skin epidermis showing epidermal cell death (B and D) epidermal denuding and ulceration (F and H), or as incidences of scab formation/outgrowths (J and L). Data presented are mean ± SEM of 3–5 animals in each group. *, $p<0.05$ compared to respective vehicle control; VC, vehicle control; NM, nitrogen mustard; e, epidermis; d, dermis; green arrows, necrosis/dead epidermal layer or epidermal denuding or scab formation.

epidermal-dermal separation [7,10]. Histopathology of skin sections from these NM-exposed mice with microblisters revealed smaller epidermal-dermal separations at 12 h post-exposure, which were more prominent after 24 h of NM exposure (Fig. 1E and G; iv-vi). Apart from epidermal-dermal separation (red arrows), NM-induced separation within the epidermis was also seen (pink arrows; Fig. 1E and G). In SKH-1 mice, 13% length of skin sections showed epidermal-dermal separation at 12 h post-NM exposure, this lesion increased to 30% after 24 h and remained equivalent thereafter at 72 and 120 h post-exposure (Fig. 1F). In C57BL/6 mice, 12 and 24 h NM exposure showed epidermal-dermal separation in less than 20% length of assessed skin sections (Fig. 1H). However, after 72 h of NM exposure, this type of lesion was maximal, which covered 50% length of the observed skin sections (Fig. 1H). Microvesication was not seen in vehicle control skin sections (Fig. 1E–H).

ii) Dead epidermal layer, epidermal denuding and ulceration, and scab formation. Skin pathology effects after 12–120 h NM (3.2 mg) exposure included erythema, broken skin (ulceration) and dead peeled skin areas [15]. Therefore, we sought to study the structural changes in the skin associated with these NM-related observations. Examination of the NM-exposed skin sections from both hairless and haired mice showed areas of partial and full thickness epidermal death (Fig. 2A and C), epidermal denuding/absence of epidermis and ulcerated skin areas (Fig. 2E and G), and scab or eschar like formation (Fig. 2I and K). NM exposure after 12–72 h in both the mouse strains resulted in a time-dependent increase in the length of examined skin sections with dead, and denuded epidermis. Less of this injury was observed at 120 h after NM exposure (Fig. 2B and D; 2F and H). At 72 h post-NM exposure, dead epidermis was maximal; 46% and 64% length of examined skin sections showed dead epidermis in SKH-1 and C57BL/6 mice, respectively (Fig. 2B and D). Similarly, a maximum of 19% and 5% of the length of these skin sections in SKH-1 and C57BL/6 mice, respectively, showed denudation of epidermis at 72 h after NM exposure (Fig. 2F and H). In addition to dead and denuded epidermal areas, NM exposure also resulted in incidences of small outgrowths/scab formation where the dead epidermal regions accumulated inflammatory cells (Fig. 2I and K; green arrows). Little scab formation was observed prior to 72 h after NM exposure; at this time point it was maximal and then decreased at 120 h post-exposure (Fig. 2J and L). None of these lesions were observed in skin tissue sections from controls (Fig. 2).

iii) Parakeratosis and hyperkeratosis. Gross examination of NM treated hairless and haired mice showed thick leathery, scaly and desquamating skin as well as pigmentation changes at 72 and 120 h post-NM exposure [15]. Parakeratosis refers to abnormal retention of nucleated keratinocytes in the stratum corneum. Hyperkeratosis is overproduction of keratin (could also cause altered pigmentation) and thickening of the stratum corneum [19]. These conditions are reported following SM exposure in mice [10,11] and could be related to the above mentioned pathological features observed in mice with NM. Accordingly, examination of skin sections from NM exposed skin revealed the occurrence of parakeratosis (Fig. 3A and C, green arrows) and hyperkeratosis (Fig. 3E and G, green arrows). A maximum quantity of parakeratosis was observed at 72 h post-NM exposure in SKH-1 mice (Fig. 3B). However, in C75BL/6 mice it took 120 h of NM exposure to induce a maximal amount of parakeratosis; at this time it occurred in 27% of the length of skin sections (Fig. 3D). A time-dependent increase in hyperkeratosis was evident in SKH-1 mice between 12–120 h post-NM exposure; the maximal length of examined skin sections with hyperkeratosis was 34% observed at 120 h post-exposure (Fig. 3F). In contrast, in C57BL/6 mice, NM-exposure (12–72 h) resulted in a time-dependent increase in the length of skin sections with hyperkeratosis, which only reached a maximum of 7% at 72 h and decreased at 120 h post-NM exposure (Fig. 3H).

iv) Acanthosis and hyperplasia. Acanthosis has been reported to be induced by SM; it is defined as diffuse hyperproliferation and thickening of the stratum spinosum with an increased size of the cells in this layer [4,8]. This lesion was observed at 72 and 120 h post-NM exposure in both SKH-1 and C57BL/6 mice skin sections (Fig. 4). A more profound NM-induced increase in length of skin sections with acanthosis was observed in SKH-1 mice as compared to C57BL/6 mice (Fig. 4B and D; green arrows). This NM-induced lesion was maximal (21% length of skin sections) at 120 h post-exposure in SKH-1 mice (Fig. 4B). However, only a maximum of 5% length of examined C57BL/6 mice skin sections showed acanthosis at 72 h post-NM exposure (Fig. 4D). Acanthosis was not observed in mice from the vehicle control group, nor from 12 and 24 h NM-exposed mice (Fig. 4).

NM Exposure causes Structural Changes in the Dermis of the Skin in SKH-1 and C57BL/6 Mice

SM exposure causes a profound inflammatory response including dermal edema, necrosis and influx of inflammatory cells in the dermis. Hence, we next assessed these changes following NM exposure in SKH-1 and C57BL/6 mice.

i) Dermal necrosis and edema. Histological analysis of NM-exposed skin tissue sections from both hairless and haired mice revealed that NM-induced dermal necrosis (dead dermal areas), which was accompanied by the presence of a large number of inflammatory cells (Fig. 5A and C). In both mouse strains, NM exposure for 12–72 h caused a time-dependent increase in the length of skin sections with dermal necrosis. Inflammation reached a maximum at 72 h and then decreased at 120 h post-exposure (Fig. 5B and D). NM exposure for 72 h resulted in dermal necrosis in 22% and 26% length of skin sections in SKH-1 and C57BL/6 mice, respectively (Fig. 5B and D). NM exposure in both the mouse strains also caused an increase in dermal thickness; this was maximal at 24 h after exposure, and decreased at 72 and 120 h post-exposure (Fig. 5E and F).

ii) Infiltration of inflammatory cells and extravasated red blood cells. NM exposure also resulted in an influx of inflammatory cells (Fig. 5G and H) and extravasated red blood

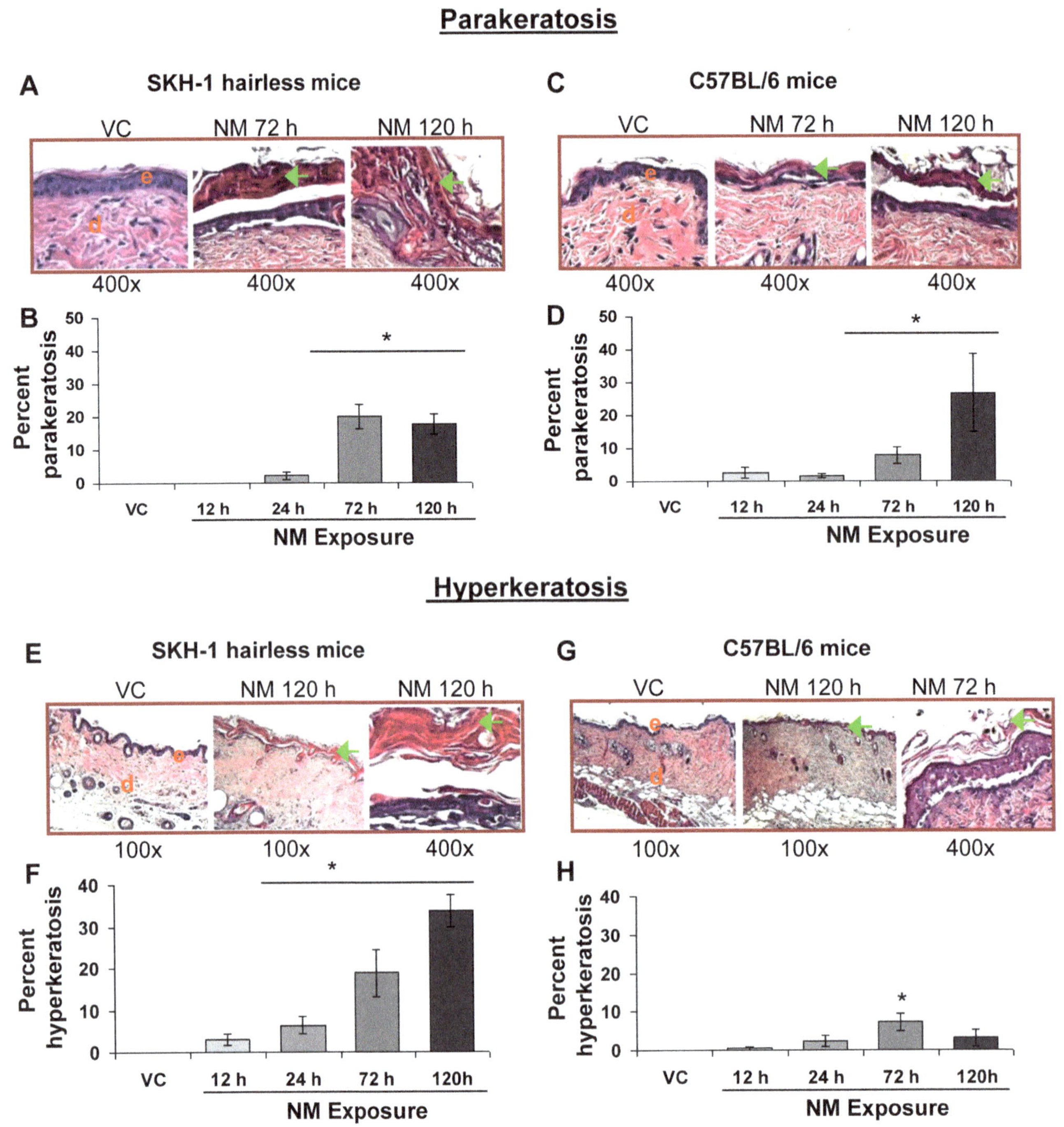

Figure 3. NM exposure causes parakeratosis and hyperkeratosis in the skin epidermis of SKH-1 and C57BL/6 mice. Dorsal skin of mice was exposed topically to either 200 μL of acetone or NM (3.2 mg) in 200 μL acetone. After 12, 24, 72 and 120 h of NM exposure, mice were sacrificed and dorsal skin tissue sections (5 μM) were processed, H&E stained and analyzed as detailed under Materials and Methods. Panels A and C (i–iii) and E and G (i–iii) are representative H&E stained skin sections (100 or 400× magnification) showing parakeratosis and hyperkeratosis, respectively, from vehicle control as well as NM exposed (72 and 120 h) skin tissue in mice. These NM-related histopathological changes were assessed as detailed under materials and methods, and calculated as percent length of mice skin epidermis showing parakeratosis (B and D) and hyperkeratosis (F and H). Data presented are mean ± SEM of 3–5 animals in each group. *, $p<0.05$ compared to respective vehicle control; VC, vehicle control; NM, nitrogen mustard; e, epidermis; d, dermis; green arrows, parakeratosis, hypercornification or acanthosis.

cells (RBCs; Fig. 5I and J) in the dermal region in both SKH-1 and C57BL/6 mice. The NM-induced increase in the inflammatory cells was scored as detailed under Materials and Methods. NM exposure-induced a profound infiltration of inflammatory cells at 12, 24 and 72 h post-exposure in SKH-1 mice, which was moderate at 120 h after exposure (Table 1). However, in C57BL/6 mice, a large number of inflammatory cells were observed only at 24 h post-NM exposure (Table 1). Similarly, a large number of extravasated RBCs were observed in the skin sections at 24, 72

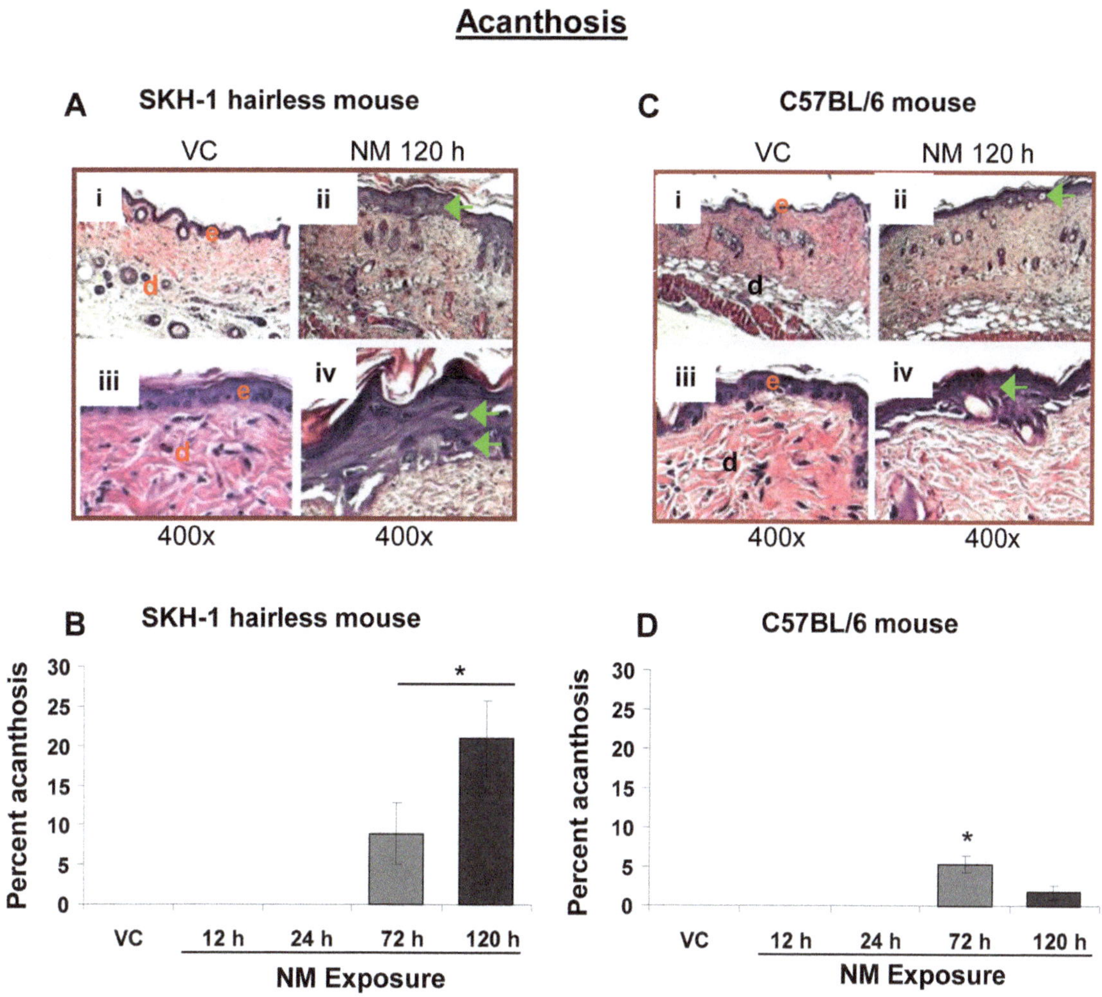

Figure 4. NM exposure causes acanthosis in the skin epidermis of SKH-1 and C57BL/6 mice. Dorsal skin of mice was exposed topically to either 200 μL of acetone or NM (3.2 mg) in 200 μL acetone. After 12, 24, 72 and 120 h of NM exposure, mice were sacrificed and dorsal skin tissue sections (5 μM) were processed, H&E stained and analyzed as detailed under Materials and Methods. Panels A and B are representative H&E stained skin sections (100 or 400× magnification) showing acanthosis from vehicle control as well as NM exposed (72 and 120 h) skin tissue in mice. This NM-related histopathological change was assessed as detailed under materials and methods, and calculated as percent length of mice skin epidermis showing acanthosis (B and D). Data presented are mean ± SEM of 3–5 animals in each group. *, $p<0.05$ compared to respective vehicle control; VC, vehicle control; NM, nitrogen mustard; e, epidermis; d, dermis; green arrows, acanthosis.

and 120 h post-NM exposure in SKH-1 mice and at 12–120 h after its exposure in C57BL/6 mice (Table 2).

Discussion

NM is an analog of SM with reported chemical properties and cutaneous toxic effects similar to SM. Thus far it has not been used as a weapon of mass destruction [14,20–22]. However, NM was stockpiled during World War II and its leakage from Tankers bombed by Germans at Bari Harbor in Italy was reported to cause injuries as well as human casualties [23]. Therefore NM poses a potential warfare and terrorist threat as does SM [21,24]. Both SM and NM are powerful vesicants and alkylating agents, which are reported to cause edema, blister formation, ulceration, necrosis and desquamation [6,14,25]. Consistent with these earlier reports, our published study examining NM exposure in both SKH-1 hairless and C57BL/6 mice identified clinical effects of NM, which are comparable to clinicopathological injuries with SM [15]. In the current study, we further evaluated the histopathological structural changes related to the clinical effects of NM exposure.

Inflammatory response in the skin is associated with an increase in epidermal thickness, which has also been reported following SM exposure [13]. In our study, NM exposure caused comparable increases in epidermal thickness in both hairless and haired mice. This NM-induced lesion could contribute to the NM-caused edema and increased skin bi-fold thickness observed in these mice in our earlier report [15]. Skin blistering is the most prominent characteristic lesion following SM exposure [3,26–28]. Normally the basal epidermal keratinocytes maintain attachment to the basement membrane through hemidesmosomes [10,28]. However, SM-induces keratinocyte cell death via apoptosis and results in protease digestion of anchoring filaments of the epidermal-dermal junction allowing blister formation [28]. Similar to the blister formation observed following SM exposure, our NM-induced microblisters show a comparable histopathology observed as epidermal-dermal separation associated with epidermal cell death. This is in agreement with reported NM-induced keratin destruc-

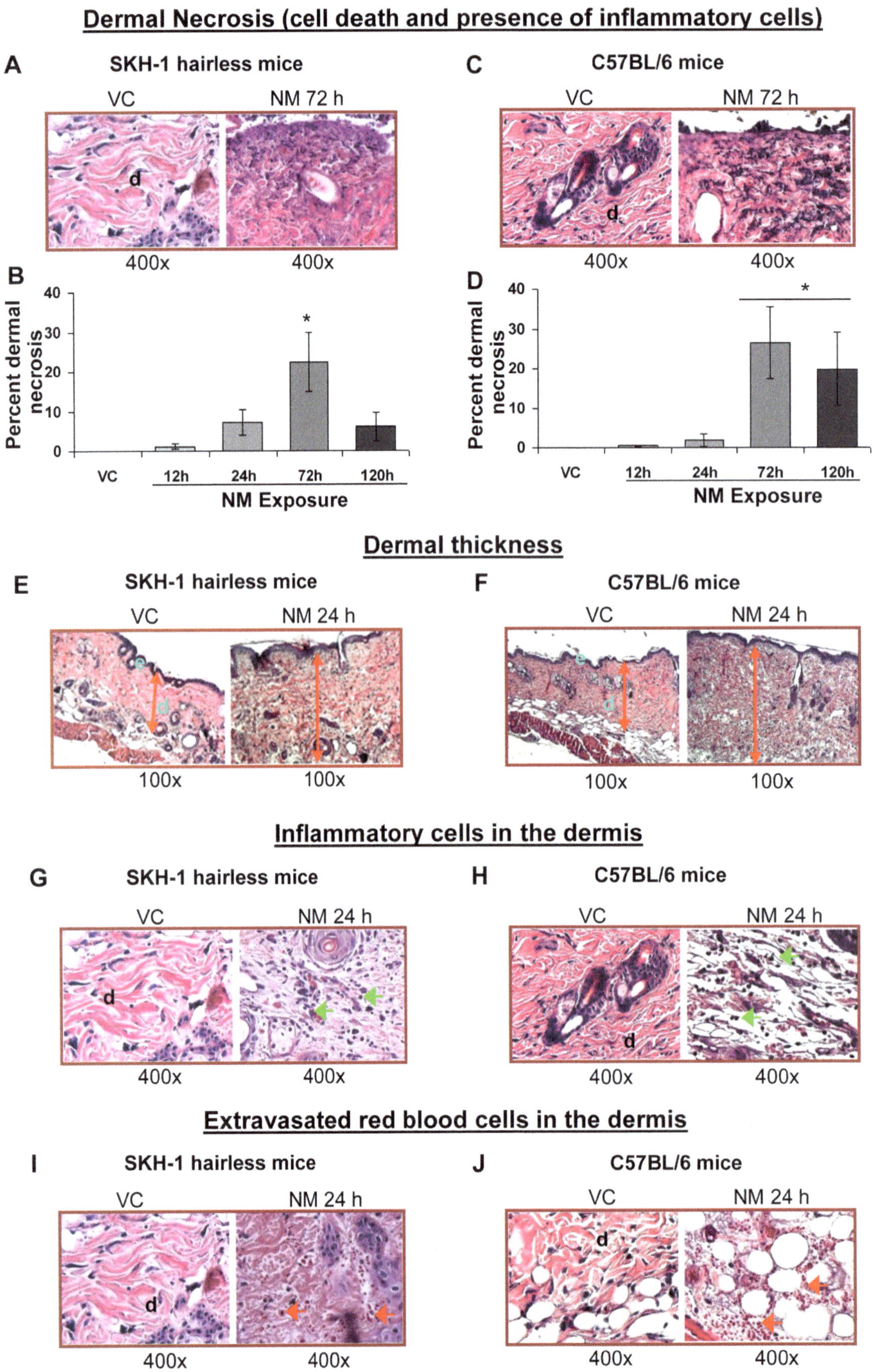
Dermal Necrosis (cell death and presence of inflammatory cells)
A
SKH-1 hairless mice
VC
NM 72 h
d
400x
400x
C
C57BL/6 mice
VC
NM 72 h
d
400x
400x
B
Percent dermal necrosis
40
30
20
10
0
*
VC
12h
24h
72h
120h
NM Exposure
D
Percent dermal necrosis
40
30
20
10
0
*
VC
12h
24h
72h
120h
NM Exposure
Dermal thickness
E
SKH-1 hairless mice
VC
NM 24 h
e
d
100x
100x
F
C57BL/6 mice
VC
NM 24 h
e
d
100x
100x
Inflammatory cells in the dermis
G
SKH-1 hairless mice
VC
NM 24 h
d
400x
400x
H
C57BL/6 mice
VC
NM 24 h
d
400x
400x
Extravasated red blood cells in the dermis
I
SKH-1 hairless mice
VC
NM 24 h
d
400x
400x
J
C57BL/6 mice
VC
NM 24 h
d
400x
400x

Figure 5. NM exposure causes necrosis, dermal thickness, recruitment of inflammatory cells and extravasated red blood cells in the dermal region of SKH-1 and C57BL/6 mice skin. Dorsal skin of mice was exposed topically to either 200 μL of acetone or NM (3.2 mg) in 200 μL acetone. After 12, 24, 72 and 120 h of NM exposure, mice were sacrificed and dorsal skin tissue sections (5 μM) were processed, H&E stained and analyzed as detailed under Materials and Methods. Panels A and C, E and F, G and H, and I and J are representative H&E stained skin sections from vehicle control as well as NM exposed skin tissue in mice for dermal necrosis (with presence of breaking down inflammatory cells, mainly neutrophils), dermal thickness, inflammatory cells, and extravasated red blood cells. These NM-related histopathological changes were assessed as detailed under materials and methods, and calculated as percent area of mice skin dermis showing necrosis (B and D), inflammatory cells (Table 1), and extravasated red blood cells (Table 2). *, $p<0.05$ compared to respective vehicle control; VC, vehicle control; NM, nitrogen mustard; d, dermis; green arrows, inflammatory cells; red arrows, extravasated red blood cells.

tion which leads to lysis of basal epidermal cells and blister formation [29]. The NM-induced epidermal-dermal separations in both SKH-1 and C57BL/6 observed in this study are consistent with those observed in SKH-1 mice with NM [30]. In addition, the NM-related epidermal-dermal separations are comparable to the SM-induced epidermal-dermal separations in human and animal (mouse and guinea pig) skin [3,4,6,8,12,28,31,32].

Following 48–72 h of cutaneous SM exposure in humans, blisters in the skin burst open causing ulceration, epidermal denudation, necrosis and finally scab or eschar like formation [9]. Similarly, histopathological examination of NM-exposed skin sections from hairless and haired mice in the present study revealed dead/necrotic epidermis, epidermal denudation and ulceration, and scab formation which was maximal at 72 h post-NM exposure. Both SM and NM target the basal epidermal keratinocytes [33], and cause apoptotic and necrotic cell death. Consistent with this, NM exposure in this study also induced necrotic/dead epidermis regions in both hairless and haired mice due to basal epidermal cell death. It is suggested that keratinocyte cell death is one of early responses to SM exposure and plays an important role in blister formation, inflammation and the wound healing process [31,34,35]. The NM-induced epidermal denuding observed in this study could contribute to the ulceration of the skin. This denudation is also comparable to the epidermal loss/desquamation observed following SM exposure in human skin, and in mouse and guinea pig models [3,13,32,36]. The SM-induced necrotic and ulcerated regions of epidermis are reported to be very sensitive to secondary infections [9]. Since NM also induced denudation of epidermis and ulcerated skin areas in mice, further studies are needed to determine whether secondary infections also occurred in these mice. SM exposure in humans causes eschar or scab formation in the skin 72 h after its exposure; a similar pathology has been reported in animal models [11,12,32,37]. The thickened area in the scab contains dead epidermal cells and an inflammatory infiltrate, mainly neutrophils [11]. Similar to SM exposure in humans, NM exposure for 72 h in hairless and haired mice induced maximal incidences of scab formation containing dead cells and inflammatory cells.

The presence of parakeratosis at 72 and 120 h post-NM exposure in our study is consistent with reports of parakeratosis in human and animal models with SM cutaneous exposure [4,11,38]. Parakeratosis refers to retention of nucleated keratinocytes in the stratum corneum, and is linked to inflammatory skin diseases like psoriasis [19]. Psoriasis, pruritus and dermatitis are reported chronic signs of SM exposure [9]; these will need to be examined in our NM-exposed mouse models. An acute complication of SM exposure in humans is hyperkeratosis [3,4,8,39]. This thickening of the stratum corneum layer was also observed following NM exposure in the mouse strains studied here, however, it was more pronounced in our SKH-1 hairless mice than C57BL/6 mice. These findings are in accord with SM-induced hyperkeratosis in animal models including SKH-1 hairless mice and guinea pigs [8,11]. A major keratin in keratinocytes, K10 (associated with epidermolytic hyperkeratosis), is reported to play an important role in SM-exposed hyperkeratosis observed in SKH-1 hairless mice [11]. The role of this keratin in NM-related hyperkeratosis could be further examined. Our study shows that acanthosis with hyperplasia, larger nuclei and areas of re-epithelialization appear in 72 and 120 h NM exposed hairless and haired mouse skin. These findings are consistent with reports that SM exposure in humans and animal models caused delayed acanthosis and hyperplasia to compensate for cell death and thus allow healing of wounds by forming a new epidermal layer [4,8,11,39,40].

Dermal changes following SM exposure in humans and animals include edema, infiltration of inflammatory cells, extravasated erythrocytes, necrosis and endothelial swelling [4,8,12,13,39]. Our assessments in this study also show increases in edema, infiltration of inflammatory cells, dermal necrosis and extravasation of RBCs following 12–120 h of NM exposure. In our study, the dermal thickness peaked at 24 h after NM exposure indicating that this is an early inflammatory response. The inflammatory cells including neutrophils, macrophages and mast cells in the dermis following SM exposure release cytokines and other inflammatory mediators

Table 1. NM exposure caused infiltration of inflammatory cells (PMNs) in the dermis of SKH-1 hairless and C57BL/6 mice following 12–120 h of its exposure.

SKH-1					
Exposure	VC	12 h NM	24 h NM	72 h NM	120 h NM
Inflammatory cells	+	+++	+++	+++	++
C57 BL/6					
Exposure	VC	12 h NM	24 h NM	72 h NM	120 h NM
Inflammatory cells	+	++	+++	++	++

+, Few (less than 100); ++, moderate (100–1000); +++, high (more than 1000) inflammatory cells per skin section (at 400×); VC, vehicle control.

Table 2. NM exposure caused an increase in the percent extravasated RBCs in the dermis of SKH-1 hairless and C57BL/6 mice following 12–120 h of its exposure.

SKH-1					
Exposure	VC	12 h NM	24 h NM	72 h NM	120 h NM
Extravasated RBCs	+	++	+++	+++	+++
C57 BL/6					
Exposure	VC	12 h NM	24 h NM	72 h NM	120 h NM
Extravasated RBCs	++	+++	+++	+++	+++

+, Few (less than 10%); ++, moderate (10–30%); +++, high (more than 30%) extravasated RBCs per skin section (at 400×); vehicle control.

to initiate healing process [4,11,17,41,42]. Neutrophils, macrophages and mast cells could also be involved in NM-related inflammatory response since NM caused profound infiltration of inflammatory cells in both the mouse strains. We then observed a maximal dermal necrosis at 72 h post-NM exposure.

According to the observation from this study, immunohistochemical analyses, and other specific assays to further investigate the NM-induced inflammatory response, epidermal cell death, and microvesication are under investigation. These studies will further help in dissecting and examining mechanisms involved in NM-induced skin injuries, which will also be useful in screening treatment agents against vesicant injuries.

In summary, this study provides a detailed assessment of NM-related structural changes in both hairless and haired mice to establish that its histopathological parameters are comparable to SM exposure in humans and other animal models. We believe this histopathological analysis will be valuable for screening and identification of therapies against skin injuries induced by both SM and NM.

Author Contributions

Conceived and designed the experiments: NTS CWW RA. Performed the experiments: NTS AKJ. Analyzed the data: NTS DO CWW RA. Wrote the paper: NTS AKJ DO CWW RA.

References

1. Balali-Mood M, Hefazi M (2005) The pharmacology, toxicology, and medical treatment of sulphur mustard poisoning. Fundam Clin Pharmacol 19: 297–315.
2. Emadi SN, Aslani J, Poursaleh Z, Izadi M, Soroush M, et al. (2012) Comparison late cutaneous complications between exposure to sulfur mustard and nerve agents. Cutan Ocul Toxicol 31: 214–219.
3. Ghabili K, Agutter PS, Ghanei M, Ansarin K, Shoja MM (2010) Mustard gas toxicity: the acute and chronic pathological effects. J Appl Toxicol 30: 627–643.
4. Naraghi ZS, Mansouri P, Mortazavi M (2005) A clinicopathological study on acute cutaneous lesions induced by sulfur mustard gas (yperite). Eur J Dermatol 15: 140–145.
5. Wormser U, Sintov A, Brodsky B, Casillas RP, Nyska A (2004) Protective effect of topical iodine containing anti-inflammatory drugs against sulfur mustard-induced skin lesions. Arch Toxicol 78: 156–166.
6. Smith KJ, Smith WJ, Hamilton T, Skelton HG, Graham JS, et al. (1998) Histopathologic and immunohistochemical features in human skin after exposure to nitrogen and sulfur mustard. Am J Dermatopathol 20: 22–28.
7. Kehe K, Balszuweit F, Steinritz D, Thiermann H (2009) Molecular toxicology of sulfur mustard-induced cutaneous inflammation and blistering. Toxicology 263: 12–19.
8. Benson JM, Seagrave J, Weber WM, Santistevan CD, Grotendorst GR, et al. (2011) Time course of lesion development in the hairless guinea-pig model of sulfur mustard-induced dermal injury. Wound Repair Regen 19: 348–357.
9. Graham JS, Schoneboom BA (2013) Historical perspective on effects and treatment of sulfur mustard injuries. Chem Biol Interact.
10. Shakarjian MP, Heck DE, Gray JP, Sinko PJ, Gordon MK, et al. (2010) Mechanisms mediating the vesicant actions of sulfur mustard after cutaneous exposure. Toxicol Sci 114: 5–19.
11. Joseph LB, Gerecke DR, Heck DE, Black AT, Sinko PJ, et al. (2011) Structural changes in the skin of hairless mice following exposure to sulfur mustard correlate with inflammation and DNA damage. Exp Mol Pathol 91: 515–527.
12. Dachir S, Cohen M, Fishbeine E, Sahar R, Brandies R, et al. (2010) Characterization of acute and long-term sulfur mustard-induced skin injuries in hairless guinea-pigs using non-invasive methods. Skin Res Technol 16: 114–124.
13. Lomash V, Deb U, Rai R, Jadhav SE, Vijayaraghavan R, et al. (2011) Designing of mouse model: a new approach for studying sulphur mustard-induced skin lesions. Burns 37: 851–864.
14. Wormser U, Brodsky B, Reich R (2002) Topical treatment with povidone iodine reduces nitrogen mustard-induced skin collagenolytic activity. Arch Toxicol 76: 119–121.
15. Tewari-Singh N, Jain AK, Inturi S, White CW, Agarwal R (2013) Clinically-Relevant Cutaneous Lesions by Nitrogen Mustard: Useful Biomarkers of Vesicants Skin Injury in SKH-1 Hairless and C57BL/6 Mice. PLoS One 8: e67557.
16. Tewari-Singh N, Rana S, Gu M, Pal A, Orlicky DJ, et al. (2009) Inflammatory biomarkers of sulfur mustard analog 2-chloroethyl ethyl sulfide-induced skin injury in SKH-1 hairless mice. Toxicol Sci 108: 194–206.
17. Jain AK, Tewari-Singh N, Orlicky DJ, White CW, Agarwal R (2011) 2-Chloroethyl ethyl sulfide causes microvesication and inflammation-related histopathological changes in male hairless mouse skin. Toxicology 282: 129–138.
18. Ghasemi H, Owlia P, Jalali-Nadoushan MR, Pourfarzam S, Azimi G, et al. (2013) A clinicopathological approach to sulfur mustard-induced organ complications: a major review. Cutan Ocul Toxicol 32: 304–324.
19. Song J, Shea CR (2010) Benign versus malignant parakeratosis: a nuclear morphometry study. Mod Pathol 23: 799–803.
20. Sharma M, Vijayaraghavan R, Agrawal OP (2010) Comparative toxic effect of nitrogen mustards (HN-1, HN-2, and HN-3) and sulfur mustard on hematological and biochemical variables and their protection by DRDE-07 and its analogues. Int J Toxicol 29: 391–401.
21. Papirmeister B, Gross CL, Meier HL, Petrali JP, Johnson JB (1985) Molecular basis for mustard-induced vesication. Fundam Appl Toxicol 5: S134–149.
22. Wang GQ, Xia ZF (2007) Tissue injury by hot fluid containing nitrogen mustard. Burns 33: 923–926.
23. Alexander SF (1947) Medical report on the Bari Harbor mustard casualties. Mil Surg 101: 1–17.
24. Watson AP, Griffin GD (1992) Toxicity of vesicant agents scheduled for destruction by the Chemical Stockpile Disposal Program. Environ Health Perspect 98: 259–280.
25. Wormser U (1991) Toxicology of mustard gas. Trends Pharmacol Sci 12: 164–167.
26. Smith KJ, Casillas R, Graham J, Skelton HG, Stemler F, et al. (1997) Histopathologic features seen with different animal models following cutaneous sulfur mustard exposure. J Dermatol Sci 14: 126–135.
27. Kehe K, Thiermann H, Balszuweit F, Eyer F, Steinritz D, et al. (2009) Acute effects of sulfur mustard injury–Munich experiences. Toxicology 263: 3–8.
28. Hayden PJ, Petrali JP, Stolper G, Hamilton TA, Jackson GR Jr, et al. (2009) Microvesicating effects of sulfur mustard on an in vitro human skin model. Toxicol In Vitro.
29. Hess JF, FitzGerald PG (2007) Treatment of keratin intermediate filaments with sulfur mustard analogs. Biochem Biophys Res Commun 359: 616–621.
30. Anumolu SS, Menjoge AR, Deshmukh M, Gerecke D, Stein S, et al. (2011) Doxycycline hydrogels with reversible disulfide crosslinks for dermal wound healing of mustard injuries. Biomaterials 32: 1204–1217.
31. Mol MA, van den Berg RM, Benschop HP (2009) Involvement of caspases and transmembrane metalloproteases in sulphur mustard-induced microvesication in adult human skin in organ culture: directions for therapy. Toxicology 258: 39–46.
32. Wormser U, Langenbach R, Peddada S, Sintov A, Brodsky B, et al. (2004) Reduced sulfur mustard-induced skin toxicity in cyclooxygenase-2 knockout and celecoxib-treated mice. Toxicol Appl Pharmacol 200: 40–47.
33. Hardej D, Billack B (2007) Ebselen protects brain, skin, lung and blood cells from mechlorethamine toxicity. Toxicol Ind Health 23: 209–221.
34. Kan RK, Pleva CM, Hamilton TA, Anderson DR, Petrali JP (2003) Sulfur mustard-induced apoptosis in hairless guinea pig skin. Toxicol Pathol 31: 185–190.
35. Kehe K, Szinicz L (2005) Medical aspects of sulphur mustard poisoning. Toxicology 214: 198–209.
36. Dorandeu F, Taysse L, Boudry I, Foquin A, Herodin F, et al. (2011) Cutaneous challenge with chemical warfare agents in the SKH-1 hairless mouse. (I) Development of a model for screening studies in skin decontamination and protection. Hum Exp Toxicol 30: 470–490.
37. Petrali JP, Oglesby-Megee S (1997) Toxicity of mustard gas skin lesions. Microsc Res Tech 37: 221–228.
38. Ghabili K, Agutter PS, Ghanei M, Ansarin K, Panahi Y, et al. (2011) Sulfur mustard toxicity: history, chemistry, pharmacokinetics, and pharmacodynamics. Crit Rev Toxicol 41: 384–403.
39. Ghanei M, Poursaleh Z, Harandi AA, Emadi SE, Emadi SN (2010) Acute and chronic effects of sulfur mustard on the skin: a comprehensive review. Cutan Ocul Toxicol 29: 269–277.
40. Poursaleh Z, Ghanei M, Babamahmoodi F, Izadi M, Harandi AA, et al. (2012) Pathogenesis and treatment of skin lesions caused by sulfur mustard. Cutan Ocul Toxicol 31: 241–249.
41. Arroyo CM, Broomfield CA, Hackley BE Jr (2001) The role of interleukin-6 (IL-6) in human sulfur mustard (HD) toxicology. Int J Toxicol 20: 281–296.
42. Sabourin CL, Danne MM, Buxton KL, Casillas RP, Schlager JJ (2002) Cytokine, chemokine, and matrix metalloproteinase response after sulfur mustard injury to weanling pig skin. J Biochem Mol Toxicol 16: 263–272.

11

Panton-Valentine Leukocidin Does Play a Role in the Early Stage of *Staphylococcus aureus* Skin Infections: A Rabbit Model

Urszula Lipinska[1]*, Katleen Hermans[1], Lieve Meulemans[1], Oana Dumitrescu[3,4,5], Cedric Badiou[3,4], Luc Duchateau[2], Freddy Haesebrouck[1], Jerome Etienne[3,4,5], Gerard Lina[3,4,5]

1 Department of Pathology, Bacteriology and Avian Diseases, Faculty of Veterinary Medicine, Ghent University, Merelbeke, Belgium, **2** Department of Physiology and Biometry, Faculty of Veterinary Medicine, Ghent University, Merelbeke, Belgium, **3** Centre National de Référence des Staphylocoques, Université Lyon 1, Lyon, France, **4** INSERM U851, IFR128, Lyon, France, **5** Hospices Civils de Lyon, Lyon, France

Abstract

Despite epidemiological data linking necrotizing skin infections with the production of Panton-Valentine leukocidin (PVL), the contribution of this toxin to the virulence of *S. aureus* has been highly discussed as a result of inconclusive results of in vivo studies. However, the majority of these results originate from experiments using mice, an animal species which neutrophils - the major target cells for PVL - are highly insensitive to the action of this leukocidin. In contrast, the rabbit neutrophils have been shown to be as sensitive to PVL action as human cells, making the rabbit a better experimental animal to explore the PVL role. In this study we examined whether PVL contributes to *S. aureus* pathogenicity by means of a rabbit skin infection model. The rabbits were injected intradermally with 10^8 cfu of either a PVL positive community-associated methicillin-resistant *S. aureus* isolate, its isogenic PVL knockout or a PVL complemented knockout strain, and the development of skin lesions was observed. While all strains induced skin infection, the wild type strain produced larger lesions and a higher degree of skin necrosis compared to the PVL knockout strain in the first week after the infection. The PVL expression in the rabbits was indirectly confirmed by a raise in the serum titer of anti-LukS-PV antibodies observed only in the rabbits infected with PVL positive strains. These results indicate that the rabbit model is more suitable for studying the role of PVL in staphylococcal diseases than other animal models. Further, they support the epidemiological link between PVL producing *S. aureus* strains and necrotizing skin infections.

Editor: Binh An Diep, University of California San Francisco, United States of America

Funding: This research was funded by the Special Research Fund of Ghent University (01J.055.06), the grant European Community (EC 222718), Pfizer, bioMerieux and Novartis. The funders had no role in study design, data collection and analysis, decision to publish, or preparation of the manuscript.

Competing Interests: Gerard Lina received grants from Pfizer and Novartis to examine the impact of their molecule on PVL production, and from bioMerieux to develop rapid test for PVL detection. There is no relationship between these projects and the manuscript.

* E-mail: urszula.lipinska@ugent.be

Introduction

Staphylococcus aureus is a potent human pathogen causing various medical conditions, from minor skin infections (i.a. pimples, impetigo, abscesses) to life-threatening diseases (i.a. bacteraemia, endocarditis and sepsis) [1]. The capacity of *S. aureus* to evoke such a wide range of clinical manifestations may be attributed to the production of numerous exoproteins. One of them, Panton-Valentine leukocidin (PVL), is a two-component (LukS-PV and LukF-PV), pore-forming toxin with affinity for neutrophils and macrophages - cells responsible for the first line defence against invading bacteria [2–5]. Epidemiologically, PVL-producing strains have been linked with necrotizing 'skin and soft tissues infections' (SSTI) already in the 1990s [6–10]. More recently, the emergence of community-associated methicillin-resistant *S. aureus* (CA-MRSA) strains containing PVL determinants and their association with a rapid growing number of skin infections [11], severe necrotising pneumonia [12] and necrotizing fasciitis [13] raised an interest in the importance of PVL in staphylococcal infections.

One of the first *in vivo* studies evaluating the role of PVL in staphylococcal skin infections showed that intradermal injection of PVL provokes widespread and infiltrated erythema followed by skin necrosis in rabbits [6]. In contrast, subsequent *in vivo* experiments using murine models failed to uniformly prove the PVL contribution to the development of staphylococcal skin infections [14–17]. The reason for this inconsistency has been linked to a species-specific susceptibility of the host cells to PVL [18,19]. Since neutrophils isolated from mice have been reported to be relatively insensitive to the leukotoxic effect of PVL in contrast to human and rabbit cells [2,18], the latter has been postulated to be a better model for studying the role of PVL [18,19].

Therefore, we employed a rabbit skin infection model in order to evaluate the contribution of PVL to the pathogenicity of the *S. aureus* USA300 strain, a predominant cause of community-associated staphylococcal infections in Northern America [20], using isogenic PVL positive and negative strains.

Materials and Methods

Bacterial strains and culture

To provide optimal conditions for the production of PVL, all strains used in this study were cultivated in CCY medium [3]. LAC is a USA300 pulsotype community-associated methicillin resistant *S. aureus* (CA-MRSA) isolate, LACΔ*pvl* is its isogenic PVL knockout strain constructed as described elsewhere [14]. LUG1515 was obtained by trans-complementation of PVL in the LACΔ*pvl* strain using a pLUG534 plasmid [21]. To support plasmid maintenance, all growth media for the LUG1515 strain were supplemented with chloramphenicol (10 µg/ml).

To prepare the bacterial inoculum, a single colony was propagated in 5 ml of casein hydrolysate and yeast extract medium (CCY) medium with constant shaking at 200 revolutions per minute (rpm) at 37°C. The overnight culture was diluted 1:200 in CCY, incubated till the mid-exponential growth phase ($OD_{600} = 0.8$) and harvested by centrifugation. The pelleted bacteria were washed once, resuspended in sterile phosphate buffered saline (PBS) to a concentration of about 2×10^9 colony-forming units (cfu) per ml and immediately used for inoculation. The exact number of bacteria used was determined by plating out serial dilutions of the inocula.

Experimental animals

Thirty-three twelve-week-old albino hybrid rabbits of either sex, weighing 2.5–3 kg, were purchased from ILVO (Melle, Belgium). These animals do not carry rabbit-associated high virulence *S. aureus* strains evoking i.a. skin lesions, as was confirmed by the absence of such strains in swab samples taken from nine different body sites from all animals [22,23]. The rabbits were divided randomly into three groups of eleven animals, which were kept in separate HEPA-filtered rooms with negative pressure and light-dark cycles of 12 h per 12 h. The rabbits were housed individually with water and feed provided *ad libitum*.

Experimental design

From each animal 4 ml of blood was collected from the marginal ear vein before the onset of the experiment. On the day of the infection, the hair on the right flank of each rabbit was shaved with electric clippers (Wella Contura Hair Clipper, Wella) and the skin was disinfected thoroughly with 70% ethanol (Chem-Lab NV, Zedelgem, Belgium). After evaporation of the ethanol, 50 µl of PBS containing 10^8 cfu of either the knockout strain LACΔ*pvl*, the PVL producing strain LAC or the complemented strain LUG1515 were injected intradermally in the right flank of the rabbits of the respective groups.

During the following 14 days the behavior of the animals and their rectal temperature were examined daily, and the appearance of the lesions was noted. Width and length of the lesions and the necrotic areas were measured, and their surface was calculated as described earlier [15], using the formula $A = \pi(l \times w)/2$, where A is a surface, l is a length and w is a width of the lesion. At day 4 after inoculation (p.i.) three randomly selected animals per group were euthanized. Skin biopsies from the inoculation site were taken aseptically and preserved until further analysis. From the remaining animals, blood samples were collected at day 21 p.i., preceding euthanasia and collection of skin biopsies.

The experimental protocol was approved by the ethical committee of the Faculties of Veterinary Medicine and Bioscience Engineering, Ghent University (permit number 2009_121). The animal studies were performed following the EU legislation being the Council Directive 86/609 EEC covering the protection of animals used for experimental and other scientific purposes. Housing and care of the rabbits was in conformity with the adapted Appendix A of the European Convention ETS 123 of the council of Europe, as approved by the multilateral consultation in 2007.

Histological analysis

Following fixation in 10% buffered formalin, the skin samples were dehydrated with increasing concentrations of ethanol, cleared with Histosolve (Thermo Shandon, Pittsburgh, PA) and embedded in paraffin. Four microns sections were used to perform hematoxylin-eosin staining. All samples were examined by light microscopy in the absence of any information about their origin.

Hematoxylin-eosin stained sections were evaluated according to the following parameters: degree of dermal necrosis, degree of dermal inflammation and inflammatory cell type, degree of fibrosis and epidermal changes present.

Detection of anti-PVL antibodies

Blood samples collected during the experiment were incubated for 30 min at room temperature in glass tubes with inert gel barrier and activated disc (Venoject VT109SAS, Terumo). Next, the sera were separated by centrifugation at 1500 rpm for 10 min and stored at −20°C until use.

Antibodies against PVL (before *S. aureus* challenge and at sacrifice) were measured in rabbit sera using an ELISA protocol adapted from Croze et al. [24], with a peroxidase-conjugated swine anti-rabbit polyvalent IgG diluted $1{:}10^3$ (DAKO). Serial dilutions of anti-LukS-PV polyclonal rabbit serum (bioMérieux) were used for calibration. The results were expressed in arbitrary units per liter (AU/L), with one arbitrary unit corresponding to the amount of anti-LukS-PV antibodies present in a $1{:}10^7$ dilution of the polyclonal rabbit reference serum.

Statistical analysis

The comparison between strains with respect to diameter of the necrotic area, diameter and surface of the lesion was based on the linear mixed model with strain, time and their interaction as categorical fixed effects and rabbit as random effect. A global significance level of 5% was used. For multiple comparisons (the comparison of the 3 strains at each of the 14 times separately), Bonferroni's adjustment technique was used leading to a comparisonwise significance level of $0.5\%/(5 \times 14) = 0.096\%$.

Antibody levels were compared pairwise between strains at 0 and 21 days after infection using a t-test.

Results

Clinical observations

The rectal temperature registered for all rabbits during the experiment was within the normal range [25], with an exception of the first day after the infection. On that day, two animals in group LACΔ*pvl* and one animal in group LUG1515 developed fever (above 40.6°C).

Despite the developing lesions and the raised temperature on day 1 p.i., all animals remained alert, showed normal grooming behavior and appetite throughout the entire experiment.

Macroscopic description of the lesion development

All 33 rabbits developed an inflammatory reaction at the site of injection of the bacteria within the first 24 h, which within the following days evolved into fully grown lesions. The lesions appeared as a central necrotic area surrounded by a region of inflamed skin. The areas of necrosis became encrusted in all animals by day 5 p.i. (photos in fig. 1 show the appearance of the

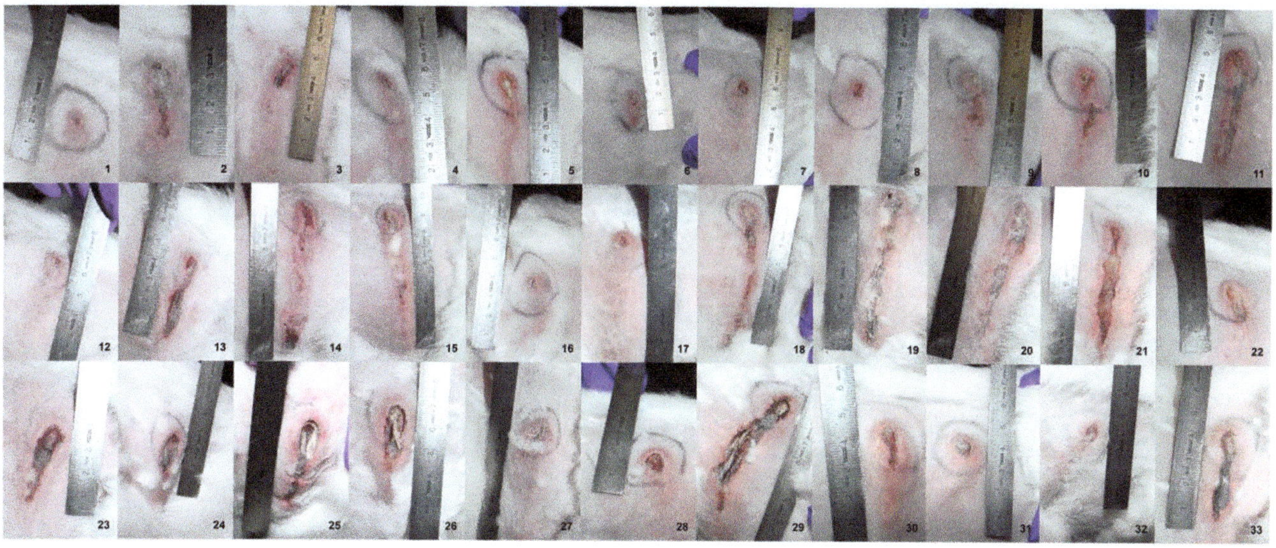

Figure 1. The appearance of lesions on day 4 after infection. The appearance of the lesions on day 4 p.i. in rabbits infected with LACΔ*pvl* (1–11), LAC (12–22) and LUG1515 (23–33). The unit of length of used measuring rod is centimetre.

lesions on day 4). The crusts in the LUG1515 group were situated deeper in the surrounding inflamed skin (fig. 1C), which was not the case in the remaining two groups. Periodic loss of the crusts in all groups revealed purulent material, whereafter a new crust was formed within the following 24 h. Before the end of the observation period (day 14 p.i.) the purulent material within the lesions was replaced by fibrotic scarring tissue.

A graphic overview of the mean surface of the lesions and necrotic areas in different groups during 14 days after infection is presented in figure 2.

The maximal mean diameter of the lesions was observed for all three infection groups on day 3 p.i. and reached 41 (range 7–75), 80 (range 38–115) and 58 mm (range 25–90) in group LACΔ*pvl*, LAC and LUG1515, respectively. On the last day of the observation the mean diameter of the lesions had decreased to 22 mm (range 10–38) in group LACΔ*pvl*, 35 mm (range 15–55) in group LAC and 30 mm (range 16–63) in group LUG1515. The mean diameter of the lesions in group LACΔ*pvl* was significantly smaller than in group LAC from day 3 till 6 p.i. ($P<0.00096$). As the surface of the lesions is a function of their diameter, a similar tendency was observed for the mean surface of the lesions, where a significant difference was observed between group LACΔ*pvl* and LAC from day 3 till 5 p.i. The difference between the surface of the lesions of group LACΔ*pvl* and LUG1515 was significant only on day 3 p.i.

The maximal mean diameter of the necrotic area was observed in group LACΔ*pvl* on day 6 p.i., in group LAC on day 2 and in group LUG1515 on day 5, reaching a diameter of 20 (range 7–47), 47 (range 6–92) and 30 mm (range 9–69), respectively. On the last day of the observation the mean diameter of the dermonecrosis had decreased to 12 mm in group LACΔ*pvl*, 23 in group LAC and 17 in group LUG1515. The mean diameter of the necrotic area in group LACΔ*pvl* was significantly smaller than in group LAC on day 2 p.i. ($P<0.00096$). For days 3–7 p.i. the results were similar, but the difference was not significant. The surface of the dermonecrosis showed a similar tendency with significant difference between LACΔ*pvl* and LAC on day 2 and 3 p.i., and similar but not significant results for days 4–6 p.i.

In the course of the experiment one animal in group LACΔ*pvl*, three in group LAC and two in group LUG1515 developed a secondary lesion on their abdomen. This was possibly a result of gravity-enhanced transport of the bacteria through the lymphatic system. Those lesions were not included in the statistical analysis as there was no physical connection of those lesions with the lesion at the original inoculation site.

Histological examination

The histopathological changes observed in skin samples collected from animals euthanized at day 4 p.i. are presented in table 1, and photos of the representative histological sections are shown in figure 3.

For rabbits euthanized at the end of the experiment (day 21 p.i.), the following histological findings were noted in the skin. In all samples from the LACΔ*pvl* and LAC inoculated groups there was a marked epidermal hyperplasia and the dermis showed moderate to marked fibrosis with mild perivascular infiltrations of mainly monocytes and lymphocytes. Similar findings were noted in the LUG1515 group, except for one biopsy where there was only a mild dermal fibrosis. In three biopsies from each group some PMNs were present as well. In four LAC, two LUG1515 and one LACΔ*pvl* inoculated skin samples, macrophages were noted. In one biopsy from the LUG1515 group, an old organised intravascular thrombus was present.

Detection of anti-PVL antibodies in the sera

The distribution of the titers of the anti-PVL antibodies detected in the sera collected from the rabbits from LACΔ*pvl*, LAC and LUG1515 group before challenge and at euthanasia are presented in figure 4.

There was no statistical difference between the groups in the titer of anti-PVL antibodies in the sera collected before challenge. While in group LACΔ*pvl* there was no statistical difference in the level of antibody before infection and at day 21 p.i., in group LAC and LUG1515 the mean antibody titers were significantly higher in the samples collected at the end of the experiment (8.4 and 19.6 times, respectively).

A

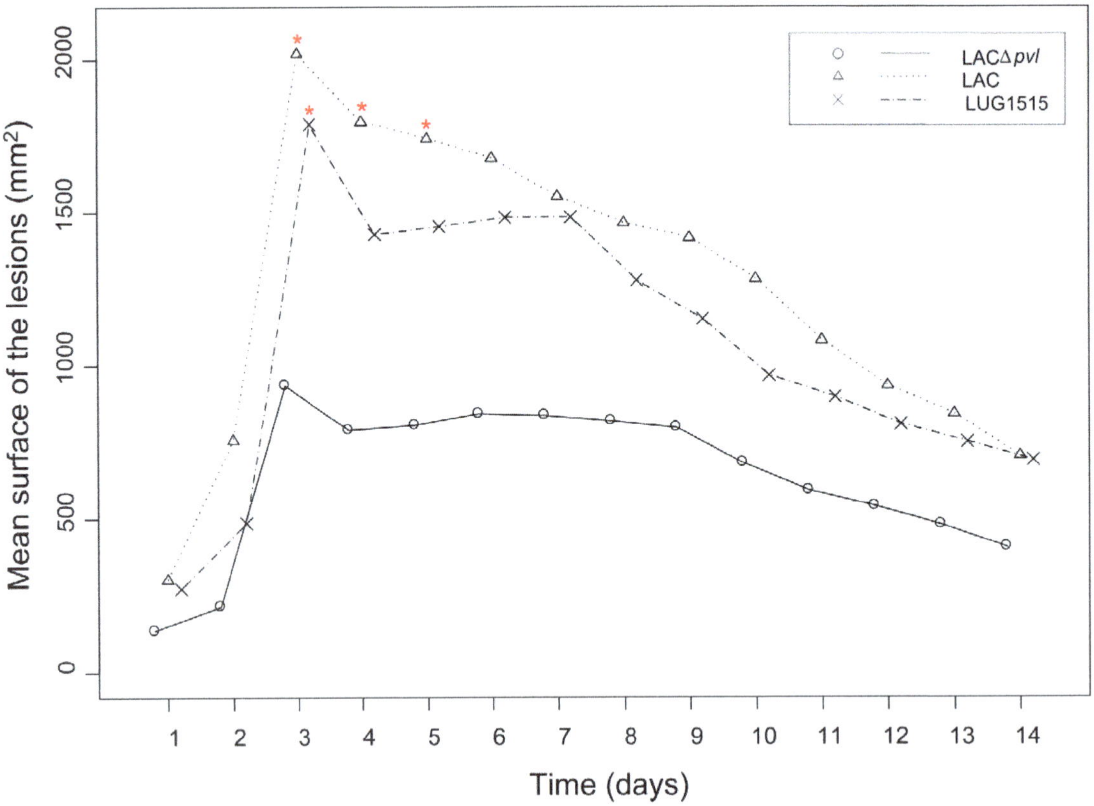
Mean surface of the lesions (mm²)
0
500
1000
1500
2000
LACΔpvl
LAC
LUG1515
1 2 3 4 5 6 7 8 9 10 11 12 13 14
Time (days)

B

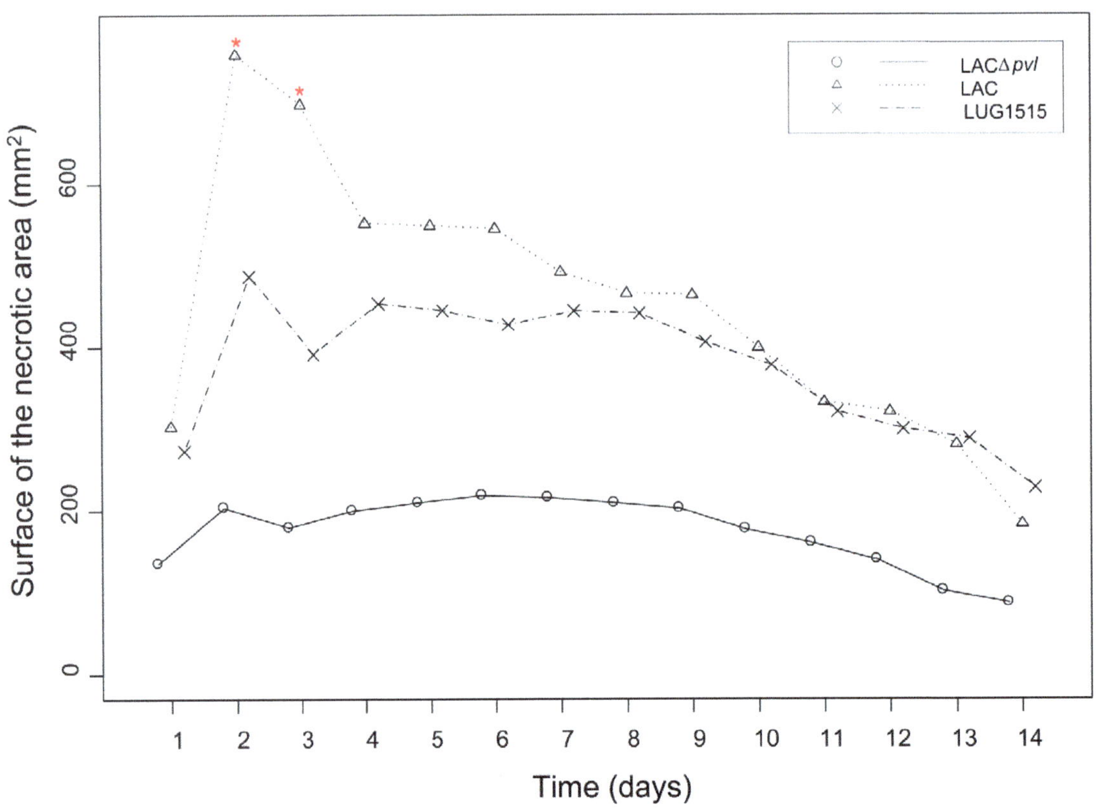
Surface of the necrotic area (mm²)
0
200
400
600
LACΔpvl
LAC
LUG1515
1 2 3 4 5 6 7 8 9 10 11 12 13 14
Time (days)

Figure 2. The size of the lesions and skin necrosis over the time. Mean surface of the lesions (a) and necrotic areas (b) evoked by intradermal injection of LAC (Δ), LACΔ*pvl* (o) and LUG1515 (x) in the rabbits. Asterisk (*) represents a statistically significant result in comparison to LACΔ*pvl* group.

Discussion

Involvement of PVL in the virulence of *S. aureus* has been a controversial topic for many scientists searching for factors responsible for the high pathogenicity of community associated *S. aureus* strains. Inasmuch as murine models have been delivering inconclusive results on the PVL contribution to the staphylococcal skin infections, we examined the role of this toxin using a rabbit - an animal species whose neutrophils are as sensitive to the action of PVL as those of humans [18]. We found that the CA-MRSA USA300 isolate expressing PVL produced lesions with significantly bigger surface than the isogenic PVL knockout strain in the first week after inoculation. Those data suggest that PVL has an impact on the early development of *S. aureus* skin infections in rabbits. In line with our results are the conclusions drawn from other studies investigating the role of PVL in rabbit models. Diep et al. depicted a modest, but measurable role of PVL in the pathogenesis during the early stages of bacteremic seeding in the kidney [26], and Cremieux et al. demonstrated PVL contribution to the local extension of osteomyelitis during the early phase of bone infection [27]. With regard to skin infections, our results are the first showing the capability of PVL producing strain to produce bigger lesions in rabbits, in comparison to their isogenic PVL knockout.

Recently, Li et al. published a study showing that rabbits infected with another USA300-type isolate produced lesions with a surface corresponding to that observed in our study in animals infected with LAC [28]. However, in the same study a PVL negative USA500 isolate evoked comparable lesions, which prompted the authors to the conclusion that PVL does not contribute to the development of skin lesions. The variation between the conclusions of the above mentioned and our study could be attributed to the study set up. While strains used in our study varied only upon PVL expression, those used by Li et al. may differ in respect to other determinants as well. Moreover, the latter failed to detect any PVL mRNA by qRT-PCR in the abscesses of PVL positive strains in their experimental model.

As the PVL determinants have been linked with necrotizing infections, the development of skin necrosis was evaluated during our study. The animals in all experimental groups initially developed necrotic lesions in the place of injection of bacteria. Interestingly, the majority of animals inoculated with the PVL knockout strain developed skin necrosis restricted to the surrounding of the inoculation spot. In contrast, the animals injected with PVL producing strains (LAC and LUG1515) developed necrotic lesions largely exceeding the inoculation area, suggesting that PVL activity accounts for development of severe

Table 1. Histopathological changes in rabbit skin produced by PVL-positive or -negative *S. aureus* strains.

Rabbit belonging to group	Necrosis		Inflammation			Remarks
	location	level	location	level	cell type	
LACΔ*pvl*	dermis	++	dermis	++	PMN ++, MF +/−, LF +/−	
	muscle	−	muscle	+	PMN +/−, MF +	
LACΔ*pvl*	dermis	+++	dermis	+++	PMN +++, MF +/−, LF +/−	
	muscle	−	muscle	+	PMN +/−, MF +	
LACΔ*pvl*	dermis	+++	dermis	+++	PMN +++, MF +, LF +	
	muscle	−	muscle	+/−	PMN +/−, MF +	
LAC	dermis	++++	dermis	++++	PMN ++++, MF +, LF +/−	bacteria observed
	muscle	+++	muscle	+++	PMN ++, MF +	
LAC	dermis	+++++	dermis	++	PMN ++, MF +	bacteria observed
	muscle	+++	muscle	+++	PMN +++	
LAC	dermis	+++++	dermis	++++	PMN +++, MF +/−, LF +/−	
	muscle	+	muscle	++	PMN +/−, MF +	
LUG1515	dermis	++++	dermis	++++	PMN +++, MF +, LF +	bacteria observed
	muscle	+++	muscle	++	PMN ++	
LUG1515	dermis	++	dermis	+++	PMN +++, MF +/−, LF +	bacteria observed
	muscle	+	muscle	+	PMN +/−, MF +	
LUG1515	dermis	+++	dermis	++++	PMN +++, MF +, LF +	
	muscle	++	muscle	+	PMN +	

From animals euthanized at day 4 p.i. lesions samples were used to prepare histological slides and the histopathological changes observed are summarized in the table. The grading system used was as follows: for necrosis (−) absent, (+) mild, (++) mild to moderate, (+++) moderate, (++++) pronounced, (+++++) severe; for inflammation (+/−) several inflammatory cells present, (+) mild, (++) moderate, (+++) pronounced and (++++) severe inflammation; presence of specific cell populations (+/−) few cells present, (+) several, (++) some, (+++) many cells present, (++++) big population of cells observed. Abbreviations: PMN = Polymorphonuclear cells; MF = macrophages; LF = lymphocytes.

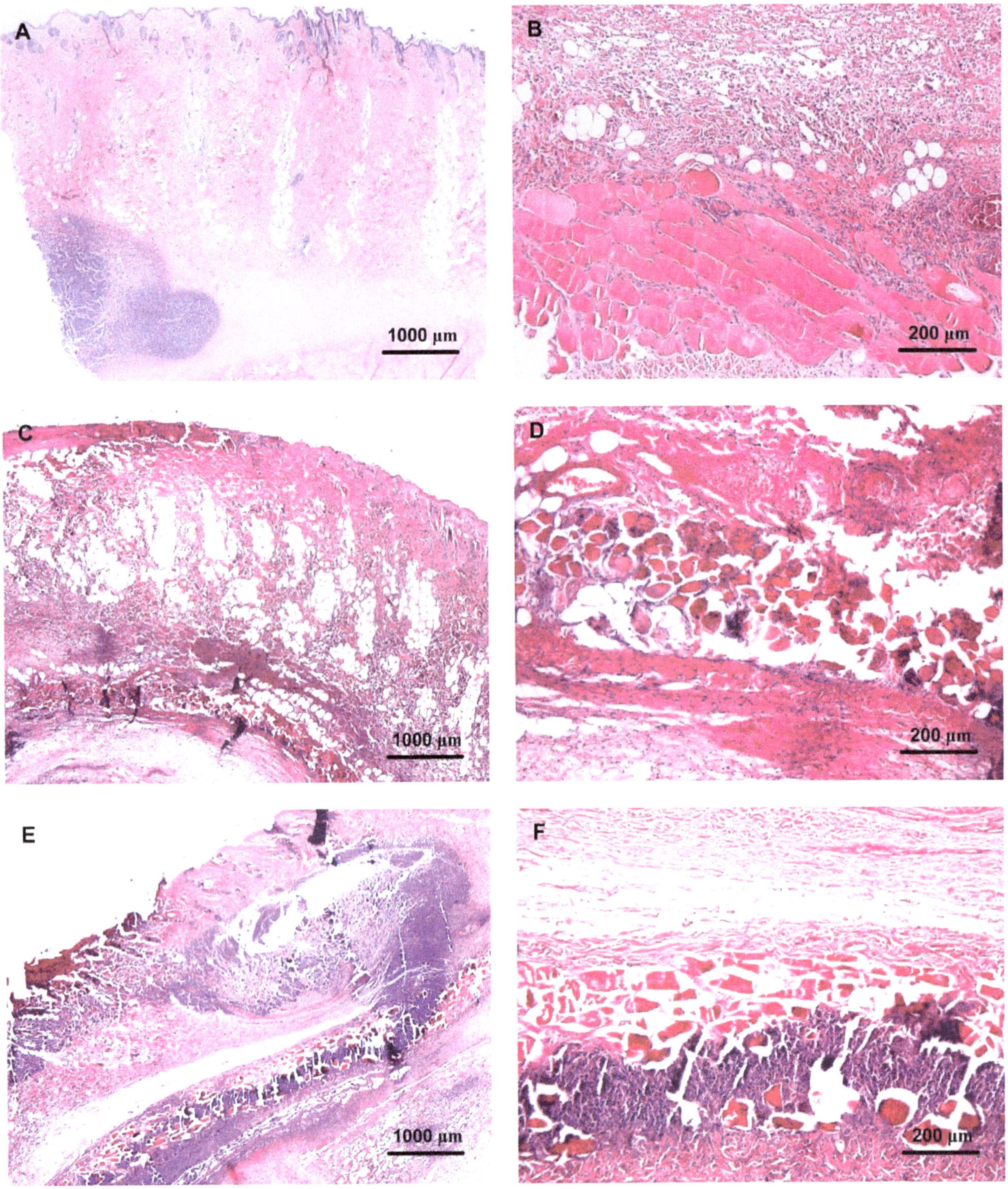

Figure 3. Microscopic appearance of skin lesions on day 4 after infection. The sections of the skin lesions collected from rabbits euthanized at day 4 p.i. were stained with hematoxylin and eosin, and observed under light microscope. A, C and E present the sections from the skin of rabbits infected with LACΔ*pvl*, LAC and LUG1515, respectively. B, D and F show the appearance of the skin muscle layer in animals inoculated with the strains mentioned above.

necrotizing lesions. Obtained results are consistent with those of Cribier et al. [6] who observed development of skin necrosis in rabbits injected with purified PVL and observations from a rabbit model of necrotizing pneumonia where a PVL-producing strain caused more lung necrosis than its PVL knockout [19]. Moreover, the histological analysis of skin biopsies collected at day 4 p.i. from

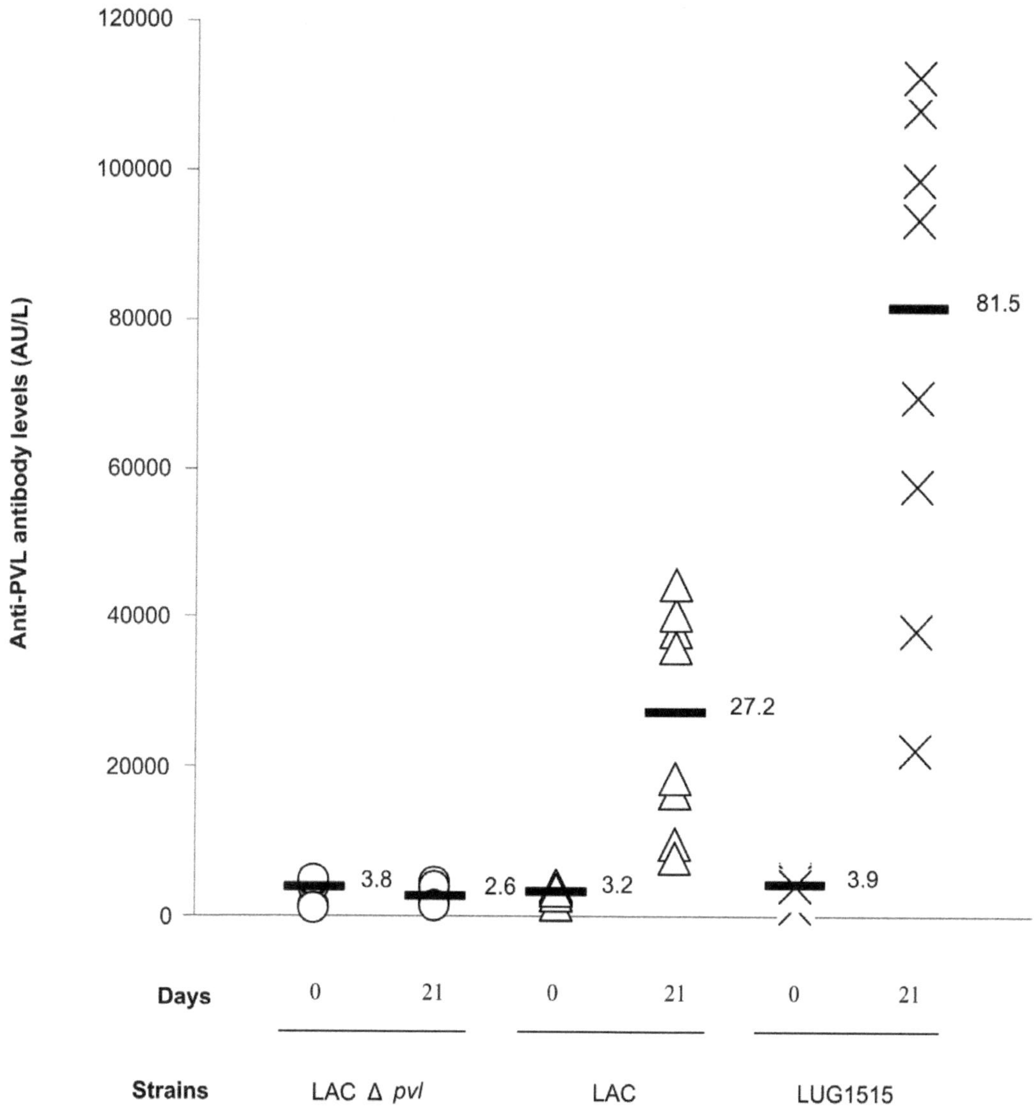

Figure 4. Production of anti-PVL antibodies. Distribution of anti-PVL antibody levels in the sera collected before challenge and at day 21 p.i. from rabbits infected with LACΔ*pvl*, LAC and LUG1515. Bars show the mean value.

the inoculation spot revealed slightly more pronounced damage and inflammatory response in animals infected with PVL positive *S. aureus* strains. The fact that some necrosis and inflammation was observed in the group infected with the PVL knockout strain indicates that other staphylococcal factors (i.e. phenol-soluble modulin, α-toxin) may contribute to the lesion development [28,29]. In conclusion, the presented results endorse the epidemiological link between PVL-producing strains and necrotizing skin infections [6–8,10].

Interestingly, while only minor histopathological differences have been noted for the dermis, necrosis of the skin muscle layer was observed for animals infected with PVL positive strains, in contrast to the PVL knockout where normal muscle was observed. Similarly, Tseng at al. observed damage of the muscle underlying inoculation spot in mice infected with high doses of PVL producing *S. aureus* [16]. Those data indicate that PVL may contribute to the damage of both the dermis and the skin muscle layer during skin infection.

To confirm the fact that differences between the wild type CA-MRSA strain and its PVL knockout could be accounted to PVL action, our study included a PVL knockout strain expressing PVL from a plasmid (LUG1515). Although the lesions produced by that strain differed macroscopically (smaller, but deeper - see fig. 1 and fig. 2a) from those evoked by the wild type strain, both strains produced bigger lesions in the early phase of infection than the PVL negative strain. Despite the fact that the PVL genes were accompanied by the original promoter and translator, the difference in the structure of the lesions produced by the wild type and the complemented strain could be result of a difference in the amount of PVL produced.

In order to confirm the *in vivo* expression of PVL, blood samples collected from the rabbits were analysed for the presence of antibodies directed against PVL. The anti-PVL antibody level in the rabbits infected with the PVL positive strains increased significantly in the course of the infection, while no shift in the titer of the antibody was observed for the rabbits infected with the PVL knockout strain. This raise in the titer of anti-PVL antibody is an indirect proof for production of this toxin during the infection. In line with our results are the observations from human patients where the anti-PVL antibody titers were demonstrated to be higher in patients with PVL positive *S. aureus* infection and to rise 4.6 times in the course of a skin infection [24].

Our results indicate that the rabbit is a better model than the mouse to study the contribution of PVL in the pathogenesis of skin infections by *S. aureus*. It is important that attention is paid to use animals free of high virulence rabbit *S. aureus* strains [30]. Those can be isolated from different body sites in carrier rabbits and can lead to the development of massive skin infection when introduced into the skin lesion. Through the collection of skin swabs from rabbits prior to the experiment, followed by bacteriological examination and molecular analysis of detected staphylococci, high virulence rabbit *S. aureus* strains can be identified [23] and their interference in the studies of human isolates can be avoided.

Although it could be remarked that the evaluation of the lesions was not performed blinded during this experiment, the significant difference in the size of the lesions evoked by wild type strain and its PVL knockout, in combination with the histological observations, indicate that PVL contributes to the severity of skin infections evoked by the CA-MRSA USA300 strain. As USA300 type isolates are epidemic in the USA and are responsible for a growing number of infections worldwide, further studies concerning community-associated staphylococcal infections should not neglect the impact of PVL.

Acknowledgments

We would like to acknowledge Dr. Frank DeLeo for providing us with *S. aureus* strains LAC and LACΔ*pvl*.

Author Contributions

Conceived and designed the experiments: UL GL KH. Performed the experiments: UL OD CB LM. Analyzed the data: UL KH GL JE FH LD. Contributed reagents/materials/analysis tools: UL OD CB. Wrote the paper: UL.

References

1. Lowy FD (1998) Medical progress - *Staphylococcus aureus* infections. New England Journal of Medicine 339: 520–532.
2. Gladstone GP, Van Heyningen WE (1957) Staphylococcal leucocidins. British Journal of Experimental Pathology 38: 123–137.
3. Woodin AM (1959) Fractionation of a leucocidin from *Staphylococcus aureus*. Biochemical Journal 73: 225–237.
4. Szmigielski S, Sobiczewska E, Prévost G, Monteil H, Colin DA, et al. (1998) Effect of purified staphylococcal leukocidal toxins on isolated blood polymorphonuclear leukocytes and peritoneal macrophages *in vitro*. Zentralblatt Fur Bakteriologie-International Journal of Medical Microbiology Virology Parasitology and Infectious Diseases 288: 383–394.
5. Hongo I, Baba T, Oishi K, Morimoto Y, Ito T, et al. (2009) Phenol-soluble modulin alpha 3 enhances the human neutrophil lysis mediated by Panton-Valentine leukocidin. Journal of Infectious Diseases 200: 715–723.
6. Cribier B, Prévost G, Couppie P, Finckbarbancon V, Grosshans E, et al. (1992) *Staphylococcus aureus* leukocidin - a new virulence factor in cutaneous infections - an epidemiologic and experimental study. Dermatology 185: 175–180.
7. Couppie P, Cribier B, Prévost G, Grosshans E, Piemont Y (1994) Leukocidin from *Staphylococcus aureus* and cutaneous infections - an epidemiologic study. Archives of Dermatology 130: 1208–1209.
8. Prévost G, Supersac G, Colin DA, Couppie P, Sire S, et al. (1994) The new family of leucotoxins from *Staphylococcus aureus* - structural and biological properties. In: Freer J, Aitken R, Alouf JE, Boulnois G, Falmagne P, et al. (1994) Bacterial Protein Toxins - Sixth European Workshop. Stuttgart 70: Gustav Fischer Verlag. pp 284–293.
9. Prévost G, Couppie P, Prévost P, Gayet S, Petiau P, et al. (1995) Epidemiologic data on *Staphylococcus aureus* strains producing synergohymenotropic toxins. Journal of Medical Microbiology 42: 237–245.
10. Lina G, Piemont Y, Godail-Gamot F, Bes M, Peter MO, et al. (1999) Involvement of Panton-Valentine leukocidin-producing *Staphylococcus aureus* in primary skin infections and pneumonia. Clinical Infectious Diseases 29: 1128–1132.
11. Diep BA, Sensabaugh GF, Somboona NS, Carleton HA, Perdreau-Remington F (2004) Widespread skin and soft-tissue infections due to two methicillin-resistant Staphylococcus aureus strains harboring the genes for Panton-Valentine leucocidin. Journal of Clinical Microbiology 42: 2080–2084.
12. Gillet Y, Issartel B, Vanhems P, Fournet JC, Lina G, et al. (2002) Association between *Staphylococcus aureus* strains carrying gene for Panton-Valentine leukocidin and highly lethal necrotising pneumonia in young immunocompetent patients. Lancet 359: 753–759.
13. Miller LG, Perdreau-Remington F, Rieg G, Mehdi S, Perlroth J, et al. (2005) Necrotizing fasciitis caused by community-associated methicillin-resistant *Staphylococcus aureus* in Los Angeles. New England Journal of Medicine 352: 1445–1453.
14. Voyich JM, Otto M, Mathema B, Braughton KR, Whitney AR, et al. (2006) Is Panton-Valentine leukocidin the major virulence determinant in community-associated methicillin-resistant *Staphylococcus aureus* disease? Journal of Infectious Diseases 194: 1761–1770.
15. Wardenburg JB, Palazzolo-Ballance AM, Otto M, Schneewind O, DeLeo FR (2008) Panton-Valentine leukocidin is not a virulence determinant in murine models of community-associated methicillin-resistant *Staphylococcus aureus* disease. Journal of Infectious Diseases 198: 1166–1170.
16. Tseng CW, Kyme P, Low J, Rocha MA, Alsabeh R, et al. (2009) *Staphylococcus aureus* Panton-Valentine leukocidin contributes to inflammation and muscle tissue injury. Plos One 4(7): e6387.
17. Brown EL, Dumitrescu O, Thomas D, Badiou C, Koers EM, et al. (2009) The Panton-Valentine leukocidin vaccine protects mice against lung and skin infections caused by *Staphylococcus aureus* USA300. Clinical Microbiology and Infection 15: 156–164.
18. Löffler B, Hussain M, Grundmeier M, Bruck M, Holzinger D, et al. (2010) *Staphylococcus aureus* Panton-Valentine leukocidin is a very potent cytotoxic factor for human neutrophils. Plos Pathogens 6(1): e1000715.
19. Diep BA, Chan L, Tattevin P, Kajikawa O, Martin TR, et al. (2010) Polymorphonuclear leukocytes mediate Staphylococcus aureus Panton-Valentine leukocidin-induced lung inflammation and injury. Proceedings of the National Academy of Sciences of the United States of America 107: 5587–5592.
20. Tenover FC, Goering RV (2009) Methicillin-resistant Staphylococcus aureus strain USA300: origin and epidemiology. Journal of Antimicrobial Chemotherapy 64: 441–446.
21. des Horts TB, Dumitrescu O, Badiou C, Thomas D, Benito Y, et al. (2010) A histidine-to-arginine substitution in Panton-Valentine leukocidin from USA300 community-acquired methicillin-resistant *Staphylococcus aureus* does not impair its leukotoxicity. Infection and Immunity 78: 260–264.
22. Hermans K, De Herdt P, Devriese LA, Hendrickx W, Godard C, et al. (1999) Colonization of rabbits with *Staphylococcus aureus* in flocks with and without chronic staphylococcosis. Veterinary Microbiology 67: 37–46.
23. Vancraeynest D, Haesebrouck F, Hermans K (2007) Multiplex PCR assay for the detection of high virulence rabbit *Staphylococcus aureus* strains. Veterinary Microbiology 121: 368–372.
24. Croze M, Dauwalder O, Dumitrescu O, Badiou C, Gillet Y, et al. (2009) Serum antibodies against Panton-Valentine leukocidin in a normal population and during *Staphylococcus aureus* infection. Clinical Microbiology and Infection 15: 144–148.
25. Harcourt-Brown F (2002) The rabbit consultation and clinical techniques. In: Textbook of rabbit medicine. London, . pp 52–93.
26. Diep BA, Palazzolo-Ballance AM, Tattevin P, Basuino L, Braughton KR, et al. (2008) Contribution of Panton-Valentine leukocidin in community-associated methicillin-resistant *Staphylococcus aureus* pathogenesis. Plos One 3(9): e3198.
27. Cremieux AC, Dumitrescu O, Lina G, Vallee C, Cote JF, et al. (2009) Panton-Valentine leukocidin enhances the severity of community-associated methicillin-resistant *Staphylococcus aureus* rabbit osteomyelitis. Plos One 4(9): e7204.
28. Li M, Cheung GY, Hu J, Wang D, Joo H, et al. (2010) Comparative analysis of virulence and toxin expression of global community-associated methicillin-resistant *Staphylococcus aureus* strains. Journal of Infectious Diseases 202: 1866–1876.
29. Wang R, Braughton KR, Kretschmer D, Bach THL, Queck SY, et al. (2007) Identification of novel cytolytic peptides as key virulence determinants for community-associated MRSA. Nature Medicine 13: 1510–1514.
30. Hermans K, Devriese LA, Haesebrouck F (2003) Rabbit staphylococcosis: difficult solution for serious problems. Veterinary Microbiology 91: 57–64.

Involvement of TNF-α Converting Enzyme in the Development of Psoriasis-Like Lesions in a Mouse Model

Kenji Sato[1,2], Mikiro Takaishi[1], Shota Tokuoka[2], Shigetoshi Sano[1]*

1 Department of Dermatology, Kochi Medical School, Kochi University, Nankoku, Japan, 2 Pharmacology Department, Drug Research Center, Kaken Pharmaceutical Co., Ltd., Kyoto, Japan

Abstract

TNF-α plays a crucial role in psoriasis; therefore, TNF inhibition has become a gold standard for the treatment of psoriasis. TNF-α is processed from a membrane-bound form by TNF-α converting enzyme (TACE) to soluble form, which exerts a number of biological activities. EGF receptor (EGFR) ligands, including heparin-binding EGF-like growth factor (HB-EGF), amphiregulin and transforming growth factor (TGF)-α are also TACE substrates and are psoriasis-associated growth factors. Vascular endothelial growth factor (VEGF), one of the downstream molecules of EGFR and TNF signaling, plays a key role in angiogenesis for developing psoriasis. In the present study, to assess the possible role of TACE in the pathogenesis of psoriasis, we investigated the involvement of TACE in TPA-induced psoriasis-like lesions in K5.Stat3C mice, which represent a mouse model of psoriasis. In this mouse model, TNF-α, amphiregulin, HB-EGF and TGF-α were significantly up-regulated in the skin lesions, similar to human psoriasis. Treatment of K5.Stat3C mice with TNF-α or EGFR inhibitors attenuated the skin lesions, suggesting the roles of TACE substrates in psoriasis. Furthermore, the skin lesions of K5.Stat3C mice showed down-regulation of tissue inhibitor of metalloproteinase-3, an endogenous inhibitor of TACE, and an increase in soluble TNF-α. A TACE inhibitor abrogated EGFR ligand-dependent keratinocyte proliferation and VEGF production in vitro, suggesting that TACE was involved in both epidermal hyperplasia and angiogenesis during psoriasis development. These results strongly suggest that TACE contributes to the development of psoriatic lesions through releasing two kinds of psoriasis mediators, TNF-α and EGFR ligands. Therefore, TACE could be a potential therapeutic target for the treatment of psoriasis.

Editor: Akihiko Yoshimura, Keio University School of Medicine, Japan

Funding: This study was funded in part by Kaken Pharmaceuticals Co. Ltd. KS, ST, SS received the funding. This study was additionally funded by grants-in-aid from the Ministry of Education, Culture, Sports, Science and Technology of Japan; and by a grant for Research on Intractable Diseases from the Ministry of Health, Labour, and Welfare of Japan. The funders had no role in study design, data collection and analysis, decision to publish, or preparation of the manuscript.

Competing Interests: The authors have read the journal's policy and have the following competing interests: KS and ST are employees of Kaken Pharmaceuticals Co. Ltd.

* Email: sano.derma@kochi-u.ac.jp

Introduction

Psoriasis is one of the most common inflammatory disorders and affects >2% of the population in Western countries. It has been demonstrated that TNF-α is involved in the development of psoriasis, as evidenced by the therapeutic efficacy of TNF-α inhibitors on psoriasis [1,2]. TNF-α has multiple functions and is one of the most important proinflammatory cytokines in psoriasis, linking innate immunity to adaptive immunity [3]. Indeed, previous studies suggested that TNF-α production from dendritic cells (DCs) is essential for activation of the pathogenic IL-23/Th17 axis in psoriasis [4].

TNF-α is produced as a membrane-bound form and is processed by TNF-α converting enzyme (TACE) to become a soluble form that exerts biological activity [5–7]. In addition to TNF-α, membrane-bound EGFR ligands, including amphiregulin, heparin-binding EGF (HB-EGF) and transforming growth factor (TGF)-α, are TACE substrates. More importantly, these EGFR ligands are known to contribute to the pathogenesis of psoriasis [8–10]. Furthermore, TACE is expressed by epidermal keratinocytes and inflammatory cells in the dermis in psoriatic lesions [11]. However, it remains unclear whether TACE is involved in the pathogenesis of psoriasis.

We previously reported that Stat3 is activated in keratinocytes in the majority of human psoriatic lesions [12]. K5.Stat3C transgenic mice, in which Stat3 is constitutively active in keratinocytes, develop psoriasis-like lesions following wounding stimuli or topical treatment with the tumor promoter 12-*O*-tetradecanoylphorbol-13-acetate (TPA), which strongly suggests that Stat3 activation is required for the development of psoriasis. The skin lesions of K5.Stat3C mice closely resemble psoriasis and provide a relevant animal model of psoriasis based on clinical, histological, immunophenotypic and biological criteria [12,13]. For example, the skin lesions in K5.Stat3C mice show epidermal hyperplasia, infiltration of immune cells into the dermis and abscess formation in the epidermis, which represent shared pathologic features with human psoriasis [12,14]. Furthermore, the skin lesions in K5.Stat3C mice are attenuated by administration of an anti-IL-17A antibody or anti-IL-12/23p40 antibody, similar to human psoriasis [14]. Therefore, K5.Stat3C mice provide a platform for screening potential therapeutic targets for the treatment of psoriasis.

Angiogenesis is a hallmark of psoriasis and the psoriasis-like skin lesions in K5.Stat3C mice [12]. VEGF plays a key role in angiogenesis and wound healing [15], and is a potential target for the treatment of psoriasis [16]. Upon wounding, keratinocytes produce VEGF, which is also strongly up-regulated in the epidermis of psoriatic lesions [17]. Previous studies have demonstrated that VEGF production by keratinocytes is regulated by TNF-α or HB-EGF [18,19]. Therefore, it is likely that TACE plays a role in VEGF production from keratinocytes not only during wound healing but also in psoriasis. In this regard, TACE is a post-translational regulator for the release of multiple soluble mediators required for psoriasis.

In the present study, we investigated the expression of TACE and its related molecules in psoriasis-like skin lesions in K5.Stat3C mice, and addressed the question as to how TACE inhibition impacts the release of cytokines/growth factors and keratinocyte proliferation. The sum of our results suggests TACE inhibition as a potential strategy for the treatment of psoriasis.

Materials and Methods

Patients and normal controls

The study protocol was conducted in accordance with the guidelines of the World Medical Association's Declaration of Helsinki and was approved by the Institute Ethical Review Board of the Kochi Medical School, Kochi University. Written informed consent was obtained from subjects after explaining the purpose of the study.

Mice

All experimental procedures performed on mice were approved by the Institutional Animal Care and Use Committee of Kochi Medical School. K5.Stat3C mice were generated as previously reported [20]. Briefly, Stat3C cDNA (a gift from Dr. J. Bromberg, Memorial Sloan Kettering Cancer Center) was ligated into the pBK5 construct, followed by digestion with EcoRI. The construct was then used to generate transgenic founder mice on an FVB/N background.

TPA-induced psoriasis-like lesions in the ears of K5.Stat3C mice

The generation of psoriasis-like lesions in the ears of K5.Stat3C mice was conducted as previously described [14,21]. In brief, the skin lesions were generated by topical application of 0.68 nmol TPA (Wako) in 20 μl acetone to all surfaces of the left and right ears at day 0 and 2. Etanercept (Pfizer) (1 mg/mouse) was intravenously injected on day 0 and 2. The dosage of etanercept was decided as previously described [22]. AG1478 (LC laboratories) was dissolved in acetone to prepare a 0.016% solution. Following this, 20 μl AG1478 solution was topically applied to all surfaces of the left and right ears twice a day. The concentration of AG1478 was decided as previously described [23]. Ear thickness was measured every day from day 0 to 3. The mice were sacrificed and ear skins were collected for gene and protein expression analysis and histological analysis. All mouse experiments were performed with strict adherence to institutional guidelines for minimizing distress.

Histology

Ear tissues were fixed in 20% formalin and then embedded in paraffin. Sections were obtained from the paraffin blocks and stained by hematoxylin and eosin (H&E) using standard methods. Epidermal thickness was measured at 12 spots in the interfollicular epidermis in each slide.

Immunohistochemical staining

Formalin-fixed slides were deparaffinized with xylene and rehydrated in an alcohol gradient. Slides were autoclaved in 10 mmol/l citrate (pH 6.0) at 115°C for 5 min to retrieve antigen, then incubated for 40 min at room temperature. Endogenous peroxidase was quenched using 3% hydrogen peroxide, then nonspecific antibody reaction was blocked using protein block serum free (DAKO) at room temperature for 30 min. Slides were incubated with specific primary antibodies, rabbit anti-human TACE antibody (QED Bioscience) or rabbit anti-human TNF-α (IHC-world), at 4°C overnight. Slides were washed with PBS and subjected to horseradish peroxidase-conjugated secondary antibody (DAKO) for 30 min at 37°C. The slides were washed with PBS, then detected by diaminobenzidine substrate kit (Life Technologies). All slides were counterstained with hematoxylin.

Quantitative real-time PCR

Ear tissues were minced with scissors into small pieces on ice, and were then disrupted by sonication in RNA lysis buffer contained in an RNA isolation kit (Promega). For some experiments, primary keratinocytes were stimulated with 20 ng/ml IL-17A (R&D Systems) and 10 ng/ml TNF-α (R&D Systems) for 24 h and peritoneal macrophages were stimulated with 100 ng/ml LPS (Sigma) for 0.5, 6 and 24 h pretreated with or without 10 μmol/l TAPI-1 (Enzo Life Sciences), for 30 min prior to stimulation. Total RNAs were extracted using an RNeasy Mini kit (Qiagen) according to the manufacturer's protocol. RNAs were reverse transcribed using M-MLV reverse transcriptase with random oligonucleotide hexamers (Life Technologies). Quantitative PCR reactions were performed using Taqman Master Mix or Power SYBR Green PCR Master Mix (Life Technologies). Amplification conditions were as follows: 50°C for 2 min, 90°C for 10 min for 1 cycle, followed by 40 cycles of 95°C for 15 sec and 60°C for 1 min. Primers used were described elsewhere [14] and those for HPRT (Mm01545399_m1), TNF-α (Mm00443258_m1), amphiregulin (Mm00437583_m1), HB-EGF (Mm00439306_m1), TGF-α (Mm00446232_m1) and TIMP-3 (Mm00441826_m1), all from Life Technologies. The quantity of each transcript was analyzed using the 7300 Fast System Software (Life Technologies) and was normalized to hypoxanthine phosphoribosyltransferase (*HPRT*), according to the ΔΔ Ct method.

Determination of TNF-α in skin samples

For measurement of TNF-α in skin, ear biopsy samples were taken using a punch (a diameter of 8 mm, Kai Industries Co. Ltd.). Ear tissues were minced with scissors into small pieces on ice in cold PBS containing protease inhibitor cocktail, phosphatase inhibitor cocktail 2 and 3 (Sigma), and were disrupted by sonication. The homogenized tissues were centrifuged at 20,000 g for 20 min at 4°C, and supernatants were harvested. TNF-α in the supernatants was measured using ELISA for TNF-α (R&D Systems).

Measurement of in vivo TACE activity

TACE activity was determined by the SensoLyte 520 TACE Activity Assay Fluorimetric Kit (AnaSpec), according to the manufacturer's instructions. In brief, Ear skins were minced with scissors into small pieces in cold assay buffer containing 0.1% TritonX-100 and were homogenized. The lysates were centrifuged at 2,000 g for 15 min at 4°C, and supernatants were harvested. TACE activity from 25 μg of total protein was measured using the kit for TACE activity.

Western blot

The protein extraction from ear skins was performed as described above. The protein concentration of each supernatant was measured with the Bio-Rad protein assay system (Bio-Rad). The supernatants were separated on 4–20% SDS/PAGE according to the method as previously described [24], under reducing conditions. Recombinant TNF-α (eBioscience) was loaded as a positive control in some experiments. Separated proteins were electrophoretically transferred to polyvinylidene difluoride membranes and blocked with 5% skim milk in TBS with 0.1% Tween 20 (TBST) for 1 h at room temperature. Membranes were incubated with specific primary antibodies, goat anti-mouse TNF-α antibody (Antigenix America) or rabbit anti-mouse TIMP-3 antibody (Millipore), at 4°C overnight. Membranes were washed with TBST and subjected to horseradish peroxidase-conjugated secondary antibodies against goat (SantaCruz) and rabbit (GE Healthcare) for 45 min at room temperature. The membranes were washed with TBST, then detection for TNF-α and TIMP-3 were performed using SuperSignal West Femto (Thermo Fisher Scientific) and ECL plus Western Blotting Detection System (GE Healthcare), respectively. The membranes were stripped by Restore Western blot stripping buffer (Thermo Fisher Scientific) and reprobed with mouse anti-mouse fiactin (Sigma) for 1 h at room temperature. The membranes were washed with TBST, then subjected to corresponding horseradish peroxidase-conjugated secondary antibodies (GE Healthcare). The membranes were washed with TBST, then detected with ECL plus Western Blotting Detection System.

Preparation of bone marrow derived dendritic cells (BMDCs), peritoneal macrophages and keratinocytes

BMDCs were generated as previously described [25]. Briefly, bone marrow cells taken from wild-type FVB/N mice were suspended in RPMI 1640 (Life Technologies) containing 10 ng/ml GM-CSF (Peprotech), antibiotic-antimycotic (Life Technologies) and 10% FBS (Nichirei Bioscience). BMDCs were harvested 9 d later and plated at 5×10^4 cells/well in 96-well plates. Peritoneal macrophages were isolated as previously described [26] with modifications. Briefly, wild-type FVB/N mice were injected i.p. with 500 µL 4% sterile thioglycolate (Becton Dickinson) solution in PBS, and cells were harvested by peritoneal lavage 4 d later. Cells were plated at 5×10^4 cells/well in 96-well plates. For gene expression analysis, cells were plated at 2.5×10^5 cells/well in 24-well plates. Primary keratinocytes were isolated from the skin of K5.Stat3C newborn mice as described [12]. In brief, epidermis was isolated by overnight digestion of dorsal skin from K5.Stat3C newborn mice with dispase (Becton Dickinson) at 4°C. The epidermis was incubated with 0.25% trypsin (Life Technologies) for 5 min at 37°C. After stopping the trypsin reaction with FBS, the keratinocyte suspension was passed through a 70 µm cell strainer. Freshly isolated primary keratinocytes were plated at 2.5×10^5 cells/well in 24-well plates for the detection TNF-ted wiamphiregulin or 1.5×10^5 cells/well in 48-well plates for the detection VEGF in DMEM-Glutamax (Life Technologies) containing antibiotic-antimycotic and 10% FBS. Three hours later, the medium and floating cells were removed, and attached cells were refed with Epilife (Life Technologies) supplemented with Hu-Media KG (Kurabo). Cells were cultured until they were subconfluent, then used for the detection of TNF-α, amphiregulin and VEGF. For the proliferation assay, freshly isolated primary keratinocytes were plated at 6×10^4 cells/well in 48-well plates. A medium change was performed as described above, then cells were cultured for 2 days.

Production of TNF-α, amphiregulin and VEGF in vitro

BMDCs and peritoneal macrophages from wild-type FVB/N mice were stimulated with 100 ng/ml LPS. Primary keratinocytes isolated from K5.Stat3C newborn mice were stimulated with 100 nmol/l TPA for 24 h. Cells were pretreated with or without TAPI-1 for 30 min prior to stimulation. The concentrations of cytokines and growth factors in the culture medium were examined by ELISA for TNF-α (eBioscience), amphiregulin (R&D Systems) and VEGF (R&D Systems).

Keratinocyte proliferation assay and Cytotoxic assay

Primary keratinocytes were treated with or without 100 µmol/l TAPI-1 or 100 nmol/l AG1478. HB-EGF (BioVision) or amphiregulin (R&D Systems) (all at 100 ng/ml) were added at 30 min after TAPI-1 or AG1478 treatment, then cultured for 3 days. Keratinocyte proliferation was assessed using 3-(4,5-dimethylthiazol-2-yl)-5-(3-carboxymethoxyphenyl)-2-(4-sulfophenyl)-2H-tetrazolium, inner salt (MTS) assay (Promega) on day 0 to 3, or bromodeoxyuridine (BrdU) ELISA (Roche) on day 2. Toxicity effects and adverse reactions to chemical compounds were assessed by measuring lactate dehydrogenase (LDH) release in the culture medium (Promega), and Triton X-100 (Wako) was used as a positive control.

Statistical analysis

Statistical differences were evaluated by Student's *t*-test, Tukey-Kramer's test or Duunett's test. *p* values less than 0.05 were considered significant.

Results

Expression of TACE and TNF-α in human psoriatic skin and in psoriasis-like skin lesions of K5.Stat3C mice

As previously described, TACE was expressed in all layers of the epidermis, blood vessels and appendages in human psoriatic lesions as well as in uninvolved human skin (Fig. 1A, middle panels) [11,27]. However, dermal inflammatory cells in psoriatic lesions strongly expressed TACE (Fig. 1A, right middle panel) [11,27]. TNF-α was expressed in the epidermis and inflammatory cell infiltrates of psoriatic lesions (Fig. 1A, right bottom panel), whereas uninvolved skin did not express TNF-α (Fig. 1A, left bottom panel) as previously reported [28]. Topical treatment with TPA resulted in the emergence of psoriasis-like lesions in K5.Stat3C mice, but not in wild-type mice (Fig. 1B–D) [14]. The histopathology of skin lesions in K5.Stat3C included epidermal hyperplasia, a number of inflammatory cell infiltrates in the dermis, and abscess formation in the epidermis, all of which resemble psoriasis (Fig. 1A–B, top panels). Similar to human psoriasis, TPA-induced psoriasis-like lesions in K5.Stat3C mice were positive for TACE in the epidermis, inflammatory cells, blood vessels and appendages (Fig. 1A–B, middle panels). It is noteworthy that the neutrophilic abscess in the epidermis showed strong TACE expression (Fig. 1B, arrow). Furthermore, as found in human psoriasis [28] (Fig. 1A, bottom panels), TNF-α was overexpressed in psoriasis-like skin lesions of K5.Stat3C mice, although virtually no TNF-α was found in untreated control skin (Fig. 1B, bottom panels). However, TPA treatment induced TNF-α expression in the epidermis of wild-type mice as well (Fig. 1C, bottom). This was supported by the results of RT-PCR (Fig. 1E) and ELISA (Fig. 1F) showing that TPA-treated skins of wild-type mice showed increased TNF-α expression as well as K5.Stat3C mice on day 3. Taken together, elevated levels and distribution of TACE and TNF-α in skin lesions of K5.Stat3C mice are similar to those in human psoriasis.

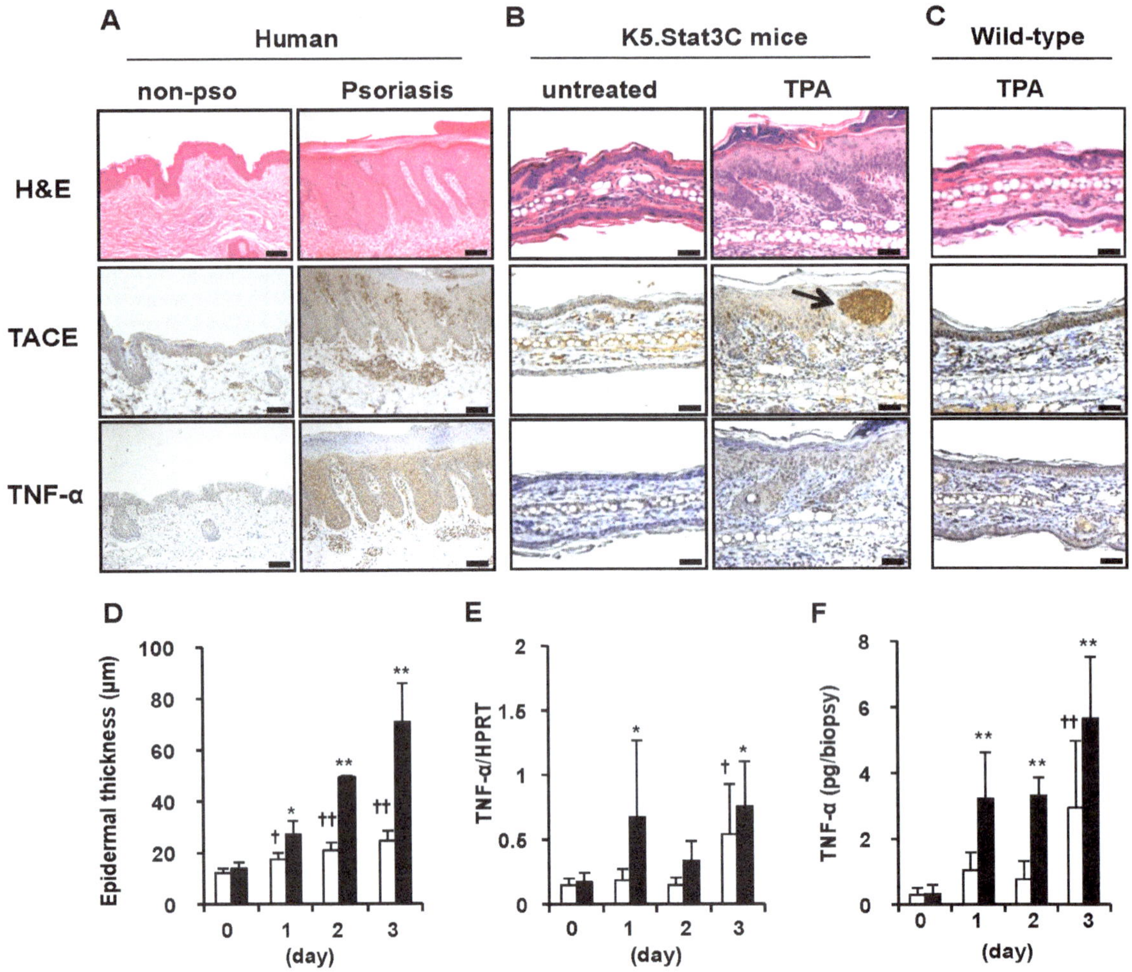

Figure 1. Expression of TACE and TNF-α in the development of psoriasis-like skin lesions in K5.Stat3C mice. (A–C), Representative histology and immunohistochemistry of human skins (A), ear skins in K5.Stat3C mice (B), and wild-type mice (C). non-pso, non-psoriasis control; TPA, TPA-treated ear skins sampled at day 3; Hematoxylin and eosin staining (H&E, top panels), Immunohistochemical staining for TACE (middle panels) and TNF-α (bottom panels). Arrow, intraepidermal pustule of neutrophils. Bars = 100 μm (human), 50 μm (mouse). (D–F), epidermal thickness (D), TNF-α mRNA expression (E) and TNF-α protein levels (F) in the TPA-treated ear skins of K5.Stat3C mice (black bars) and wild-type mice (white bars). Data represent means ± SD of 3 to 8 mice. **p*<0.05, ***p*<0.01, versus K5.Stat3C mice at day 0, †*p*<0.05, ††*p*<0.01, versus wild-type mice at day 0, by Dunnett's test.

TNF-α is involved in the development of psoriasis-like skin lesions in K5.Stat3C mice

To examine whether TNF-α is involved in the development of skin lesions, we intravenously injected a TNF-α inhibitor, etanercept, to K5.Stat3C mice before topical TPA application. Etanercept attenuated the TPA-induced thickening of ear skins (Fig. 2A) as well as epidermal hyperplasia (Fig. 2B–C). In addition, etanercept lowered the TPA-induced gene expression of IL-17A and IL-12/23p40 in the skin lesions (Fig. 2D–E). These results suggest that the inhibition of TNF-α signaling attenuates the psoriasis-like phenotype in K5.Stat3C mice through down-regulation of the IL-23/Th17 axis as found in patients with psoriasis treated with TNF-α inhibitors [4]. These results suggest that the inhibition of TNF-α attenuates the psoriasis-like phenotype in K5.Stat3C mice as occurs in patients with psoriasis treated with TNF-α inhibitors.

EGFR signaling is involved in the development of skin lesions in K5.Stat3C mice

EGFR ligands, including amphiregulin, HB-EGF and TGF-α, all of which are TACE substrates, have been shown to be up-regulated in psoriatic lesions [29]. We analyzed the gene expression of EGFR ligands during the development of psoriasis-like skin lesions in K5.Stat3C mice. Transcriptional levels of amphiregulin, HB-EGF and TGF-α were increased at day 1, and remained elevated until day 3, whereas the increase in levels of those genes in wild-type mouse skin was much less pronounced during 3 days of topical TPA application (Fig. 3A). This result indicated that up-regulation of EGFR ligands was associated with Stat3 activation in keratinocytes [13]. To assess whether EGFR signaling is involved in TPA-induced psoriasis-like skin lesions, we topically treated K5.Stat3C mice with AG1478, an EGFR inhibitor. AG1478 attenuated the epidermal thickness (Fig. 3B–C), which suggests that the EGFR signaling by the aforementioned EGFR ligands contributed, at least in part, to the generation of lesions in K5.Stat3C mice.

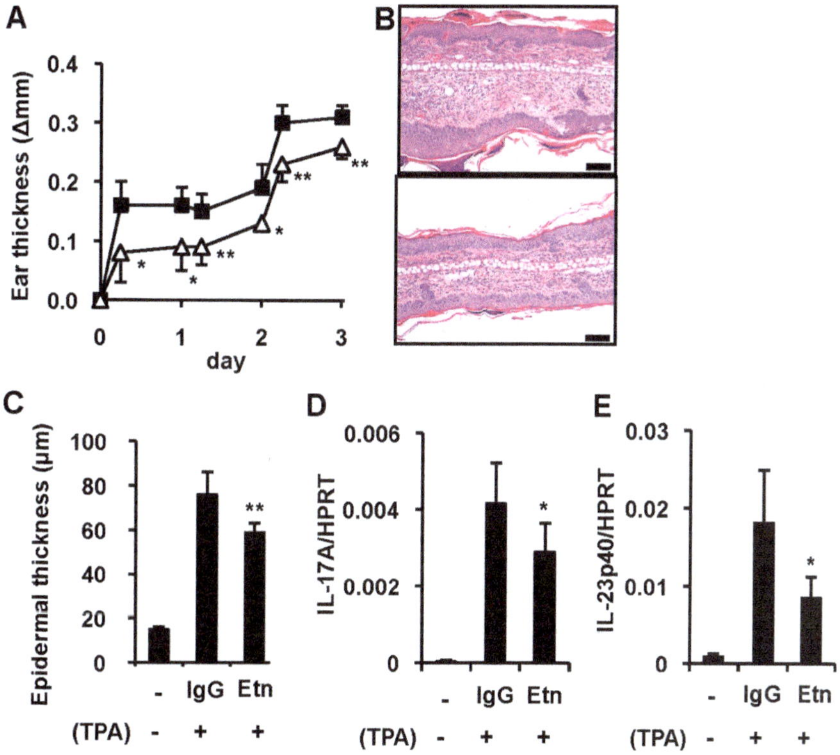

Figure 2. Involvement of TNF-α in the development of psoriasis-like skin lesions in K5.Stat3C mice. (A), Ear thickness (Δmm) ± SD following topical TPA in mice treated with control IgG (n = 6, squares) and etanercept (n = 6, triangles). *$p<0.05$, **$p<0.01$, versus control IgG, by Student's *t*-test. (B), Representative histology of ear skins from K5.Stat3C mice treated with control IgG (top) and etanercept (bottom). H&E staining. Bar = 100 μm. (C–E), Inhibitory effect of etanercept (Etn) on TPA-induced epidermal hyperplasia (C), gene expression of IL-17A (D), and IL-12/23p40 (E) in ear skins. Data represent means ± SD of 3 to 6 mice. *$p<0.05$, **$p<0.01$, versus control IgG, by Student's *t*-test.

Down-regulation of TIMP-3, an endogenous TACE inhibitor, and increased TACE enzymatic activity in psoriasis-like skin lesions of K5.Stat3C mice

Tissue inhibitor of metalloproteinase-3 (TIMP-3) has been reported as the negative regulator of the enzymatic activity of TACE [30–32]. Gene expression of TIMP-3 in the ear skin of K5.Stat3C mice was decreased in a time-dependent manner during the generation of TPA-induced lesions (Fig. 4A, black bars), while this decline was much less pronounced in wild-type mice (Fig. 4A, white bars). Strikingly, Western blot analysis revealed that TIMP-3 protein levels in the ear skin of K5.Stat3C mice were almost completely abrogated as early as 6 h of TPA application (Fig. 4B), and in turn, soluble TNF-α emerged around 17 kDa of molecular weight (Fig. 4C), through TACE-mediated processing of its membrane-bound form. In contrast, soluble TNF-α was hardly detected from the lysates of wild-type mice at this early time point (Fig. 4C). However, the gene expression of TACE was not different between wild-type mice and K5.Stat3C mice, or not increased by TPA treament (data not shown), suggesting that the post-transcriptional function of TACE might be enhanced likely by down-regulation of TIMP-3. Indeed, the skin of K5.Stat3C mice at baseline showed higher enzymatic activity of TACE than wild-type mice, and it was further increased following TPA treatment (Fig. 4D). Taken collectively, these results implicated that TACE was favorably activated in the skin of K5.Stat3C mice, at least in part, due to down-modulation of TIMP-3, leading to lesion development.

TACE releases TNF-α from various cells

TNF-α is produced by various cells in psoriasis, including keratinocytes, dendritic cells, macrophages and lymphocytes [33,34]. To assess whether TACE plays a role in releasing TNF-α from these cells, we added a relatively selective inhibitor of TACE, TAPI-1 [35], to an in vitro culture of bone marrow-derived dendritic cells (BMDCs), peritoneal macrophages and primary keratinocytes. TAPI-1 significantly and dose-dependently suppressed the LPS- or TPA-induced release of TNF-α from BMDCs and macrophages from wild-type FVB/N mice and keratinocytes of K5.Stat3C newborn mice, respectively (Fig. 5A–C). The release of TNF-α from T lymphocytes was also abrogated by TAPI-1 (data not shown). It should be noted that TNF-α mRNA levels in macrophages were increased by LPS stimulation but not affected by TAPI-1 treatment (Fig. S1), verifying that TAPI-1 inhibited the release of TNF-α post-transcriptionally. Collectively, these results clearly indicate that the release of soluble TNF-α from a variety of cells is dependent on TACE activity.

TACE induces the release of EGFR ligands from keratinocytes

EGFR ligands are produced by keratinocytes, and thereby an auto-stimulation loop is formed to generate psoriatic changes in an autocrine and paracrine fashion [10,36]. To assess whether TACE activity is required for the release of EGFR ligands as well as TNF-α, we evaluated the effects of TAPI-1 using primary cultured keratinocytes isolated from K5.Stat3C mice. Like TNF-α, amphiregulin was released by TACE from keratinocytes in response to TPA, since it was significantly suppressed by TAPI-1

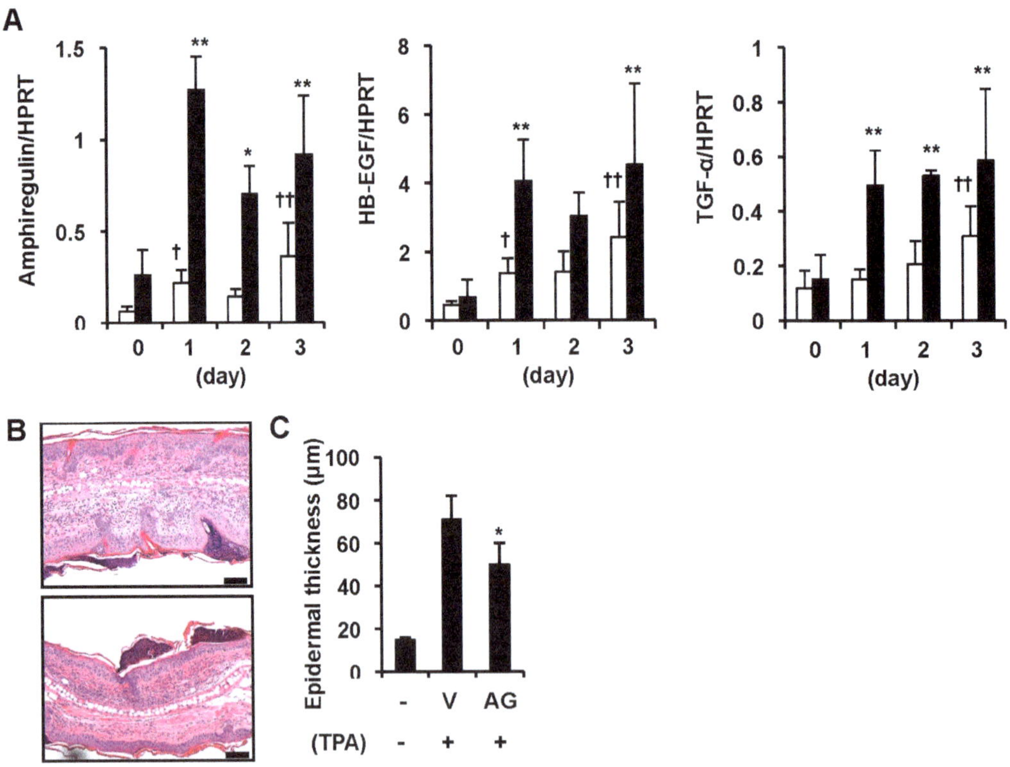

Figure 3. Involvement of EGFR signaling in the development of psoriasis-like skin lesions in K5.Stat3C mice. (A), Gene expression of amphiregulin, HB-EGF and TGF-α in the TPA-treated ear skins of K5.Stat3C mice (black bars) and wild-type mice (white bars). Data represent means ± SD of 3 to 8 mice. *$p<0.05$, **$p<0.01$, versus K5.Stat3C mice at day 0, $^{\dagger}p<0.05$, $^{\dagger\dagger}p<0.01$, versus wild-type mice at day 0, by Dunnett's test. (B), Representative histology of ear skins from K5.Stat3C mice treated with vehicle alone (top) and AG1478 (bottom). Bars = 100 µm. (C), Suppression of TPA-induced epidermal hyperplasia by treatment with AG1478 (AG) at day 3. Data represent means ± SD of 3 to 5 mice, *$p<0.05$ versus vehicle alone (V) by Student's *t*-test.

in a dose-dependent manner (Fig. 5D). EGFR stimulation leads to keratinocyte proliferation, and contributes to epidermal hyperplasia in psoriasis [29,37] and the skin phenotypes of K5.Stat3C mice as well (Fig. 3). We next examined whether TACE is directly required for keratinocyte proliferation in response to the endogenous EGFR ligands. In vitro keratinocyte proliferation was suppressed by TAPI-1 and AG1478 (Fig. 5E). The inhibitory effects of both reagents on cell proliferation were confirmed using a BrdU incorporation assay (Fig. S2A). TAPI-1 or AG1478 did not raise lactate dehydrogenase levels in the culture supernatants compared with the vehicle control, thus ruling out cytotoxicity as a possible cause of impaired keratinocyte proliferation (Fig. S2B). The suppression of keratinocyte proliferation by TAPI-1 was reversed by the addition of amphiregulin, suggesting that TACE is involved in keratinocyte proliferation via EGFR stimulation with soluble amphiregulin (Fig. 5E). Although the underlying mechanism is not known, HB-EGF seemed to augment the TAPI-1-induced suppression of keratinocyte proliferation. VEGF is an angiogenetic factor, and is involved in the pathogenesis of psoriasis [17,38,39]. Psoriatic lesions in K5.Stat3C mice showed increased levels of VEGF [12] (Fig. S3). Furthermore, TAPI-1 and AG1478 inhibited the TPA-induced VEGF production from K5.Stat3C keratinocytes to a similar extent (Fig. 5F). Suppression of VEGF production by TAPI-1 was reversed by the addition of HB-EGF, but not by amphiregulin (Fig. 5F). These results demonstrate that TACE-dependent HB-EGF stimulation leads to VEGF production by K5.Stat3C keratinocytes. Taken together, TACE is required for the release of soluble EGFR ligands from keratinocytes, thereby promoting keratinocyte proliferation and VEGF production, which are required for the development of psoriasis.

Discussion

The auto-stimulation loop of cytokine/growth factors within the epidermis and its bidirectional interaction with immunocytes play critical roles in the development of psoriasis. One of the proinflammatory cytokines, TNF-α, and growth factors of the EGFR ligand family represent essential mediators for the pathogenesis of psoriasis. TNF-α and EGFR ligands are overexpressed in plaque psoriasis compared with uninvolved skin or healthy control skin [28,29]. Our current study highlights the role of TACE, by which both TNF-α and growth factors for EGFR are shed to form soluble ligands. Here we took advantage of K5.Stat3C mice, which develop skin lesions that closely resemble human psoriasis with respect to clinical features, histopathology, immunological abnormalities and sensitivities to biologics [12,14,40].

The role for TNF-α in psoriasis has been well documented, and is supported by a number of studies showing successful therapeutic effects of its inhibitors [1,2]. It was suggested that TNF-α stimulation of DCs results in IL-23 production, which is required for Th17 cell activation [4,41]. Indeed, a comparison of gene expression in psoriasis patients between responders to etanercept,

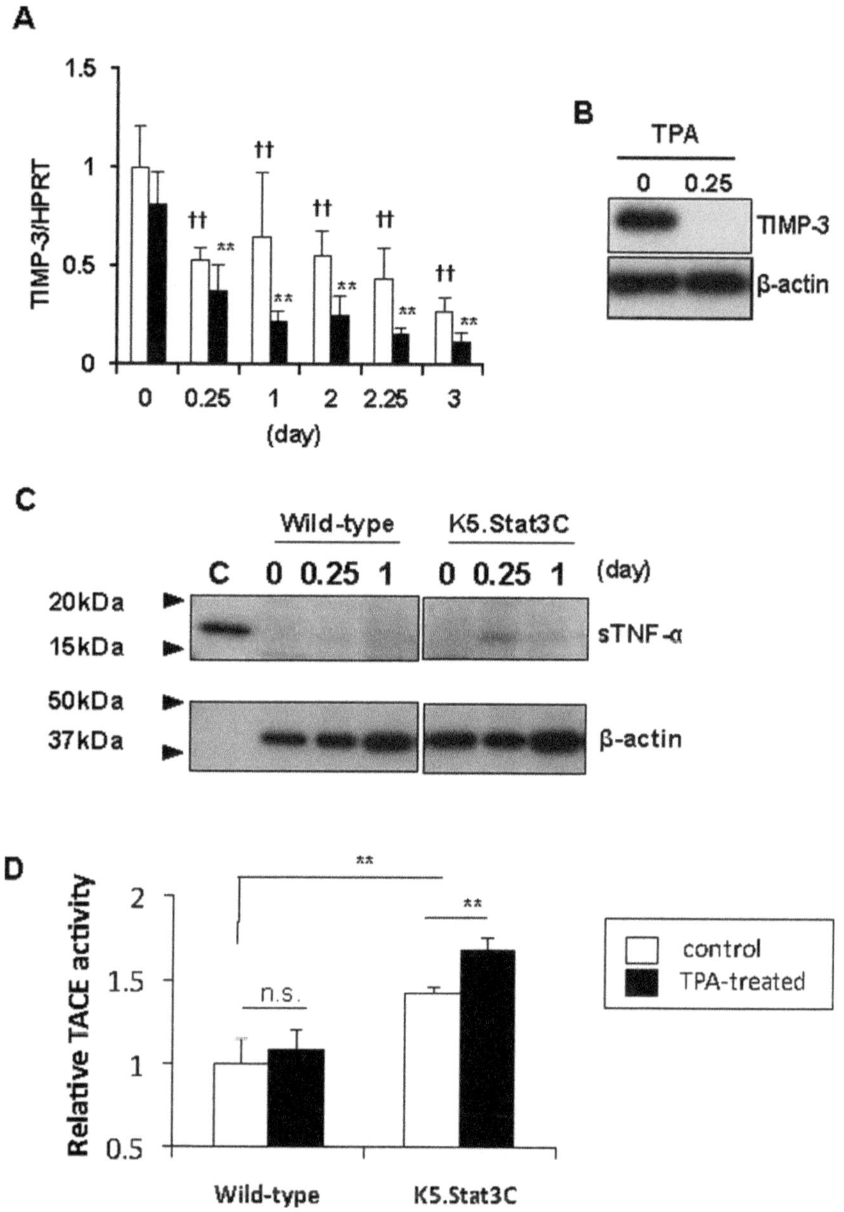

Figure 4. Down-regulation of TIMP-3, an endogenous TACE inhibitor, and TACE enzymatic activity in the development of psoriasis-like skin lesions. (A), Gene expression of TIMP-3 in the TPA-treated ear skins of K5.Stat3C mice (black bars) and wild-type mice (white bars). Data represent means ± SD of 3 to 8 mice. $^{**}p<0.01$, versus K5.Stat3C mice at day 0, $^{\dagger\dagger}p<0.01$, versus wild-type mice at day 0, by Dunnett's test. (B), Western blot analysis of TIMP-3 in ear skins of K5.Stat3C mice collected before TPA application (0) or 6 h (0.25) after TPA application. (C), Western blot analysis of soluble TNF-α (sTNF-α), which is around 17 kDa of molecular size, in the lysates from ear skins of K5.Stat3C mice compared with wild-type mice. The ear skins were collected before TPA application (0) or at 6 h (0.25) and 1 day (1) after TPA application. C, Control of soluble TNF-α. (D), Enzymatic activity of TACE in ear skins of K5.Stat3C mice versus wild-type mice; untreated control (white bars) and TPA-treated at 6h of the second TPA application (black bars). Enzymatic activity in skins was indicated as ratio to that in untreated wild-type skins. Data represent means ± SD of 4 to 5 mice, $^{**}p<0.01$; n.s., not significant by Tukey-Kramer's test.

a TNF-α inhibitor, and non-responders revealed that the responsiveness is dependent on inactivation of the Th17 immune response [42]. We showed that TNF-α stimulation enhances the production of IL-12/IL-23p40, one of the IL-23 subunits, from murine bone marrow-derived DCs (BMDCs) (data not shown). TNF-α inhibition also abrogates Th17 differentiation in vitro [43]. Furthermore, TNF-α synergistically augments IL-17A stimulation of gene expression by keratinocytes, including IL-24 (a member of IL-20 subfamily cytokines), IL-17C, TNF-α, HB-EGF, TGF-α, S100A7, S100A8, S100A9, β-defensin-3 and β-defensin-14 (Fig. S4). Thus, TNF-α stimulation impacts a variety of cells that release mediators required for the pathogenesis of psoriasis. In the experimental setting of the present study, however, treatment with etenercept (Etn) resulted in significant but insufficient attenuation of psoriatic phenotype of K5.Stat3C mice. The incomplete in vivo effect of Etn might be due to insufficient local concentrations of Etn in the skin lesions or lymphoid organs, where TNF-α was required for immune cell activation to drive psoriatic change.

EGFR signaling participates in psoriasis through its promotion of keratinocyte proliferation [44,45], and production of growth

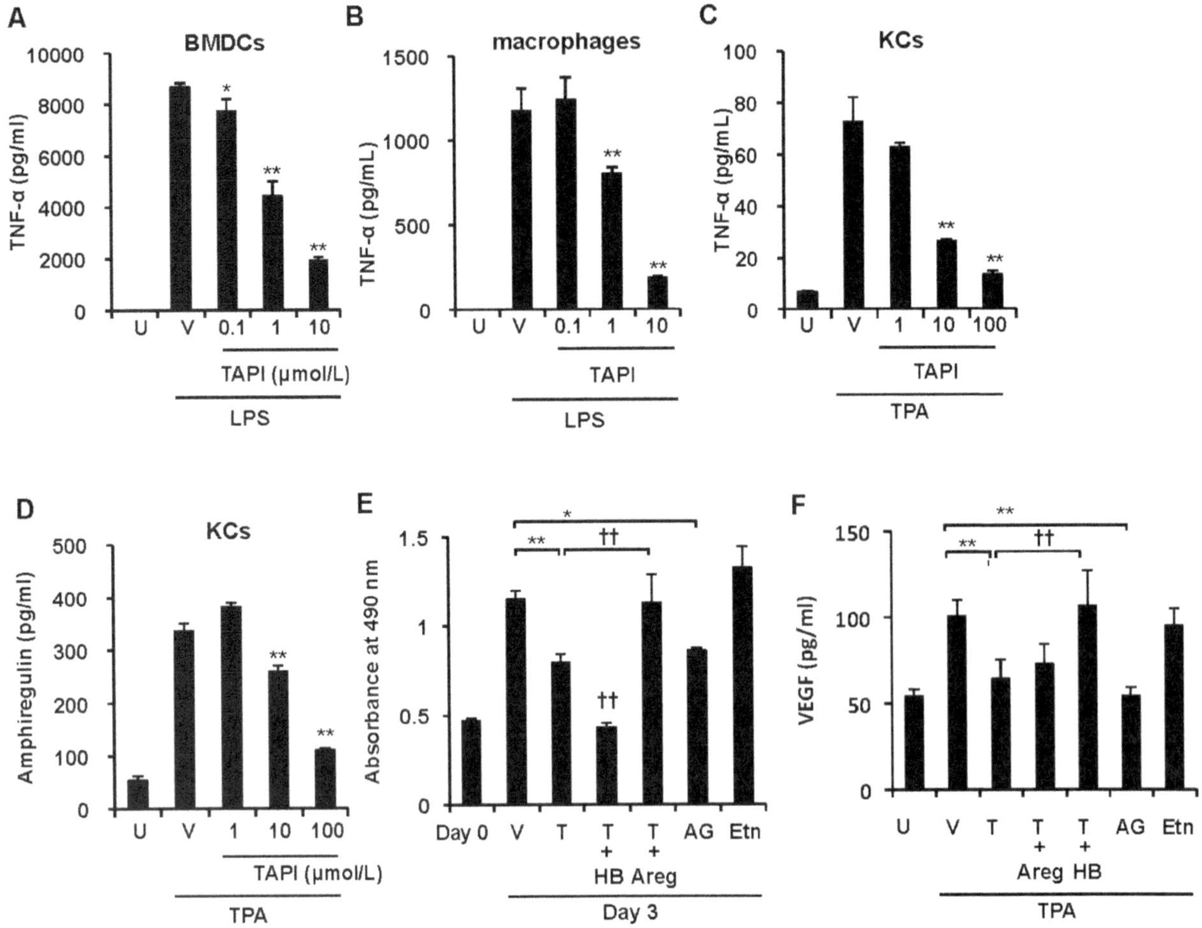

Figure 5. Contribution of TACE to the production of soluble TNF-α and EGFR ligands from murine cells. (A–C), TNF-α proteins in the 24 h culture supernatants of cells pretreated with or without TAPI-1 (TAPI) at the indicated concentrations. LPS-stimulated bone marrow derived dendritic cells (BMDCs) from wild-type FVB/N mice (A), LPS-stimulated thioglycolate-elicited peritoneal macrophages from wild-type FVB/N mice (B), and TPA-stimulated primary keratinocytes from K5.Stat3C newborn mice (C). Cells were pretreated with or without TAPI-1 (TAPI) for 30 min prior to stimulation. (D), Production of amphiregulin from TPA-treated primary keratinocytes of K5.Stat3C newborn mice for 24 h. Cells were pretreated with or without TAPI-1 (TAPI) at the indicated concentrations for 30 min prior to stimulation. U, unstimulated control. V, vehicle alone. Data represent means ± SD of triplicate wells. *$p<0.05$, **$p<0.01$, versus vehicle alone by Dunnett's test. (E), Keratinocyte proliferation evaluated by MTS assay with absorbance at 490 nm. Cells were untreated or treated with TAPI-1 (100 μmol/l) (T) and cultured in the absence or presence of HB-EGF (HB), amphiregulin (Areg), AG1478 (AG) or etanercept (Etn) for 3 days. (F), VEGF production from primary keratinocytes. Cells were stimulated with TPA for 24 h treated with or without reagents as described. Data represent means ± SD from triplicate wells. *$p<0.05$, **$p<0.01$ versus vehicle alone, $^{††}p<0.01$ versus TAPI-1 alone by Tukey-Kramer's test.

factors such as VEGF [18,19]. Indeed, EGFR inhibitors improve lesions in patients with psoriasis [46,47], as also shown in skin lesions of K5.Stat3C mice in the present study. Previous studies demonstrated that topical TPA application led to EGFR activation followed by Stat3 activation in keratinocytes [48]. Therefore, it was suggested that EGFR signaling was involved in the amplification of Stat3 signaling and contributed to the development of the skin lesions in this murine model. Similar to previous studies showing that amphiregulin promotes human keratinocyte proliferation [36,37], we showed here that the TACE inhibitor-induced attenuation of murine keratinocyte proliferation was reversed by the inclusion of amphiregulin but not by HB-EGF. Specifically, HB-EGF-mediated EGFR triggering led to VEGF production by HaCat cells [19]. VEGF plays a critical role in angiogenesis of psoriatic lesions [15], which are attenuated by treatment with an anti-VEGF antibody [39]. Likewise, we confirmed the role of HB-EGF-mediating EGFR signaling in inducing VEGF production by keratinocytes from K5.Stat3C mice, since TACE inhibition reduced the production of VEGF, which was reversed by the addition of recombinant HB-EGF, but not by amphiregulin. Thus, EGFR-mediated biological outcomes were determined by distinct ligands, all of which were sensitive to TACE inhibition. Therefore, results in the present study is, at least in part, reproduced previous studies demonstrating that TACE mediated context-dependent function of amphiregulin and HB-EGF; cell proliferation and migration possibly through VEGF signaling, respectively [37,49].

Psoriatic lesions both in humans and in K5.Stat3C mice demonstrated a similar distribution pattern of TACE and its substrate TNF-α. Interestingly, an endogenous TACE inhibitor, TIMP-3 was found to be decreased in psoriatic lesions compared with uninvolved skin and healthy control skin [50]. It was demonstrated that mice lacking Jun-B/c-Jun in the epidermis showed a down-regulation of TIMP-3, resulting in the generation of a psoriasis-like phenotype through massive TNF-α shedding by TACE activation [32]. Likewise, TIMP-3 expression in the skin of

K5.Stat3C mice was attenuated as the psoriasis-like lesions developed by TPA application. TACE enzymatic activity was elevated in the skin of K5.Stat3C mice at baseline, compared with wild-type mice, and it was further increased by TPA treatment. Since TACE mRNA levels were not elevated in K5.Stat3C mice, this finding suggested that Stat3 signaling contributed to enhanced TACE activity via post-transcriptional regulation. Most recently, it has been reported that microRNA-21 (miR-21) targeted *TIMP-3* and was functionally involved in the pathogenesis of psoriasis [51]. Most interestingly, miR-21 expression was up-regulated by the Stat3 signaling [52], supporting our data using K5.Stat3C keratinocytes, which showed acute decline of *TIMP-3* upon TPA treatment, thereby TACE activity might be elevated, followed by release of the TACE substrates. In other words, Stat3 is not only a transcriptional but post-transcriptional regulator for TACE ligands.

The results of the present study strongly suggest that TACE is involved in the pathogenesis of psoriasis through the release of TNF-α and EGFR ligands. Therefore, TACE inhibitors in clinical use may be relevant to both TNF-α and EGFR inhibitors. Our preliminary data showed that topical treatment with TAPI-1 mildly but significantly attenuated skin lesion development in K5.Stat3C mice. We are now under seeking for more potent and specific TACE inhibitors than TAPI-1, so that they should be relevant to clinical use for treatment of psoriasis.

Supporting Information

Figure S1 Effect of TAPI-1 treatment on TNF-α gene expression in LPS-stimulated peritoneal macrophages. Cells were pretreated with or without 10 μM TAPI-1 (TAPI) for 30 min prior to 100 ng/ml LPS stimulation and harvested at 0.5, 6 and 24 h. Data represent means ± SD of triplicate wells.

Figure S2 Inhibition of keratinocyte proliferation by TAPI-1. (A) BrdU incorporation of primary keratinocytes from K5.Stat3C mice. (B) LDH assay using keratinocyte culture supernatants. Cells were treated with or without 100 μmol/l TAPI-1 (TAPI), 100 nmol/l AG1478 (AG) or 1% TritonX-100 (Triton) and cultured for 2 days. BrdU incorporation was quantified by ELISA. Data represent means ± SD of triplicate wells. $^{**}p<0.01$, versus vehicle alone (V), by Dunnett's test. n.s., not significant.

Figure S3 VEGF production in the skin lesions of K5.Stat3C mice. VEGF production was determined by ELISA using untreated or TPA treated ear skins. TPA treated skins were sampled at day 3. Data represent means ± SD of 4 to 5 mice. $^{**}p<0.01$, versus the untreated group, by Student's *t*-test.

Figure S4 Expression of psoriasis-related genes in primary murine keratinocytes by synergistic stimulation with TNF-α and IL-17A. Primary keratinocytes were stimulated with 20 ng/ml IL-17A and 10 ng/ml TNF-α for 24 h. Data represent means ± SD of triplicate wells. $^{**}p<0.01$, by Tukey-Kramer's test.

Acknowledgments

We thank Kimiko Nakajima for helpful discussion; Reiko Kamijima, Chisa Fujimoto and Tomoko Nagayama for technical assistance; Keiko Udaka and Toshihiro Komatsu for technical advice for BMDC preparation.

Author Contributions

Conceived and designed the experiments: KS ST SS. Performed the experiments: KS MT. Analyzed the data: KS MT SS. Contributed reagents/materials/analysis tools: ST SS. Contributed to the writing of the manuscript: KS SS.

References

1. Menter A, Feldman SR, Weinstein GD, Papp K, Evans R, et al. (2007) A randomized comparison of continuous vs. intermittent infliximab maintenance regimens over 1 year in the treatment of moderate-to-severe plaque psoriasis. J Am Acad Dermatol 56: 31 e31–15.
2. Gordon K, Papp K, Poulin Y, Gu Y, Rozzo S, et al. (2012) Long-term efficacy and safety of adalimumab in patients with moderate to severe psoriasis treated continuously over 3 years: results from an open-label extension study for patients from REVEAL. J Am Acad Dermatol 66: 241–251.
3. Gaspari AA (2006) Innate and adaptive immunity and the pathophysiology of psoriasis. J Am Acad Dermatol 54: S67–80.
4. Zaba LC, Cardinale I, Gilleaudeau P, Sullivan-Whalen M, Suarez-Farinas M, et al. (2007) Amelioration of epidermal hyperplasia by TNF inhibition is associated with reduced Th17 responses. J Exp Med 204: 3183–3194.
5. Black RA, Rauch CT, Kozlosky CJ, Peschon JJ, Slack JL, et al. (1997) A metalloproteinase disintegrin that releases tumour-necrosis factor-alpha from cells. Nature 385: 729–733.
6. Moss ML, Jin SL, Milla ME, Bickett DM, Burkhart W, et al. (1997) Cloning of a disintegrin metalloproteinase that processes precursor tumour-necrosis factor-alpha. Nature 385: 733–736.
7. Blaydon DC, Biancheri P, Di WL, Plagnol V, Cabral RM, et al. (2011) Inflammatory skin and bowel disease linked to ADAM17 deletion. N Engl J Med 365: 1502–1508.
8. Vassar R, Fuchs E (1991) Transgenic mice provide new insights into the role of TGF-alpha during epidermal development and differentiation. Genes Dev 5: 714–727.
9. Cook PW, Piepkorn M, Clegg CH, Plowman GD, DeMay JM, et al. (1997) Transgenic expression of the human amphiregulin gene induces a psoriasis-like phenotype. J Clin Invest 100: 2286–2294.
10. Piepkorn M, Pittelkow MR, Cook PW (1998) Autocrine regulation of keratinocytes: the emerging role of heparin-binding, epidermal growth factor-related growth factors. J Invest Dermatol 111: 715–721.
11. Kawaguchi M, Mitsuhashi Y, Kondo S (2005) Overexpression of tumour necrosis factor-alpha-converting enzyme in psoriasis. Br J Dermatol 152: 915–919.
12. Sano S, Chan KS, Carbajal S, Clifford J, Peavey M, et al. (2005) Stat3 links activated keratinocytes and immunocytes required for development of psoriasis in a novel transgenic mouse model. Nat Med 11: 43–49.
13. Sano S, Chan KS, DiGiovanni J (2008) Impact of Stat3 activation upon skin biology: a dichotomy of its role between homeostasis and diseases. J Dermatol Sci 50: 1–14.
14. Nakajima K, Kanda T, Takaishi M, Shiga T, Miyoshi K, et al. (2011) Distinct roles of IL-23 and IL-17 in the development of psoriasis-like lesions in a mouse model. J Immunol 186: 4481–4489.
15. Ferrara N (2004) Vascular endothelial growth factor: basic science and clinical progress. Endocr Rev 25: 581–611.
16. Weidemann AK, Crawshaw AA, Byrne E, Young HS (2013) Vascular endothelial growth factor inhibitors: investigational therapies for the treatment of psoriasis. Clin Cosmet Investig Dermatol 6: 233–244.
17. Detmar M, Brown LF, Claffey KP, Yeo KT, Kocher O, et al. (1994) Overexpression of vascular permeability factor/vascular endothelial growth factor and its receptors in psoriasis. J Exp Med 180: 1141–1146.
18. Frank S, Hubner G, Breier G, Longaker MT, Greenhalgh DG, et al. (1995) Regulation of vascular endothelial growth factor expression in cultured keratinocytes. Implications for normal and impaired wound healing. J Biol Chem 270: 12607–12613.
19. Nakai K, Yoneda K, Moriue T, Igarashi J, Kosaka H, et al. (2009) HB-EGF-induced VEGF production and eNOS activation depend on both PI3 kinase and MAP kinase in HaCaT cells. J Dermatol Sci 55: 170–178.
20. Sano S, Chan KS, Kira M, Kataoka K, Takagi S, et al. (2005) Signal transducer and activator of transcription 3 is a key regulator of keratinocyte survival and proliferation following UV irradiation. Cancer Res 65: 5720–5729.
21. Hirai T, Kanda T, Sato K, Takaishi M, Nakajima K, et al. (2013) Cathepsin K is involved in development of psoriasis-like skin lesions through TLR-dependent Th17 activation. J Immunol 190: 4805–4811.

22. Murakawa M, Yamaoka K, Tanaka Y, Fukuda Y (2006) Involvement of tumor necrosis factor (TNF)-alpha in phorbol ester 12-O-tetradecanoylphorbol-13-acetate (TPA)-induced skin edema in mice. Biochem Pharmacol 71: 1331–1336.
23. Chun KS, Lao HC, Trempus CS, Okada M, Langenbach R (2009) The prostaglandin receptor EP2 activates multiple signaling pathways and beta-arrestin1 complex formation during mouse skin papilloma development. Carcinogenesis 30: 1620–1627.
24. Laemmli UK (1970) Cleavage of structural proteins during the assembly of the head of bacteriophage T4. Nature 227: 680–685.
25. Feng T, Qin H, Wang L, Benveniste EN, Elson CO, et al. (2011) Th17 cells induce colitis and promote Th1 cell responses through IL-17 induction of innate IL-12 and IL-23 production. J Immunol 186: 6313–6318.
26. Gais P, Tiedje C, Altmayr F, Gaestel M, Weighardt H, et al. (2010) TRIF signaling stimulates translation of TNF-alpha mRNA via prolonged activation of MK2. J Immunol 184: 5842–5848.
27. Kawaguchi M, Mitsuhashi Y, Kondo S (2004) Localization of tumour necrosis factor-alpha converting enzyme in normal human skin. Clin Exp Dermatol 29: 185–187.
28. Terajima S, Higaki M, Igarashi Y, Nogita T, Kawashima M (1998) An important role of tumor necrosis factor-alpha in the induction of adhesion molecules in psoriasis. Arch Dermatol Res 290: 246–252.
29. Johnston A, Gudjonsson JE, Aphale A, Guzman AM, Stoll SW, et al. (2011) EGFR and IL-1 signaling synergistically promote keratinocyte antimicrobial defenses in a differentiation-dependent manner. J Invest Dermatol 131: 329–337.
30. Lee MH, Verma V, Maskos K, Becherer JD, Knauper V, et al. (2002) The C-terminal domains of TACE weaken the inhibitory action of N-TIMP-3. FEBS Lett 520: 102–106.
31. Mohammed FF, Smookler DS, Taylor SE, Fingleton B, Kassiri Z, et al. (2004) Abnormal TNF activity in Timp3−/− mice leads to chronic hepatic inflammation and failure of liver regeneration. Nat Genet 36: 969–977.
32. Guinea-Viniegra J, Zenz R, Scheuch H, Hnisz D, Holcmann M, et al. (2009) TNFalpha shedding and epidermal inflammation are controlled by Jun proteins. Genes Dev 23: 2663–2674.
33. Lowes MA, Russell CB, Martin DA, Towne JE, Krueger JG (2013) The IL-23/T17 pathogenic axis in psoriasis is amplified by keratinocyte responses. Trends Immunol 34: 174–181.
34. Johansen C, Funding AT, Otkjaer K, Kragballe K, Jensen UB, et al. (2006) Protein expression of TNF-alpha in psoriatic skin is regulated at a posttranscriptional level by MAPK-activated protein kinase 2. J Immunol 176: 1431–1438.
35. Kim S, Beyer BA, Lewis C, Nadel JA (2013) Normal CFTR inhibits epidermal growth factor receptor-dependent pro-inflammatory chemokine production in human airway epithelial cells. PLoS One 8: e72981.
36. Stoll SW, Johnson JL, Li Y, Rittie L, Elder JT (2010) Amphiregulin carboxy-terminal domain is required for autocrine keratinocyte growth. J Invest Dermatol 130: 2031–2040.
37. Stoll SW, Johnson JL, Bhasin A, Johnston A, Gudjonsson JE, et al. (2010) Metalloproteinase-mediated, context-dependent function of amphiregulin and HB-EGF in human keratinocytes and skin. J Invest Dermatol 130: 295–304.
38. Xia YP, Li B, Hylton D, Detmar M, Yancopoulos GD, et al. (2003) Transgenic delivery of VEGF to mouse skin leads to an inflammatory condition resembling human psoriasis. Blood 102: 161–168.
39. Akman A, Yilmaz E, Mutlu H, Ozdogan M (2009) Complete remission of psoriasis following bevacizumab therapy for colon cancer. Clin Exp Dermatol 34: e202–204.
40. Miyoshi K, Takaishi M, Nakajima K, Ikeda M, Kanda T, et al. (2011) Stat3 as a therapeutic target for the treatment of psoriasis: a clinical feasibility study with STA-21, a Stat3 inhibitor. J Invest Dermatol 131: 108–117.
41. Gottlieb AB, Chamian F, Masud S, Cardinale I, Abello MV, et al. (2005) TNF inhibition rapidly down-regulates multiple proinflammatory pathways in psoriasis plaques. J Immunol 175: 2721–2729.
42. Zaba LC, Suarez-Farinas M, Fuentes-Duculan J, Nograles KE, Guttman-Yassky E, et al. (2009) Effective treatment of psoriasis with etanercept is linked to suppression of IL-17 signaling, not immediate response TNF genes. J Allergy Clin Immunol 124: 1022–1010 e1021–1395.
43. Sugita S, Kawazoe Y, Imai A, Yamada Y, Horie S, et al. (2012) Inhibition of Th17 differentiation by anti-TNF-alpha therapy in uveitis patients with Behcet's disease. Arthritis Res Ther 14: R99.
44. Peus D, Hamacher L, Pittelkow MR (1997) EGF-receptor tyrosine kinase inhibition induces keratinocyte growth arrest and terminal differentiation. J Invest Dermatol 109: 751–756.
45. Tokumaru S, Higashiyama S, Endo T, Nakagawa T, Miyagawa JI, et al. (2000) Ectodomain shedding of epidermal growth factor receptor ligands is required for keratinocyte migration in cutaneous wound healing. J Cell Biol 151: 209–220.
46. Neyns B, Meert V, Vandenbroucke F (2008) Cetuximab treatment in a patient with metastatic colorectal cancer and psoriasis. Curr Oncol 15: 196–197.
47. Oyama N, Kaneko F, Togashi A, Yamamoto T (2012) A case of rapid improvement of severe psoriasis during molecular-targeted therapy using an epidermal growth factor receptor tyrosine kinase inhibitor for metastatic lung adenocarcinoma. J Am Acad Dermatol 66: e251–253.
48. Chan KS (2004) Epidermal Growth Factor Receptor-Mediated Activation of Stat3 during Multistage Skin Carcinogenesis. Cancer Research 64: 2382–2389.
49. Maretzky T, Evers A, Zhou W, Swendeman SL, Wong PM, et al. (2011) Migration of growth factor-stimulated epithelial and endothelial cells depends on EGFR transactivation by ADAM17. Nat Commun 2: 229.
50. Zibert JR, Lovendorf MB, Litman T, Olsen J, Kaczkowski B, et al. (2010) MicroRNAs and potential target interactions in psoriasis. J Dermatol Sci 58: 177–185.
51. Guinea-Viniegra J, Jimenez M, Schonthaler HB, Navarro R, Delgado Y, et al. (2014) Targeting miR-21 to Treat Psoriasis. Sci Transl Med 6: 225re221.
52. Iliopoulos D, Jaeger SA, Hirsch HA, Bulyk ML, Struhl K (2010) STAT3 activation of miR-21 and miR-181b-1 via PTEN and CYLD are part of the epigenetic switch linking inflammation to cancer. Mol Cell 39: 493–506.

13

IL-17 Induces an Expanded Range of Downstream Genes in Reconstituted Human Epidermis Model

Andrea Chiricozzi[1,2,3]*, Kristine E. Nograles[1,2], Leanne M. Johnson-Huang[1], Judilyn Fuentes-Duculan[1], Irma Cardinale[1], Kathleen M. Bonifacio[1], Nicholas Gulati[1], Hiroshi Mitsui[1], Emma Guttman-Yassky[1,2,4], Mayte Suárez-Fariñas[1,2¶], James G. Krueger[1,2¶]

1 Laboratory for Investigative Dermatology, The Rockefeller University, New York City, New York, United States of America, **2** Center for Clinical and Translational Science, The Rockefeller University, New York City, New York, United States of America, **3** Department of Dermatology, University of Rome "Tor Vergata", Rome, Italy, **4** Department of Dermatology, Mount Sinai School of Medicine, New York City, New York, United States of America

Abstract

Background: IL-17 is the defining cytokine of the Th17, Tc17, and $\gamma\delta$ T cell populations that plays a critical role in mediating inflammation and autoimmunity. Psoriasis vulgaris is an inflammatory skin disease mediated by Th1 and Th17 cytokines with relevant contributions of IFN-γ, TNF-α, and IL-17. Despite the pivotal role IL-17 plays in psoriasis, and in contrast to the other key mediators involved in the psoriasis cytokine cascade that are capable of inducing broad effects on keratinocytes, IL-17 was demonstrated to regulate the expression of a limited number of genes in monolayer keratinocytes cultured in vitro.

Methodology/Principal Findings: Given the clinical efficacy of anti-IL-17 agents is associated with an impressive reduction in a large set of inflammatory genes, we sought a full-thickness skin model that more closely resemble in vivo epidermal architecture. Using a reconstructed human epidermis (RHE), IL-17 was able to upregulate 419 gene probes and downregulate 216 gene probes. As possible explanation for the increased gene induction in the RHE model is that C/CAAT-enhancer-binding proteins (C/EBP) -β, the transcription factor regulating IL-17-responsive genes, is expressed preferentially in differentiated keratinocytes.

Conclusions/Significance: The genes identified in IL-17-treated RHE are likely relevant to the IL-17 effects in psoriasis, since ixekizumab (anti-IL-17A agent) strongly suppressed the "RHE" genes in psoriasis patients treated in vivo with this IL-17 antagonist.

Editor: Akihiko Yoshimura, Keio University School of Medicine, Japan

Funding: These authors have no support or funding to report.

Competing Interests: The authors have read the journal's policy and have the following conflict: the authors do not have any conflict of interest related to this work, with the exception of JGK who has been consultant to Eli Lilly (company developing ixekizumab) and Amgen (company developing etanercept).

* E-mail: chiricozziandrea@gmail.com

¶ These authors are joint senior authors on this work.

Introduction

Psoriasis is a chronic inflammatory skin disorder characterized by a dense dermal inflammatory infiltrate and altered keratinocyte (KC) differentiation [1]. Leukocytes that infiltrate the dermis produce many pro-inflammatory mediators that set up the cycle of pathogenic inflammation. Interleukin (IL)-17 has emerged as one of the most crucial players in the current model of psoriasis pathogenesis. IL-17 was thought to be produced mainly by Th17 cells, a subset of CD4+ T helper cells that is distinct from the Th1 and Th2 lineages [2,3], but it is becoming increasingly appreciated that it is also produced by CD8+ T cells (Tc1) and $\gamma\delta$ T cells [4,5], and potentially by some non-T cells, including mast cells and neutrophils [6]. IL-17 signaling activates the Nuclear factor kappa-light-chain-enhancer of activated B cells (NF-κB) pathway and the C/CAAT-enhancer-binding proteins (C/EBP) family, particularly C/EBPβ and C/EBPδ [7,8] to enhance expression of pro-inflammatory cytokines and chemokines, intercellular adhesion molecules, and anti-microbial peptides (AMPs) by numerous cell types, including granulocytes, chondroblasts, fibroblasts, and epithelial cells (keratinocytes, endothelial cells, and mucosal epithelial cells) [9–16].

A crucial role of IL23/Th17 axis in the pathogenesis of psoriasis was proposed based on several recent studies: (i) dermal IL-17-producing CD4+ T cell and $\gamma\delta$ T cell infiltrate as well as (ii) IL-17-producing CD8+ T cells within psoriatic epidermis; (iii) high expression levels of IL-23, IL-17, and IL-22 in psoriatic lesional skin; (iv) high serum levels of IL-22 and IL-17 that correlated with disease severity score [4,5,17–21]. Moreover, some of the Th17 pathway-related genes, IL-23A subunit, IL-23R, IL23B subunit, have been identified as psoriasis susceptibility genes [22–24]. Responses to tumor necrosis factor (TNF)α-blocking therapy and narrow-band ultraviolet B light therapy are correlated with the suppression of Th17 pathway [20,25–27]. More recently, therapeutic approaches suppressing the IL-23/Th17 axis have proved highly effective in the treatment of psoriasis [28–33].

Keratinocytes are the key-responding cells to the psoriatic pro-inflammatory and pro-proliferative microenvironment since they bear receptors for key inflammatory cytokines, including IL-17 [12,34,35]. Surprisingly, although anti-IL-17 therapies showed astonishing clinical efficacy in improving psoriasis, in vitro studies of cultured monolayer keratinocytes identified a restricted number of genes induced by IL-17 [10,12]. This discrepancy between the biological effects of neutralizing IL-17 and the IL-17–induced gene expression is even more pronounced considering other key-cytokines, such as TNFα and interferon (IFN)-γ, are capable of broadly regulating genomic expression in keratinocytes (502 and 3549 gene transcripts induced by TNFα and IFN-γ, respectively) [12]. Hence, in order to investigate this discrepancy further, we analyzed expression of C/EBPβ, a downstream signaling molecule of IL-17, and found that it localizes to the uppermost layers of the human epidermis in non-lesional and lesional psoriatic skin, indicating that perhaps only mature keratinocytes fully respond to IL-17 stimulation. We, therefore, sought to create in vitro conditions that could more closely mimic the in vivo epidermal architecture. Using Reconstructed Human Epidermis (RHE), a 3D epidermal skin model composed of a keratinocyte multi-layer supported by connective tissue, we evaluated the genomic response to IL-17.

Our results suggest IL-17 acts as a regulator of inflammatory gene expression preferentially in differentiated keratinocytes and induced genes include many psoriasis-related transcripts.

Results

Increased expression of the IL-17-specific transcription factor, C/EBPβ, by terminally differentiated keratinocytes

Normal human keratinocytes were found to constitutively bear the IL-17 receptor (IL-17R) and they are able to produce several IL-17-induced inflammatory and immune-related mediators implicated in psoriasis pathogenesis (e.g. IL-8, CCL20, S100A12, CXCL1, and CXCL2).

Unlike the constitutively expressed IL-17R, C/EBPβ, a critical transcriptional factor in the IL-17 signaling cascade, was detected only within more mature keratinocytes localized to the upper spinous-granular layers of the epidermis (Figure 1). C/EBPβ staining showed a nuclear pattern that was slightly detectable in the uppermost layers of the epidermis in normal skin, while it was very evident in the epidermis of non-lesional and lesional psoriatic skin. In addition to C/EBPβ, IL-17-regulated proteins, such as human β-defensin 2 (HBD2) and lipocalin 2 (LCN2), also localized to the outermost spinous-granular layers (Figure 1). Immunofluorescence staining further illustrated the co-localization of C/EBPβ and HBD2 in psoriatic skin (Figure S1).

In order to verify whether this staining pattern was specific for C/EBPβ, we examined the expression patterns of additional epidermal transcriptional factors: RFX5, which is not usually overexpressed in lesional psoriatic skin, and STAT (Signal Transducers and Activators of Transcription) −1, a crucial mediator of IFN-γ signaling that has also been implicated in psoriasis pathogenesis. In contrast to the localization C/EBPβ to the spinous-granular layers of the epidermis, RFX5 was only localized to the basal layer of the epidermis (Figure S2). On the other hand, STAT1 was expressed by all viable keratinocytes as shown by pan-epidermal staining (Figure S2). These distinct staining patterns suggest that transcription factors may be activated in different types of KCs (e.g. basal KCs versus granular KCs).

As further confirmation of increased expression of C/EBPβ in differentiated keratinocytes, we accessed data from a new study that measured mRNAs in human dermis, basal epidermis, and suprabasal epidermis after laser-capture microdissection [36] C/EBPβ mRNA was increased about 4–fold in suprabasal epidermis compared to the basal layer (Figure S3).

Furthermore, attempting to fully differentiate monolayer *in vitro* normal human epidermal keratinocytes (NHEKs) using different calcium concentrations, we obtained a significantly higher C/EBPβ expression in high-calcium-treated NHEKs compared to low-calcium condition. Together with C/EBPβ, we tested the expression of some keratinocyte-terminal differentiation genes such as involucrin (IVL), transglutaminase-1 (TGM1), and filaggrin-2 (FLG2). Keratinocytes differentiated after culturing in high Ca^{++} plus 2% fetal bovine serum (FBS) medium, showed enhanced expression of C/EBPβ ($p = 0.03$) as well as high expression of FLG2, TGM1, and IVL mRNAs ($p<0.002$ for all) (Figure S4).

IL-17 induces a large number of genes in RHE

The fact that C/EBPβ and some IL-17-regulated proteins are expressed mainly by terminally differentiated KCs may explain why IL-17 induces such a limited number of genes in primary KCs cultured in vitro, as these KCs maintain a more undifferentiated, basal phenotype.

Therefore, in order to fully characterize the genes induced by IL-17 in KCs, we used a Reconstructed Human Epidermis (RHE) model, a full thickness epidermal skin structure, consisting of normal human-derived epidermal KCs organized into basal, spinous, granular, and cornified layers, analogously to those found in vivo. This epidermal structure is supported by connective tissue including fibroblasts. RHE was incubated with IL-17 (200 ng mL−1), IL-22 (200 ng mL−1), or IFN-γ (20 ng mL−1) for 48 hours and the cytokine-induced gene expression levels were measured with AffymetrixU133A Plus 2.0 arrays. In order to align the gene array analysis with the previously published data [12], we compared gene expression levels in IL-17-treated RHE versus untreated RHE using the selection criteria of fold change (FCH) >1.5 and false discovery rate (FDR)<0.1 that were used for the monolayer KC gene expression analysis [12]. In contrast to monolayer KCs [12] in which IL-17 altered the expression of only 65 probe-sets (60 unique differentially expressed gene, DEGs, using ENTREZ identifiers), in RHE, IL-17 induced the expression of many more genes (641 probe-sets, representing 490 DEGs) (Table S1), of which 425 probe-sets (322 DEGs) resulted upregulated and 216 probe-sets (168 DEGs) downregulated (Figure 2).

To demonstrate that the IL-17 response in RHE did not merely represent the sum of the genes induced by IL-17 in fibroblasts and KCs, the RHE gene set was compared to gene sets obtained from in vitro cultured KCs or fibroblasts treated with IL-17. Differential expression induced by IL-17 in KCs or fibroblasts was compared to the respective untreated conditions. A subset of transcripts (323 probe-sets) was only detected in RHE with U133A plus 2.0 arrays, as these probe-sets were not present on the U133A 2.0 arrays, which were used for treated fibroblasts and KCs (Figure 2, semi-circle). Even when the analysis was restrictedly performed with U133A 2.0 arrays, the number of upregulated RHE gene transcripts (227 probe-sets) resulted about 3-fold and 4-fold higher than the number of upregulated gene detected in fibroblasts and KCs, respectively. There was very little overlap in the IL-17-regulated genes between the three conditions (9 DEGs were detected in both RHE and fibroblasts and 18 DEGs in both KCs and RHE). While there were some KC or fibroblast-specific genes,

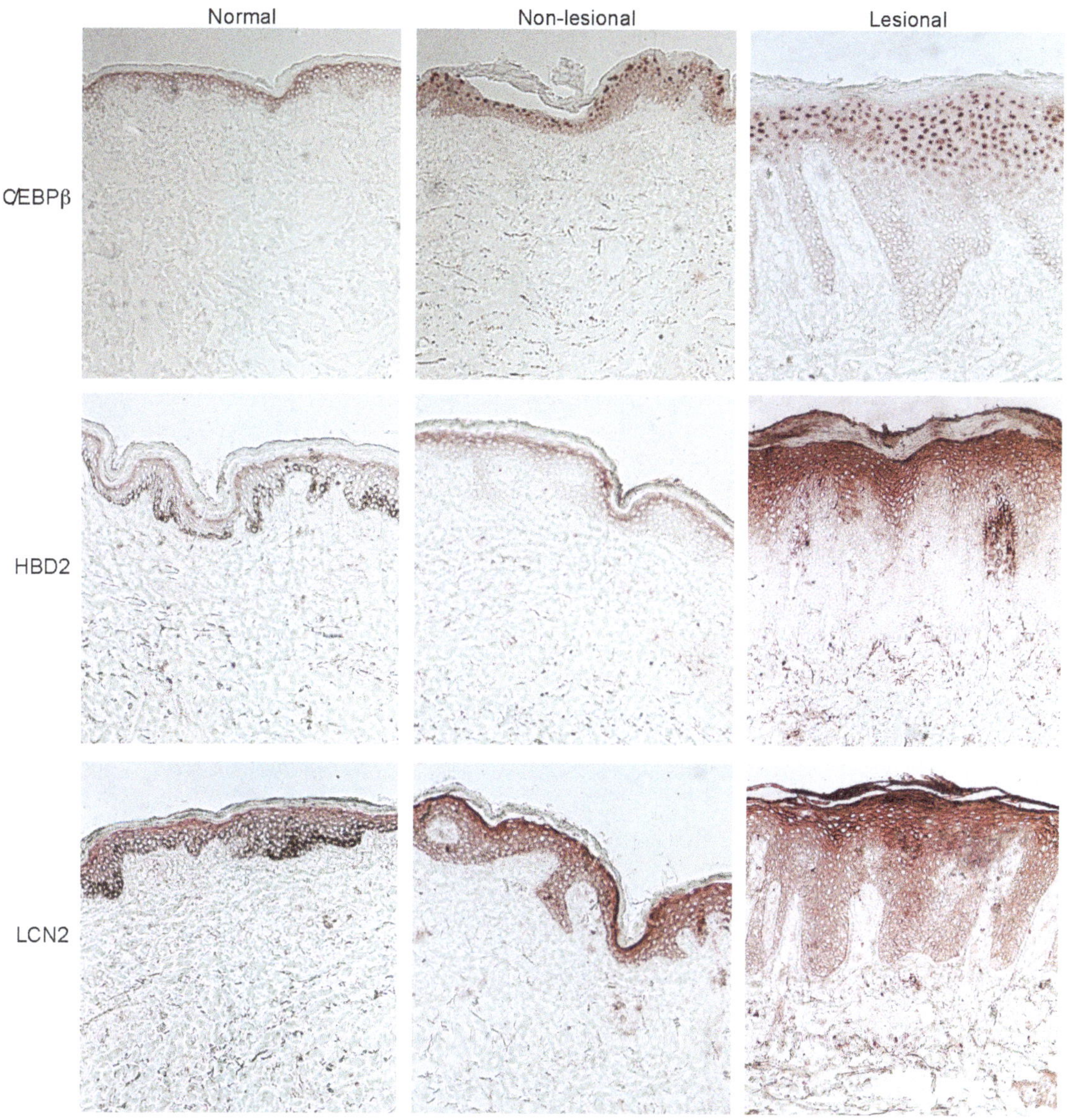

Figure 1. IL-17-regulated C/EBPβ, human β-defensin 2, and lipocalin are expressed by terminally differentiated keratinocytes. Immunohistochemistry for C/EBPβ (top), human β-defensin 2 (HBD2, middle), and lipocalin (LCN-2, bottom) in normal, non-lesional or lesional psoriatic skin showing predominant expression in the spinous-granular layer of the epidermis.

a large number of genes were uniquely expressed in RHE (Figure 2 and Table S1).

IL-17 induces the expression of C/EBPβ and many inflammatory genes in RHE

We also verified the expression of C/EBPβ in RHE model, eventually reflecting the *in vivo* condition. In the IL-17-treated RHE compared with untreated RHE, we detected an upregulation of C/EBPβ gene transcripts by polymerase chain reaction (PCR), and also, protein expression of C/EBPβ within the granular layer cells by immunohistochemistry (Figure S5). The expression of C/EBPβ induced by IL-17 in RHE correlates with the upregulation of Th17 pathway genes, such as IL23A, STAT3, and DEFB4 (Table 1 and Table S1). IL-17 also induced a number of anti-microbial peptides, including S100A12, S100A7A, SERPINB4, SERBINB3, which are highly expressed in psoriasis (Table 1) [37], as has been described previously [12]. Some other characteristic IL-17-regulated genes, such as IL8, IL6, CCL20, CXCL2, CXCL3, CXCL5, and LCN2 were up-regulated to a lesser extent (1.3–2.3 fold induction), but these elevations did not pass significance thresholds (Table S1). Interestingly, IL-1 family members, IL1A, IL1B, IL1F8, and IL1F9 were significantly activated by IL-17 in this model (Table 1). Signaling through these cytokines activates NF-κB, which may synergize with IL-17-induced C/EBPs to enhance transcription of many IL-17-regulated genes, further amplifying the inflammatory loops in psoriasis. In addition, there was up-regulation of cytokines, which limit NF-κB activation, such as IL1F5 and IL11, suggesting that IL-17 may also induce control mechanisms to prevent excessive inflammation [38,39].

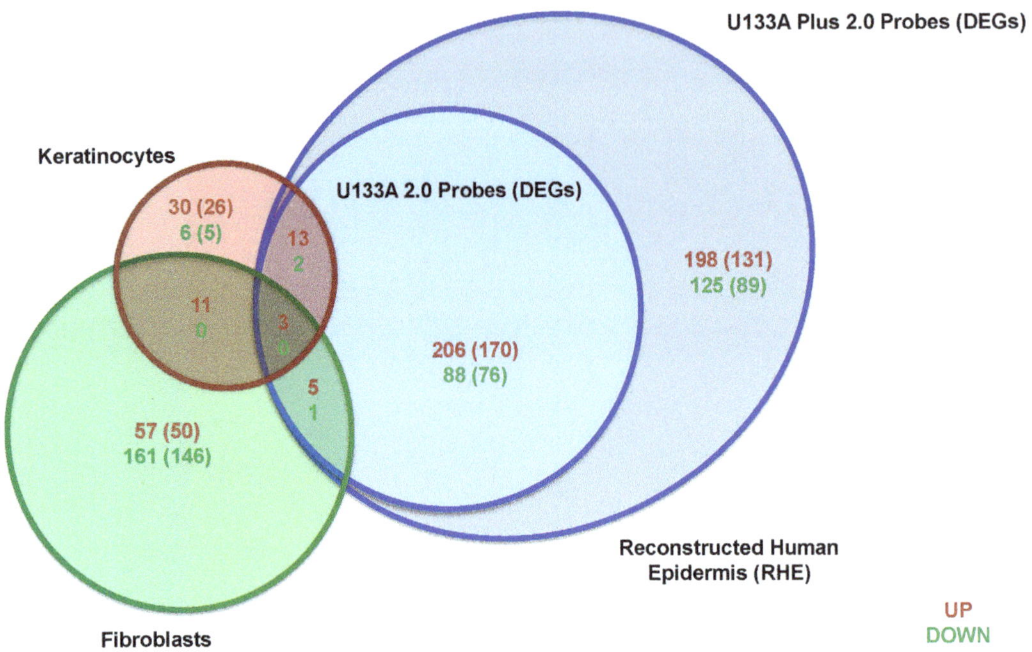

Figure 2. IL-17 induces a large number of genes in RHE. Venn diagram illustrates the number of up-regulated (red) and down-regulated (green) probe-sets with the number of unique DEGs in parentheses of IL-17-treated keratinocytes, fibroblasts or RHE compared to the respective untreated conditions. U133A 2.0 arrays were used for KC and fibroblasts, while U133A Plus 2.0 arrays were used for RHE (FCH >1.5 and FDR<0.1 were used for all arrays). The additional semi-circle of RHE genes represents the probe-sets (DEGs) that were not present in the U133A 2.0 arrays.

IL-17 modulates keratinocyte mitogens and cell-cycle genes

Intriguingly, we observed an induction of cytokines that induce epidermal hyperplasia, including IL19 and heparin-binding EGF-like growth factor (HBEGF). Thus, IL-17 might indirectly stimulate KC proliferation and epidermal hyperplasia via paracrine cytokine secretion. There was also over-expression of cell cycle-related genes, such as cyclin E1 (CCNE1), cell division cycle associated 5 (CDCA5), and cell division cycle 25 homolog A (CDC25A). IL-17 likely stimulates epidermal keratinocyte differentiation, modulating the expression of KC differentiation genes including transglutaminase (TGM)-1, TGM3, small proline-rich protein 2C and 4 (SPRR2C, SPRR4), kallikrein-related peptidase 6, 10, and 13 (KLK6, KLK10, KLK13), and cornifelin (CNFN). Furthermore, IL-17 also modulates the expression of genes, including sphingomyelin phosphodiesterase 1, acid lysosomal (SMPD1) and serine palmitoyltransferase, long chain base subunit 2(SPTLC2), which are related to lamellar bodies and epidermal lipid barrier formation (Table 2).

RHE showed a specific genomic response to IL-17 stimulation

To verify whether the RHE genomic response to IL-17 stimulation was specific to IL-17, we stimulated RHE with IFN-γ or IL-22, cytokines thought to be involved in the psoriasis inflammatory cascade. The IL-22 response in KCs or RHE was minimal with only 35 probe-sets induced in RHE and 23 in KCs (data not shown). The response to IFN-γ was strong, with upregulation of 294 transcripts (Figure S6). As illustrated in Figure S6A, there was minimal overlap in the genes induced by IL-17 or IFN-γ. Furthermore, scatter plots comparing the genes induced in RHE versus *in vitro* cultured KCs showed that IL-17 induced a large number of genes only in RHE, while on the contrary, IFN-γ, induced a larger number of genes in monolayer KCs compared to RHE (Figure S6B), consistent with the constitutive expression of STAT1 by all KCs at all stages of differentiation (Figure S2).

As confirmation of the specific RHE response to cytokine stimulation, we performed Reverse transcriptase-PCR (RT-PCR) (Figure S6C) testing some genes including IL23A, S100A7A, IL19, and IL1F8, which appeared to be upregulated by IL-17 in RHE, as listed in Table S1. We also correlated RHE gene expression induced by IL-17, IL-22, or IFN-γ with various gene sets using gene set enrichment analysis (GSEA) (Figure 3A). The phenotype induced by IL-17 on RHE (as defined by the FCH between IL17 treated vs. control), was strongly enriched of genes in the psoriasis transcriptomes, and, to a lesser strength, with additive and synergistic TNF-α/IL-17 KC genes. RHE profile response to IL-22 or IFN-γ showed lower normalized enrichment scores (NESs), compared to IL-17 stimulation.

In order to determine if this IL-17 response is a reasonable model for the in vivo role of IL-17 in psoriasis, we compared the transcriptome of RHE treated with IL-17 to a previously published MAD-3 psoriasis transcriptome [40]. As shown in Figure 3B, half of the genes induced by IL-17 in RHE are also included in the psoriasis transcriptome, indicating that the response of RHE to IL-17 may reflect gene activation common in psoriasis lesion.

We next examined to what extent IL-17 blockade suppressed the genes highly induced by IL-17 in RHE. We hypothesized that if the genes regulated by IL-17 in the RHE model are relevant to psoriasis, then there should be a corresponding reduction in the same genes after therapeutic blockade of IL-17. Therefore, we compared the transcriptome of IL-17-treated RHE with the transcriptome of lesional skin two weeks after treatment with ixekizumab, an anti-IL-17 antibody [29] (Figure 3B). We have previously defined a "residual disease genomic profile," which included the genes that do not improve by at least 75% compared to NL levels by the end of successful treatment [40]. In the recent

Table 1. Selected immune-related genes expressed in IL-17-treated RHE.

Symbol	Description	FCH[1]	FDR[2]
DEFB4A	defensin, beta 4A	24.37	0.005
IL1F9	interleukin 1 family, member 9	16.37	0.001
IL19	interleukin 19	12.82	0.007
S100A7A	s100 calcium binding protein A7A	12.70	0.011
IL23A	interleukin 23, alpha subunit, p19	11.53	0.001
SERPINB4	serpin peptidase inhibitor, clade B, member 4	7.03	0
TGFA	transforming growth factor, alpha	5.04	0.035
S100A12	s100 calcium binding protein A12	4.85	0.013
IL1F8	interleukin 1 family, member 8 (eta)	4.34	0.086
C/EBPA	CCAAT/enhancer binding protein (C/EBP), alpha	4.28	0.006
IL1B	interleukin 1, beta	3.94	0.013
IL1B	interleukin 1, beta	3.89	0.038
RNASE7	ribonuclease, RNase A family, 7	3.48	0.005
IL11	interleukin 11	3.42	0.045
RNASE7	ribonuclease, RNase A family, 7	3.23	0.013
SERPINA1	serpin peptidase inhibitor, clade A, member 1	3.08	0.058
SERPINA1	serpin peptidase inhibitor, clade A, member 1	2.88	0.089
TGFA	transforming growth factor, alpha	3.08	0.046
IL1A	interleukin 1, alpha	2.85	0.038
IL1F5	interleukin 1 family, member 5 (delta)	2.68	0.01
MAP3K9	mitogen-activated protein kinase kinasekinase 9	2.58	0.044
RNASE7	ribonuclease, RNase A family, 7	2.30	0.031
STAT3	signal transducer and activator of transcription 3	2.18	0.021
MAP2K3	mitogen-activated protein kinase kinase 3	1.97	0.03
SERPINB3	serpin peptidase inhibitor, clade B, member 3	1.88	0.01

[1]FCH, fold change;
[2]FDR, false discovery rate.

ixekizumab study, 72.5% of the 95 genes in the IL-17 treated RHE model that were also part of the MAD-3 psoriasis transcriptome improved by over 75% at two weeks post-treatment compared with 68% of all psoriasis genes (Figure 3C) [41]. For comparison, only 31% of either the RHE genes or the psoriasis genes had recovered with etanercept at the same time point. There was a 3.45 FCH (1,79 log2) average expression of these RHE genes towards recovery with ixekizumab at two weeks, compared with 1.62 FCH (0.70 log2) for etanercept and no change (1.01 FCH, 0.01 log2) with placebo (Figure 3D). Overall, these results suggest that IL-17-induced genes in the RHE model coincide with genes that are suppressed *in vivo* by blocking IL-17 signaling with a neutralizing antibody to IL-17A.

Discussion

Previous experiments have shown a limited number of genes induced by IL-17 in KCs despite ubiquitous epidermal expression of the IL-17 receptor [10,12,42]. In this study, we found that the distinct expression pattern of C/EBPβ, a crucial IL-17-related transcriptional factor, in the upper spinous-granular layers composed of more differentiated keratinocytes, may explain why undifferentiated, monolayer KCs respond less to IL-17 stimulation. Thus, in order to more fully investigate the genomic effects of IL-17 on KCs, we used a full-thickness skin model that more closely mimicked epidermal architecture and KC differentiation process. Using RHE, we identified a much larger number of genes induced by IL-17.

IL-17 elicits its pro-inflammatory effects in RHE, stimulating the expression of several genes including IL23A, IL1β, and IL36B (IL1F8) that have been implicated in psoriasis pathogenesis and found to be over-expressed in psoriatic lesional skin. The production of inflammatory cytokines by epidermal KCs likely perpetuates and sustains skin inflammation driven by T cells, especially given the essential roles of IL-23 and IL-1β in stimulating IL-17 production. Moreover, as key-regulator of innate immunity, IL-17 was shown to modulate antimicrobial peptides (AMPs) such as S100A7A, DEFB4, RNASE7, and Serpins A1, B3, and B4. Johnston *et al.* [43], demonstrated that IL-1F8 significantly induced several AMPs in an RHE model, including LCN2, defensins, HBD-2 and HBD-3, CAMP, elafin, serpinB1, and IL-8, and thus, the IL-1F8 expression induced by IL-17 stimulation may lead to a feed-forward loop amplifying AMP expression, which represents a distinct feature of lesional psoriatic skin.

Many abnormalities in keratinocyte differentiation are highly evident in psoriasis, including the expansion of the spinous-granular layer of the epidermis and alterations in terminal differentiation of KCs leading to a defective epidermal barrier with increased transepidermal water loss. Expression of the IL-17-specific transcription factor, C/EBPβ, in the spinous-granular layer may implicate IL-17 in these processes. Along these lines, Rizzo *et al.* [44], showed that IL-17A, like IL-22, was a downstream mediator of the changes induced by IL-23 injection in murine skin, and that both of these Th17 cytokines are necessary to produce IL-23–mediated psoriasis-like skin pathology. Indeed, the blockade of IL-17 or IL-22 in this model inhibits epidermal hyperplasia, indicating that either IL-17 or IL-22 can increase keratinocyte proliferation. Accordingly, in RHE, IL-17 induced IL19, a pro-proliferative cytokine belonging to IL-10 family, that is overexpressed in lesional psoriatic skin and has been implicated in epidermal hyperplasia [45]. Moreover, IL-17 induced several genes involved in terminal differentiation, including S100 proteins, S100A12 and S100A7A, and transglutaminases, TGM1 and TGM3, suggesting a role for IL-17 in this process. Additionally, the up-regulation of cell cycle-related genes such as CCNE1, CDCA5, and CDCA25A, suggests a direct contribution of IL-17 to epidermal KC proliferation. Therefore, the results of the current study suggest that IL-17 may have a much broader role than previously thought in stimulating the epidermal changes seen in psoriasis.

We defined the *in vivo* correlations of the novel gene set induced by IL-17 in RHE by analyzing the results of a recent clinical trial in psoriasis patients with a potent IL-17A antagonist, ixekizumab. IL-17 blockade is highly effective in reversing psoriasis, impressively resolving clinical, histological, and genomic facets of the disease [29]. Our results suggest that the genes regulated by IL-17 in RHE are likely relevant to the effects of IL-17 in psoriasis, since ixekizumab strongly suppressed these "RHE" genes in psoriasis patients treated in vivo with this IL-17 antagonist.

Psoriasis is thought to develop and be maintained as a result of cooperative efforts of several T cell cytokines in addition to IL-17, namely IFN-γ and IL-22, which augments cellular recruitment through chemokine induction and stimulates epidermal hyperplasia, respectively. However, the complete reversal of the psoriasis phenotype by ixekizumab and other IL-17 antagonists [29], suggests that this model may need to be revised to account for the centrality of IL-17 in driving the inflammatory circuits in psoriasis. While epidermal acanthosis is not highly evident in histological

Table 2. Selected genes involved in keratinocyte proliferation and differentiation.

Symbol	Description	FCH[1]	FDR[2]	Biological Function
IL19	interleukin 19	12.82	0.01	Epidermal hyperplasia inducers
HBEGF	herparin-binding EGF-like growth factor	3.29	0.03	
SPRR2C	smallproline-rich protein 2C (pseudogene)	27.07	0.00	
TGM3	transglutaminase 3	7.15	0.01	
SPRR4	smallproline-rich protein 4	5.21	0.01	
KLK13	kallikrein-related peptidase 13	4.75	0.10	
KLK13	kallikrein-related peptidase 13	4.57	0.08	KC differentiation-related genes
TGM1	transglutaminase 1	3.01	0.02	
KLK6	kallikrein-related peptidase 6	2.89	0.04	
CNFN	cornifelin	2.80	0.05	
KLK10	kallikrein-related peptidase 10	2.13	0.01	
SMPD1	sphingomyelinphosphodiesterase 1, acid lysosomal	2.61	0.01	Laminar bodies/extra-cellular lipids formation
SPTLC2	serinepalmitoyltransferease, long chain base subunit 2	2.54	0.08	
CCNE1	cyclin E1	2.50	0.02	
CDCA5	cell division cycle associated 5	1.88	0.04	Cell cycle-related genes
CDC25A	cell division cycle 25 homolog A (S. pombe)	1.68	0.01	

[1]FCH, fold change;
[2]FDR, false discovery rate.

sections of IL-17 treated RHE, many cyclins associated with increased cell proliferation are elevated in IL-17 treated cultures and growth factors associated with keratinocyte proliferation, e.g. IL-19, TGFα, HBEGF, are increased. Thus, IL-17 might contribute to epidermal hyperplasia in vivo through indirect effects on keratinocytes. In addition, leukocytes that are recruited by cytokines induced in keratinocytes by IL-17 could also be important in producing epidermal hyperplasia in vivo, either through elaborated interleukins or by migration through the epithelium [38,43,45–47]. Furthermore, the induction of genes such as CCL20 (a chemoattractant for CCR6-bearing cells, such as Th17 cells), IL1β, and IL23 (both involved in the Th17 differentiation process) suggests that IL-17 may create feed-forward loops that perpetuate Th17-polarized inflammatory processes. Along these lines, the induction of anti-microbial peptides may also sustain inflammation as IL-17-induced cathelicidin (LL-37) has been shown to complex with nucleic acids to activate DC stimulation of broader and more non-specific T cell activation [48,49]. Overall, these data strongly implicate IL-17 as a central player in the pathogenic mechanism underlying the pathogenesis of psoriasis. Additionally, this study provides insight into the IL-17-induced expression of inflammatory genes belonging to damage-associated molecular pattern molecules (DAMP) or inflammasome that could be potentially identified as novel therapeutic targets. Indeed, the blockade of these IL-17-downstream genes may represent a further step in the therapeutic strategy to be more selective in inhibiting the inflammatory cascade.

IL-17 is most closely associated with the pathogenesis of psoriasis, but it could also contribute to other inflammatory skin disease, e.g., atopic dermatitis (AD). Significant IL-17 expression is seen in skin lesions of intrinsic AD (low IgE sub-type) and increased expression of several S100A genes (S100A7, S100A8, S100A9, S100A12), that are synergistically regulated by IL-17 and IL-22 is also detected [50].

Additionally, relative to normal skin, AD lesions have increased expression of AMPs (LCN, β-defensins, etc.) that are IL-17-regulated, although the measured levels are much lower than seen in psoriasis. Since the range of products regulated by IL-17 in AD are largely overexpressed in the upper spinous and granular layers of AD epidermis, the selective expression of C/EBPβ in more differentiated KCs is also likely to be relevant to AD pathogenesis.

Materials and Methods

Skin samples

Skin punch biopsies (6 mm diameter) were obtained from normal volunteers and patients with moderate-to-severe chronic plaque psoriasis under a Rockefeller University Institutional Review Board-approved protocol. Written, informed consent was obtained from all subjects, and adhered to the Declaration of Helsinki Principles.

The biopsy specimens were frozen in OTC (Sakura, Torrance, CA, U.S.A.) and stored at −80°C for immunohistochemistry and immunofluorescence.

Immunohistochemistry and Immunofluorescence

Frozen tissue sections of psoriatic lesional, non-lesional, and normal skin were stained using standard procedures for both IHC and IF as previously described [51].

Immunohistochemistry. Staining was performed with antibody targeting C/EBPβ, LCN2, HBD2, STAT1, RFX5 (Table S2). According to the primary antibody species, either biotin-labeled horse anti-mouse antibodies (Vector Laboratories, Burlingame, CA, U.S.A.) or biotin-labeled rabbit anti-goat antibodies (Vector Laboratories, Burlingame, CA, U.S.A.) were amplified with avidin-biotin complex (Vector Laboratories) and developed

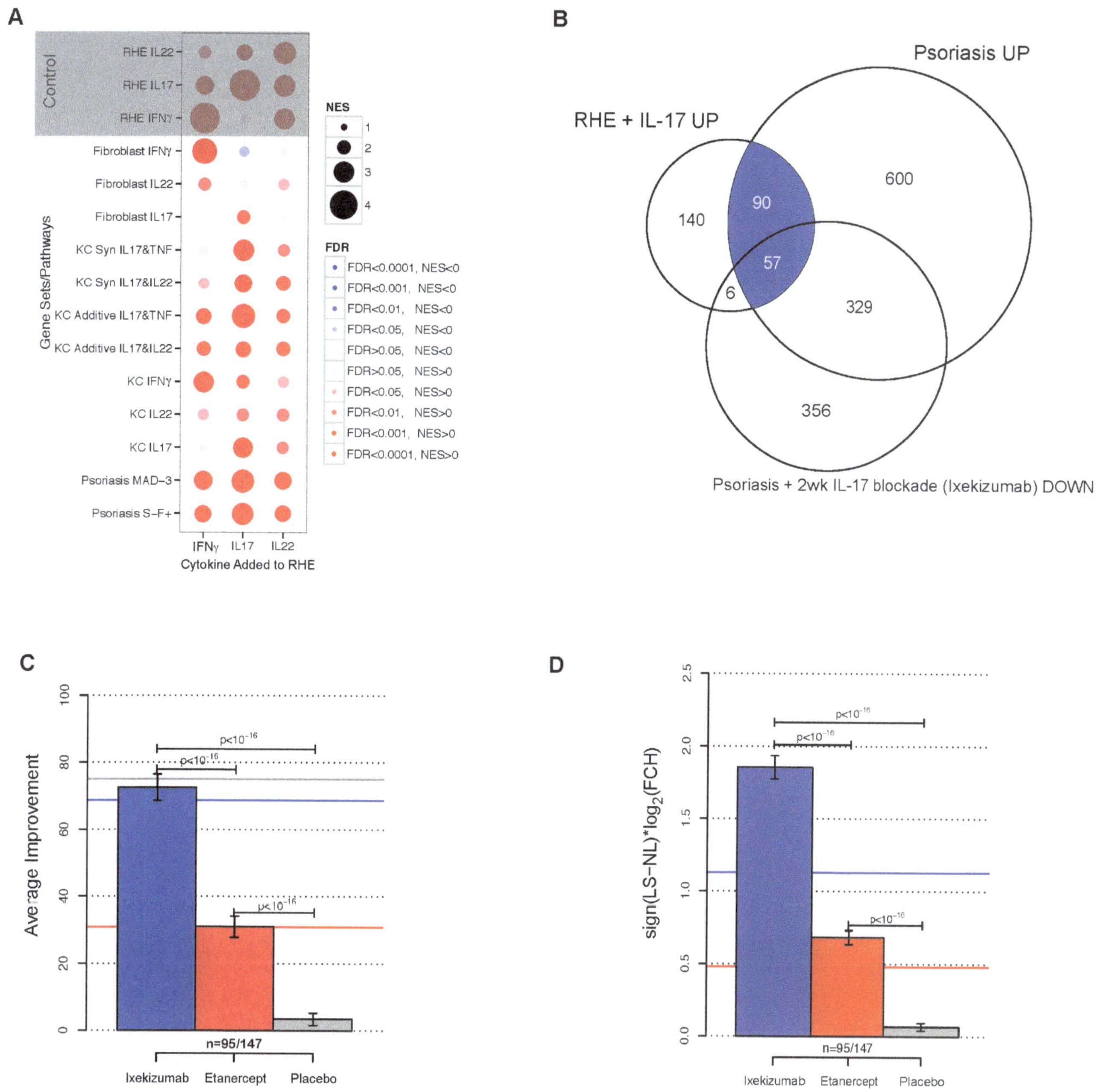

Figure 3. Improvement of psoriasis with IL-17 blockade is associated with reduced expression of IL-17-induced RHE genes. (A) Correlation between various gene sets and RHE gene profile response to cytokine stimulation (IL-17, IFN-γ, or IL-22) using GSEA. NES: normalized enrichment score; FDR: false discovery rate. **(B)** Venn diagram summarizing the number of DEGs among those in the psoriasis transcriptome or IL-17-treated RHE with improvement of at least 75% at two weeks post-ixekizumab. **(C)** Proportion of genes in IL-17-treated RHE that were differentially regulated in psoriasis (blue shaded area of **(A)**) and on the U133A 2.0 arrays (n = 95 out of 147 total DEGs which included additional genes only seen on the U133A Plus 2.0 arrays) that responded to treatment with IL-17 blockade (Ixekizumab, blue), TNF blockade (etanercept, red) or placebo (gray) at 2 weeks. Colored lines are changes in all MAD-3 psoriasis genes after both treatments. **(D)** The average change in expression (log_2FCH) of RHE+IL-17 genes toward recovery with ixekizumab, etanercept, or placebo at 2 weeks.

using chromogen 3-amino-9-ethylcarbazole (Sigma Aldrich, St Louis, MO, U.S.A.). For the staining in the RHE, a black line denotes the dermoepidermal junction. Appropriate negative controls were used.

Immunofluorescence. Frozen skin sections from non-lesional and lesional psoriasis patients were fixed with acetone and blocked in 10% normal chicken serum (Vector Laboratories) for 30 minutes. Primary antibodies for C/EBPβ and HBD2 (Table S2) were incubated overnight at 4°C and amplified with the appropriate secondary antibody goat anti-mouse IgG1 conjugated to Alexa Fluor 488 and chicken anti-goat Alexa Flour 594 (Invitrogen, Eugene, OR) respectively, for 30 minutes.

IF images were acquired using the appropriate filters of a Zeiss Axioplan 2 wide-field fluorescence microscope (Thornwood, NY) with a Plan Neofluar 20×0.7 numerical aperture lens and a Hamamatsu Orca Er-cooled charge-coupled device camera

(Bridgewater, NJ), controlled by the METAVUE software (MDS Analytical Technologies, Downington, PA). Images in each figure are presented both as single-color stains (green and red) located above the merged image, so that localization of two markers on similar or different cells can be appreciated. Cells that co-express the two markers in a similar location are yellow in color. A white line denotes the dermoepidermal junction. Dermal collagen fibers gave green autofluorescence, and antibodies conjugated with a fluorochrome often gave background epidermal fluorescence.

Cell cultures

We cultivated primary human skin fibroblast lines (HF40 and HFF-1) (n = 2 each) that were obtained from the American Type Culture Collection (ATCC, Manassas, VA) and cultivated in Dulbecco's minimum essential medium supplemented with 10% fetal calf serum and, when confluent, medium was supplemented with or without recombinant human (rh)-IL-17 (R&D System, Minneapolis, MN) of 200 ng ml^{-1} (same IL-17 source and concentration used in prior experiments with human keratinocytes) [10,12]. After 24-hour incubation, fibroblasts were harvested for further analyses.

We also cultivated NHEKs obtained from PromoCell, in the Keratinocyte Growth Medium 2 supplemented with 0.004 ml/ml BPE, 0.125 ng/ml EGF, 5 ug/ml Insulin, 0.33 ug/ml Hydrocortisone, 0.39 ug/ml Epinephrine, 10 ug/ml Transferrin, and 0.06 mM Ca++ (all items purchased from PromoCell GmbH, Heidelberg, Germany). The experiment was performed in triplicate.

Once 70–80% confluent, the medium was changed with full media containing 0.06 mM Ca++, 1.2 mM Ca++, or 1.2 mM Ca++ plus 2.0% FBS, for 24 and 48 hours before harvesting for other analyses.

Human full-thickness skin model (RHE)

Full-thickness human skin models (MatTek Corp., Ashland, MA, U.S.A.) (n = 4) were incubated in assay media (MatTek Corp.) supplemented with or without rh-IL-17 (R&D Systems, Minneapolis, MN, U.S.A.) 200 ng mL^{-1}, rh-IL-22 (Peprotech Inc., Rocky Hill, NJ, U.S.A.) 200 ng mL^{-1} 200, or rh-IFN-γ (R&D Systems, Minneapolis, MN, U.S.A.) 20 ng mL^{-1}, for 2 days. On day 2, the skin models were harvested for microarray analyses. The same concentrations used for treating *in vitro* monolayer keratinocytes were applied for RHE, as they were proved effective in gene modulation as previously described by our group [12].

Gene array

RNA was extracted from RHE using the RNeasy Mini Kit (Qiagen, Valencia, CA, U.S.A.) and on-column DNAse digestion (RNAse-free DNAse Set, Qiagen), for either gene array or RT-PCR procedures.

For each Affymetrix genechip, 4 μg total RNA was reverse transcribed, amplified, and labeled as described previously using BioArray High Yield RNA Transcription Labeling Kit (Enzo Biochem Inc., Farmingdale, NY, U.S.A.) [52]. Fifteen micrograms of the biotinylated cRNA were then hybridized to Affymetrix Human Genome U133A Plus 2.0 Array (Affymetrix, Santa Clara, CA, U.S.A.). The chips were washed, stained with streptavidin-phycoerythin, and scanned with a Hewlett-Packard HP GeneArray Scanner (Hewlett-Packard, Palo Alto, CA, U.S.A.).

Reverse transcriptase–polymerase chain reaction

To perform RT-PCR, the RNA extracted from fibroblasts and RHE model was processed using EZ PCR core reagents, primers, and probes (Applied Biosystems, Foster City, CA) as previously published [53], whilst total RNA was extracted from NHEKs using RNeasy micro kit (QIAGEN Inc, Valencia, CA).

The following sequences of primers and probes were used in this study: IL-19 (Hs00604655_m1), C/EBPβ (Hs 00270923_s1), S100A7A (Hs00752780_s1), IL-1F8 (Hs00758166_m1), IL-23A (Hs00372324_m1). The data were analyzed by the Applied Biosystems PRISM 7700 software (Sequence Detection Systems, ver. 1.7) and normalized to human acidic ribosomal protein (hARP) housekeeping gene (primer sequences Forward: CGCTGCTGAACATGCTCAA, Reverse: TGTCGAACACCT-GCTGGATG, Probe: 6-FAM-TCCCCCTTCTCCTTTGGGC-TGG- TAMRA).

Statistical analysis

Preprocessing and statistical analysis was conducted in R (http://www.rproject.org/).

Microarray GeneChip CEL data files were scanned for spatial artifacts using Harshlight package (http://asterion.rockefeller.edu/Harshlight/index2.html) [54]. Expression values were pre-processed using GCRMA algorithm [55]. ArrayQualityControl was used for standard QC.

Probes with at least one sample showing expression values greater than 3 and SD >0.1 were selected for further analyses.

Significance of cytokine induction in RHE gene expression was assessed by using a moderated paired t-test, comparing untreated RHE with cytokine-treated RHE. Subsequently, p-values were adjusted using Benjamini-Hochberg correction, which controls the FDR.

Genes were considered DEGs if FDR>0.1 and FCH>1.5, accordingly to the same cut-offs used for gene array data derived from previous IL-17/keratinocyte experiments [12]. IL-17 effects on gene expression was evaluated in RHE and compared with keratinocyte [12] and fibroblast responses to IL-17 exposure. These data are available in the Gene Expression Omnibus (GEO) repository under accession No. GSE52361.

To assess the biological meaning of IL-17-induced RHE genes in psoriasis, a comparison with the MAD-3 psoriasis transcriptome (defined by a meta-analysis of 3 published transcriptomes) [40] was performed. To evaluate the effect of antipsoriatic therapies on RHE genes induced by IL-17, previously published genomic responses to different therapeutic agents, namely ixekizumab [29] and etanercept [27], were analyzed. Comparisons included only IL17-induced RHE probe sets in hgu133a2 chips, since the gene array data for both treatments were performed using the same kind of chips. For those probes, whose expression differed after 2-week treatment compared to baseline, the mean variation was calculated. Similarly, the improvement at 2 weeks of treatment under both treatments was summarized, meaning as improvement the treatment effect divided by the level of disregulation at baseline, which was measured as LS vs NL differences estimated through the MAD-3 transcriptome.

Gene Set Enrichment Analysis (GSEA) was used to evaluate the enrichment of various gene sets in the gene response profile of the RHE treated with IL-17, IL-22, or IFN-γ [56].

Supporting Information

Figure S1 Co-localization of C/EBPβ and HBD2 in psoriatic skin. Immunofluorescence staining for IL-17 transcription factor, C/EBPβ (green), and downstream target, human β-defensin 2 (HBD2, red), in non-lesional (left) or lesional (right) psoriatic skin. Both proteins are localized to the spinous-granular layer, which is especially evident in non-lesional skin.

Figure S2 Distinct staining patterns of epidermal transcription factors. Immunohistochemistry for transcription factors, RFX-5 and STAT1, in normal, non-lesional, and lesional psoriatic skin. RFX5 stains basal keratinocytes, while STAT1 has pan-epidermal expression.

Figure S3 C/EBPβ gene expression in normal skin. C/EBPβ gene expression in reticular dermis, basal epidermis, and suprabasal epidermis, obtained by laser capture microdissection of normal human skin (Gulati et al., 2013).

Figure S4 Expression levels of terminal differentiation genes in monolayer *in vitro* NHEKs. Increased expression of terminal differentiation genes was detected in high-calcium-treated NHEKs: (A) C/EBPβ, (B) FLG2, (C) TGM1, (D) IVL. Differences with low-calcium condition were statistically significant. Gene expression was normalized by hARP.

Figure S5 C/EBPβ expression in RHE model. Differential C/EBPβ expression in untreated RHE (**A**) versus IL-17-treated RHE (**B**). Black line shapes the dermoepidermal junction, while arrows mark the light staining displayed in differentiated keratinocytes localized in the upper layers of the epidermis. (**C**) Detection of C/EBPβ gene expression in untreated and IL-17-treated-RHE by PCR.

Figure S6 IL-17, IL-22, and IFN-γ induce unique RHE gene signatures. (**A**) Venn diagram illustrates the number of probe-sets regulated in RHE by IL-17, IL-22, or IFN-γ treatment. (**B**) Scatter plots comparing the genes induced in RHE versus *in vitro* cultured KCs showing that IL-17 induced a large number of genes only in RHE, while IFN-γ induced a larger number of genes in monolayer KCs compared to RHE. (**C**) Gene expression levels of some IL-17 signature genes detected by RT-PCR, confirmatory of the gene array results.

Table S1 Differentially expressed genes in IL-17-treated keratinocytes and/or RHE and/or fibroblasts.

Table S2 Antibodies used for immunohistochemistry and immunofluorescence.

Acknowledgments

We thank Artemis Khatcherian and Inna Cueto for the precious support in immunohistochemical procedures. Andrea Chiricozzi is supported by Leo-Pharma Research Foundation Silver Award 2012.

Author Contributions

Conceived and designed the experiments: AC KEN JGK. Performed the experiments: AC KEN JFD IC KMB NG HM. Analyzed the data: MSF. Contributed reagents/materials/analysis tools: JFD IC HM. Wrote the paper: AC LMJH EGY MSF JGK. Support for immunohistochemical procedures: IC.

References

1. Lowes MA, Russell CB, Martin DA, Towne JE, Krueger JG (2013) The IL-23/T17 pathogenic axis in psoriasis is amplified by keratinocyte responses. Trends Immunol 34: 174–81.
2. Harrington LE, Hatton RD, Mangan PR, Turner H, Murphy TL, et al. (2005) Interleukin 17-producing CD4+ effector T cells develop via a lineage distinct from the T helper type 1 and 2 lineages. Nat Immunol 6: 1123–32.
3. Park H, Li Z, Yang XO, Chang SH, Nurieva R, et al. (2005) A distinct lineage of CD4 T cells regulates tissue inflammation by producing interleukin 17. Nat Immunol 6: 1133–41.
4. Cai Y, Shen X, Ding C, Qi C, Li K, et al. (2011) Pivotal role of dermal IL-17-producing gamma/delta T cells in skin inflammation. Immunity 35: 596–610.
5. Ortega C, Fernandez AS, Carrillo JM, Romero P, Molina IJ, et al. (2009) IL-17-producing CD8+ T lymphocytes from psoriasis skin plaques are cytotoxic effector cells that secrete Th17-related cytokines. J Leukocyte Biol 86: 435–43.
6. Lin AM, Rubin CJ, Khandpur R, Wang JY, Riblett M, et al. (2011) Mast cells and neutrophils release IL-17 through extracellular trap formation in psoriasis. J Immunol 187: 490–500.
7. Gaffen SL (2009) Structure and signalling in the IL-17 receptor family. Nat Rev Immunol 9: 556–67.
8. Ruddy MJ, Wong GC, Liu XK, Yamamoto H, Kasayama S, et al. (2004) Functional cooperation between interleukin-17 and tumor necrosis factor-alpha is mediated by CCAAT/enhancer-binding protein family members. J Biol Chem 279:2559–67.
9. Albanesi C, Cavani A, Girolomoni G (1999) IL-17 is produced by nickel-specific T lymphocytes and regulates ICAM-1 expression and chemokine production in human keratinocytes: synergistic or antagonist effects with IFN-gamma and TNF-alpha. J Immunol 162: 494–502.
10. Chiricozzi A, Guttman-Yassky E, Suarez-Farinas M, Nograles KE, Tian S, et al. (2011) Integrative Responses to IL-17 and TNF-alpha in Human Keratinocytes Account for Key Inflammatory Pathogenic Circuits in Psoriasis. J Invest Dermatol 131: 677–87.
11. Laan M, Lotvall J, Chung KF, Linden A (2001) IL-17-induced cytokine release in human bronchial epithelial cells in vitro: role of mitogen-activated protein (MAP) kinases. Br J Pharmacol 133: 200–6.
12. Nograles KE, Zaba LC, Guttman-Yassky E, Fuentes-Duculan J, Suarez-Farinas M, et al. (2008) Th17 cytokines interleukin (IL)-17 and IL-22 modulate distinct inflammatory and keratinocyte-response pathways. Br J Dermatol 159: 1092–102.
13. Pickens SR, Volin MV, Mandelin AM 2nd, Kolls JK, Pope RM, et al. (2010) IL-17 contributes to angiogenesis in rheumatoid arthritis. J Immunol 184: 3233–41.
14. Roussel L, Houle F, Chan C, Yao Y, Berube J, et al. (2010) IL-17 promotes p38 MAPK-dependent endothelial activation enhancing neutrophil recruitment to sites of inflammation. J Immunol 184: 4531–7.
15. Ruddy MJ, Shen F, Smith JB, Sharma A, Gaffen SL (2004) Interleukin-17 regulates expression of the CXC chemokine LIX/CXCL5 in osteoblasts: implications for inflammation and neutrophil recruitment. J Leukocyte Biol 76: 135–44.
16. Shen F, Ruddy MJ, Plamondon P, Gaffen SL (2005) Cytokines link osteoblasts and inflammation: microarray analysis of interleukin-17- and TNF-alpha-induced genes in bone cells. J Leukocyte Biol 77: 388–99.
17. Arican O, Aral M, Sasmaz S, Ciragil P (2005) Serum levels of TNF-alpha, IFN-gamma, IL-6, IL-8, IL-12, IL-17, and IL-18 in patients with active psoriasis and correlation with disease severity. Mediators Inflamm 2005:273–9.
18. Lee E, Trepicchio WL, Oestreicher JL, Pittman D, Wang F, et al. (2004) Increased Expression of Interleukin 23 p19 and p40 in Lesional Skin of Patients with Psoriasis Vulgaris. J Exp Med 199:125–30.
19. Lowes MA, Kikuchi T, Fuentes-Duculan J, Cardinale I, Zaba LC, et al. (2008) Psoriasis vulgaris lesions contain discrete populations of Th1 and Th17 T cells. J Invest Dermatol 128: 1207–11.
20. Zaba L, Cardinale I, Gilleaudeau P, Sullivan-Whalen M, Suárez-Fariñas M, et al. (2007) Amelioration of epidermal hyperplasia by TNF inhibition is associated with reduced Th17 responses. J Exp Med 204: 3183–94.
21. Caproni M, Antiga E, Melani L, Volpi W, Del Bianco E, et al (2009) Serum levels of IL-17 and IL-22 are reduced by etanercept, but not by acitretin, in patients with psoriasis: a randomized-controlled trial. J Clin Immunol 29:210–4.
22. Capon F, Di Meglio P, Szaub J, Prescott NJ, Dunster C, et al. (2007) Sequence variants in the genes for the interleukin-23 receptor (IL23R) and its ligand (IL12B) confer protection against psoriasis. Hum Genet 122: 201–6.
23. Cargill M, Schrodi SJ, Chang M, Garcia VE, Brandon R, et al. (2007) A large-scale genetic association study confirms IL12B and leads to the identification of IL23R as psoriasis-risk genes. Am J Hum Genet 80: 273–90.
24. Nair RP, Ruether A, Stuart PE, Jenisch S, Tejasvi T, et al. (2008) Polymorphisms of the IL12B and IL23R genes are associated with psoriasis. J Invest Dermatol 128: 1653–61.
25. Johnson-Huang LM, Suarez-Farinas M, Sullivan-Whalen M, Gilleaudeau P, Krueger JG, et al (2010) Effective narrow-band UVB radiation therapy suppresses the IL-23/IL-17 axis in normalized psoriasis plaques. J Invest Dermatol 130: 2654–63.
26. Piskin G, Tursen U, Sylva-Steenland RM, Bos JD, Teunissen MB (2004) Clinical improvement in chronic plaque-type psoriasis lesions after narrow-band

UVB therapy is accompanied by a decrease in the expression of IFN-gamma inducers – IL-12, IL-18 and IL-23. Exp Dermatol 13: 764–72.
27. Zaba LC, Suarez-Farinas M, Fuentes-Duculan J, Nograles KE, Guttman-Yassky E, et al. (2009) Effective treatment of psoriasis with etanercept is linked to suppression of IL-17 signaling, not immediate response TNF genes. J Allergy Clin Immunol 124: 1022–10.
28. Hueber W, Patel DD, Dryja T, Wright AM, Koroleva I, et al. (2010) Effects of AIN457, a fully human antibody to interleukin-17A, on psoriasis, rheumatoid arthritis, and uveitis. Sci Transl Med 2: 52ra72.
29. Krueger JG, Fretzin S, Suarez-Farinas M, Haslett PA, Phipps KM, et al. (2012) IL-17A is essential for cell activation and inflammatory gene circuits in subjects with psoriasis. J Allergy Clin Immunol 130: 145–54.
30. Leonardi C, Matheson R, Zachariae C, Cameron G, Li L, et al. (2012) Anti-interleukin-17 monoclonal antibody ixekizumab in chronic plaque psoriasis. N Engl J Med 366: 1190–9.
31. Leonardi CL, Kimball AB, Papp KA, Yeilding N, Guzzo C, et al. (2008) Efficacy and safety of ustekinumab, a human interleukin-12/23 monoclonal antibody, in patients with psoriasis: 76-week results from a randomised, double-blind, placebo-controlled trial (PHOENIX 1). Lancet 371: 1665–74.
32. Papp KA, Langley RG, Lebwohl M, Krueger GG, Szapary P, et al. (2008) Efficacy and safety of ustekinumab, a human interleukin-12/23 monoclonal antibody, in patients with psoriasis: 52-week results from a randomised, double-blind, placebo-controlled trial (PHOENIX 2). Lancet 371: 1675–84.
33. Papp KA, Leonardi C, Menter A, Ortonne JP, Krueger JG, et al. (2012) Brodalumab, an anti-interleukin-17-receptor antibody for psoriasis. N Engl J Med 366:1181–9.
34. Scheynius A, Fransson J, Johansson C, Hammar H, Baker B, et al. (1992) Expression of interferon-gamma receptors in normal and psoriatic skin. J Invest Dermatol 98: 255–8.
35. Trefzer U, Brockhaus M, Loetscher H, Parlow F, Kapp A, et al. (1991) 55-kd tumor necrosis factor receptor is expressed by human keratinocytes and plays a pivotal role in regulation of human keratinocyte ICAM-1 expression. J Invest Dermatol 97: 911–6.
36. Gulati N, Krueger JG, Suárez-Fariñas M, Mitsui H (2013) Creation of Differentiation-Specific Genomic Maps of Human Epidermis Through Laser Capture Microdissection. J Invest Dermatol. 133: 2640–2.
37. Morizane S, Gallo RL (2012) Antimicrobial peptides in the pathogenesis of psoriasis. J Dermatol 39: 225–30.
38. Blumberg H, Dinh H, Trueblood ES, Pretorius J, Kugler D, et al. (2007) Opposing activities of two novel members of the IL-1 ligand family regulate skin inflammation. J Exp Med 204: 2603–14.
39. Trepicchio WL, Ozawa M, Walters IB, Kikuchi T, Gilleaudeau P, et al. (1999) Interleukin-11 therapy selectively downregulates type I cytokine proinflammatory pathways in psoriasis lesions. J Clin Invest 104: 1527–37.
40. Tian S, Krueger JG, Li K, Jabbari A, Brodmerkel C, et al. (2012) Meta-analysis derived (MAD) transcriptome of psoriasis defines the "core" pathogenesis of disease. PloS One 7: e44274.
41. Suarez-Farinas M, Fuentes-Duculan J, Lowes MA, Krueger JG (2011) Resolved psoriasis lesions retain expression of a subset of disease-related genes. J Invest Dermatol 131: 391–400.
42. Nograles KE, Suarez-Farinas M, Shemer A, Fuentes-Duculan J, Chiricozzi A, et al. (2010) Atopic dermatitis keratinocytes exhibit normal T(H)17 cytokine responses,J Allergy Clin Immunol 125: 744–6, 6 e1–6 e2.
43. Johnston A, Xing X, Guzman AM, Riblett M, Loyd CM, et al. (2011) IL-1F5, -F6, -F8, and -F9: a novel IL-1 family signaling system that is active in psoriasis and promotes keratinocyte antimicrobial peptide expression. J Immunol 186: 2613–22.
44. Rizzo HL, Kagami S, Phillips KG, Kurtz SE, Jacques SL, et al. (2011) IL-23-mediated psoriasis-like epidermal hyperplasia is dependent on IL-17A. J Immunol 186: 1495–502.
45. Sa SM, Valdez PA, Wu J, Jung K, Zhong F, et al. (2007) The effects of IL-20 subfamily cytokines on reconstituted human epidermis suggest potential roles in cutaneous innate defense and pathogenic adaptive immunity in psoriasis. J Immunol 178: 2229–40.
46. Muhr P, Zeitvogel J, Heitland I, Werfel T, Wittmann M (2011) Expression of interleukin (IL)-1 family members upon stimulation with IL-17 differs in keratinocytes derived from patients with psoriasis and healthy donors. Br J Dermatol 165: 189–93.
47. Tohyama M, Hanakawa Y, Shirakata Y, Dai X, Yang L, et al. (2009) IL-17 and IL-22 mediate IL-20 subfamily cytokine production in cultured keratinocytes via increased IL-22 receptor expression. Eur J Immunol 39: 2779–88.
48. Ganguly D, Chamilos G, Lande R, Gregorio J, Meller S, et al. (2009) Self-RNA-antimicrobial peptide complexes activate human dendritic cells through TLR7 and TLR8. J Exp Med 206: 1983–94.
49. Lande R, Gregorio J, Facchinetti V, Chatterjee B, Wang YH, et al. (2007) Plasmacytoid dendritic cells sense self-DNA coupled with antimicrobial peptide. Nature 449: 564–9.
50. Suárez-Fariñas M, Dhingra N, Gittler J, Shemer A, Cardinale I, et al. (2013) Intrinsic atopic dermatitis shows similar TH2 and higher TH17 immune activation compared with extrinsic atopic dermatitis. J Allergy Clin Immunol. 132: 361–70.
51. Zaba LC, Fuentes-Duculan J, Steinman RM, Krueger JG, Lowes MA (2007) Normal human dermis contains distinct populations of CD11cBDCA-1 dendritic cells and CD163FXIIIA macrophages. J Clin Invest 117: 2517–2525.
52. Zhou X, Krueger JG, Kao MC, Lee E, Du F, et al. (2003) Novel mechanisms of T-cell and dendritic cell activation revealed by profiling of psoriasis on the 63,100-element oligonucleotide array. Physiol Genomics 13: 69–78.
53. Chamian F, Lowes MA, Lin SL, Lee E, Kikuchi T, et al. (2005) Alefacept reduces infiltrating T cells, activated dendritic cells, and inflammatory genes in psoriasis vulgaris. Proc Natl Acad Sci U S A. 102: 2075–80.
54. Suárez-Fariñas M, Pellegrino M, Wittkowski KM, Magnasco MO (2005) Harshlight: a "corrective make-up" program for microarray chips. BMC Bioinformatics 6: 294.
55. Wu Z, Irizarry RA, Gentleman R, Martinez-Murillo F, Spencer F. (2004) A Model-Based Background Adjustment for Oligonucleotide Expression Arrays. J Am Stat Assoc 99: 909–917.
56. Suarez-Farinas M, Lowes MA, Zaba LC, Krueger JG (2010) Evaluation of the psoriasis transcriptome across different studies by gene set enrichment analysis (GSEA). PLoS One 5:e10247.

14

Skin Regeneration in Adult Axolotls: A Blueprint for Scar-Free Healing in Vertebrates

Ashley W. Seifert[1]*, James R. Monaghan[1], S. Randal Voss[2,3], Malcolm Maden[1]

1 Department of Biology, University of Florida, Gainesville, Florida, United States of America, 2 Department of Biology, University of Kentucky, Lexington, Kentucky, United States of America, 3 Spinal Cord and Brain Injury Research Center, University of Kentucky, Lexington, Kentucky, United States of America

Abstract

While considerable progress has been made towards understanding the complex processes and pathways that regulate human wound healing, regenerative medicine has been unable to develop therapies that coax the natural wound environment to heal scar-free. The inability to induce perfect skin regeneration stems partly from our limited understanding of how scar-free healing occurs in a natural setting. Here we have investigated the wound repair process in adult axolotls and demonstrate that they are capable of perfectly repairing full thickness excisional wounds made on the flank. In the context of mammalian wound repair, our findings reveal a substantial reduction in hemostasis, reduced neutrophil infiltration and a relatively long delay in production of new extracellular matrix (ECM) during scar-free healing. Additionally, we test the hypothesis that metamorphosis leads to scarring and instead show that terrestrial axolotls also heal scar-free, albeit at a slower rate. Analysis of newly forming dermal ECM suggests that low levels of fibronectin and high levels of tenascin-C promote regeneration in lieu of scarring. Lastly, a genetic analysis during wound healing comparing epidermis between aquatic and terrestrial axolotls suggests that matrix metalloproteinases may regulate the fibrotic response. Our findings outline a blueprint to understand the cellular and molecular mechanisms coordinating scar-free healing that will be useful towards elucidating new regenerative therapies targeting fibrosis and wound repair.

Editor: Zhongjun Zhou, The University of Hong Kong, Hong Kong

Funding: The Ambystoma Affymetrix Genechips were designed from a transcript assembly funded by NIH-NCRR (R24-RR016344). Most of the transcripts were generated under the NIH-NCRR grant and an Army Research Office grant (MURI: W911NF-09-1-0305) to Ken Muneoka, David Gardiner, and SRV. Additional transcripts were provided by Elly Tanaka through funding from the DFG Center for Regenerative Therapies, and Bernd Fritsch through funding from NIH-NIDCD (R01-DC005590-07S1). The axolotls were obtained from the Ambystoma Genetic Stock Center at the University of Kentucky, which is funded by the National Science Foundation (DBI-0951484). This study was supported by NIH 5RC2NS069480 to MM and AWS is funded by NIH-NIDDK 5T32DK074367. Publication of this article was funded in part by the University of Florida Open-Access Publishing Fund. The funders had no role in study design, data collection and analysis, decision to publish, or preparation of the manuscript.

Competing Interests: The authors have declared that no competing interests exist.

* E-mail: seifert@ufl.edu

Introduction

Among its many functions, the skin is primarily responsible for maintaining the structural and physiological barrier between an organism's internal and external environment. As the first line of defense against external insult the skin is injured more frequently than any other tissue and resulting damage, while repairable, leads to permanent scarring in mammals [1]. At least 100 million people in the developed world acquire scars each year in response to trauma and surgery and the result is a spectrum of pathologies from thin line surgical scars to hypertrophic and chronic non-healing wounds [2,3,4]. Adding to this medical burden, burn injuries, which often elicit an over-exuberant fibrotic response, result in hypertrophic scarring with treatment costs in the US alone accounting for $4 billion annually [5]. While not as complex as regenerating a human digit or limb, the ability to develop regenerative strategies that lead to scar-free healing in adult skin remain tantalizingly out of reach. Understanding how to coax the natural wound repair process towards a regenerative outcome remains the grail of wound healing research.

Our knowledge of the molecular and cellular events during mammalian tissue repair is extensive (see refs [1,6,7,8]) and yet, even with such broad understanding of the wound repair process, regenerative medicine has failed to develop therapies that can perfectly regenerate skin. This stems partly from the dynamic reciprocity of cellular interactions and signaling pathways and partly from a lack of appropriate models to observe these interactions in a regenerative environment [9]. While wound repair in fetal mammals [10,11,12,13,14] and marsupials [15] has provided insight into the cellular and molecular regulation of scar-free healing, comparisons of wound repair between fetal mammals and adults has limitations, both biological and practical [16]. The developing fetus, at the time when it heals scar-free, has an immature endocrine system, is immuno-incompetent, is contained in a moist sterile environment, and its cells are in a state of chronic hypoxia [16]. Adult skin is more completely differentiated and adult wounds are open to desiccation and infection, two factors that seriously complicate wound repair. Other promising models of scar-free healing, such as the MRL mouse, which share the ability to regenerate ear punches with rabbits, hares, pikas, cows, pigs and cats [17,18,19] has proven less than perfect when challenged to heal excisional skin wounds [20,21] casting doubt on the special regenerative powers of this inbred mouse model.

Compared to other vertebrates, urodeles possess the amazing capacity to regenerate their limbs, hearts, lenses, spinal cords, tails, internal organs and joints. Observations from studies examining limb regeneration have been extrapolated to the skin, but direct comparisons to the processes of cutaneous wound repair have rarely been made [22]. Studies examining limb wounds have yielded insight into the process of re-epithelialization [23,24,25,26] and regeneration of the basement membrane [27,28], but the dynamics of dermal regeneration have remained obscure. Direct study of wound repair in urodele skin outside of regeneration fields like the limb and tail, however, has not been undertaken.

Given their seemingly absolute powers of regeneration, a recurring question has been whether wounds made outside of regenerating structures (e.g. limbs and tails) in adult urodeles are capable of scar-free healing or, like adult anurans, heal with a scar [29]. In this study we examined full thickness excisional (FTE) wound healing of dorsal back skin in adult axolotls. Using an established mammalian excisional wound model to directly characterize cutaneous wound healing in adult axolotls, we examined hemostasis, inflammation, new tissue formation and remodeling processes. Additionally, we induced metamorphosis in adult axolotls to test the hypothesis that loss of larval skin characters and transition to a terrestrial form results in fibrotic scarring following FTE flank wounds. Here we demonstrate that both aquatic and terrestrial axolotls are capable of perfect, scar-free skin regeneration. We discuss these findings in the context of mammalian wound repair and present a blueprint for investigating the cellular and molecular mechanisms that regulate scar-free skin healing in adult vertebrates.

Results

Full Thickness Excisional Flank Wounds are Perfectly Regenerated in Adult Axolotls

Adult axolotls (*Ambystoma mexicanum*) are aquatic and paedomorphic, exhibiting several juvenile features as adults (e.g. retention of leydig cells, pseudo-stratified epidermis, external gills). Although the dermis of adult axolotl skin is typical for amphibians, the epidermis is pseudo-stratified and lacks a well-defined stratum corneum (Figure 1A, B). Above the stratum germinativum, epithelial cells are interspersed with leydig cells (specialized cells containing highly granulated cytoplasm) that are characteristic of larval amphibian skin (Figure 1B and [30,31]). The dermis contains epidermally-derived mucous and granular glands that are embedded within the stratum spongiosum, a loose network of thin collagen fibers and fibroblasts that lies above the stratum compactum (Figure 1A, B and Figure S1A, B). The stratum compactum forms a thickened sheet of compressed collagen fibers that sits atop hypodermis and separates the skin from the underlying muscle (Figure 1A).

It has been reported that wounds made outside of regeneration fields (i.e. limbs, tail, head) heal with a scar [32] and to date, this controversy remains unresolved. To directly test the hypothesis that axolotls can perfectly regenerate (i.e. heal scar-free) full thickness excisional (FTE) wounds, we made circular 4mm FTE wounds through the dermis into the dorsal flank muscle ($n = 12$) and observed the wound healing process over 180 days (Figure 1C-H, Figure 2, Figures S2). In response to injury blood flowed into the wound bed, clotted, but did not form a scab (Figure 2). Epithelial cells from the wound margins migrated across the underlying muscle and accumulated plasma and completely re-epithelialized the wound within 24hrs (Figure 1C, green arrows indicate plasma). Following re-epithelialization numerous blood cells (leukocytes and erythrocytes) were apparent in the wound bed and the neoepidermis remained in close proximity with the underlying muscle and plasma over the next 7–10 days (Figure 1D). Fourteen days post injury we observed dermal fibroblasts in the wound bed and Masson's Trichrome staining revealed newly deposited extracellular matrix (ECM) (Figure 1E). Twenty-one days post injury muscle fibers continued to fragment liberating mono-nucleate cells into the surrounding tissue and a robust ECM formed between the epidermis and muscle (Figure 1E, F). Forty-seven days post-injury new epidermal organs were present in the regenerated stratum spongiosum (Figure 1G and Figure S2A). The stratum compactum, however, had not completely regenerated and this was clearly evident at its margins (Figure 1G and Figure S2B). Although the timing to regeneration varied among individuals, full thickness skin, including epidermal organs and underlying muscle, was completely regenerated by 80 days (Figure 1H and Figure 2). Maturation and development of glands and the stratum compactum continued over the next 100 days (Figure S2C).

New ECM Deposition Corresponds with Formation of the Lamina Densa

Previous work in regenerating newt limbs suggested that reformation of the basement membrane (BM) facilitates dermal regeneration and its delayed formation permits blastema formation [28]. We followed BM regeneration after re-epithelialization and asked whether it occurred prior to the onset of dermal regeneration in excisional flank wounds. In uninjured skin the BM is visible as a thick fibrous band separating epidermis from dermis and is continuous except where mucous glands interject into the epidermis (Figure 3A). Following re-epithelialization histological staining revealed a thin, immature structure beneath the new epidermis (Figure 3A). The BM continued to mature and was completely regenerated at least 47 days after wounding (Figure 3A; yellow arrows D47). Interestingly, complete regeneration of the BM corresponded to regeneration of the dermis (except for stratum spongiosum) (Figure 3A and Figure 1G).

In order to test if assembly and maturation of the BM corresponded to the onset of ECM deposition we analyzed formation of the lamina lucida and lamina densa using antibodies that recognize laminin (lamina lucida) and collagen type IV (lamina densa) (Figure 3B). Both proteins were detectable in the BM of uninjured skin, and surrounding glands and muscle fibers (Figure 3B). Following re-epithelialization, basal epidermal cells were negative for both laminin and collagen IV (Figure 3B; white arrows). We detected strong and continuous laminin staining beneath the epidermis 7 days post injury indicating lamina lucida reformation (Figure 3B). Collagen IV was not detected continuously beneath the epidermis until D14 (corresponding to the onset of ECM deposition) (Figure 3B).

In addition to protein localization we tracked epidermal gene expression of the BM components *collagen type IV* and *laminin alpha 1* (*Lama1*), *laminin beta 1* (*Lamb1*), *laminin gamma 1* (*Lamc1*), which together form the protein laminin-111 (Table S1). Expression of all three laminin-111 subunits was unchanged during re-epithelialization (Table S1). Expression of both *alpha-1* and *beta-1* components of laminin-111 increased 5.6-fold and 4.1-fold respectively between D1 and D3, and continued increasing at D7 post injury (Table S1). In the skin basement membrane of humans and mice, two hetero-trimeric collagen type IV molecules consisting of alpha1(IV)$_2$/alpha2(IV) and alpha5(IV)$_2$/alpha6(IV) chains exist [33]. We examined expression of each of these alpha chains following injury and found that expression of *alpha1* and *alpha2* chains were down regulated following injury, remained below baseline levels until D3, after which they returned to baseline levels at D7 post injury (Table S1). Whereas expression of the *alpha6* chain remained unchanged, the *alpha5* chain was upregulated 4.9-fold at D1 and sustained through D7 (Table S1).

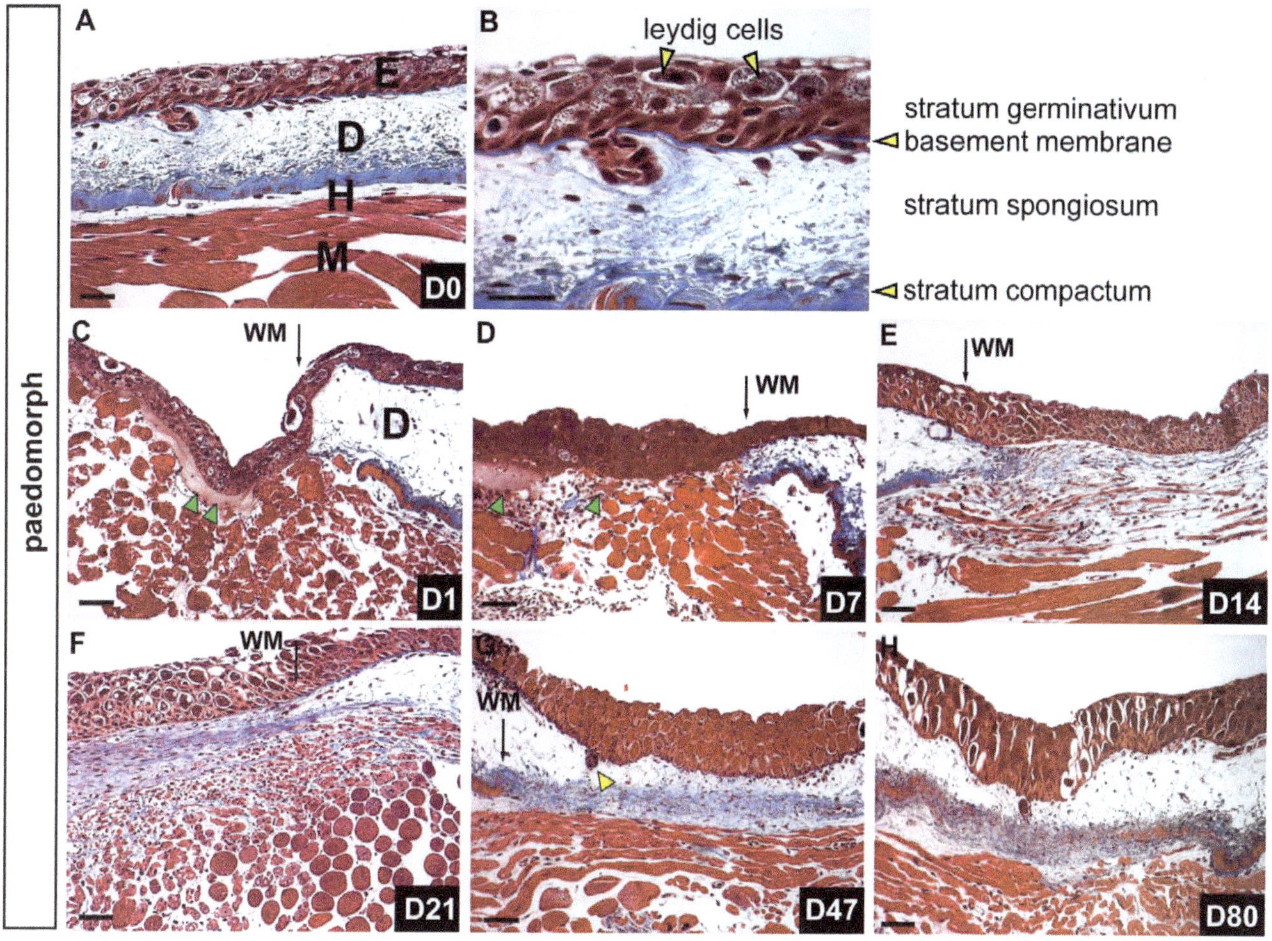

Figure 1. Scar-free healing of full thickness excisional wounds in adult axolotls. A) Masson's trichrome staining of uninjured dorsal flank skin in axolotls showing epidermis (E), dermis (D), hypodermis (H) and underlying muscle (M). B) Magnified image of epidermis and dermis. The epidermis is pseudo-stratified and contains epithelial cells and leydig cells (yellow arrows) while the dermis is divided into the stratum spongiosum (containing glands and dermal fibroblasts) atop the densely compacted ECM of the stratum compactum. C-H) Scar-free healing over 80 day period following full thickness excisional wounding. C) One day post injury (dpi) the wound bed is completely re-epithelialized. Some blood plasma has accumulated beneath the neoepidermis (green arrows) (wound margin = WM). D) Seven dpi there is little evidence of a fibrin clot between the epidermis and underlying muscle and no new ECM has been deposited. Green arrows depict residual blood plasma. E) Fourteen dpi fibroblasts are visible beneath the epidermis where new ECM is deposited (blue staining) and muscle cells are fragmenting into individual myoblasts. F) Twenty-one dpi a thick band of transitional matrix is visible beneath the epidermis. Collagen is visible within the regenerating muscle. G) Forty-seven dpi the underlying muscle has completely regenerated and is devoid of collagen. Skin glands (yellow arrow) have regenerated and descended from the epidermis. The dermal stratum spongiosum has reformed and the stratum compactum is coalescing. H) Eighty dpi all skin layers have regenerated. Scale bars = 100 μm.

Taken together, these results demonstrate that regeneration of the BM proceeds through formation of the lamina lucida followed by production of the lamina densa and that complete lamina densa formation corresponds to the onset of ECM production in the wound bed.

Metamorphic Axolotls Exhibit a Delay in Skin Regeneration Compared to Paedomorphic Axolotls

While adult mammals are incapable of regenerating full thickness skin wounds, fetal mammals exhibit scarless healing of similar type wounds [12]. Similarly, while pre-metamorphic anurans heal scar-free, post-metamorphic anurans have been documented to heal flank wounds through scar formation [29]. Adult axolotls retain several larval skin features (e.g. leydig cells, pseudo-stratified epithelium), thus we asked if these characteristics facilitate their ability to heal wounds scar-free. To test this hypothesis we exploited the fact that normally aquatic axolotls retain the ability to undergo metamorphosis to a terrestrial form through administration of thyroxine and we induced metamorphosis in adult axolotls (controlling for age and size with sibling paedomorphs). Comparing uninjured epidermis between both forms we noted two major differences; first, granular glands that occupied relatively little space in the paedomorph dermis were greatly enlarged and occupied most of the stratum spongiosum while mucous glands appeared similar in form between morphs (Figure 4A and Figure S3A). Second, the epidermis no longer contained leydig cells and had transitioned to a completely stratified epithelium exhibiting a well-defined stratum germinativum, stratum spinosum, stratum granulosum and stratum corneum (Figure 4B).

We next examined wound repair in metamorphs following 4mm full thickness excisional wounds over 180 days (Figure 4C-H

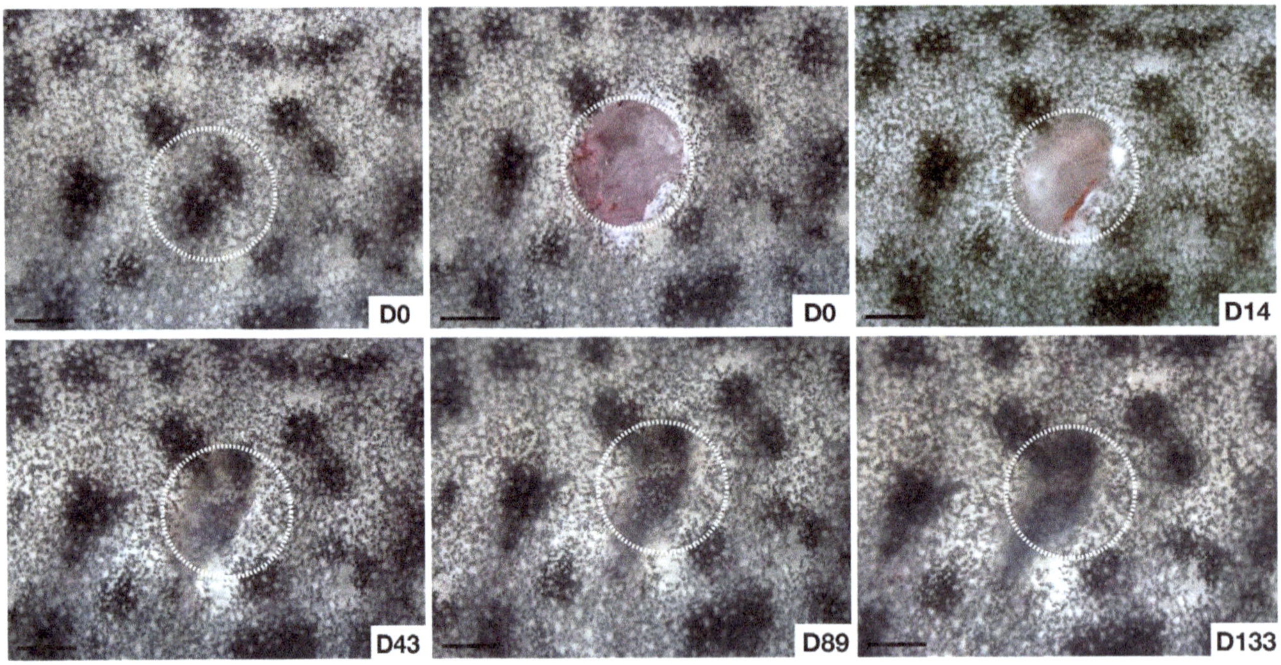

Figure 2. Scar-free healing in adult axolotls. Regeneration of dorsal flank skin following 4 mm full thickness biopsy punch wounding. White circles depict area of original injury. Individual pigment cells are visible at D14 in the overlying epithelium. Regeneration and scar-free healing at D89. Contraction is evident at the wound edges after D14. Scale bars = 2.0 mm.

and Figure S3B-E). Twenty-four hours post injury re-epithelialization was not complete and the leading edge of migrating epidermal cells was visible both macroscopically and in section (Figure 4C). Re-epithelialization was complete by 72hours post injury and the epidermis had re-stratified to establish apical/basal polarity along the regenerating basement membrane (Figure 4D). Seven days post injury the wound bed contained plasma beneath the epidermis and within the fragmented muscle, along with large numbers of erythrocytes and leukocytes (Figure 4D). ECM deposition began as it had in the paedomorph approximately 10–14 days post injury and we noted that it appeared to extend deep into the muscle (Figure 4E). Twenty-one days post injury the ECM was dense within the wound bed, new vasculature was present in both the epidermis and ECM, muscle fibers continued to fragment and aggregations of cells appeared in the epidermis suggesting glands were beginning to regenerate (Figure 4F and Figure S3B).

Complete dermal regeneration was delayed in metamorphs (compare Figure 1G and Figure 4G). While epidermal organs regenerated in both forms after 40 days, the wound bed and underlying muscle still contained densely compacted extracellular matrix in metamorphs (Figure 4G and Figure S3C). After 80+ days the stratum spongiosum had regenerated but the stratum compactum remained incomplete (Figure 4H). After 120 days, the wound site resembled an 80-day regenerating wound in paedomorphs and a few collagen deposits still persisted in the underlying muscle (Figure S3D). Fibrosis was not resolved until at least 148 days and while mucous glands regenerated to pre-wound size, granular glands remained small even after 148 days (Figure S3E). Taken together these findings suggest that flank skin in adult metamorphic axolotls can completely regenerate following FTE wounding, but the time required to regenerate both the stratum compactum and mature granular glands is lengthened compared to paedomorphs.

The Rate of Re-epithelialization is Slower in Metamorphs

Following injury, re-epithelialization of the wound bed is necessary to re-establish epidermal integrity. In various rodent species, untreated FTE wounds re-epithelialize between 3 and 7 days (personal obser.). In contrast, aquatic axolotls re-epithelialize 4mm flank wounds in ~18hrs (Figure 1C and Figure S4). We compared the rate of re-epithelialization between paedomorphs and metamorphs to test whether the completely stratified epidermis of terrestrial axolotls affected its ability to cover the wound bed. Using an antibody to a wide-spectrum of cytokeratins we labeled the epidermis 24 and 72hrs after injury (Figure 5). Compared to the completely re-epithelialized wound bed of paedomorphs, wound edge epithelial cells in metamorphs had just begun migrating 24 hrs after injury (Figure 5A, B). Metamorph re-epithelialization was complete by 72 hrs (Figure 5C). Examination of the wound epidermis in paedomorphs showed leydig cells present in the new epidermis (Figure 5D). The leading edge of metamorph epidermis appeared pseudo-stratified (reminiscent of paedomorph epidermis without leydig cells) and moved as a sheet of cells with a single cell at the leading edge (Figure 5E). Following re-epithelialization, the wound epidermis re-established a stratified epithelial morphology (Figure 5F). In conjunction with this delay in re-epithelialization we observed a concomitant delay in appearance of the BM components laminin and collagen type IV reflecting the dependency of BM reassembly on the timing of complete re-epithelialization (data not shown). We examined the expression of the same molecular components of laminin and collagen type IV as we did for paedomorphs and did not detect a significant increase in expression prior to D7 (Table S1). These results show that stratified epidermis in metamorphs requires an extended activation period (relative to paedomorphs) before migration begins and this delay contributes to a slower rate of re-epithelialization.

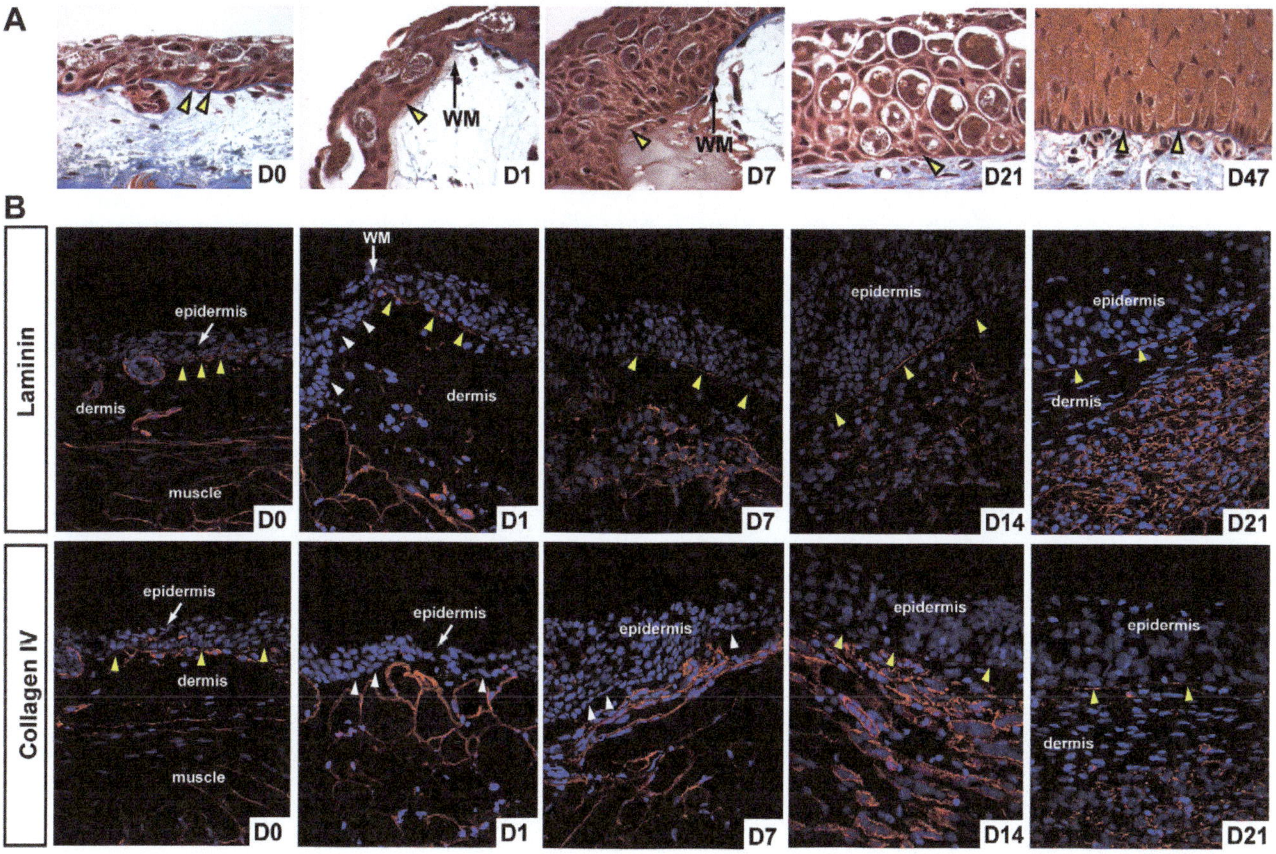

Figure 3. Lamina lucida and lamina densa regenerate before new ECM deposition. A) Histological examination of basement membrane (BM) regeneration in axolotls. The uninjured BM is visible as a thick blue-stained fibrous band (yellow arrows). An immature BM has begun to reform (yellow arrow D1) after re-epithelialization and is visible at the wound margin (WM) in contrast to the uninjured BM. The regenerated BM is visible at D47. Yellow arrows at D7 and D21 indicate reforming BM. B) Examination of lamina lucida (laminin) and lamina densa (collagen type IV) during basement membrane regeneration. The uninjured BM is positive for laminin and collagen type IV (yellow arrows) as are the basement membranes surrounding glands and muscle fibers. Following re-epithelialization the basal lamina of the epidermis is negative for laminin and collagen type IV (white arrows) and this is clearly evident at the wound margin (WM). Seven days post injury the BM stains strongly for laminin indicating reformation of the lamina lucida, while staining for collagen type IV is punctuated. The lamina densa is regenerated by D14 based on continuous collagen type IV staining and persists during dermal regeneration.

Migrating Keratinocytes and Neoepidermis Express High MMP Levels

Epidermal expression and enzymatic activity of serine proteinases and matrix metalloproteinases has been shown to affect keratinocyte migration and ECM degradation during the early stages of mammalian wound healing [1]. In order to begin addressing the role these enzymes play during skin regeneration in axolotls we analyzed the expression of the serine proteinase *plasminogen tissue activator* (*PLAT*), matrix metalloproteinase (*MMP*) family members and the *tissue inhibitors of metalloproteinases* (*TIMP 1–4*) in migrating and neoepidermis following excisional wounding at D1, D3 and D7 in paedomorphs and metamorphs (Table S1). *PLAT* functions to convert plasminogen to plasmin and consistent with the absence of a fibrin clot was not expressed either in uninjured axolotl skin or following injury in the epidermis (Table S1).

During skin regeneration in axolotls we found a strong *MMP* response to injury in both migrating keratinocytes and neoepidermis in paedomorphs and metamorphs (Table S1). For all *MMPs* demonstrating significant changes in gene expression following injury, the expression kinetics generally followed two patterns; (1) a strong upregulation at D1 followed by an equally strong decrease at D3 and a continued decrease or leveling off at D7 and (2) a strong upregulation at D1 which remained higher than baseline at D3 and then was downregulated at D7 (Figure 6).

The collagenases *MMP1* and *axCOL* (an amphibian specific collagenase orthologous to newt *nCOL*) followed the first pattern with *MMP1* exhibiting a particularly strong response, increasing 425-fold (paedomorphs) and 502-fold (metamorphs) at D1, while remaining 88-fold (paedomorphs) and 61-fold elevated (metamorphs) at D7 (Table S1). The stromelysin *MMP3/10a* exhibited a similar expression profile as the collegenases except D7 levels returned near baseline (Figure 6). *MMP3/10b* levels, while exhibiting strong upregulation at D1, exhibited a slow decreasing rate of expression (pattern 2) compared to *MMP3/10a* and remained elevated at D7 (Figure 6). While *MMP19* and *MMP28* followed expression pattern 1 for paedomorphs, expression of both genes remained high in metamorphs mirroring the lag time in the metamorphic re-epithelialization rate (Figure 6). The gelatinase *MMP9* exhibited pattern 1 expression kinetics and responded 2-fold greater in metamorphs. *MMP2* was the one exception to the generally observed patterns. *MMP2* was effectively turned off at D1, remained off at D3 and then was upregulated in both paedomorphs and metamorphs (Figure 6). Given the strong

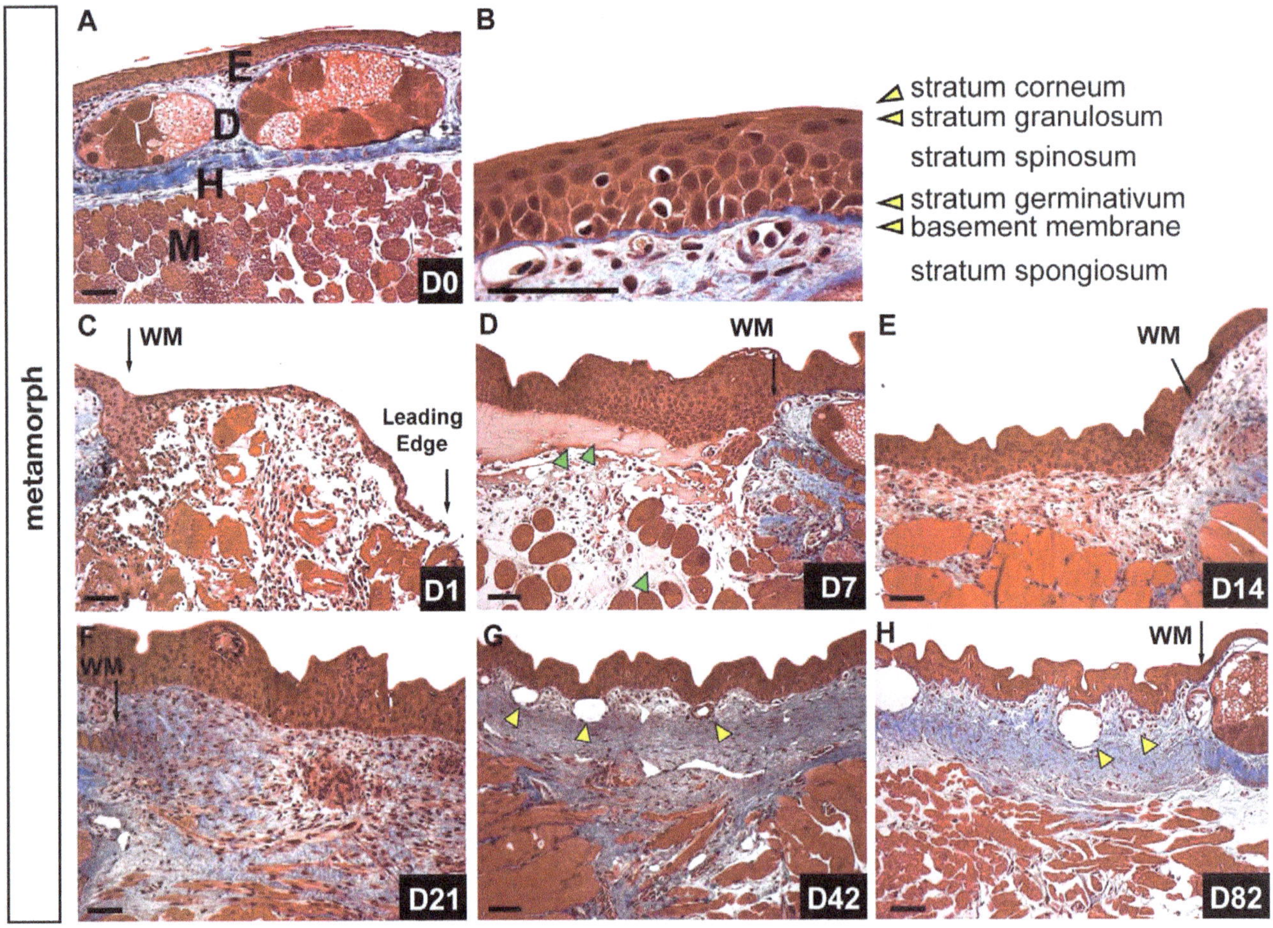

Figure 4. Metamorphic axolotl skin heals scar-free but slower compared to paedomorphs. A–B) Morphology of uninjured axolotl skin after metamorphosis. A) Masson's trichrome staining showing epidermis (E), dermis (D) containing enlarged granular glands in stratum spongiosum atop stratum compactum, hypodermis (H) and muscle (M). B) High magnification of epidermis showing stratified epithelium. Leydig cells have disappeared and the epidermis now contains a well-defined stratum spinosum, granulosum and corneum. C-H) Wound healing following FTE wounds over 82-day period. C) One day post injury (dpi) epithelial cells have begun to migrate but the wound is not re-epithelialized. Erythrocytes are visible in the wound bed and between muscle fibers undergoing histolysis. D) Re-epithelialization is complete 3 dpi and at 7 dpi coagulated plasma (green arrows), erythrocytes and leukocytes are visible in the wound bed. E) Fourteen dpi fibroblasts are visible in the wound bed and new ECM is deposited (blue staining). The wound margin (WM) is still clearly visible. F) The wound bed 21 dpi is rich in ECM. This ECM extends deep into the underlying muscle fibers which are fragmenting into myoblasts. G). Regenerating glands (yellow arrows) are present in the dermis 42 dpi and the stratum spongiosum is beginning to develop. The underlying muscle continues to remain damaged with deep pockets of collagen persisting beneath the wound. H) Eighty dpi the dermis is partially regenerated but the stratum compactum has not coalesced. Some collagen still persists deep in the muscle and both mucous and granular glands have regenerated (yellow arrows). Scale bars = 100 μm.

response to injury reflected in *MMP* levels, we also analyzed expression levels for the *tissue inhibitors of MMPs* (*TIMPs*) (Table S1). Only *TIMP1* changed significantly, with paedomorphs exhibiting pattern 1 expression and metamorphs exhibiting pattern 2. Interestingly, axolotls appear to have two copies of *TIMP1* based on sequence analysis and this second copy did not change in either morph following injury (data not shown). Previous experiments during newt limb regeneration have shown that *MMP* transcription correlates well with their enzymatic activity [34] and the high sequence similarity between newt and axolotl *MMP* sequences strongly supports MMP orthology. We conducted gelatin zymography during paedomorphic tail regeneration and found that transcription and activity of MMP9 were well correlated, thus supporting this association in axolotl (Figure S5 A-C). This confirms recent work during axolotl limb regeneration demonstrating the activity of axolotl MMP [35]. Taken together these results suggest MMPs may play a key role during keratinocyte migration and regeneration, and suggest that sustained activity may control the timing of ECM deposition.

Metamorphic Axolotls Exhibit Increased Leukocyte Infiltration

During wound repair, adult mammals exhibit a stereotypical inflammatory response characterized by infiltration and subsequent removal of leukocytes [36]. The trade-off between regeneration and fibrosis has been postulated to result from a weak inflammatory response with greater inflammation contributing to increased fibrosis [37]. In order to characterize the inflammatory response during skin regeneration, we assayed the wound bed for L-plastin positive cells, a pan-leukocytic marker conserved in vertebrates. To control for individual variation we harvested wound tissue from the same animal (4 wounds per animal) at D0, D1, D3, D7 and D14 from paedomorphs (n = 4)

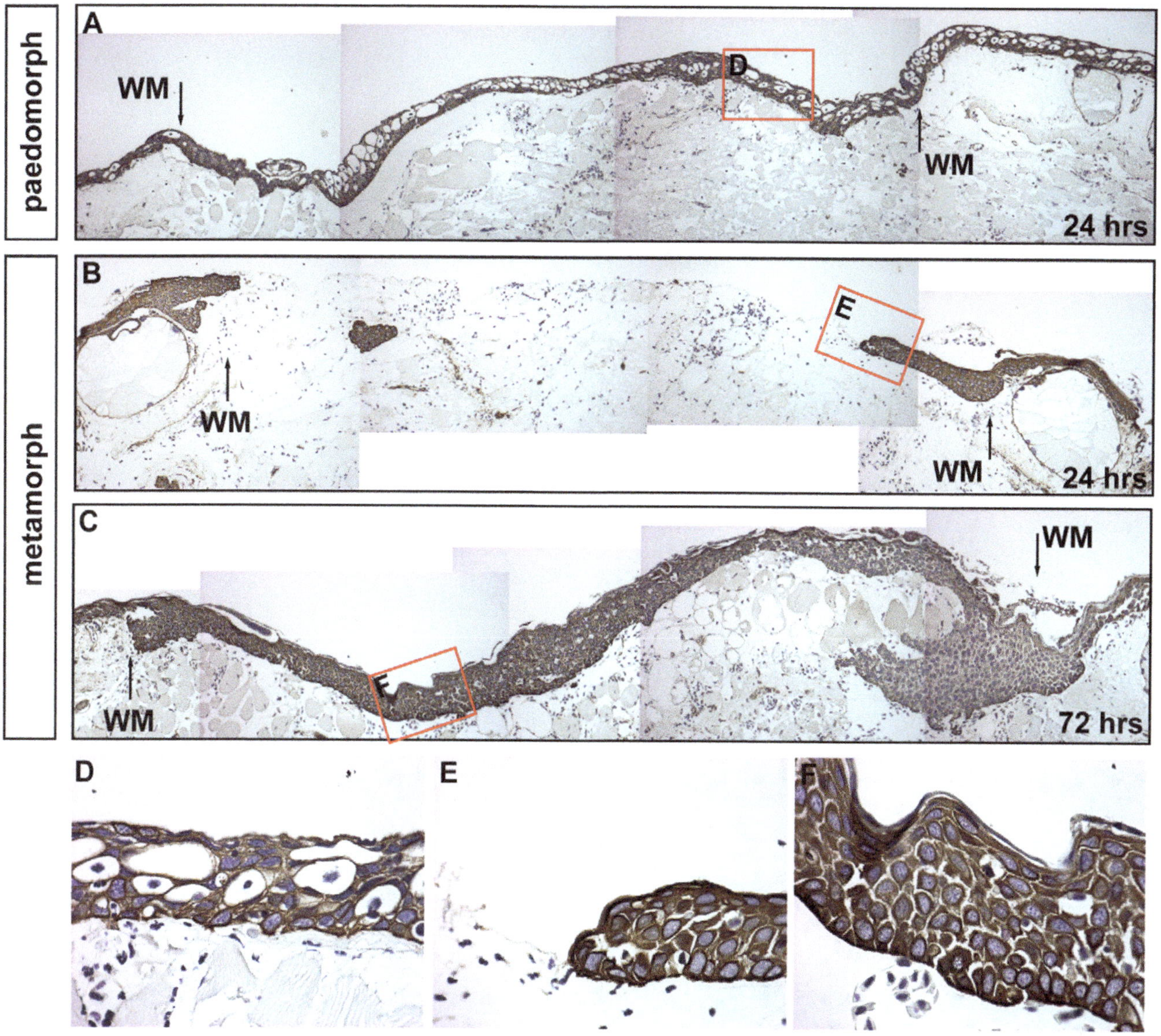

Figure 5. The rate of re-epithelialization is slower in metamorphs compared to paedomorphs. Epidermis was labeled with a pan-cytokeratin antibody. A) The wound bed is completely re-epithelialized 24 hrs after injury in paedomorphs. The wound margins (WM) are visible where the stratum compactum is disrupted. B, C) Wound edge keratinocytes have just begun migrating 24 hrs dpi and re-epithelialization is complete by 72 hrs dpi in metamorphs. D) Leydig cells are present in the paedomorph neoepidermis. E) The leading edge of migrating metamorph keratinocytes. The epidermal cells appear to move as a group of cells with one cell at the leading edge. F) After re-epithelialization is complete in metamorphs the epidermis becomes re-stratified.

and metamorphs ($n=4$). Examining the number of L-plastin positive cells we found both morphs exhibited a robust infiltration of leukocytes into the wound bed (Figure 7A and Figure S6A). We used a 2-way ANOVA to examine the effects of morph (metamorph vs paedomorph) and day post injury on total leukocyte numbers (with individual as a random effect to allow for repeated sampling). This analysis yielded a small p-value for the effect of morph ($F=3.05$, $p=0.095$). An examination of each individual over time showed that one paedomorph exhibited much higher levels of L-plastin positive cells (suggesting chronic stress or sickness) compared with the other three individuals (Figure S6B, C; paed 4). Therefore we analyzed the data without this individual and found that metamorphs had a significantly higher number of leukocytes following injury ($F=5.32$, $p=0.032$) (Figure 7A). This difference was most pronounced between D1 and D3 (Figure 7A) when re-epithelialization was complete in paedomorphs but not in metamorphs.

In order to further quantify the inflammatory response we examined neutrophil infiltration in paedomorphs and metamorphs. Using a polyclonal antibody to myloperoxidase (MPO) we counted all neutrophils in 5μm sections of the wound bed between the epidermis and underlying muscle following injury (Figure 7B). Neutrophils were present in low numbers following injury (compared to mammals) and were not significantly different between paedomorphs ($n=8$) and metamorphs ($n=8$) ($F=2.50$, $p=0.136$). Examining MPO positive cells across all axolotls ($n=16$) the effect of days post injury approached significance ($F=3.04$, $p=0.058$) and post-hoc comparisons

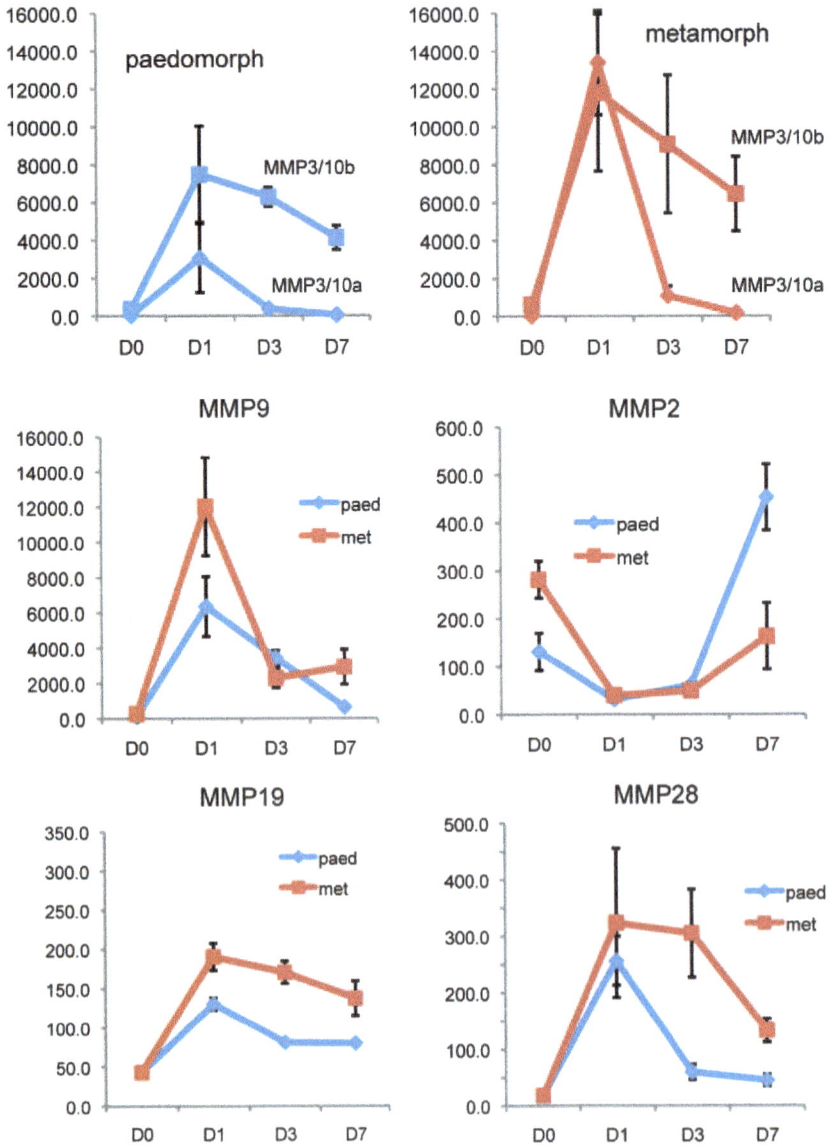

Figure 6. ***Matrix metalloproteinase (MMP)* expression during re-epithelialization and new tissue formation.** Expression values (y-axis) reflect absolute expression values from Affymetrix axolotl genechips (see Table S1 for exact values). Error bars represent standard error. Blue lines represent paedomorphs and red lines represent metamorphs. Expression kinetics for selected *MMPs* generally followed two patterns; (1) a strong upregulation at D1 followed by an equally strong decrease at D3 and a continued decrease or leveling off at D7 [*MMP3/10a, MMP9*] and (2) a strong upregulation at D1 which remained high at D3 and then downregulated at D7 [*MMP3/10b, MMP19*]. For *MMP28* the kinetics followed pattern 1 for paedomorphs and pattern 2 for metamorphs suggesting that *MMP28* expression was highly connected to re-epithelialization. The expression profile for *MMP2* was unique in that is was downregulated following injury and was upregulated after re-epithelialization was complete.

revealed a significant decrease in neutrophil levels at D7 ($t = 2.014$, $p = 0.0226$).

In mammalian wounds, neutrophils represent the majority of leukocytes present during the early inflammatory response and comprise approximately 59% of circulating leukocytes [38]. Our data suggested that neutrophils comprised a relatively small fraction of infiltrating leukocytes in axolotls after injury, and we asked if this was due in part to low levels in circulation. Using a modified Wright's stain to identify leukocytes and Sudan Black to accurately identify the neutrophil population, we calculated leukocyte profiles (percentage of total leukocytes) for both paedomorphs ($n = 5$) and metamorphs ($n = 5$) (Figure 7C and Table S2). We found that leukocytes comprise approximately 4% of circulating blood cells with neutrophils accounting for ~21% of the leukocyte population in both forms (Table S2). Comparing paedomorphs and metamorphs we found significantly higher eosinophil levels in paedomorphs ($t = 2.49$, $p = 0.043$) and significantly higher lymphocyte levels in metamorphs ($t = 3.96$, $p = 0.004$). Taken together, these results show that axolotls display an influx of leukocytes following full thickness excisional wounding demonstrating an inflammatory response to wounding. However, relative to mammals, neutrophils comprise a smaller fraction of inflammatory cells at the wound site, and this correlates with their relatively lower representation in circulating blood.

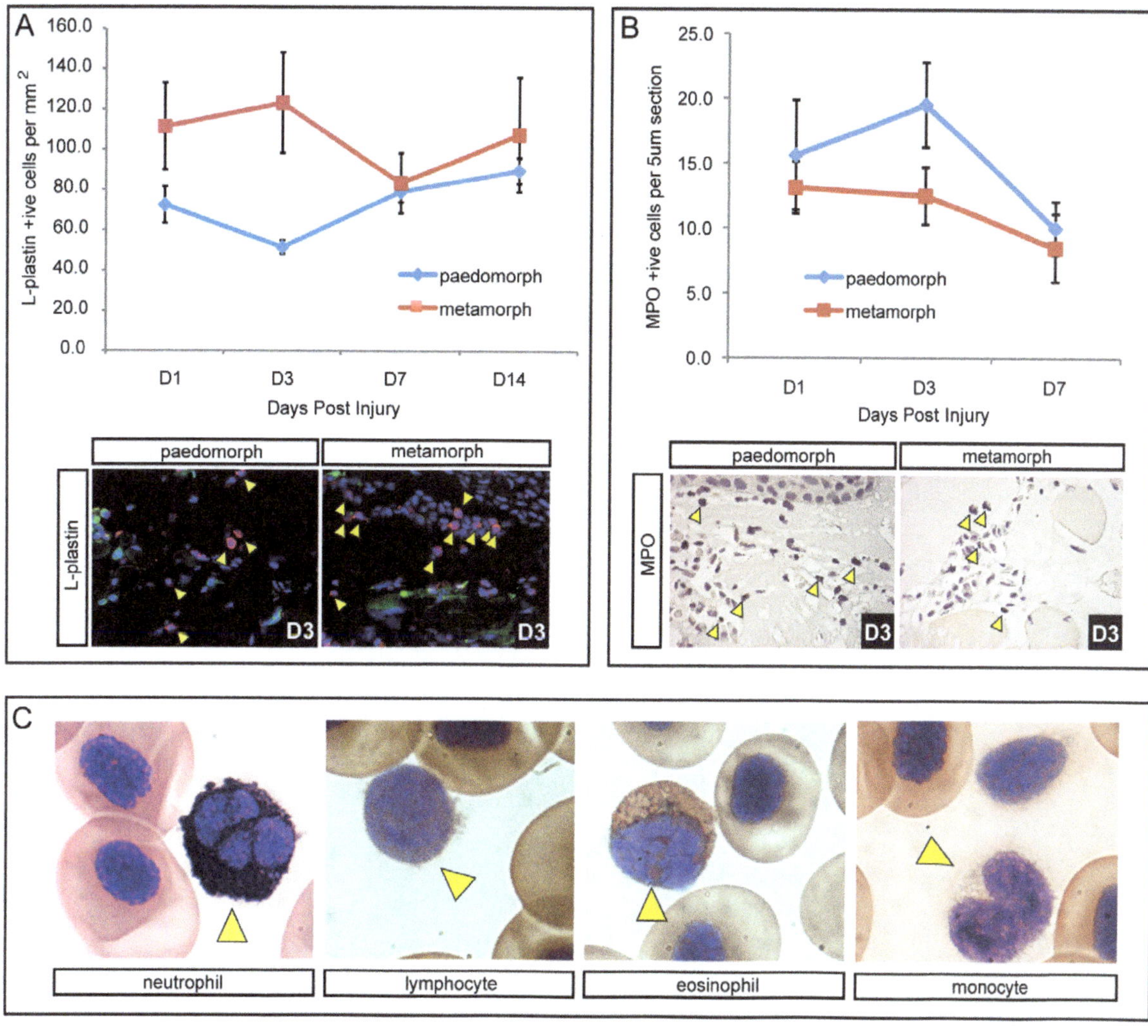

Figure 7. Higher initial leukocyte levels are present in terrestrial axolotls coincident with slower re-epithelialization, but neutrophil levels are not different between morphs. L-plastin was used as a pan-leukocytic marker to quantify total leukocyte levels following injury. A) Total leukocytes counted per mm^2 in the wound bed at 1, 3, 7 and 14 dpi (n = 4 for each morph). L-plastin positive cells are red (yellow arrows), nuclei are stained blue (Hoescht) and green fluorescence was used to account for autofluorescencing erythrocytes that were excluded as leukocytes. An influx of leukocytes was observed 24 hrs dpi, with higher numbers present in terrestrial axolotls. Leukocyte levels dropped in metamorphs at D7 and converged with paedomorph levels. Levels for paedomorphs were not significantly changed after D1. B) All neutrophils present in the wound bed (yellow arrows) were counted on 5 µm sections above the muscle using myloperoxidase (n = 8 for each morph; see Figure S6 for positive control staining in liver). Neutrophil levels were generally low and were not significantly different between paedomorphs and metamorphs, although they did drop significantly at D7. C) Modified Wright-Giemsa stain used to indentify individual leukocytes in circulating axolotl blood. Sudan black was used to stain neutrophils. Yellow arrows indicate the specific leukocyte type.

Percent Wound Closure Mimics Contraction Rates During Healing of Human Skin Wounds

Wound contraction is an important component of the repair process and is an important metric when comparing wound repair across taxa [39]. In humans and pigs, contraction of circular wounds accounts for less than 50% of wound closure, while in rodents contraction accounts for ~90% of repair [39]. Following excisional wounding, the wound area increased slightly in metamorphs while remaining constant in paedomorphs and after 24hrs the wounds in both groups contracted at approximately the same rate (Figure 8A). Quantifying the rate of wound contraction between paedomorphs and metamorphs, we found that percent contraction was significantly greater in paedomorphs and resulted in a greater degree of wound closure (paedomorphs = 67% ± 4.4% and metamorphs = 37.9% ± 9%) (Figure 8B). In fact, our analysis shows that metamorphic axolotls contract their wounds to approximately the same degree as human skin after wounding.

Prior to wound contraction, some dermal fibroblasts in the granulation tissue and at the wound margins begin to express smooth muscle actin and are responsible for generating contractile forces that pull the wound margins together [40,41]. We also examined localization of alpha-smooth muscle actin (alpha-SMA) (a marker of myofibroblasts) in paedomorphs and compared its distribution to mice at similar time points after wounding (Fig. 8C). Approximately 10 days after injury, mice showed a high number of alpha-SMA positive cells at the wound margins when the wound area begins to rapidly contract (Figure 8C; white circled area). In contrast, we did not detect many alpha-SMA positive cells in axolotls at the wound margins or in the wound bed at D10, although the basement membrane beneath the wound epidermis

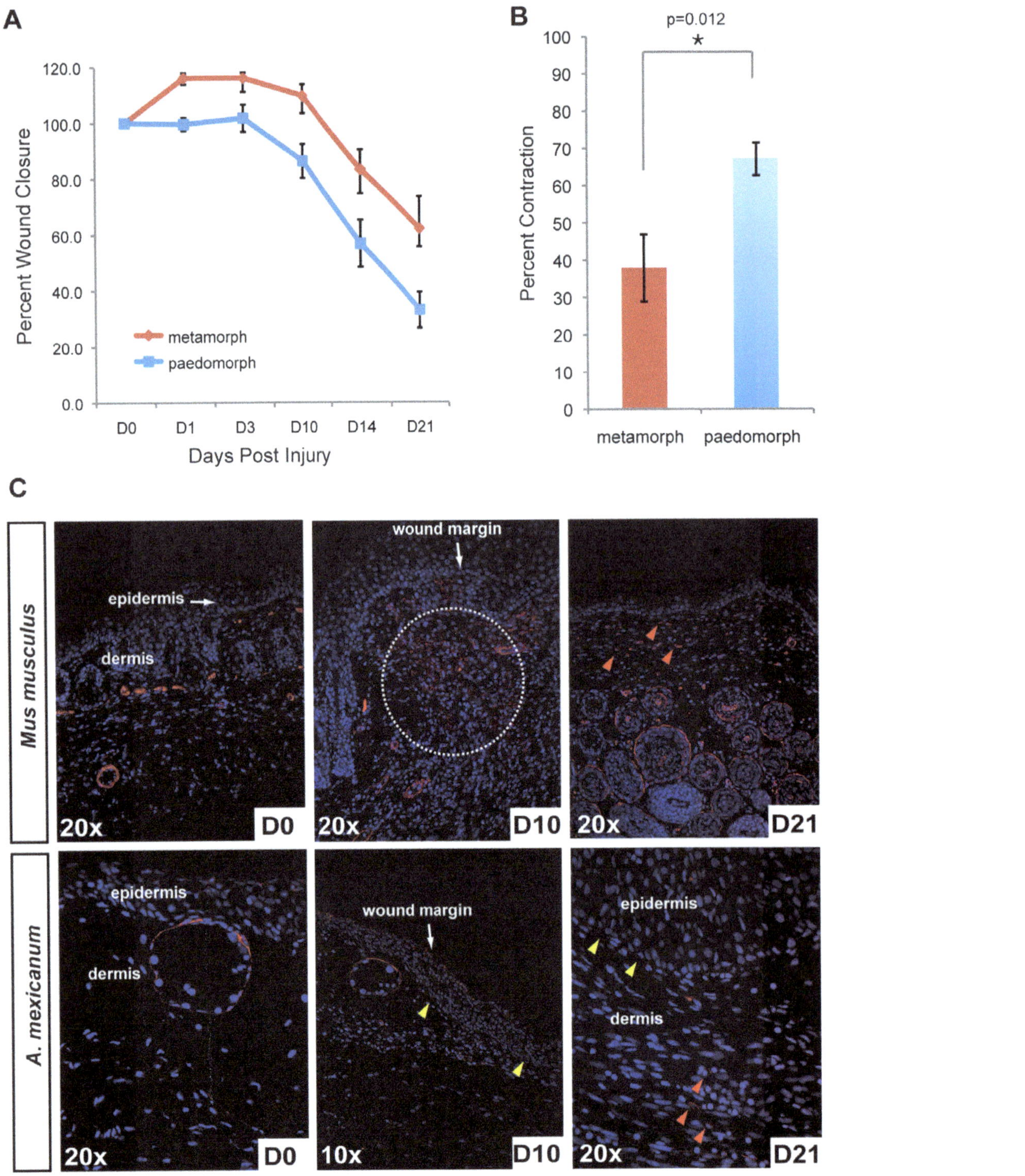

Figure 8. Contraction during scar-free healing in axolotls is similar to tight-skinned mammals. A) Percent wound closure in paedomorphs and metamorphs over 21 days (when contraction is complete). Metamorph wounds expanded by 10% following wounding and wounds contracted at about the same rate in both morphs. B) Paedomorph wounds contracted ~27% more than metamorph wounds with contraction accounting for 37.9% of wound closure in metamorphs. C) Alpha-smooth muscle actin (alpha-SMA) localization in unwounded skin and during wound repair in *Mus musculus* and axolotls (*A. mexicanum*) to identify myofibroblasts. Alpha-SMA localized to blood vessels and a few cells in mouse skin and around glands and the stratum compactum in axolotl skin. Ten days post injury (dpi), when contraction rates are highest in mouse wounds, alpha-SMA positive cells are detected at high levels at the wound margins (white dotted circle). In contrast, we detected very few alpha-SMA positive cells ten days after wounding in axolotl tissue. We did, however, detect alpha-SMA in the regenerating basement membrane (yellow arrows). Twenty-one dpi we detected a high number of myofibroblasts in mouse tissue (red arrows). We detected a few myofibroblasts in axolotl tissue at D21 (red arrows) near the underlying muscle.

appeared positive for alpha-SMA (Figure 8C). We observed numerous alpha-SMA positive cells at D21 in mouse granulation tissue compared with relatively few in axolotl provisional matrix. Taken together, these data show that wound contraction in axolotls mimic wound contraction in human skin, although there are relatively few myofibroblasts present during axolotl skin regeneration.

Dermal regeneration is Characterized by High Levels of Tenascin-C

The process of dermal repair in mammals (which ultimately results in a scar) proceeds via production of a fibrin clot, (referred to as the provisional extracellular matrix), degradation and replacement of provisional matrix by granulation tissue, and remodeling of granulation tissue into a fibrotic scar [1]. Following re-epithelialization in paedomorphs (D1) and metamorphs (D3), the wound bed was rich in blood cells and plasma but no scab formed (Figure 2). Provisional matrix in mammals is rich in fibronectin and thrombospondin [1] and along with plasma we detected low levels of fibronectin at the wound margins and beneath the wound epidermis at D7 in both morphs (Figure 9A). In contrast, we were unable to detect appreciable collagen deposition at D7 using histochemical techniques (Figure 1 and Figure 3). During mammalian wound healing, deposition of granulation tissue matrix proceeds in the stereotypical sequence of fibronectin, collagen type III and collagen type I [42]. At D14 fibronectin was present in low concentrations in granulation tissue in both morphs (Figure 9A). Using picrosirius red to detect both collagen type III and collagen type I, we predominantly observed collagen type III beneath the epidermis at D14 (Figure 10). As collagen synthesis continued collagen type III was replaced with collagen type I and as new dermis became progressively acellular, the density and diameter of collagen type I fibers increased (Figure 10). Fibronectin remained detectable in granulation tissue (D21), albeit at very low levels (Figure 9A).

While high levels of fibronectin and collagen are present in granulation tissue and also fibrotic scar tissue, the appearance of tenascin-C (TN-C) during mammalian wound healing is normally restricted to the wound margins and thought to stimulate cell migration. Concomitant with these observations we found intense TN-C protein localization at the wound margins and beneath the epidermis at D7 (Figure 9B). However, as dermal regeneration proceeded, TN-C persisted in high amounts throughout the wound bed and within regenerating muscle (Figure 9B). This association was particularly striking in the underlying muscle where TN-C formed a sharp boundary between regenerating and undamaged muscle (Figure 9B). TN-C levels remained high until the dermis had regenerated (Figure 9B). Taken together these findings suggest that collagen synthesis during axolotl scar-free healing proceeds similarly to that which is observed during mammalian wound repair and low levels of fibronectin and persistent high levels of TN-C characterize the anti-scarring matrix.

Discussion

Although many salamanders are capable of complete appendage regeneration (e.g. limb, tail), a recurring question is whether wounds made on the body heal with a scar or instead, heal scar-free [32]. In this study we demonstrate complete and perfect regeneration of adult axolotl skin following full thickness excisional (FTE) wounding to the dorsal flank. Additionally, we tested the hypothesis that loss of larval skin characters in metamorphic axolotls results in scarring following FTE wounding. Instead, we find that metamorphic axolotls are capable of scar-free healing. To our knowledge, this is the first demonstration of perfect scar-free healing of non-limb FTE wounds in an aquatic or terrestrial adult vertebrate. Comparing skin regeneration in paedomorphic (aquatic) and metamorphic (terrestrial) axolotls, metamorphic axolotls exhibited slower re-epithelialization, increased numbers of leukocytes during the early inflammatory response, increased deposition of extracellular matrix (ECM) and an almost doubling in the time required for complete skin regeneration. Compared to mammalian wound repair, terrestrial axolotls exhibited a reduced hemostatic response, lower neutrophils levels, similar duration of inflammation, faster time to complete re-epithelialization, a delay in new transitional matrix production and differences in the relative composition of the new ECM (Figure 11). These data suggest that further exploration of FTE wounding in axolotls is an excellent model to investigate the cellular and molecular regulation of scar-free healing.

Hemostasis

Wound healing in mammals proceeds along a stereotypical timeline consisting of repair processes that overlap in time and space and these processes have generally been included within three general phases; inflammation, new tissue formation and tissue remodeling [1,6,43]. Wound healing begins immediately after injury through the extravasation of blood products and activation of the coagulation cascade. In mammals, subsequent hemostasis is achieved through formation of a thick clot formed from platelets and plasma derived fibrin. This clot acts as a temporary plug and as a reservoir of growth factors, while the fibrin matrix acts as a scaffold for infiltrating inflammatory cells. In aquatic axolotls, the hemostatic response appeared limited with a thin layer of coagulated plasma at the wound site that was mostly devoid of cells. Following re-epithelialization, the neoepidermis was in close proximity to the underlying muscle with little evidence of a persistent fibrin clot prior to new ECM production. The presence of a clot in terrestrial axolotls was more pronounced, but was still greatly reduced compared to mammals. Erythrocytes and plasma formed the majority of material above the fragmenting muscle and it was unclear to what extent fibrin contributed to the loosely aggregated clot matrix. Following re-epithelialization, some blood plasma, erythrocytes and leukocytes were observed above and within the fragmenting muscle fibers, but the extent of a clot remained minimal and the epidermis remained in close proximity to the underlying muscle. Taken together, these findings show that axolotls restore hemostasis quickly and without formation of an extensive fibrin clot.

During mammalian wound healing, platelets degranulate, initiate the coagulation cascade and provide a wealth of growth factors and chemokines (e.g. PDGF, TGFß, VEGF, EGF, and IGF) that activate mesenchymal cells and attract inflammatory cells to the wound site [7,44]. Although some evidence suggests that platelets are not required during wound healing in mammals [45], all of these molecules have been shown to play a role during wound repair [46]. The degranulating action of amphibian platelets (thrombocytes) during injury is poorly understood, as are the growth factors produced during hemostasis. Future studies investigating the relative complement of chemoattractants and mitogens present in the clot matrix during scar-free healing in axolotls will shed light on how this molecular cocktail might direct the early events of wound healing towards regeneration in lieu of scarring.

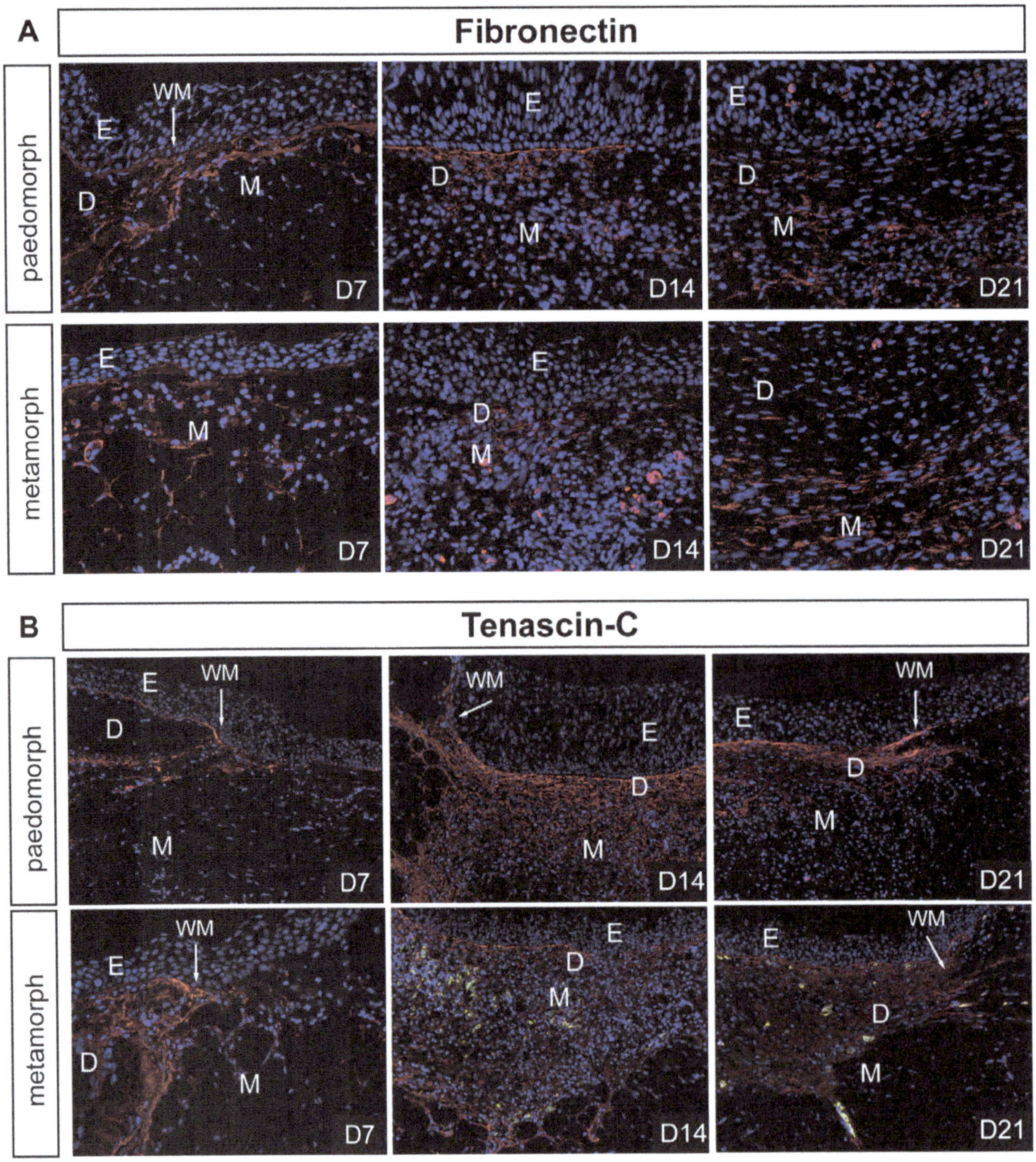

Figure 9. Regenerative ECM in axolotl wounds is characterized by high levels of tenascin-C. A-B) Fibronectin (FN) and tenascin-C (TN-C) levels were detected during scar-free healing in paedomorphs and metamorphs using an antibody to axolotl fibronectin and a polyclonal antibody to chick tenascin-C. We detected low levels of FN in the basement membrane at D7, and at the wound margins in both morphs. FN was present during ECM deposition at D14 in the center of the wound bed, but in relatively small amounts. By D21 little FN persisted in the regenerating dermis. B) TN-C was detected at the wound margins, in the basement membrane and surrounding some cells at D7. Fourteen days post injury we detected high levels of TN-C throughout the wound bed and in regenerating muscle. A sharp boundary formed between intact muscle and regenerating muscle. These high levels of TN-C persisted during dermis regeneration. Green fluorescence was used to detect autofluorescing erythrocytes. Epidermis (E), dermis (D), muscle (M), wound margin (WM).

Inflammation

Including hemostasis, the sequential influx and action of neutrophils, macrophages and lymphocytes constitutes the inflammatory phase of wound repair. In mammalian wounds, neutrophils are the predominant cell type present immediately after injury and are necessary to destroy bacteria and combat infection. The recruitment of neutrophils occurs passively (through plasma aggregation) and via chemotaxis in response to the activation of complement, degranulating platelets, and from bacterial degradation. Neutrophils in turn have the capacity to attract additional inflammatory cells and amplify the inflammatory response. Monocytes arrive at the wound site 2–3 days after injury and transform into macrophages. Macrophages serve to remove neutrophils and cellular debris, which helps to resolve inflamma-

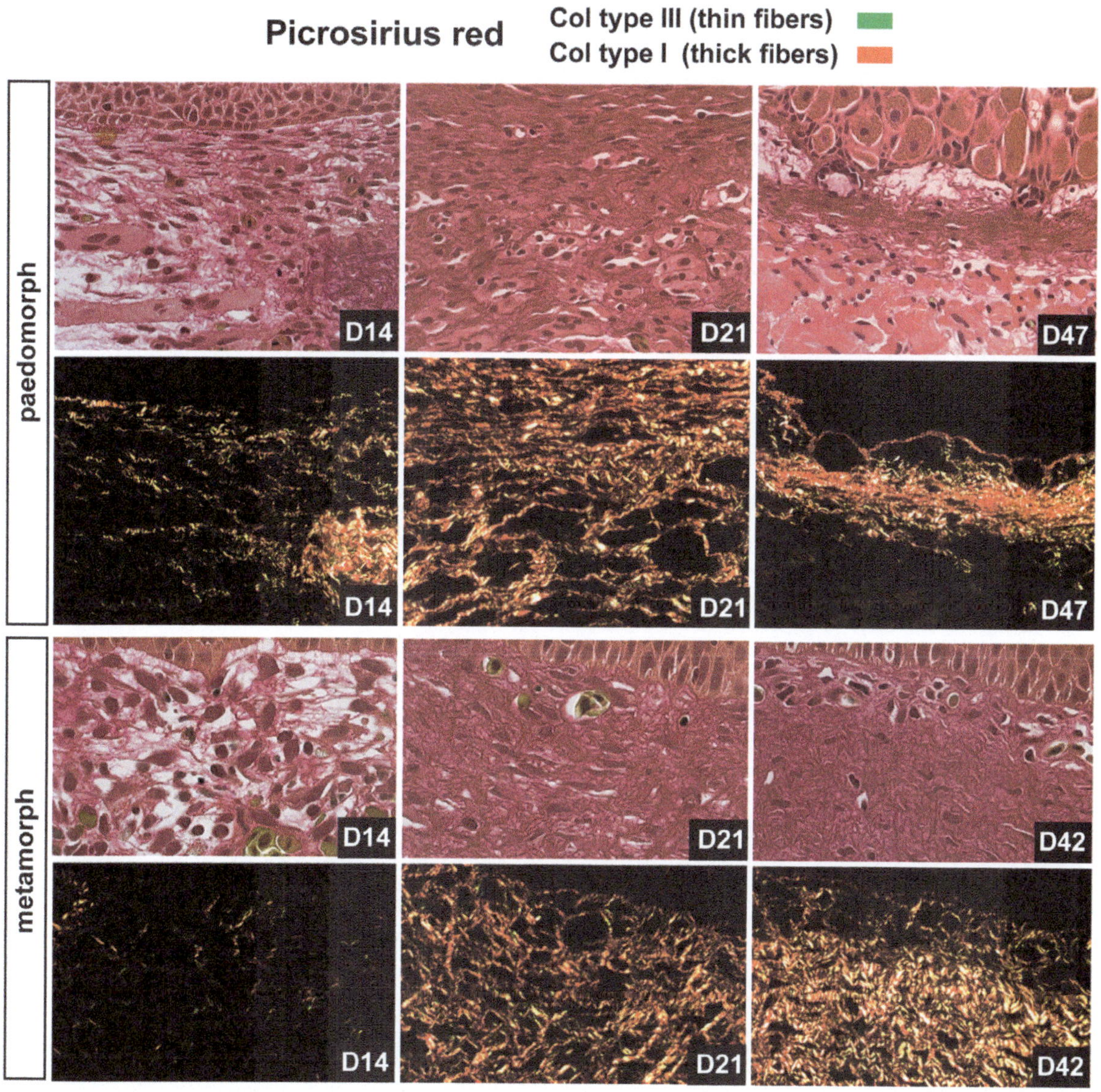

Figure 10. Collagen type III predominates early during new tissue formation and is slowly replaced by collagen type I during scar-free healing. Picrosirius red staining was used to detect collagen type III and collagen type I during scar-free healing in the wound bed. Using polarized light to detect bifringence, collagen type III (green fibers) was deposited first during new ECM deposition in both morphs. As the dermis regenerated, collagen type III was slowly replaced by collagen type I (red fibers) in both morphs.

tion, and also are thought to assist later during new tissue formation to regulate the balance between fibrosis and scarring [36]. Following FTE wounding in aquatic and terrestrial axolotls we detected neutrophils 24 hrs after injury. Neutrophil levels, however, were reduced compared to equal size FTE wounds in mammals suggesting a reduction through passive aggregation or chemotaxis [47]. Compared to mammals, which maintain ~60% of their circulating leukocytes as neutrophils, we found axolotls maintain approximately ~21% of their circulating leukocytes as neutrophils and this suggests that low neutrophil numbers at the wound site result partly from low numbers in circulation. In support of this finding, a recent study in larval axolotls found very few neutrophils in partial thickness tail wounds (which incur very little bleeding), while stab wounds made into the tail muscle, led to greater numbers at the wound site [26]. Neutrophil depletion studies in mammals have shown that as long as conditions remain sterile, neutrophils are not required during wound healing, and their loss may actually increase the rate of re-epithelialization [48,49]. Our findings show that their presence, albeit in low numbers, is compatible with scar-free healing and is coincident with a faster rate of re-epithelialization compared to mammalian wounds.

Although we did not examine additional individual leukocytic lineages, comparing L-plastin positive cells (a pan-leukocytic marker) in aquatic and terrestrial axolotls, we found higher total leukocyte numbers persisting in terrestrial animals while the wound bed remained exposed. Following re-epithelialization, total leukocyte numbers converged for both morphs suggesting that the early influx of inflammatory cells may not significantly influence the subsequent arrival of inflammatory cells. Together, our finding that total leukocyte levels remain high at least 14 days post injury

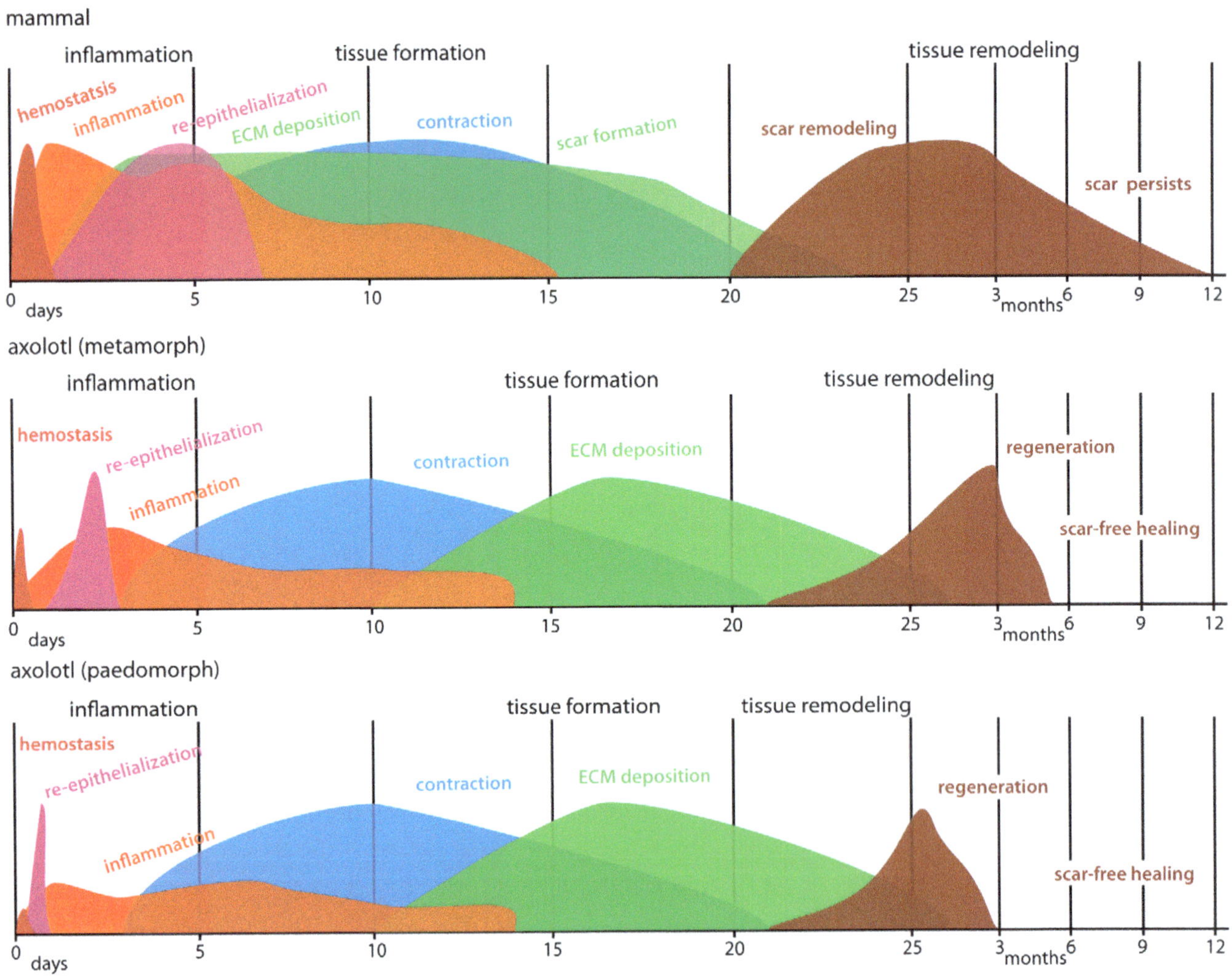

Figure 11. Summary of wound healing processes comparing axolotls and mammals. The x-axis represents time and the y-axis represents percent maximal response for each process. Information for mammals has been approximated from the literature and from our own experiments with 4mm FTE wounds in mice. Colors represent individual processes overlapping across the three phases of wound healing; inflammation, new tissue formation and tissue remodeling. Comparing paedomorphic and metamorphic axolotls, metamorphs exhibited an increased hemostatic response, slower re-epithelialization, increased early inflammatory response, increased and prolonged deposition of extracellular matrix (ECM) and an almost doubling in the time required for complete skin regeneration. Comparing scar-free healing in terrestrial axolotls to scar formation in mammals, terrestrial axolotls exhibited a reduced hemostatic response, lower neutrophil levels, faster re-epithelialization rate, delay in ECM production, differences in the relative composition of the new ECM, regeneration of glands and dermis regeneration instead of scarring. Schematic for mammals is adapted from Mikael Häggström.

supports the role of an active inflammatory phase during scar-free healing in axolotls.

The notion that reduced inflammation promotes regeneration in lieu of scarring has been popular, but evidence from mammals and amphibians remains inconclusive [50,51]. Aspects of limb regeneration in adult anurans, which lose the ability for limb regeneration following metamorphosis, can be stimulated through tissue aggravation [52] and chemical irritation [53], suggesting that prolonging tissue inflammation can prime a dormant regenerative response. On the other hand, scar-free healing in fetal mammals is correlated with reduced inflammation prior to their development of a mature immune system (compared to scarring in adults) [10,54]. Data from adult mammals suggests platelets [45], neutrophils [48] and macrophages [55] are dispensable for wound repair, but their removal does not lead to scar-free healing suggesting that reducing inflammation alone will not induce a regenerative response. The existing data from chronic and hypertrophic wounds support the hypothesis that too much inflammation promotes excessive fibrosis, and in the context of our results, it is likely that inflammation must not exceed a threshold level for scar-free healing to occur [7,56]. A recent study designed to increase inflammation in axolotls by injecting bleomycin following partial thickness tail wounds, found evidence of increased fibrosis following thirty days of administering the drug during the healing process [26]. While it is tempting to speculate that this exposure might lead to scarring, given the continuous exposure to bleomycin prior to tissue harvest it is difficult to interpret their results as they relate to heightened inflammation early during the healing process. Future experiments over-stimulating inflammation in our terrestrial FTE model of scar-free healing through chemical and molecular methods during the naturally occurring window of inflammation will allow us to examine the cellular and molecular mechanisms that connect inflammation and fibrosis. Our findings reinforce the idea that inflammation is not altogether anti-regenerative and support a role for an active inflammatory response during scar-free healing.

Re-epithelialization

As the inflammatory phase begins to wind down, keratinocytes at the wound-edge migrate to re-epithelialize the wound bed and restore the physical barrier separating the external environment. Concomitantly, granulation tissue (transitional matrix) is produced to replace the fibrin clot and together these processes will contribute to new tissue formation at the wound site. We found that adult paedomorphic axolotls completely re-epithelialized 4mm wounds 18–24 hrs post injury, while terrestrial axolotls exhibited slower re-epithelialization. In terrestrial axolotl skin, wound edge keratinocytes migrated after a delay period of ~24 hrs and complete re-epithelialization occurred up to 3 days after injury. This finding suggests that the transition from a pseudo-stratified to stratified epidermis following metamorphosis prevents rapid re-epithelialization in response to injury. Previous research in newt limbs suggested that epidermal keratinocytes are constitutively active and thus are primed to migrate following injury [24]. Our finding in paedomorphs supports this conclusion, while the observed delay in terrestrial axolotls demonstrates the need for keratinocyte activation as occurs in mammalian wound healing [57]. Interestingly, the onset of keratinocyte migration in mammals occurs after a delay period of 18–24 hrs [57,58], which is identical to what we observe in terrestrial axolotls. FTE wounds made in fetal rats that heal scar-free (E16), or result in scarring (E19), both re-epithelialize in 72hrs and together with our data in terrestrial axolotls, suggest that the speed of re-epithelialization cannot alone explain the ability to perfectly regenerate skin [13]. Our results suggest that rapid re-epithelialization reduces the time required to regenerate skin, and may contribute to reduced inflammation. Once activated, terrestrial axolotl keratinocytes appeared to migrate rapidly across the wound bed and it would be interesting to compare the rate of re-epithelial migration to similar sized mammalian wounds where moisture prevents scab formation. Comparing epidermal cells between these two morphs during wound healing will provide a powerful model to identify the molecular control of keratinocyte activation and will be useful in identifying new molecules that might stimulate keratinocyte migration in non-healing chronic wounds.

ECM Production and New Tissue Formation

While a dampened hemostatic response, reduced inflammation and quicker rate of re-epithelialization likely contributes to scar-free healing in axolotls (compared to scarring in adult mammals), the slow deposition of new extracellular matrix (ECM) and its unique molecular composition suggests newly synthesized axolotl ECM may antagonize fibrosis and promote regeneration (Figure 11). Shortly after re-epithelialization begins during mammalian wound repair, the provisional matrix, which is rich in cross-linked plasma fibronectin, is replaced by granulation tissue rich in macrophages, fibroblasts, newly synthesized ECM molecules and neovasculature [59]. Within this granulation tissue, fibroblasts secrete fibronectin, collagen type III and collagen type I, and this matrix will form the transitional ECM that will ultimately be remodeled into dermal scar tissue [1,60]. Although fibronectin and collagen are the most abundant ECM molecules in mammalian granulation tissue, tenascin-C is also deposited, first at the wound margins, then at the epidermal-dermal junction of migrating keratinocytes, and finally, within the granulation tissue itself [61]. During scar-free healing in terrestrial axolotls the wound bed at the epidermal-dermal junction contained little new ECM for 10 days after re-epithelialization. This delay period was striking in its duration and our finding that the neoepidermis was a potent source of several matrix metalloproteinases (MMPs) suggests an active inhibition of new ECM production. While we found strong and rapid upregulation of several *MMPs* (*MMP1, axCol, MMP3/10a,b, MMP19, MMP28, MMP9*) prior to, and during re-epithelialization, most of these returned near baseline levels following re-epithelialization supporting their role during keratinocyte migration [25]. However, *MMP3/10b* and *MMP9* persisted at relatively high levels in the neoepidermis, and *MMP2* levels began increasing after re-epithelialization. All three of the homologous mammalian proteinases can degrade fibronectin, and MMP3 and MMP2 are capable of degrading collagen type III and type I [62,63]. Together these data suggest that during scar-free healing in axolotls, persistently high MMP levels may act after re-epithelialization to prevent new ECM production as resident tissue undergoes histolysis and the wound bed is prepared for deposition of the regenerative matrix. Supporting this notion, broad inhibition of MMPs during newt limb regeneration can lead to acellular scar tissue formation and studies during scar-free healing in fetal wounds have observed higher MMP levels compared to adult wounds [13,34]. Ongoing studies in our laboratory are targeting these individual MMPs and their specific activities towards understanding how they regulate both re-epithelialization and the fibrotic response during scar-free healing.

The role of other proteinases such as the ADAMs and ADAMTSs during mammalian wound healing is poorly understood, while their role during fetal wound healing is completely unknown. Their ability to cleave membrane-bound domains of a host of different proteins (e.g. cytokines, growth factors, cytokine and growth factor receptors) thus releasing them into the extracellular space, has driven speculation that these factors may play an important role during wound healing, although direct studies are lacking [64]. Only ADAM9 and ADAMTS1 have been found to have a direct role during wound healing, with faster re-epithelialization occurring in mouse knockout studies of both individual genes [65,66]. During scar-free healing in axolotls we found a small but significant increase in *ADAM9* following injury but did not detect changes above baseline in any of the other *ADAM* or *ADAMTS* genes. Together, our findings suggest that ADAMs may not play a vital role during scar-free healing, although they are likely to work synergistically during keratinocyte migration.

Comparing our ECM data with that acquired from studies on scar-free healing in fetal mammals, both similarities and differences can be noted. Although there has been considerable controversy surrounding the production of collagens in fetal wounds, owing to the variety of species, wound models and fetal age, it is generally accepted that collagens are produced during fetal wound healing and are produced more rapidly compared to adult wounds [67,68]. While collagen fibrils are deposited in dense bundles parallel to the wound bed, fetal collagen fibrils appear to be deposited in a reticular fashion, almost identical to the surrounding dermis [68]. This contrasts with the situation during scar-free healing in axolotls where collagen deposition was delayed (as in adult mammals) and also occurred in dense bundles throughout the wound bed. Thus our data suggests that the pattern of collagen deposition observed during adult scarring is not technically incongruent with regeneration and may suggest the lack of later remodeling events or differences in the structural composition of the collagen deposited.

The appearance of new ECM during axolotl wound healing was coincident with fibroblast infiltration beginning at D14, and small amounts of fibronectin production. Similarly, fibronectin is recognized as a prominent component of the provisional matrix during adult and fetal wound healing, appearing early associated with the fibrin clot and then slowly disappearing concomitant with the deposition of collagen [60,68]. It is expressed earlier in fetal wounds compared to adult wounds and its disappearance is correlated with the onset of collagen deposition. It is also present at high levels in unwounded fetal skin compared to adults [69]. In contrast to mammalian wounds, axolotl transitional matrix was highly enriched with tenascin-C. Fibronectin appeared transiently with collagen type III in the wound bed while tenascin-C persisted through D42 as collagen type I was produced and the dermis regenerated. The role of tenascin-C during fetal wound healing has been poorly studied, although in the same study that examined fibronectin distribution during incisional healing in the lip [68] tenascin-C levels were found to be slightly higher in the fetal versus the adult. Some data suggests that tenascin-C can antagonize certain functions of fibronectin including T-cell activation [70] and in the context of fetal scar-free healing and axolotl scar-free healing suggests that the relative concentration of each in the extracellular matrix might act to regulate an adaptive immune response. Tenascin-C is thought to behave as an anti-adhesive molecule promoting proliferation and migration over differentiation and as such, is a transient molecule during mammalian wound healing [1]. Tenascin-C can disrupt cell-matrix interactions and has been speculated to maintain monocytes and blastemal cells in a de-differentiated state during salamander limb regeneration [23,71,72]. These data suggest that the composition of ECM produced during a regenerative response may have an anti-fibrotic effect that helps to recapitulate embryonic development and promote a regenerative response.

Remodeling and Regeneration

The evolutionary process that has led to wound repair while efficient, is not functionally perfect. Epidermal appendages do not regenerate and the uninjured dermal architecture is replaced by dense parallel bundles of collagen that reduce the mechanical properties of normal skin. While the wound bed ECM during mammalian wound repair will eventually result in a fibrotic scar, we observed complete regeneration of not only dermal layers but of epithelial derived glands. The regeneration of hair follicles has been observed in rabbit wounds and ear punches and in very large wounds made on young mice [73,74,75]. Other than these reports, the regeneration of epithelial-derived structures in adult vertebrates has not been observed. Although hair follicle and gland development is well understood in mammals, it is poorly understood at the molecular level in amphibians. Ongoing experiments in our laboratory examining the molecular control of gland development are underway and it will be interesting to determine how regeneration of these structures is controlled following scar-free healing [76]. Specifically, it will be of interest to determine the location of inductive signals that lead to the specification of new glands and whether these signals are localized or ubiquitous during the regenerative process.

Axolotl Model of Scar-free Healing

The data in this paper establishes a novel, adult model of perfect skin regeneration in which to test hypotheses about the molecular regulation of fibrosis and more generally, the underlying genetic control of scar-free healing. As such, we have developed an FTE wound model in both aquatic and terrestrial axolotls and characterized their ability to perfectly regenerate all damaged tissues. To date no *adult* animal model has been described that is capable of perfectly healing FTE wounds and underlying muscle (outside of the limb and tail). While numerous studies have described healing without scarring in fetal mammals and marsupials [10], the fetal model provides a number of drawbacks that the axolotl model overcomes. First, the fetus is still developing in the womb and this creates both biological and practical complications. The developing fetus, at the time when it heals scar-free, has an immature endocrine system, is immunoincompetent, is contained in a moist sterile environment, and its cells are in a state of chronic hypoxia [16]. In contrast to fetal models, terrestrial axolotls are fully developed, sexually mature, have a fully developed immune system (albeit not as sophisticated as adult mammals), and their FTE wounds are desiccating and open to infection. From a practical standpoint, "in utero" surgery is not required, up to six 4 mm FTE wounds can be made on the dorsal skin and pharmacologic drugs and chemicals can be easily delivered to antagonize or agonize signaling pathways. In combination with their ability to perfectly regenerate all tissues damaged in these wounds (e.g. epidermis, dermis, glands, nerves, muscle) this model shifts experimentation into a system where the ultimate clinical outcome actually occurs.

This new animal model will provide investigators a new paradigm in which to address the multiple processes of wound repair (e.g. hemostasis, inflammation, keratinocyte activation and migration, ECM formation, tissue remodeling) in a truly scar-free healing adult, while also providing a tractable genetic system to investigate the cellular and molecular mechanisms that regulate these processes. Given the considerable body of literature on the molecular pathways and cellular processes involved during normal wound repair, understanding how these conserved molecular players operate in a pro-regenerative environment will lead to development of new therapies that target downstream effectors for testing in established mammalian models.

Materials and Methods

Animals and Wound Model

Ethics Statement. All procedures were conducted in accordance with, and approved by, the University of Florida Institutional Animal Care and Use Committee (IACUC Study #201101534 and #200903505).

Animals. *Ambystoma mexicanum* (Mexican axolotl) were acquired from the Ambystoma Genetic Stock Center (AGSC, Lexington KY) and bred in captivity. Animals were housed individually in Aquatic Habitats® (Aquatic Habitats Inc., Apopka, FL) flow-through systems at 21–23°C in Holtfreter's Solution and maintained on California blackworms (*Lumbriculus sp.*, J.F. Enterprises, Oakdale, CA). Animals were deemed adults after reaching sexual maturity (>9 months) and measured between 12–15 cm total length. Metamorphic (terrestrial) axolotls were acquired either directly from AGSC or transformed at the University of Florida through treatment with thyroxine [77]. In both cases metamorphosis occurred after animals had reached sexual maturity. Terrestrial axolotls were housed individually in 10-liter containers containing moist paper towels and fed nightcrawlers. Mice used in this study were Swiss Webster (Charles River) approximately 6-months old.

Full thickness excisional (FTE) wounding. Adult axolotls were anesthetized by full submersion in Benzocaine (Sigma) 0.01% (aquatic) or 0.02% (terrestrial). Sterile 4mm biopsy punches were used to create FTE wounds through the skin into the dorsal back muscle. In this way, 6 wounds were created on the dorsal surface posterior to the forelimbs and anterior to the hindlimbs. In order to harvest wound tissue at specific time-points, animals were anesthetized as above and the entire wound was harvested using a

6mm biopsy punch and iridectomy scissors. FTE wounds in mice (through the panniculus carnosus) were made with 4mm biopsy punches through the dorsal skin posterior to the forelimbs and anterior to the hindlimbs.

Histology and Immunohistochemistry

For histological and immunohistochemical analysis, harvested tissues were fixed in 10% NBF at 4°C for 16–24hr, washed in PBS and dehydrated to 70% EtOH. Samples were stored at 4°C and processed for paraffin embedding. Samples were cut at 5μm. For frozen sections, samples were fixed for 1hr in 10%NBF at 4°C, washed in PBS, equilibrated in sucrose and OCT freezing medium and frozen in OCT. Frozen sections where cut at 12μm. For histological analysis, paraffin sections were stained with one of the following: Masson's Trichrome (Richard Allen Scientific) or Picrosirius Red (American Mastertech). For blood smears, blood was collected from limb amputations and air-dried on slides. Slides were stained with Sudan Black [78] to detect neutrophils and counterstained with a modified Wright-Giemsa Stain (Kodak).

Immunohistochemistry. Slides were rehydrated, antigen retrieval performed if necessary (see below for each antibody), washed in TBS, blocked for streptavidin and biotin (Vector Labs), and incubated with 1° antibody (see below) overnight at 4°C. The following day, slides were washed in TBS, incubated with biotinylated 2° antibody (Vector Labs) and subsequently incubated with streptavidin conjugated horseradish peroxidase antibody (Vector Labs) and visualized using DAB (3,3–diaminobenzidine) (Vector Labs) or incubated with a streptavidin conjugated Alexa-Flour 594 (Invitrogen). Images were captured on a Nikon Eclipse 6600 upright compound microscope using a Cool-Snap Pro true color camera (light microscopy) or an Olympus inverted microscope (IX81) with fluorescence using a Leica DFC310 FX (fluorescence microscopy).

Antibodies. For paraffin sections; Widespectrum Cytokeratin (DAKO; Z0622) 1:500, *Ambystoma* Fibronectin (gift of Thierry Darribere) 1:1000, Tenascin-C (Millipore, AB19013) 1:500, Collagen type IV (Rockland, 600-401-106-0.1) 1:450, alpha-smooth muscle actin (Abcam, ab5694) 1:100, Laminin (DAKO, Z0097) 1:500. For frozen sections; Myloperoxidase (Thermo, RB-373-A) 1:100, L-plastin (gift of Paul Martin) 1:2000. Antigen retrievals used were; microwave and Citrate Buffer (pH. 6.0) (Cytokeratin, Myloperoxidase, L-plastin, Tenascin-C, alpha-smooth muscle actin) or Proteinase-K treatment (DAKO) for 2 mins (Collagen type IV, Fibronectin, Laminin). Negative controls used isotyped IgG at the same concentration as the 1° antibody. A GFP filter was used to detect autofluorescence of erythrocytes.

Microarray Analysis

Epidermal tissue was harvested using a 4mm biopsy punch. Two wounds were made along the flank and posterior to the forelimbs. Harvested epidermis was pooled for each animal. Four biological replicates were collected from uninjured epidermis (D0) and at 1, 3, and 7 days post injury. RNA was isolated using Trizol Reagent (Invitrogen) followed by Qiagen RNeasy Clean-up columns (Qiagen). RNA quality was assessed on an Agilent 2100 Bioanalyzer (Agilent). RNA processing for Affymetrix microarray analysis was performed at the University of Kentucky Microarray Core Facility and hybridized to 32, AMBY_002a520748F 2nd Generation Axolotl Affymetrix microarrays (Affymetrix) [79]. Microarray data was tested for quality control and analyzed in the software system R using the Bioconductor package and oneChannelGUI [80,81,82]. Microarray data was preprocessed, and normalized using RMA and a linear model testing the effect of time for each morph type was fit for each gene across all 32 GeneChips using limma [83,84]. Thus, two gene lists were produced containing significantly changed genes over time in paedomorphic or metamorphic animals. In these analyses, contrasts were made between each time point and a t-statistic was produced for each contrast. The moderated F-statistic calculated by the eBayes limma function [85] was used as an overall test for significance across time, similar to ANOVA. A gene was considered statistically significant if it had an FDR adjusted p-value <0.05 and changed at least 2 fold between any two time points. The microarray data is MIAME compliant and the CEL files are available on Sal-Site (www.ambystoma.org). In addition, the raw data is available through the public NCBI GEO database (accession number: GSE35255).

Statistics

For quantification of inflammation we used a 2-way ANOVA to examine the effects of morph (metamorph versus paedomorph) and day post injury on total leukocyte numbers (with individual as a random effect to allow for repeated sampling). For all other statistical analyses we used a Student's T-test.

Supporting Information

Figure S1 Axolotl (paedomorph) skin glands. A) Granular gland. B) Mucous gland.

Figure S2 Detailed aspects of dermis and gland regeneration. A) High magnification image of a gland regenerating and descending from the epidermis 44 dpi. B) Detail of wound margin (WM) showing the edge of the injured stratum compactum which is normally densely compacted and the loose collagen fibers beginning to coalesce in the wound bed. C) Detail of wound bed 180 dpi showing mature mucous gland and regenerated stratum compactum. Hypodermis (H) and dermis (D). Scale bars = 100 μm.

Figure S3 Detailed aspects of metamorphic axolotl skin regeneration over 147 days. A) Granular and mucous glands (yellow arrows) present in the stratum spongiosum. Collagen fibers are present between the glands. B) Some cellular aggregations in the epidermis appear to be early stages of regenerating glands (yellow arrows). C) Regenerated glands within densely compacted collagenous ECM beneath the epidermis. D) Stratum compactum is beginning to coalesce as the rest of the dermis has regenerated. Some fibrotic tissue remains within the regenerated muscle. E) Complete scar-free skin regeneration at D147 dpi. All tissue layers are present. Granular glands remain immature compared to uninjured skin. Scale bars = 100 μm.

Figure S4 Visualizing the rate of re-epithelialization in paedomorphic axolotls using GFP transplanted skin. 1.5 cm×1.5 cm squares of dermis and epidermis from ubiquitously expressing GFP axolotls were transplanted to same size explanted areas on the tail of adult white axolotls. After transplants had healed 4mm FTE biopsy punches were made through the transplanted tissue and GFP-labeled epidermis was observed and photographed migrating to cover the wound bed over 18hrs. Migration was observed beginning 3hrs post injury and was complete between 18 and 24hrs.

Figure S5 *MMP* transcription and activity are correlated during tail regeneration in paedomorphs. A) Axolotl *MMP9* expression (semi-quantitative PCR) from tail tissue following amputation and through D14 post-amputation. Expression is downregulated 7 days post injury. B) Gelatin zymography was used to assess MMP activity over 21 days post injury. Red arrow points to tentatively assigned MMP9 position based on size (~85 kDa) from previously published work in newt and axolotl (Vinarasky et al. 2005, Santosh et al. 2011). C) Gelatinase activity lags behind transcriptional upregulation and peaks at D7. For quantification of activity, gel images were inverted, mean optical density of individual black bands were calculated on an Gel Logic gel imaging system (Kodak) and light was blocked to calculate a baseline (black) reference for each measurement. Standard errors are reported. Regenerating tail tissue and tissue 0.5mm rostral to the amputation plane was collected at 0hrs, 3hrs, 6hrs, 12hrs, 24hrs, 7 d, 14 d, and 21 d after injury (n = 3 per time point), snap frozen on dry ice, and stored at −80°C. Tissues were homogenized for 10 minutes on ice in 1:4 (w:v) homogenization solution [50 mol/L Tris-Cl (pH 7.6), 150 mol/L NaCl, 1% (v/v) Triton-X100, 10 mol/L EDTA, 1 mol/L PMSF], sonicated, set on ice for 10 minutes, and spun at 14 000×*g* for 10 minutes at 4°C. Supernatants were decanted off, quantified using a BCA protein assay kit (Pierce), and stored at −80°C. 25 µg total protein was diluted in zymogram sample buffer (Bio-Rad) and electrophoresed on Ready Gel zymogram polyacrylimide gels containing gelatin (Bio-Rad). MMP proteins were re-natured by washing gels in zymogram renaturation buffer (Bio-Rad) for 30 minutes and incubated for 16 hrs at 37°C in development buffer (Bio-Rad). Gels were stained with 0.5% (w/v) Coomassie Blue R-250 (Bio-Rad) for 30 minutes and de-stained with an acetic acid, methanol, and dH20 solution (1:5:4) until clear bands were visible.

Figure S6 Individual variation in leukocyte numbers during scar-free healing. A) Total leukocyte numbers based on L-plastin staining for paedomorphs and metamorphs (n = 4 for each morph). Because multiple wounds were made on the same animals the inflammatory response could be tracked per individual. B) One paedomorph exhibited an unusually high inflammatory response (paed 4) and we removed it from our analysis. C) Variation across metamorphs revealed no outliers. D) Control staining for myloperoxidase in axolotl liver section.

Table S1 Axolotl gene identifications based on first homologous human gene hit in BLAST. Expression values reflect absolute expression on genechip (max expression value = 30 k; expression values <100 = no expression). N = 4 animals per time point. D0P = day 0 paedomorph, etc. D0M = day 0 metamorph.

Table S2 Leukocyte profiles for *Ambystoma mexicanum* (paedomorph and metamorph). Numbers for each particular leukocyte type represented as a percentage of total leukocytes (thrombocytes were not counted).

Acknowledgments

We thank Sri Putta for help with bioinformatics, Marda Jorgenson for histological assistance and Ashley Stuart for animal care.

Author Contributions

Conceived and designed the experiments: AWS MM. Performed the experiments: AWS JRM MM. Analyzed the data: AWS JRM SRV MM. Wrote the paper: AWS. Commented and edited the manuscript: JRM SRV MM.

References

1. Clark RAF (1996) The molecular and cellular biology of wound repair. New York: Plenum Press. xxiii, 611 p., [611] leaf of plates p.
2. Bayat A, McGrouther DA, Ferguson MW (2003) Skin scarring. BMJ 326: 88–92.
3. Brown BC, McKenna SP, Siddhi K, McGrouther DA, Bayat A (2008) The hidden cost of skin scars: quality of life after skin scarring. J Plast Reconstr Aesthet Surg 61: 1049–1058.
4. Sund B (2000) New developments in wound care. London: PBJ Publications. pp 1–255.
5. Aarabi S, Longaker MT, Gurtner GC (2007) Hypertrophic scar formation following burns and trauma: new approaches to treatment. PLoS Med 4: e234.
6. Gurtner GC, Werner S, Barrandon Y, Longaker MT (2008) Wound repair and regeneration. Nature 453: 314–321.
7. Martin P, Leibovich SJ (2005) Inflammatory cells during wound repair: the good, the bad and the ugly. Trends Cell Biol 15: 599–607.
8. Schultz GS, Davidson JM, Kirsner RS, Bornstein P, Herman IM (2011) Dynamic reciprocity in the wound microenvironment. Wound Repair Regen 19: 134–148.
9. Namazi MR, Fallahzadeh MK, Schwartz RA (2011) Strategies for prevention of scars: what can we learn from fetal skin? Int J Dermatol 50: 85–93.
10. Adzick NS, Longaker MT (1992) Fetal wound healing. New York: Elsevier. xv, 341 p., [348] p. of plates p.
11. Armstrong JR, Ferguson MW (1995) Ontogeny of the skin and the transition from scar-free to scarring phenotype during wound healing in the pouch young of a marsupial, Monodelphis domestica. Dev Biol 169: 242–260.
12. Bullard KM, Longaker MT, Lorenz HP (2003) Fetal wound healing: current biology. World J Surg 27: 54–61.
13. Dang CM, Beanes SR, Lee H, Zhang X, Soo C, et al. (2003) Scarless fetal wounds are associated with an increased matrix metalloproteinase-to-tissue-derived inhibitor of metalloproteinase ratio. Plast Reconstr Surg 111: 2273–2285.
14. Lin RY, Sullivan KM, Argenta PA, Meuli M, Lorenz HP, et al. (1995) Exogenous transforming growth factor-beta amplifies its own expression and induces scar formation in a model of human fetal skin repair. Ann Surg 222: 146–154.
15. Ferguson MWJ, Howarth GF (1991) Marsupial models of scarless fetal wound healing. In: Adzick NS, Longaker MT, eds. Fetal Wound Healing. 1st ed. Holland: Elsevier. pp 92–125.
16. Mast BA, Diegelmann RF, Krummel TM, Cohen IK (1992) Scarless wound healing in the mammalian fetus. Surg Gynecol Obstet 174: 441–451.
17. Metcalfe AD, Willis H, Beare A, Ferguson MW (2006) Characterizing regeneration in the vertebrate ear. J Anat 209: 439–446.
18. Goss RJ (1987) Why mammals don't regenerate -- or do they? News in the physiological sciences 2: 112–115.
19. Clark LD, Clark RK, Heber-Katz E (1998) A new murine model for mammalian wound repair and regeneration. Clin Immunol Immunopathol 88: 35–45.
20. Beare AH, Metcalfe AD, Ferguson MW (2006) Location of injury influences the mechanisms of both regeneration and repair within the MRL/MpJ mouse. J Anat 209: 547–559.
21. Colwell AS, Krummel TM, Kong W, Longaker MT, Lorenz HP (2006) Skin wounds in the MRL/MPJ mouse heal with scar. Wound Repair Regen 14: 81–90.
22. Wallace H (1981) Vertebrate Limb Regeneration: John Wiley and Sons.
23. Donaldson DJ, Mahan JT, Yang H, Crossin KL (1991) Tenascin localization in skin wounds of the adult newt Notophthalmus viridescens. Anat Rec 230: 451–459.
24. Donaldson DJ, Mahan JT, Yang H, Yamada KM (1995) Integrin and phosphotyrosine expression in normal and migrating newt keratinocytes. Anat Rec 241: 49–58.
25. Ferris DR, Satoh A, Mandefro B, Cummings GM, Gardiner DM, et al. (2010) Ex vivo generation of a functional and regenerative wound epithelium from axolotl (Ambystoma mexicanum) skin. Dev Growth Differ 52: 715–724.
26. Levesque M, Villiard E, Roy S (2010) Skin wound healing in axolotls: a scarless process. J Exp Zool B Mol Dev Evol 314: 684–697.
27. Neufeld DA, Day FA (1996) Perspective: a suggested role for basement membrane structures during newt limb regeneration. Anat Rec 246: 155–161.
28. Neufeld DA, Day FA, Settles HE (1996) Stabilizing role of the basement membrane and dermal fibers during newt limb regeneration. Anat Rec 245: 122–127.

29. Yannas IV, Colt J, Wai YC (1996) Wound contraction and scar synthesis during development of the amphibian Rana catesbeiana. Wound Repair Regen 4: 29–39.
30. Jarial MS (1989) Fine structure of the epidermal Leydig cells in the axolotl Ambystoma mexicanum in relation to their function. J Anat 167: 95–102.
31. Kelly DE (1966) Leydig Cell in Larval Amphibian Epidermis - Fine Structure and Function. Anatomical Record 154: 685–&.
32. Ferguson MW, O'Kane S (2004) Scar-free healing: from embryonic mechanisms to adult therapeutic intervention. Philos Trans R Soc Lond B Biol Sci 359: 839–850.
33. Hasegawa H, Naito I, Nakano K, Momota R, Nishida K, et al. (2007) The distributions of type IV collagen alpha chains in basement membranes of human epidermis and skin appendages. Arch Histol Cytol 70: 255–265.
34. Vinarsky V, Atkinson DL, Stevenson TJ, Keating MT, Odelberg SJ (2005) Normal newt limb regeneration requires matrix metalloproteinase function. Dev Biol 279: 86–98.
35. Santosh N, Windsor LJ, Mahmoudi BS, Li B, Zhang W, et al. (2011) Matrix metalloproteinase expression during blastema formation in regeneration-competent versus regeneration-deficient amphibian limbs. Dev Dyn 240: 1127–1141.
36. Stramer BM, Mori R, Martin P (2007) The inflammation-fibrosis link? A Jekyll and Hyde role for blood cells during wound repair. J Invest Dermatol 127: 1009–1017.
37. Mescher AL, Neff AW (2005) Regenerative capacity and the developing immune system. Adv Biochem Eng Biotechnol 93: 39–66.
38. Davis AK, Maney DL, Maerz JC (2008) The use of leukocyte profiles to measure stress in vertebrates: a review for ecologists. Functional Ecology 22: 760–772.
39. Yannas IV (2001) Tissue and Organ Regeneration in Adults: Springer.
40. Grinnell F (1994) Fibroblasts, myofibroblasts, and wound contraction. J Cell Biol 124: 401–404.
41. Gross J, Farinelli W, Sadow P, Anderson R, Bruns R (1995) On the mechanism of skin wound "contraction": a granulation tissue "knockout" with a normal phenotype. Proc Natl Acad Sci U S A 92: 5982–5986.
42. Kurkinen M, Vaheri A, Roberts PJ, Stenman S (1980) Sequential appearance of fibronectin and collagen in experimental granulation tissue. Lab Invest 43: 47–51.
43. Martin P (1997) Wound healing--aiming for perfect skin regeneration. Science 276: 75–81.
44. Eppley BL, Woodell JE, Higgins J (2004) Platelet quantification and growth factor analysis from platelet-rich plasma: implications for wound healing. Plast Reconstr Surg 114: 1502–1508.
45. Szpaderska AM, Egozi EI, Gamelli RL, DiPietro LA (2003) The effect of thrombocytopenia on dermal wound healing. J Invest Dermatol 120: 1130–1137.
46. Schultz GS, Wysocki A (2009) Interactions between extracellular matrix and growth factors in wound healing. Wound Repair Regen 17: 153–162.
47. Mori R, Shaw TJ, Martin P (2008) Molecular mechanisms linking wound inflammation and fibrosis: knockdown of osteopontin leads to rapid repair and reduced scarring. J Exp Med 205: 43–51.
48. Dovi JV, He LK, DiPietro LA (2003) Accelerated wound closure in neutrophil-depleted mice. J Leukoc Biol 73: 448–455.
49. Simpson DM, Ross R (1972) The neutrophilic leukocyte in wound repair a study with antineutrophil serum. J Clin Invest 51: 2009–2023.
50. Godwin JW, Brockes JP (2006) Regeneration, tissue injury and the immune response. J Anat 209: 423–432.
51. Mescher AL, Neff AW (2006) Limb regeneration in amphibians: immunological considerations. ScientificWorldJournal 6 Suppl 1: 1–11.
52. Polezhaev LV (1972) Organ Regeneration in Animals. Recovery of Organ Regeneration Ability in Animals. Springfield: Charles C. Thomas. 190 p.
53. Rose SM (1944) Methods of initiating limb regeneration in adult Anura. Journal of Experimental Zoology 95: 149–170.
54. Adzick NS, Harrison MR, Glick PL, Beckstead JH, Villa RL, et al. (1985) Comparison of fetal, newborn, and adult wound healing by histologic, enzyme-histochemical, and hydroxyproline determinations. J Pediatr Surg 20: 315–319.
55. Martin P, D'Souza D, Martin J, Grose R, Cooper L, et al. (2003) Wound healing in the PU.1 null mouse--tissue repair is not dependent on inflammatory cells. Curr Biol 13: 1122–1128.
56. Dovi JV, Szpaderska AM, DiPietro LA (2004) Neutrophil function in the healing wound: adding insult to injury? Thromb Haemost 92: 275–280.
57. Coulombe PA (1997) Towards a molecular definition of keratinocyte activation after acute injury to stratified epithelia. Biochem Biophys Res Commun 236: 231–238.
58. Grinnell F (1992) Wound repair, keratinocyte activation and integrin modulation. J Cell Sci 101(Pt 1): 1–5.
59. Grinnell F, Billingham RE, Burgess L (1981) Distribution of fibronectin during wound healing in vivo. J Invest Dermatol 76: 181–189.
60. Clark RA (1990) Fibronectin matrix deposition and fibronectin receptor expression in healing and normal skin. J Invest Dermatol 94: 128S–134S.
61. Mackie EJ, Halfter W, Liverani D (1988) Induction of tenascin in healing wounds. J Cell Biol 107: 2757–2767.
62. Okada Y, Morodomi T, Enghild JJ, Suzuki K, Yasui A, et al. (1990) Matrix metalloproteinase 2 from human rheumatoid synovial fibroblasts. Purification and activation of the precursor and enzymic properties. Eur J Biochem 194: 721–730.
63. Werb Z (1997) ECM and cell surface proteolysis: regulating cellular ecology. Cell 91: 439–442.
64. Toriseva M, Kähäri VM (2009) Proteinases in cutaneous wound healing. Cellular and Molecular Life Sciences 66: 203–224.
65. Annis DS, Murphy-Ullrich JE, Mosher DF (2006) Function-blocking antithrombospondin-1 monoclonal antibodies. J Thromb Haemost 4: 459–468.
66. Mauch C, Zamek J, Abety AN, Grimberg G, Fox JW, et al. (2010) Accelerated wound repair in ADAM-9 knockout animals. J Invest Dermatol 130: 2120–2130.
67. Frantz FW, Diegelmann RF, Mast BA, Cohen IK (1992) Biology of fetal wound healing: collagen biosynthesis during dermal repair. J Pediatr Surg 27: 945–948; discussion 949.
68. Whitby DJ, Ferguson MW (1991) The extracellular matrix of lip wounds in fetal, neonatal and adult mice. Development 112: 651–668.
69. Coolen NA, Schouten KC, Middelkoop E, Ulrich MM (2010) Comparison between human fetal and adult skin. Arch Dermatol Res 302: 47–55.
70. Hemesath TJ, Marton LS, Stefansson K (1994) Inhibition of T cell activation by the extracellular matrix protein tenascin. J Immunol 152: 5199–5207.
71. Calve S, Odelberg SJ, Simon HG (2010) A transitional extracellular matrix instructs cell behavior during muscle regeneration. Dev Biol 344: 259–271.
72. Onda H, Goldhamer DJ, Tassava RA (1990) An extracellular matrix molecule of newt and axolotl regenerating limb blastemas and embryonic limb buds: immunological relationship of MT1 antigen with tenascin. Development 108: 657–668.
73. Billingham RE, Russell PS (1956) Incomplete wound contracture and the phenomenon of hair neogenesis in rabbits' skin. Nature 177: 791–792.
74. Breedis C (1954) Regeneration of hair follicles and sebaceous glands from the epithelium of scars in the rabbit. Cancer Res 14: 575–579.
75. Ito M, Yang Z, Andl T, Cui C, Kim N, et al. (2007) Wnt-dependent de novo hair follicle regeneration in adult mouse skin after wounding. Nature 447: 316–320.
76. Kumar A, Nevill G, Brockes JP, Forge A. A comparative study of gland cells implicated in the nerve dependence of salamander limb regeneration. J Anat 217: 16–25.
77. Page RB, Voss SR (2009) Induction of metamorphosis in axolotls (Ambystoma mexicanum). Cold Spring Harb Protoc 2009: pdb prot5268.
78. Sheehan HL, Storey GW (1947) An Improved Method of Staining Leucocyte Granules with Sudan Black-B. Journal of Pathology and Bacteriology 59: 336–&
79. Huggins P, Johnson CK, Schoergendorfer A, Putta S, Bathke AC, et al. Identification of differentially expressed thyroid hormone responsive genes from the brain of the Mexican Axolotl (Ambystoma mexicanum). Comp Biochem Physiol C Toxicol Pharmacol.
80. Gautier L, Cope L, Bolstad BM, Irizarry RA (2004) affy--analysis of Affymetrix GeneChip data at the probe level. Bioinformatics 20: 307–315.
81. Gentleman RC, Carey VJ, Bates DM, Bolstad B, Dettling M, et al. (2004) Bioconductor: open software development for computational biology and bioinformatics. Genome Biol 5: R80.
82. Sanges R, Cordero F, Calogero RA (2007) oneChannelGUI: a graphical interface to Bioconductor tools, designed for life scientists who are not familiar with R language. Bioinformatics 23: 3406–3408.
83. Irizarry RA, Hobbs B, Collin F, Beazer-Barclay YD, Antonellis KJ, et al. (2003) Exploration, normalization, and summaries of high density oligonucleotide array probe level data. Biostatistics 4: 249–264.
84. Smyth GK, Michaud J, Scott HS (2005) Use of within-array replicate spots for assessing differential expression in microarray experiments. Bioinformatics 21: 2067–2075.
85. Smyth GK (2004) Linear models and empirical bayes methods for assessing differential expression in microarray experiments. Stat Appl Genet Mol Biol 3: Article3.

15

Iontophoresis of Endothelin Receptor Antagonists in Rats and Men

Matthieu Roustit[1,2,3*], Sophie Blaise[2,3,4], Claire Arnaud[2,3], Marcin Hellmann[1,3], Claire Millet[1,2,3], Diane Godin-Ribuot[2,3], Boris Dufournet[1], Jean Boutonnat[3,5], Christophe Ribuot[2,3], Jean-Luc Cracowski[1,2,3]

1 Clinical Pharmacology Unit, Inserm CIC03, Grenoble University Hospital, Grenoble, France, **2** Laboratoire HP2 - U1042, Inserm, Grenoble, France, **3** Joseph Fourier University, Grenoble, France, **4** Vascular Medicine Department, Grenoble University Hospital, Grenoble, France, **5** TIMC UMRCNRS 5525, Grenoble, France

Abstract

Introduction: The treatment of scleroderma-related digital ulcers is challenging. The oral endothelin receptor antagonist (ERA) bosentan has been approved but it may induce liver toxicity. The objective of this study was to test whether ERAs bosentan and sitaxentan could be locally delivered using iontophoresis.

Methods: Cathodal and anodal iontophoresis of bosentan and sitaxentan were performed on anaesthetized rat hindquarters without and during endothelin-1 infusion. Skin blood flow was quantified using laser-Doppler imaging and cutaneous tolerability was assessed. Iontophoresis of sitaxentan (20 min, 20 or 100 μA) was subsequently performed on the forearm skin of healthy men (n = 5).

Results: In rats neither bosentan nor sitaxentan increased skin blood flux compared to NaCl. When simultaneously infusing endothelin-1, cathodal iontophoresis of sitaxentan increased skin blood flux compared to NaCl (AUC_{0-20} were 44032.2±12277 and 14957.5±23818.8 %BL.s, respectively; P = 0.01). In humans, sitaxentan did not significantly increase skin blood flux as compared to NaCl. Iontophoresis of ERAs was well tolerated both in animals and humans.

Conclusions: This study shows that cathodal iontophoresis of sitaxentan but not bosentan partially reverses endothelin-induced skin vasoconstriction in rats, suggesting that sitaxentan diffuses into the dermis. However, sitaxentan does not influence basal skin microvascular tone in rats or in humans.

Editor: Luis Eduardo M. Quintas, Universidade Federal do Rio de Janeiro, Brazil

Funding: This work was funded by the patients' association "Association des Sclérodermiques de France" and the "Groupe Français de Recherche sur la Sclérodermie". Actelion Pharmaceuticals and Pfizer Inc provided the drugs. The funders had no role in study design, data collection and analysis, decision to publish, or preparation of the manuscript.

Competing Interests: MR and JLC received unrestricted research grants from Pfizer, Actelion, and GlaxoSmithKline for other studies. JLC reports being a consultant for Actelion. Actelion Pharmaceuticals and Pfizer Inc provided the drugs for the present study. None of the sponsors have any involvement in the design and conduct of the present study; nor in the preparation, review, or approval of the present manuscript.

* E-mail: MRoustit@chu-grenoble.fr

Introduction

Systemic sclerosis (SSc) is a rare disease affecting digital microcirculation, leading to finger ulcers and in some cases to amputation [1]. Therapy of SSc-related ulcers is challenging. Bosentan, a non specific endothelin receptor antagonist (ERA), has been indicated to prevent digital ulcers in patients at risk, but it has no efficacy on existing ulcers [2]. Elevated aminotransferase levels is the main adverse effect of bosentan, with an annual rate of 10.1%, leading to therapy discontinuation in 3.2% of bosentan-naive patients [3]. Prostacyclin (PGI_2) analogues are used intravenously [4], but their therapeutic effect is counterbalanced by potentially serious vasodilatation-induced side effects (e.g. severe headaches, flushing, tachycardia and hypotension).

The topical administration of these drugs may be a way of avoiding the toxicity of systemic treatments. Iontophoresis is a simple, non-invasive transdermal drug delivery method using a low-intensity electric current [5]. Some authors have highlighted the potential interest of iontophoresis of vasodilating drugs as a treatment for digital ulcers in SSc [6,7] and previous work from our laboratory has suggested that PGI_2 analogues are appropriate candidates [8]. Iontophoresis of ERAs could also be interesting but, to our knowledge, it has never been tested either in animals or in humans.

We conducted a laboratory and a clinical study to address this question. The main objective of the animal study was to assess whether iontophoretically-administered ERAs, bosentan and sitaxentan, increase cutaneous blood flux in rats. As a secondary objective, we tested the toxicity of the iontophoresis of ERAs. In a second study, we tested the effect of the iontophoresis of sitaxentan on human skin blood flux as well as cutaneous and systemic tolerability.

Materials and Methods

1. Animal Study

Animals. Thirty-two male Wistar rats (eight-weeks old, 295–380 g; CERJ, Le Genest-St-Isle, France) were housed in controlled conditions conforming to the current French legislation and provided with standard rat chow. The protocol was approved by the Rhone Alpes Region Animal Ethics Committee (number 309). Rats were kept in a day/night cycle of 12 h/12 h with food and water at will. Preparation of the animals for iontophoresis has been previously described [8].

Drugs. Bosentan sodium salt (Actelion Pharmaceuticals, Allschwil, Switzerland) (MW 573.6 g.mol^{-1}) and sitaxentan sodium salt (Pfizer Inc, Groton, CT, USA) (MW 476.9 g.mol^{-1}) were used for iontophoresis, and isotonic sodium chloride (NaCl 0.9%) (Aguettant, Lyon, France) was used as a control. Solutions were prepared extemporaneously by diluting 20 mg of bosentan or sitaxentan in 3.6 mL and 4.4 mL of NaCl 0.9%, respectively, to obtain 10^{-2} M solutions. These solutions were subsequently diluted with NaCl 0.9% to obtain 10^{-3} and 10^{-4} M solutions. The pH of all solutions was determined before iontophoresis using a microprocessor-based pH meter (pH 210, Hanna Instruments, Woonsocket, RI, USA). The solutions were pH 5.5 to 6.5, which is suitable for epidermal application. Endothelin-1 (Sigma-Aldrich, Saint-Quentin Fallavier, France) (MW 2491.9 g.mol^{-1}) was diluted in water for injection to obtain 0.5 10^{-5} M, 0.5 10^{-6} M, 0.5 10^{-7} M, 0.5 10^{-8} M and 0.5 10^{-9} M solutions. In order to assess the concentration of endothelin needed to decrease skin blood flux, dose-response was assessed with 0.5 10^{-9} to 0.5 10^{-5} M solutions (n = 3). Only endothelin at 0.5 10^{-5} M decreased skin blood flux. This concentration was then used throughout the study.

Laboratory experimental procedures. The rats were anesthetized with sodium pentobarbital (50 mg.kg^{-1} i.p.) and were maintained in the prone position for the duration of the whole experiment, with the back uppermost. Experiments were performed in a temperature controlled room, and the rats were placed on a thermal pad, the temperature being maintained at 37.5°C (Harvard apparatus).

Experiment 1: Iontophoresis of bosentan, sitaxentan and NaCl (20 min, 100 µA) were simultaneously performed in the same animal using cathodal or anodal current (n = 9 for each series). Mean arterial blood pressure was measured by plethysmography using the tail cuff method, before and immediately after iontophoresis. Before iontophoresis each rat was inspected to ensure that the hairless skin in the back and the hind legs was intact. Photographs were taken before iontophoresis, immediately after and 3 days later. A cutaneous score was used to assess skin tolerability, based on the International Contact Dermatitis Research Group scoring [9]. Negative reactions were coded grade 0; weak reactions (grade 1) are characterized by non-vesicular erythema. Strong positive reactions (grade 2) are characterized by erythema associated with vesicles. Extreme positive reactions (grade 3) are bullous reactions. Irritant reactions (that we coded grade 4) are characterized by necrosis.

Experiment 2: Catheters were inserted in both carotid arteries. Arterial pressure (Powerlab, ADInstrument) was recorded through the first catheter and endothelin (5 nmol.kg^{-1} i.a. bolus followed by 0.5 µL.min^{-1} infusion) was administered through the second catheter. We chose i.a. rather than i.v. endothelin infusion due to its removal in the pulmonary circulation [10]. Moreover, prolonged endothelin infusion was not possible through the catheter used to record arterial pressure. This invasive procedure led to significant hemodynamic instability in four animals in which iontophoresis was not performed. Iontophoresis of bosentan, sitaxentan and NaCl (20 min, 100 µA) were then simultaneously performed in the same animal using cathodal (n = 8) or anodal (n = 6) currents. Histopathologic examination of full-thickness skin biopsies from bosentan, sitaxentan, NaCl treated areas and from one non-treated skin area was realized 15 min after the end of iontophoresis (n = 9:5 after cathodal and 4 after anodal iontophoresis). The thirty-six biopsies were fixed in AFA fluid (5% acetic acid, 75% absolute ethyl alcohol, and 18% water; Carlo Erba) paraffin-embedded and stained with hematoxylin, eosin, and safran. In order to evaluate the effect of the treatment on the skin, various features were sought in the different skin layers [the histopathologic examination procedure has been previously described [8]].

Skin blood flux measurement and data analysis. Three 1.2 cm^2 circular iontophoresis electrodes (PeriIont System, Perimed, Järfälla, Sweden) containing bosentan, sitaxentan or NaCl were placed on the hairless skin of the lower back/hind legs. Passive electrodes were placed on the back of the neck, as previously described [8]. Skin blood flux was continuously recorded with laser Doppler imaging (LDI; PeriScan PIM 3, Perimed, Järfälla, Sweden). The laser head was placed 20 cm above the skin. The resolution was 2 mm step length and LDI scans were taken every minute.

In experiment 1, iontophoresis was started after a 5-min baseline (BL) recording. Skin blood flux was then recorded during iontophoresis and during the 20 min following the end of iontophoresis, and expressed as arbitrary perfusion units (PU). In order to take into account inter-individual BL variations, data were subsequently expressed as a percentage change from BL (%BL). Then, a minute by minute analysis was performed to calculate the area under the curve during iontophoresis (AUC_{0-20}, in %BL.s) and during the whole recording (AUC_{0-40}).

In experiment 2, the skin blood flux was recorded for 5-min under resting conditions. Iontophoresis was performed 5 min after endothelin infusion started, time for blood flux to decrease and reach a plateau (baseline). Data were expressed as percentage change between baseline and the iontophoresis plateau (averaged over 10 min) (expressed as %BL). Then, $AUC_{PU\ 0-20}$ was calculated as described above and expressed as %BL.s. In order to take into account endothelin-induced variations in blood pressure, we expressed data as cutaneous vascular conductance (CVC), i.e. flux divided by arterial pressure averaged over 1 min (in mV.mm Hg^{-1}) [11,12], to subsequently calculate $AUC_{CVC\ 0-20}$ (expressed as %BL.s).

2. Clinical Study

Study population. We recruited healthy men through the Clinical Research Centre database. Inclusion criteria were an age of 18–65 years with no significant medical history. Non-inclusion criteria included any allergies to local anaesthetics, cigarette smoking or dermatologic disease on the arm or forearm. Any abnormal liver enzyme level was also an exclusion criterion. Grenoble Institutional Review Board (IRB n°6705) approval was obtained in September 2009 and each volunteer gave written informed consent before participation.

Study design. This was an open-label pharmacology study. Upon arrival at the centre volunteers were placed in a temperature-controlled room (23+/−1°C) during 1 hour for acclimatization. They remained supine for the whole experiment.

Three consecutive visits were planned for each volunteer, separated by 7 days +/− 3. Visit 1 was the initial enrolment visit. During visit 2, iontophoresis of sitaxentan 10^{-2} M and NaCl 0.9% were performed. Volunteers arrived fasted for at least 6 hours and

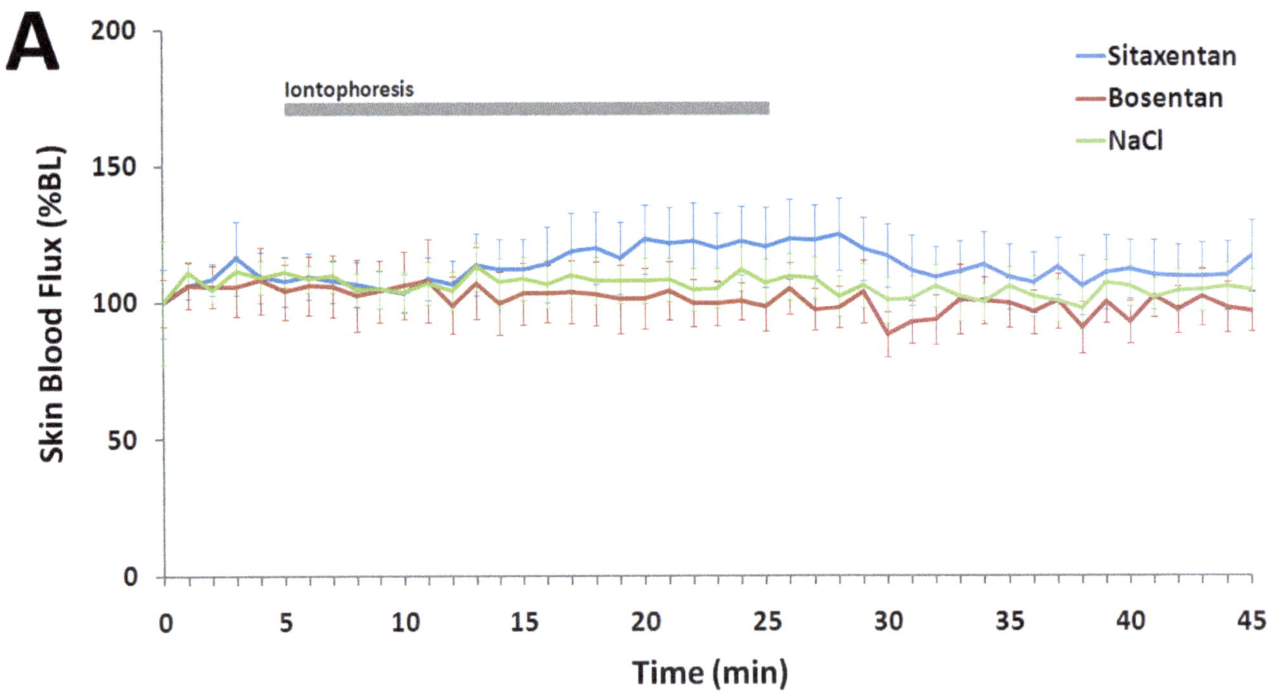

Figure 1. Effect of iontophoresis of bosentan 10^{-2} M, sitaxentan 10^{-2} M and NaCl 0.9 % on skin blood flux in rats, expressed as mean (± SEM) percentage change from baseline (%BL), in the cathodal direction (Fig. 1A) and the anodal direction (Fig. 2B).

were allowed to eat only after the end of the experiment. Visit 3 was a safety monitoring clinical visit. Skin photographs were taken before the start of iontophoresis and immediately after iontophoresis (visit 2), and 7 days later (visit 3). Liver enzyme levels were assessed at visits 1 and 3.

Iontophoresis protocol and skin blood flux measurement. Four iontophoresis skin sites were randomly chosen on the ventral side of the right forearm, more than 5 cm from the elbow and the prominence of the wrist, avoiding visible veins. Two of them were pre-treated with 1 g of lidocaine/prilocaine cream (5 g tubes containing 125 mg lidocaine and 125 mg prilocaine, Anesderm®, Pierre Fabre, Boulogne, France) in order to attenuate axon reflex-induced hyperaemia [13]. An occlusive transparent dressing was placed over the cream to

Table 1. Effect of cathodal and anodal iontophoresis of bosentan and sitaxentan on skin blood flux recorded on the back and the hind legs of rats.

Polarity		NaCl	Bosentan	P-value*	Sitaxentan	P-value*
Cathodal (n = 9)	AUC_{0-20}	9598±23693	5061±39161	0.44	13553±33368	0.86
	AUC_{0-40}	15142±48007	2717±64048	0.44	32534±74077	0.51
Anodal (n = 9)	AUC_{0-20}	15123±26678	1090±40367	0.24	20851±39909	0.80
	AUC_{0-40}	32436±55790	4215±71472	0.11	20286±64462	0.51

Data are expressed as area under the curve of the percentage change from baseline (expressed as %BL.s) during the 20-min iontophoresis (AUC_{0-20}) and during the whole recording (AUC_{0-40}).
*vs NaCl (Wilcoxon rank test).

enhance cutaneous diffusion. Each anesthetized area was larger than the area of the iontophoresis chambers.

One hour after lidocaine/prilocaine application (corresponding to the acclimatization period) the cream was removed with a cotton swab. The two pre-treated skin sites were then equipped with 1.2 cm^2 circular iontophoresis chambers (PeriIont System, Perimed, Järfälla, Sweden) containing sitaxentan or NaCl. After a 5-min baseline recording, cathodal iontophoresis was simultaneously performed for 20 minutes with a current intensity set at 20 µA. After iontophoresis, skin blood flux was recorded for an additional 20 min. During the experiment, the two remaining skin sites were pre-treated with local anaesthetic cream for one hour. The same protocol as described above was then performed on these skin sites, the only difference being the current intensity set at 100 µA.

Skin blood flux was recorded throughout with laser-Doppler imaging (PeriScan PIM 3, Perimed, Järfälla, Sweden). The resolution was 1 mm step length and LDI scans were taken every 30 seconds. Before recording, the arm was immobilized with a vacuum cushion to decrease artefacts related to arm movement. Baseline and maximal skin blood flux were averaged over 5 min. Data were subsequently expressed as a percentage change from BL (%BL) and AUC_{0-40} were calculated (expressed as %BL.s).

3. Statistical Analysis

Categorical data were reported as frequency and percentage and continuous data as mean and standard deviation. Two-sided nonparametric tests were used throughout (Friedman test, and Wilcoxon test for paired comparisons). We considered p values <0.05 as significant, corrected by Bonferroni's method for multiple comparisons. Statistical analysis was performed with SPSS 13.0 for Windows (SPSS Inc, Chicago IL, USA).

Results

1. Animal Study

Effect of iontophoresis of bosentan and sitaxentan on skin blood flux. Neither cathodal nor anodal iontophoresis of bosentan 10^{-2} M or sitaxentan 10^{-2} M induced any significant change in skin blood flux compared to NaCl (Table 1; Figure 1). Iontophoresis did not significantly affect blood pressure (87.5±17.9 mmHg before and 90.6±10.2 mmHg after iontophoresis; P = 0.7). Similarly, we observed no significant effect of bosentan or sitaxentan at 10^{-3} M or 10^{-4} M (data not shown for clarity).

Effect of cathodal and anodal iontophoresis of bosentan and sitaxentan after administration of endothelin. Resting skin blood flux before cathodal iontophoresis at bosentan, sitaxentan and NaCl skin areas were 91.5±25 PU, 116.7±48.8 PU and 102.2±32.1 PU, respectively (P = 0.2). Endothelin decreased skin blood flux to 57.8±17.4 PU, 65.1±31.6 PU and 59.4±17.7 PU, respectively (P = 0.7). We observed an initial transient decrease in blood pressure immediately after endothelin infusion was started, followed by a sustained increase (Figure 2). Cathodal iontophoresis of sitaxentan significantly increased skin blood flux compared to NaCl. However, we observed no significant difference between bosentan and NaCl (Table 2; Figure 3A).

Resting skin blood flux before anodal iontophoresis for bosentan, sitaxentan and NaCl skin areas were 88.3±16.1 PU, 106.9±39.1 PU and 98.1±21.7 PU, respectively (P = 0.3). Endothelin infusion decreased skin blood flux to 59.7±33.8 PU, 55.1±26.5 PU and 47.5±18.8 PU, respectively (P = 0.5). Anodal iontophoresis of bosentan or sitaxentan did not significantly increase skin blood flux compared to NaCl (Table 2; Figure 3B).

Skin tolerability of the iontophoresis of bosentan and sitaxentan. No skin side-effects were observed. In experiment 1, all the cutaneous scores were 0 both immediately after the procedure and at day 3. In experiment 2, no abnormal histopathologic features (e.g. perivascular inflammatory infiltration in the papillary dermis; dissociation of keratinocytes due to epidermal edema; migration of inflammatory cells from the dermis to the epidermis) were found in any of the skin biopsies.

2. Clinical Study

Study population. Six male volunteers were enrolled in the study. One of them did not attend visits 2 and 3 and was excluded. The characteristics of the population were: mean age 22.8±1.9 years and body mass index 22.1±1.5 kg/m^2. Mean systolic/diastolic arterial pressure at inclusion was 115±7.4 / 77±10.9 mm Hg.

Effect of cathodal iontophoresis of sitaxentan on skin blood flux. Neither sitaxentan nor NaCl increased skin blood flux when the iontophoresis current intensity was 20 µA (AUC_{0-40} were −2785±35811 %BL.s and −3315±42523 %BL.s, respectively; P = 0.69). Cathodal iontophoresis of sitaxentan induced an inconsistant increase in skin blood flux when the current intensity was set at 100 µA (AUC_{0-40} was 289409±348171 %BL.s). However, a similar increase was observed with NaCl (AUC_{0-40} was 236430±348333 %BL.s; P = 0.22). Individual tracings show the high heterogeneity in the response to iontophoresis (Figure 4).

Tolerability. No side-effect occurred. We observed no significant change in mean arterial pressure during iontophoresis of sitaxentan. No squamous, vesicular or bullous lesions were observed at the end of the experiment or at the safety visit. Erythema was observed in one participant. It was localized to the area surrounding the anesthetized area and was attributed to

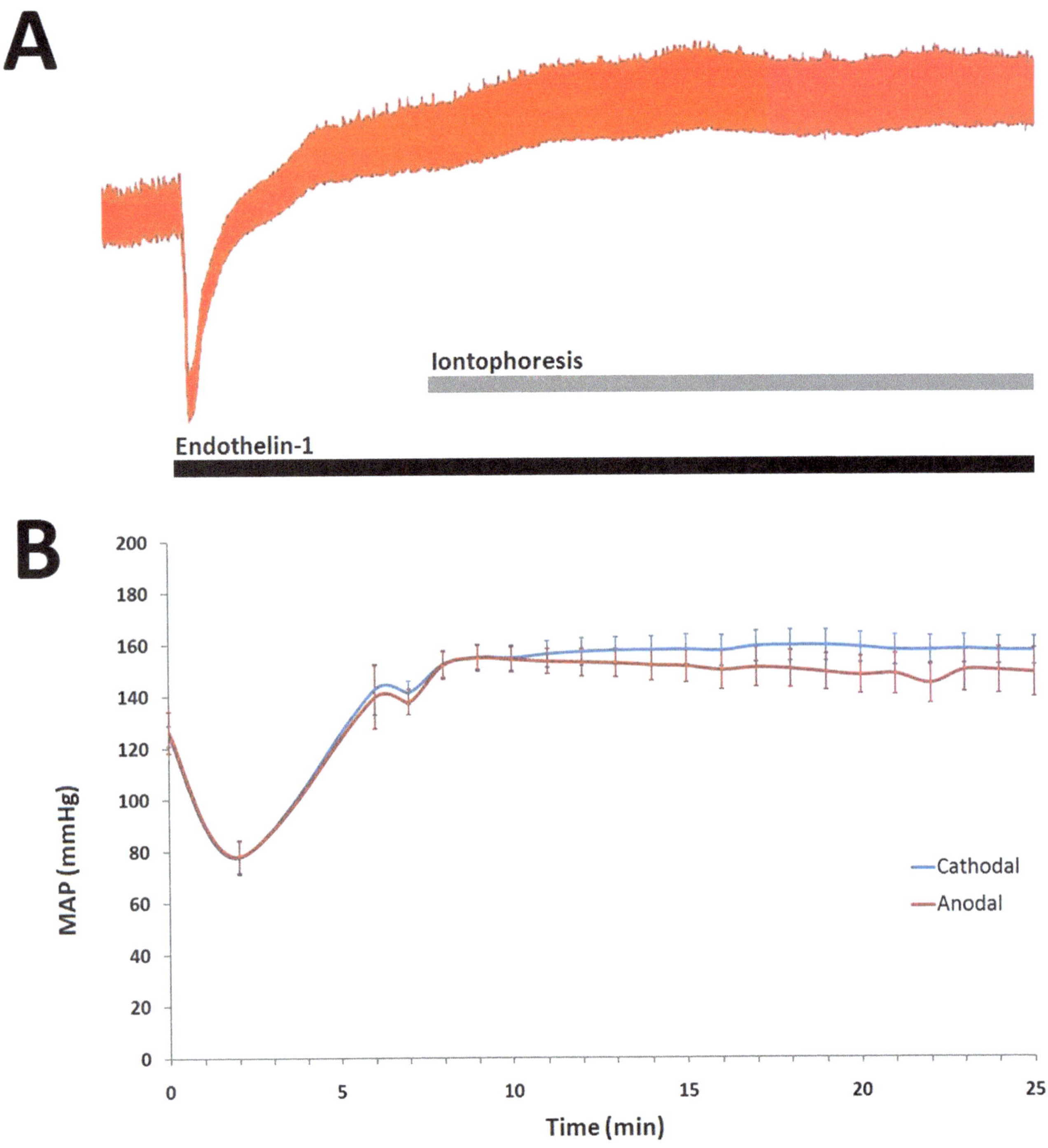

Figure 2. Typical tracing of the effect of i.a. endothelin 0.5 10^{-5} M on arterial pressure in rats: the initial transient decrease of arterial pressure is followed by a sustained increase (Fig 2A). Mean (± SEM) arterial pressure during i.a. endothelin perfusion and iontophoresis of bosentan or sitaxentan in the cathodal (blue line) and anodal (red line) directions in rats (Fig. 2B).

hypersensitivity to the adhesive of the dressing. Aspartate transaminase (AST)/alanine transaminase (ALT) at visit 1 and visit 3 for each volunteer were: 34/17 and 36/14 UI.L^{-1}, 18/27 and 21/21 UI.L^{-1}; 16/15 and 20/12 UI.L^{-1}; 30/25 and 31/25 UI.L^{-1}; 30/18 and 26/29 UI.L^{-1}.

Discussion

This study showed that in basal conditions iontophoresis of bosentan (in rats) or sitaxentan (in rats and humans) did not increase skin blood flux. However, after endothelin infusion, iontophoresis of sitaxentan significantly increased cutaneous blood flux in rats, suggesting that the absence of effect initially observed was due to low endothelin-dependent basal skin microvascular

Table 2. Effect of cathodal and anodal iontophoresis of bosentan and sitaxentan on skin blood flux recorded on the back and the hind legs of rats during endothelin infusion.

		NaCl	Bosentan	P-value*	Sitaxentan	P-value*
Cathodal (n = 8)	%BL	8.21±20	19.3±23.1	0.4	34.3±15.5	0.02
	$AUC_{PU\ 0-20}$	14957±23818	27569±25533	0.26	44032±12277	0.01
	$AUC_{CVC\ 0-20}$	3687±26073	12370±24147	0.33	27835±18050	0.01
Anodal (n = 6)	%BL	18.7±24.4	21.4±26.2	0.75	26.4±24.2	0.92
	$AUC_{PU\ 0-20}$	29513±34899	31898±30426	0.92	24747±28687	0.6
	$AUC_{CVC\ 0-20}$	19792±37485	19063±16564	0.75	13405±34335	0.75

Data are expressed as percentage change between baseline and iontophoresis plateau (%BL), and as the area under the curve (AUC_{0-20}) of the percentage change from baseline (expressed as %BL.s), whether calculated from arbitrary perfusion units (PU) or from cutaneous vascular conductance (CVC) in order to take into account variations in arterial blood pressure.
*vs NaCl (Wilcoxon rank test).
P-values <0.025 were considered as significant.

tone rather than the absence of diffusion of the antagonist into the skin. However, no effect was seen with bosentan. Iontophoresis of ERAs was well tolerated both in animals and humans.

Iontophoretic transport is influenced by several parameters, including drug concentration, molecular weight, ionization and solution pH or current strength and skin hydration and resistance [14]. Bosentan and sitaxentan are small molecules with isoelectric points (pI) at 2.64 and 4.57, respectively. These chemical properties make these ERAs appropriate candidates for cathodal iontophoresis, being negatively charged at neutral pH. However, in basal conditions, we were not able to see any effect of the iontophoresis of bosentan or sitaxentan on skin blood flux in rats (experiment 1). In order to test whether the absence of effect was related to low endothelin-dependent vascular tone in the skin of healthy rats or to the absence of iontophoretic transport into the dermis, we repeated the experiment while infusing endothelin (experiment 2). The results of this series suggest that the cathodal iontophoresis of sitaxentan enabled the drug to be locally administered in sufficient concentration to partially reverse the sustained effect of endothelin on the skin microcirculation. However, such an effect was not observed with bosentan, suggesting that we were unable to reach sufficient skin concentration to reverse endothelin vasoconstriction. It is of interest that we obtained similar results when data were expressed as cutaneous vascular conductance, to take into account the effect of endothelin on arterial blood pressure. The effect of endothelin on blood pressure was comparable to that previously described: an initial transient decrease in blood pressure immediately after endothelin infusion was started was followed by a prolonged increase [10].

The relationship between the pharmacodynamic effect of ERAs on microvascular function and their efficacy in the prevention of digital ulcers in patients at risk remains uncertain. Two groups have studied the effect of the systemic administration of bosentan on skin blood flux in patients with SSc [15,16]. Hettema *et al* did not show any difference in blood flux during acetylcholine and sodium nitroprusside iontophoresis, used as pharmacological tests of microvascular endothelium-dependent and endothelium-independent function, respectively [17]. Conversely, Rosato *et al* showed an increase in skin perfusion 8 weeks after bosentan therapy was started in SSc patients with SSc and pulmonary hypertension. In SSc patients without pulmonary hypertension however, there was no significant difference [15]. These discrepancies could be due to higher endothelin-dependent vascular tone in patients with pulmonary hypertension.

Insufficient diffusion of ERAs into the skin after oral administration is another hypothesis. Indeed, when administered directly into the dermis BQ-123 (an ET_A receptor antagonist) significantly increased skin blood flux in healthy volunteers [18]. Interestingly, intradermal BQ-788 (an ET_B receptor antagonist) also increased blood flow [18], suggesting that both ET_A and ET_B contribute to endothelin-mediated basal microvascular tone in the human skin. On the other hand, although both ET_A and ET_B mediate vasoconstriction in rat skin [19], injection of BQ-123 and bosentan (non specific ET_A and ET_B antagonist) did not alter basal skin blood flow in rats but reversed the effects of endothelin [20], which is consistent with our findings.

Therefore, iontophoresis probably did not allow sufficient concentrations of ERAs to be reached in human skin to be able to show any effect on the microvasculature. We did not use intradermal injections or microdialysis as these methods would be too far removed from the initial therapeutic objective, i.e. iontophoresis in physiological conditions.

In healthy participants, we did not observe any increase in skin blood flux for either sitaxentan or NaCl when the current intensity was 20 µA (as previously described [13]), whereas it was inconsistent at 100 µA. Indeed, one of the main issues when performing iontophoresis is the non specific effect of the current itself, often referred to as "current-induced vasodilation". The amplitude of this vasodilation depends on the delivered electrical charge (i.e. the product of current intensity by duration of application) [21], which may explain the discrepancy. As the neural axon reflex has been suggested to be involved in current-induced vasodilation [21], we pre-treated the skin sites with a local anaesthetic (lidocaine/prilocaine). However, this did not abolish current-induced vasodilation in all subjects when the current intensity was 100 µA, suggesting the involvement of pathways other than sensory nerve-dependent mechanisms.

In humans, individual data showed comparable skin blood flow for sitaxentan and NaCl in each participant (individual data not shown for clarity). The highly variability observed at 100 µA is due to major current-induced vasodilation in two participants (at all sites), whereas in the three other subjects we only observed a weak or even no effect at all. This difference could be due to inter-individual differences in skin resistance, which was not recorded at this early stage. Nonetheless, it is unlikely to have a major impact on the conclusion of these experiments as each subject was his own control. Indeed, the iontophoresis were

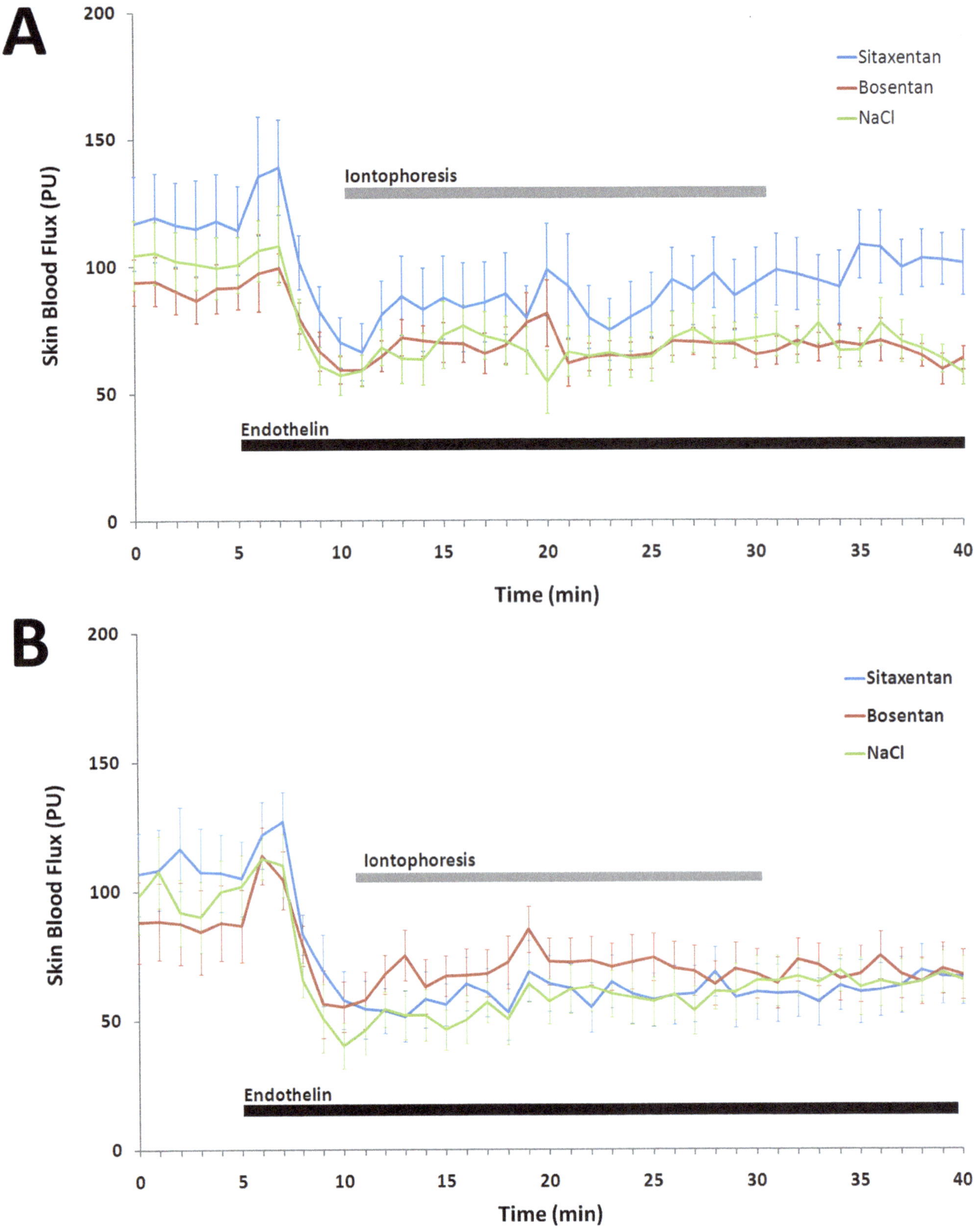

Figure 3. Effect of iontophoresis of bosentan 10^{-2} M, sitaxentan 10^{-2} M and NaCl 0.9% on skin blood flux during infusion of i.a. endothelin 0.5 10^{-5} M in rats, expressed as arbitrary perfusion units mean (mean±SEM), in the cathodal direction (Fig 3A) and anodal direction (Fig. 3B).

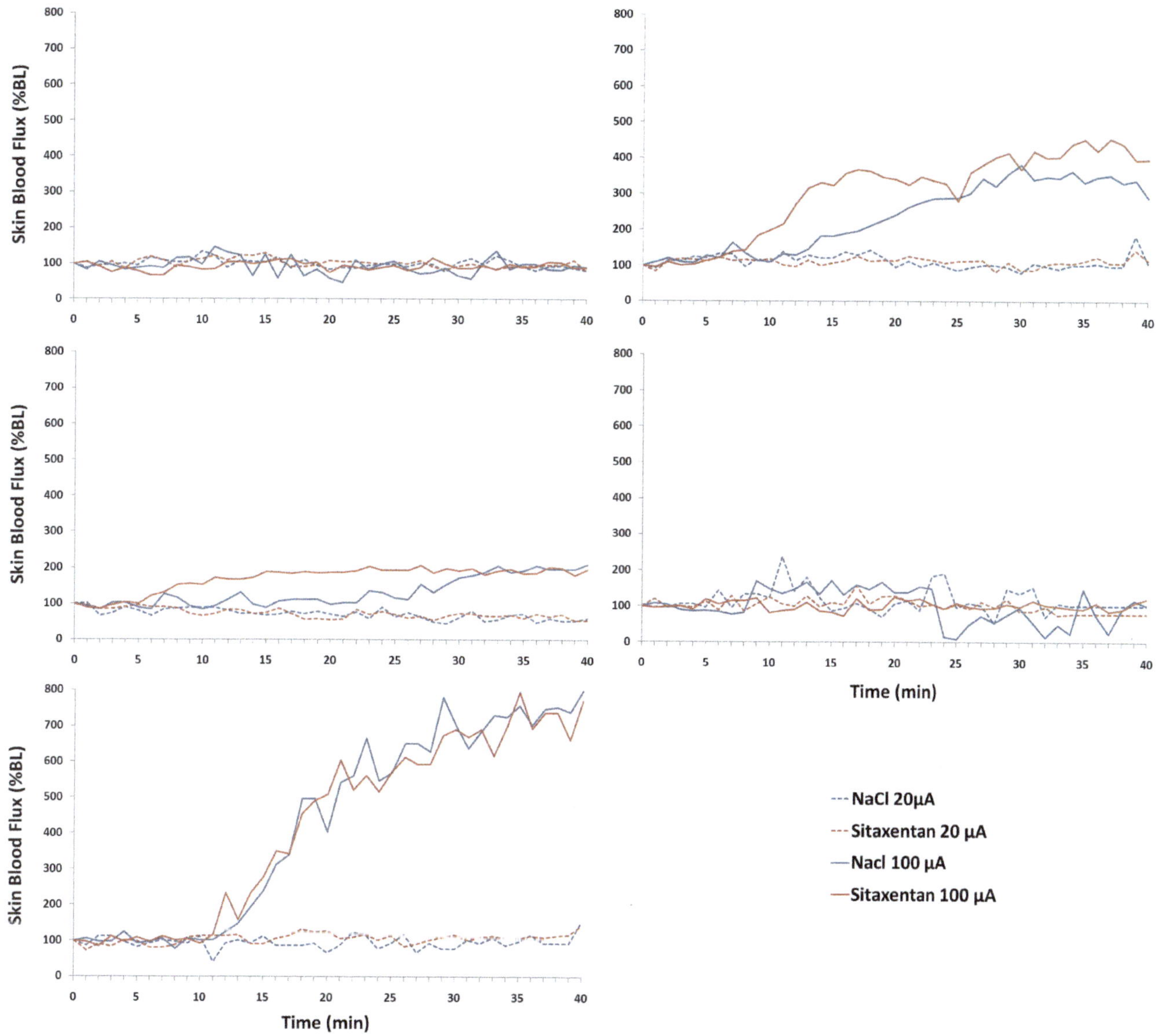

Figure 4. Effect of iontophoresis of sitaxentan 10^{-2} M (red lines) and NaCl 0.9 % (blue lines) on skin blood flux, expressed as a percentage change from baseline (%BL), in the forearm skin of five healthy volunteers. Current intensity was set at 20 µA (dashed lines) or 100 µA (solid lines).

simultaneously performed at both sites with the same distance between electrodes.

The clinical study was prematurely stopped after the manufacturer decided to discontinue all ongoing clinical trials with sitaxentan and to withdraw the commercial drug, because of several cases of fatal liver injury [22]. Nonetheless, despite the small sample size, there was no effect of iontophoresis of sitaxentan at 20 µA in any of the five participants, whereas in our experience with other molecules this current intensity leads to sustained vasodilation in humans [23]. There was an inconsistant effect at 100 µA, which is more difficult to interpret considering the small sample size and the large variability of the response. Altogether, and considering the elevated concentration used in the clinical study, our data suggest that iontophoresis is not an appropriate route of administration for sitaxentan.

Of note, we observed a difference (although not significant) in the response to NaCl between cathodal and anodal iontophoresis, the response being more pronounced in the anodal direction. This might be surprising as Durand previously showed that current-induced vasodilation was higher with cathodal iontophoresis [21]. Nonetheless, several differences should be pointed out: Durand used tap water whereas we used NaCl (which is known to make a significant difference [24]); their study was in humans, ours was in rats; they showed a marked difference, ours is modest considering the variability and does not reach significance.

It should be noted that the iontophoresis of ERAs was well tolerated both in animals and humans. No change in arterial blood pressure was observed and skin tolerance was excellent, although the skin biopsies only permitted us to detect immediate skin toxicity. Finally, it did not induce any significant increase in aspartate transaminase or alanine transaminase in humans.

In conclusion, this study shows that cathodal iontophoresis of sitaxentan but not bosentan partially reverses endothelin-induced skin vasoconstriction in rats, suggesting that sitaxentan diffuses into the dermis. Nevertheless, although the clinical study with sitaxentan had to be interrupted, we did not observe any effect of iontophoresis at 20 μA on skin blood flow in humans, and no clear-cut effect at 100 μA. Iontophoresis of other ERAs such as ambrisentan or macitentan could be an interesting alternative that remains to be explored.

Acknowledgments

We thank Sandrine Cachot, Kristen Weersink and Florence Gaillard-Bigot for technical support and Dr Alison Foote for editing the manuscript.

Author Contributions

Conceived and designed the experiments: MR SB CA DGR JLC. Performed the experiments: MR SB MH CM BD JB CR . Analyzed the data: MR MH BD JLC. Contributed reagents/materials/analysis tools: JB. Wrote the paper: MR JLC .

References

1. Herrick AL (2000) Vascular function in systemic sclerosis. Curr Opin Rheumatol 12: 527–533.
2. Korn JH, Mayes M, Matucci Cerinic M, Rainisio M, Pope J, et al. (2004) Digital ulcers in systemic sclerosis: prevention by treatment with bosentan, an oral endothelin receptor antagonist. Arthritis Rheum 50: 3985–3993.
3. Humbert M, Segal ES, Kiely DG, Carlsen J, Schwierin B, et al. (2007) Results of European post-marketing surveillance of bosentan in pulmonary hypertension. Eur Respir J 30: 338–344.
4. Wigley FM, Seibold JR, Wise RA, McCloskey DA, Dole WP (1992) Intravenous iloprost treatment of Raynaud's phenomenon and ischemic ulcers secondary to systemic sclerosis. J Rheumatol 19: 1407–1414.
5. Kalia YN, Naik A, Garrison J, Guy RH (2004) Iontophoretic drug delivery. Adv Drug Deliv Rev 56: 619–658.
6. Murray AK, Herrick AL, Gorodkin RE, Moore TL, King TA (2005) Possible therapeutic use of vasodilator iontophoresis. Microvasc Res 69: 89–94.
7. Murray AK, Moore TL, King TA, Herrick AL (2008) Vasodilator iontophoresis a possible new therapy for digital ischaemia in systemic sclerosis? Rheumatology (Oxford) 47: 76–79.
8. Blaise S, Roustit M, Millet C, Ribuot C, Boutonnat J, et al. (2011) Cathodal iontophoresis of treprostinil and iloprost induces a sustained increase in cutaneous flux in rats. Br J Pharmacol 162: 557–565.
9. Fregert S (1981) Manual of Contact Dermatitis. Copenhagen: Munskgaard.
10. de Nucci G, Thomas R, D'Orleans-Juste P, Antunes E, Walder C, et al. (1988) Pressor effects of circulating endothelin are limited by its removal in the pulmonary circulation and by the release of prostacyclin and endothelium-derived relaxing factor. Proc Natl Acad Sci U S A 85: 9797–9800.
11. Cracowski JL, Minson CT, Salvat-Melis M, Halliwill JR (2006) Methodological issues in the assessment of skin microvascular endothelial function in humans. Trends Pharmacol Sci 27: 503–508.
12. O'Leary DS (1991) Regional vascular resistance vs. conductance: which index for baroreflex responses? Am J Physiol 260: H632–637.
13. Blaise S, Hellmann M, Roustit M, Isnard S, Cracowski JL (2010) Oral sildenafil increases skin hyperaemia induced by iontophoresis of sodium nitroprusside in healthy volunteers. Br J Pharmacol 160: 1128–1134.
14. Dixit N, Bali V, Baboota S, Ahuja A, Ali J (2007) Iontophoresis - an approach for controlled drug delivery: a review. Curr Drug Deliv 4: 1–10.
15. Rosato E, Molinaro I, Borghese F, Rossi C, Pisarri S, et al. (2010) Bosentan improves skin perfusion of hands in patients with systemic sclerosis with pulmonary arterial hypertension. J Rheumatol 37: 2531–2539.
16. Hettema ME, Zhang D, Stienstra Y, Smit AJ, Bootsma H, et al. (2009) No effects of bosentan on microvasculature in patients with limited cutaneous systemic sclerosis. Clin Rheumatol 28: 825–833.
17. Hettema ME, Zhang D, Bootsma H, Kallenberg CG (2007) Bosentan therapy for patients with severe Raynaud's phenomenon in systemic sclerosis. Ann Rheum Dis 66: 1398–1399.
18. Leslie SJ, Rahman MQ, Denvir MA, Newby DE, Webb DJ (2004) Endothelins and their inhibition in the human skin microcirculation: ET[1–31], a new vasoconstrictor peptide. Br J Clin Pharmacol 57: 720–725.
19. Lawrence E, Siney L, Wilsoncroft P, Knock GA, Terenghi G, et al. (1995) Evidence for ETA and ETB receptors in rat skin and an investigation of their function in the cutaneous microvasculature. Br J Pharmacol 115: 840–844.
20. Lawrence E, Brain SD (1994) Effect of BQ-123 and Ro 47-0203 (bosentan) on endothelin-induced vasoconstriction in the rat skin. Eur J Pharmacol 260: 103–106.
21. Durand S, Fromy B, Bouye P, Saumet JL, Abraham P (2002) Current-induced vasodilation during water iontophoresis (5 min, 0.10 mA) is delayed from current onset and involves aspirin sensitive mechanisms. J Vasc Res 39: 59–71.
22. Galie N, Hoeper MM, Gibbs JS, Simonneau G (2011) Liver toxicity of sitaxentan in pulmonary arterial hypertension. Eur Respir J 37: 475–476.
23. Blaise S, Roustit M, Hellmann M, Millet C, Cracowski JL (2012) Cathodal Iontophoresis of Treprostinil Induces a Sustained Increase in Cutaneous Blood Flux in Healthy Volunteers. J Clin Pharmacol.
24. Roustit M, Cracowski JL (2012) Non-invasive assessment of skin microvascular function in humans: an insight into methods. Microcirculation 19: 47–64.

Atomic Hydrogen Surrounded by Water Molecules, $H(H_2O)_m$, Modulates Basal and UV-Induced Gene Expressions in Human Skin *In Vivo*

Mi Hee Shin[1,2,3], Raeeun Park[4], Hideo Nojima[4], Hyung-Chel Kim[4], Yeon Kyung Kim[1,2,3], Jin Ho Chung[1,2,3]*

1 Department of Dermatology, Seoul National University College of Medicine, Seoul, Korea, **2** Laboratory of Cutaneous Aging Research, Biomedical Research Institute, Seoul National University Hospital, Seoul, Korea, **3** Institute of Human-Environment Interface Biology, Medical Research Center, Seoul National University, Seoul, Korea, **4** R&D Team, Samsung Electronics CO., LTD, Suwon, Korea

Abstract

Recently, there has been much effort to find effective ingredients which can prevent or retard cutaneous skin aging after topical or systemic use. Here, we investigated the effects of the atomic hydrogen surrounded by water molecules, $H(H_2O)_m$, on acute UV-induced responses and as well as skin aging. Interestingly, we observed that $H(H_2O)_m$ application to human skin prevented UV-induced erythema and DNA damage. And $H(H_2O)_m$ significantly prevented UV-induced MMP-1, COX-2, IL-6 and IL-1β mRNA expressions in human skin *in vivo*. We found that $H(H_2O)_m$ prevented UV-induced ROS generation and inhibited UV-induced MMP-1, COX-2 and IL-6 expressions, and UV-induced JNK and c-Jun phosphorylation in HaCaT cells. Next, we investigated the effects of $H(H_2O)_m$ on intrinsically aged or photoaged skin of elderly subjects. In intrinsically aged skin, $H(H_2O)_m$ application significantly reduced constitutive expressions of MMP-1, IL-6, and IL-1β mRNA. Additionally, $H(H_2O)_m$ significantly increased procollagen mRNA and also decreased MMP-1 and IL-6 mRNA expressions in photoaged facial skin. These results demonstrated that local application of $H(H_2O)_m$ may prevent UV-induced skin inflammation and can modulate intrinsic skin aging and photoaging processes. Therefore, we suggest that modifying the atmospheric gas environment within a room may be a new way to regulate skin functions or skin aging.

Editor: Makoto Kanzaki, Tohoku University, Japan

Funding: This study was supported by a grant from the National Research Foundation of Korea (NRF) grant funded by the Korea government (MEST) (No. 2011-0029819), and research agreement with Samsung Electronics CO., LTD. The funders had no role in study design, data collection and analysis, decision to publish, or preparation of the manuscript.

Competing Interests: The authors have the following interests. Raeeun Park, Hideo Nojima and Hyung-Chel Kim are employed by Samsung Electronics CO., LTD. Part of this study was supported by a research agreement with Samsung Electronics CO., LTD. Samsung Electronics CO. LTD. is named in a patent application for the use of SPi device (atmospheric pressure plasma device releasing atomic hydrogen) as the type of air cleaner (patent actual). There are no further patents, products in development or marketed products to declare.

* E-mail: jhchung@snu.ac.kr

Introduction

Acute exposure to ultraviolet (UV) radiation leads to inflammatory responses such as skin erythema and sunburn, whereas chronic exposure to UV causes carcinogenesis and photoaging of the skin. UV stimulates the expression of a wide variety of proinflammatory mediators, including tumor necrosis factor (TNF)-α, interleukin (IL)-1β, IL-6 and IL-8. It is also known that cyclooxygenase (COX)-2 plays important roles in UV-induced acute inflammation [1,2,3,4,5]. In fact, inflammation is known to accelerate the aging process, as it is associated with the generation of free radicals and activation of various signaling pathways [6,7,8,9].

Activation of cell surface receptors, such as epidermal growth factor receptor, by UV stimulates mitogen-activated protein kinase (MAPK) signal transduction pathways [10]. Three families of MAPK exist in mammalian cells: extracellular signal-regulated kinase (ERK), c-Jun amino-terminal kinase (JNK) and p38 kinase, and each MAPK form a signaling module. It is reported that MAPKs are involved in the regulation of matrix metalloproteases (MMPs) [11,12]. MAPKs activation induces both c-Jun and c-Fos, which comprise the transcription factor activator protein (AP)-1 [13,14]. Many studies have indicated that UV exposure of human skin causes extracellular matrix degradation via induction of transcription factor AP-1 and subsequently by increased MMP production [10,15]. Another important transcription factor activated in response to UV irradiation is nuclear factor kappa B (NF-κB) [16]. Activation of the NF-κB pathway by UV stimulates inflammatory cytokine expression, and contributes to UV-induced skin damage, such as photoaging.

In addition, human skin is constantly exposed to reactive oxygen species (ROS) from the environment, such as air, solar radiation, ozone and other airborne pollutants, or from the normal metabolism. Accumulated ROS has been suggested to play important roles in the intrinsic aging and photoaging of human skin *in vivo* [17] and is associated with upregulation of MMPs and decreased collagen synthesis [18,19,20]. Oxidative stress is thought to play a central role in initiating and driving the signaling events that lead to cellular responses following UV exposure [21,22,23,24]. ROS influences MAPK signaling and thereby contributes to the AP-1-induced up-regulation of MMP-1 [25]. It has been shown that UV-induced ROS production causes skin

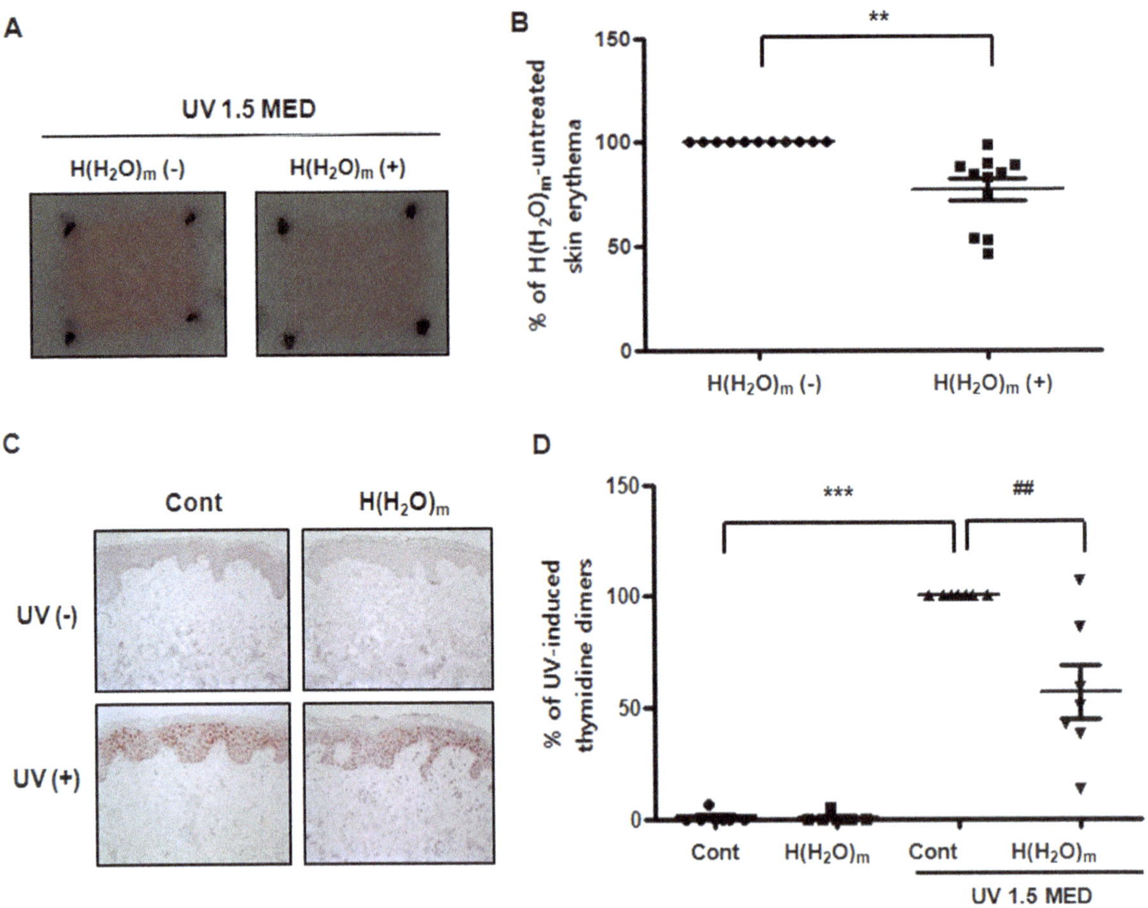

Figure 1. $H(H_2O)_m$ prevents UV-induced erythema and thymidine dimers in young human skin *in vivo*. Skin from young human buttocks was irradiated with UV light and then locally treated with or without $H(H_2O)_m$ for 2 hr. Twenty-four hours after irradiation, erythema index was measured and then skin was biopsied. (**A**) The photographs of erythema are representative of the subjects. (**B**) Erythema-index measurements are shown as means ± SEM with scatter plots (n = 11). (**C**) Immunohistochemical staining was performed using anti-thymidine dimer antibody. The figures shown are representative of seven subjects. (**D**) Results are expressed as means ± SEM with scatter plots (n = 7), *** $p<0.001$ versus the control, ## $p<0.01$ versus UV-irradiated skin.

photoaging and induces the synthesis of MMPs. Thus, strategies to counteract ROS production may be useful for preventing photoaging.

It was found that molecular hydrogen (H_2) can alleviate $^{\bullet}OH$-induced cytotoxicity, and that H_2 has potential as an antioxidant for preventive and therapeutic applications [26]. Actually, inhaled hydrogen molecule gas and hydrogen rich-saline has protective effects on oxidative organ damage, including damaged lung and brain [27,28,29,30]. Inhalation of H_2 has already been used for the prevention of decompression sickness in divers and has shown a good safety profile [26,31]. Recently, Nojima et. al reported that atomic hydrogen surrounded by water molecules ($H(H_2O)_m$), released from a novel atmospheric pressure plasma device is effective not only for deactivation of airborne indoor microbial-contaminants but also for neutralization of the OH radicals in the air [32].

In the present study, 1) we demonstrated that local application of $H(H_2O)_n$ gas to human skin could modulate UV-induced skin responses, including sunburn response and DNA damage such as thymidine dimers formation. 2) We also demonstrated that $H(H_2O)_m$ has an anti-oxidant effect and can prevent UV-induced expression of MMP-1, COX-2, IL-6 and IL-1β in human skin *in vivo* and in HaCaT cells. 3) Furthermore, we found that local application of $H(H_2O)_m$ could regulate constitutive expression of genes related to intrinsic aging and photoaging in human skin. 4) Finally, our results indicate that $H(H_2O)_m$ treatment may regulate skin aging process in human skin.

Results

$H(H_2O)_m$ treatment prevented UV-induced erythema and thymidine dimers formation in young human skin *in vivo*

To investigate whether $H(H_2O)_m$ could prevent UV-induced skin erythema in human skin, the buttocks of young subjects were irradiated with UV (1.5MED), and then treated with $H(H_2O)_m$ for 2 hr. Twenty-four hours after UV irradiation, we observed, interestingly, that UV-induced erythema was reduced in $H(H_2O)_m$-treated skin, compared with control fan-treated skin (Figure 1A). Erythema-index measurements showed that $H(H_2O)_m$ decreased UV-induced erythema by 22.8±5.8%, compared with control skin (Figure 1B). However, we found that UV-induced erythema was not significantly changed by 30 min or 1 hr treatment of $H(H_2O)_m$ (data not shown). These data indicate that $H(H_2O)_m$ has an anti-inflammatory effect against UV-induced sunburn response in human skin. Then, we investigated the effect of $H(H_2O)_m$ on UV-induced DNA damage in human skin *in vivo*.

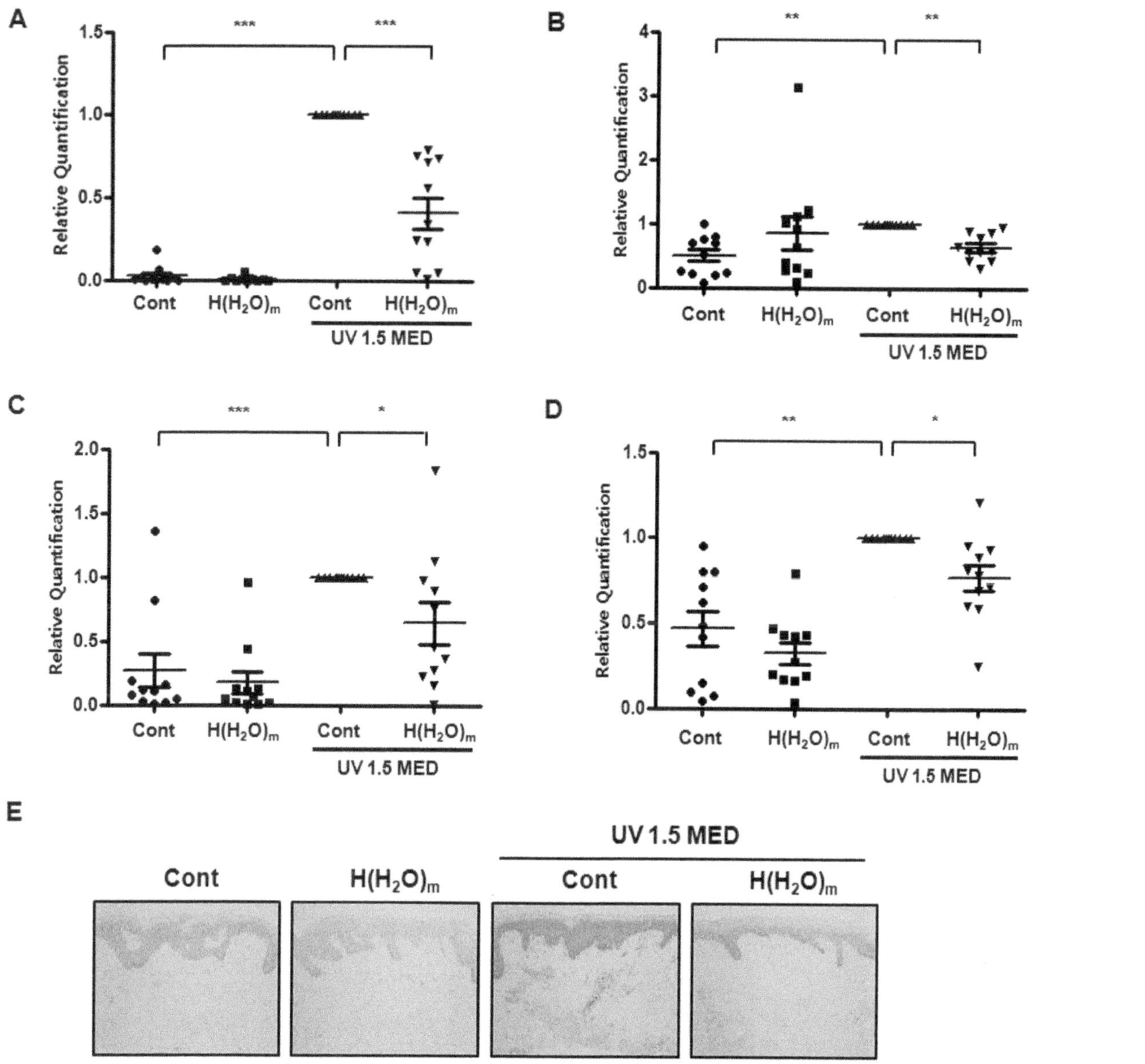

Figure 2. $H(H_2O)_m$ prevents and UV-induced MMP-1, COX-2, IL-6 and IL-1β mRNA expression in young human skin *in vivo*. Skin from young human buttocks was irradiated with UV light and then locally treated with or without $H(H_2O)_m$ for 2 hr. Twenty-four hours after irradiation, and then skin was biopsied. (A) MMP-1, (B) COX-2, (C) IL-6 and (D) IL-1β mRNA expressions were determined by real time RT-PCR. Results are expressed as means ± SEM with scatter plots (n = 11), * $p<0.05$, ** $p<0.01$, *** $p<0.001$. **(E)** Immunohistochemical staining was performed using anti-human MMP-1 antibody. The figures shown are representative of eleven subjects.

The buttocks of young subjects were irradiated with UV (1.5MED), and then treated with $H(H_2O)_m$ for 2 hr. Twenty-four hours after UV irradiation, we observed UV irradiation of human skin induces DNA damage such as thymidine dimer formation, as shown in figure 1C. Interestingly, local application of $H(H_2O)_m$ significantly decreased UV-induced thymidine dimers formation by 56.7±11.8% compared with UV-irradiated skin (Figure 1C and D).

$H(H_2O)_m$ treatment prevented UV-induced MMP-1, COX-2, IL-6 and IL-1β in young human skin *in vivo*

Next, by real-time RT-PCR, we demonstrated that $H(H_2O)_m$ prevented UV-induced expressions of MMP-1, COX-2, IL-6 and IL-1β mRNA significantly by 58.9±8.1, 36.1±7.6, 35.4±17.1 and 23.7±9.2%, respectively, compared with UV-irradiated skin (Figure 2A, B, C and D). COX-2 mRNA expression tended to be increased in unirradiated $H(H_2O)_m$, although it was not statistically significant. This tendency seems to be due to unexpected increase of COX-2 mRNA in unirradiated $H(H_2O)_m$ in 2 out of 11 volunteers. However, $H(H_2O)_m$ did not prevent UV-induced decreases in type I procollagen expression (data not shown). Also, similar to UV-induced erythema, we found that UV-induced expression of MMP-1, COX-2, IL-6 and IL-1β mRNA were not significantly changed after 30 min or 1 hr treatments of $H(H_2O)_m$ (data not shown). Immunohistochemical staining revealed that UV induced MMP-1 protein expression throughout the epidermis and

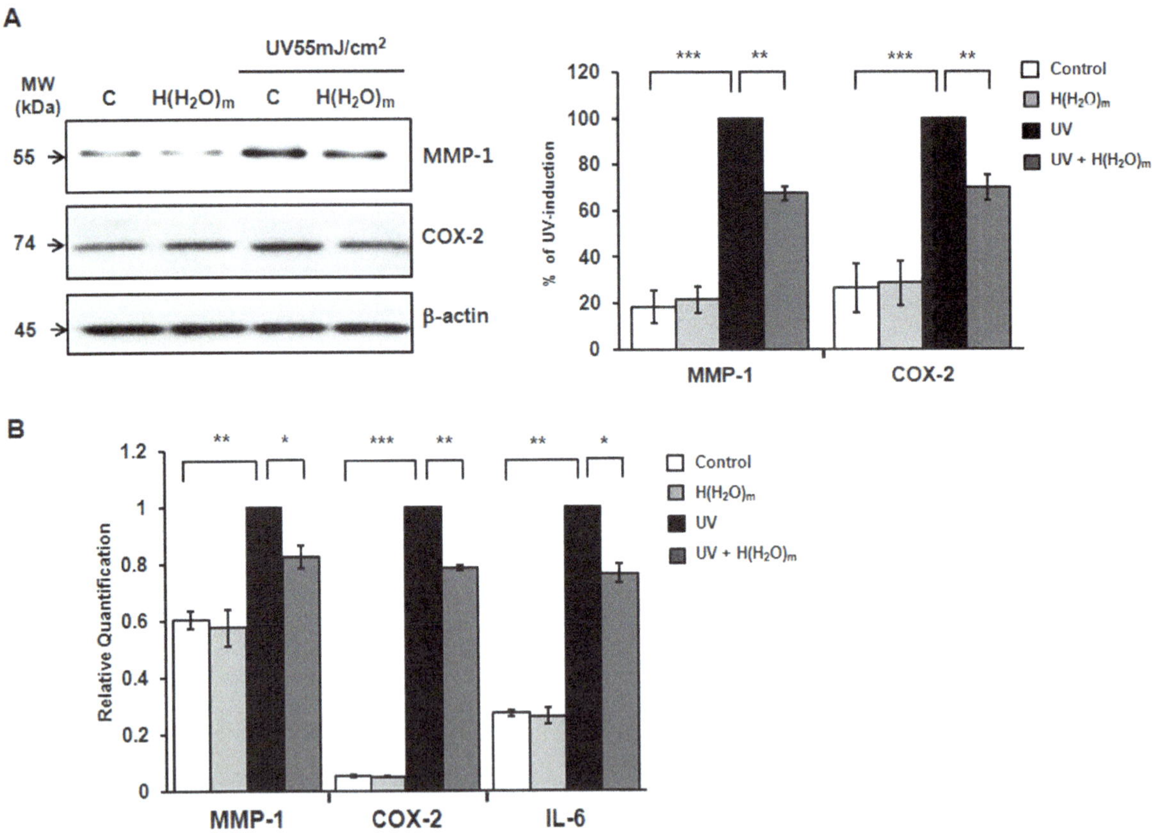

Figure 3. $H(H_2O)_m$ prevents UV-induced MMP-1, COX-2 and IL-6 mRNA expression in HaCaT cells. (**A**) Cells were pre-treated with $H(H_2O)_m$ for 15 min, then irradiated with UV (55 mJ/cm^2) and post-treated with $H(H_2O)_m$ for 15 min in PBS. After incubation for 48 hr with serum-free DMEM, MMP-1 expression was determined in culture media and COX-2 and β-actin expression were determined in cell lysates by Western blotting. The bands are representative of results from three independent experiments. Results are expressed as means ± SEM (n = 6). (**B**) Cells were treated with $H(H_2O)_m$ and UV as described above. After incubation for 24 hr with serum free DMEM, MMP-1, COX-2 and IL-6 mRNA expressions were determined by real-time RT-PCR. Results are expressed as means ± SEM (n = 3), * $p<0.05$, ** $p<0.01$, *** $p<0.001$.

that $H(H_2O)_m$ substantially inhibited UV-induced MMP-1 expression versus fan-treated, UV-irradiated skin (Figure 2E). These results suggest that $H(H_2O)_m$ may prevent acute UV-induced skin responses.

$H(H_2O)_m$ prevented UV-induced MMP-1, COX-2 and IL-6 expressions, and inhibited UV-induced SEK1/JNK activation and c-Jun phosphorylation in HaCaT cells

To confirm and investigate the action mechanisms of $H(H_2O)_m$ on UV-induced skin inflammation in human skin *in vivo*, we used HaCaT cells for the next experiments. Cells were irradiated with 55 mJ/cm^2 of UV with or without $H(H_2O)_m$ treatment. By western blotting, we demonstrated that $H(H_2O)_m$ significantly prevented up-regulation of MMP-1 and COX-2 expression by UV (Figure 3A). Real-time PCR reveals that UV-induced MMP-1, COX-2 and IL-6 mRNA expression was inhibited by $H(H_2O)_m$ in a pattern similar to the Western blotting results (Figure 3B). From these results, we demonstrated that $H(H_2O)_m$ decreased the UV-induced MMP-1, COX-2 and IL-6 in human keratinocyte.

In HaCaT cells, MAPKs were activated by UV within 30 min after UV irradiation and then declined to basal levels (Figure 4A). To investigate the roles of MAPKs in UV-induced MMP-1 expression, cells were pretreated with U0126 (10 μM; MEK1-inhibitor), SP600125 (10 μM; JNK-inhibitor), or SB203580 (10 μM; p38-inhibitor) for 1 hr and then irradiated with UV. UV-induced MMP-1 expression was inhibited by pretreating with U0126 and SP600125, but not by SB203580 (Figure 4B). These results suggest that the activation of the ERK and JNK pathways mediates UV-induced MMP-1 expression in HaCaT cells.

As ERK and JNK activation are required for UV-induced MMP-1 expression in HaCaT cells, we investigated the effects of $H(H_2O)_m$ on UV-induced ERK and JNK activation. Treatment with $H(H_2O)_m$ significantly inhibited JNK phosphorylation without altering total JNK levels (Figure 5A and B). But, UV-induced ERK activation was not inhibited by $H(H_2O)_m$ treatment. We also found that $H(H_2O)_m$ significantly inhibited the UV-induced phosphorylation of SEK1, which is the upstream kinase of JNK (Figure 5A and B). These results suggest that inhibition of SEK1/JNK pathways by $H(H_2O)_m$ might attenuate UV-induced MMP expression.

AP-1 is known to play a critical role in MMP-1 expression by UV [33,34,35]. The transcriptional activity of AP-1 is also dependent on the degree of phosphorylation of c-Jun. Therefore, we investigated the effect of $H(H_2O)_m$ on UV-induced c-Jun phosphorylation in HaCaT cells. UV was found to increase the level of phosphorylated c-Jun and $H(H_2O)_m$ inhibited UV-induced phospho-c-Jun expression significantly (Figure 5A and B). In addition, although UV irradiation increased the expression of c-Fos, $H(H_2O)_m$ did not inhibit UV-induced c-Fos expression. In the result of immunofluorescence staining, UV-induced phospho-c-Jun expression was decreased by $H(H_2O)_m$ (Figure 5C). These

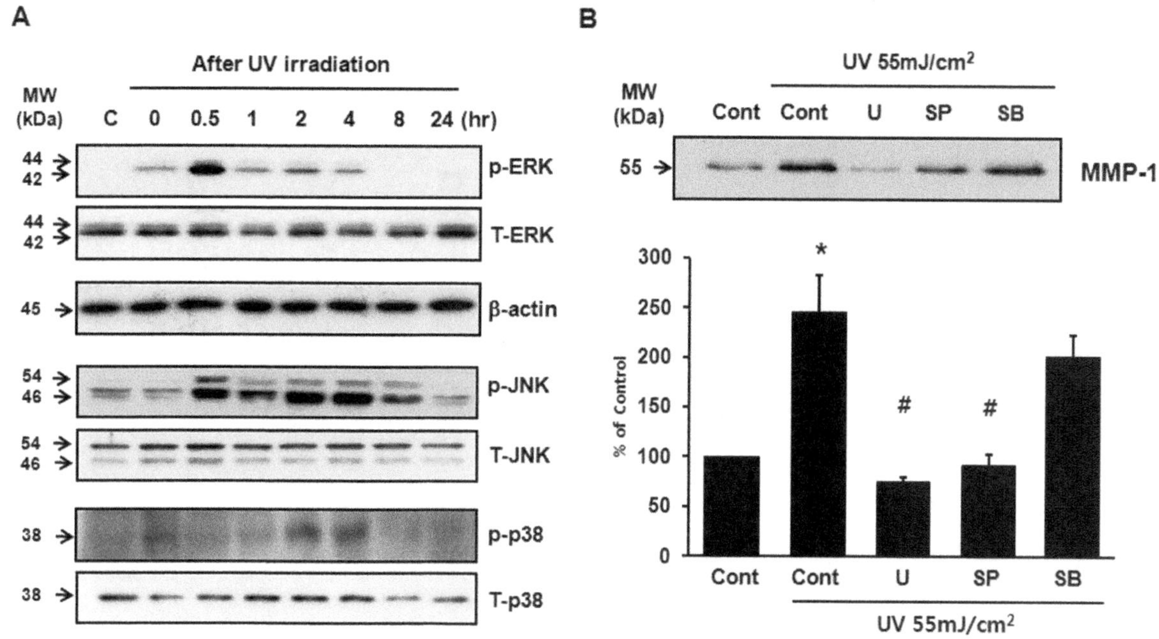

Figure 4. UV-induced MMP-1 expression is mediated by ERK and JNK activation but not by p38 activation in HaCaT cells. (**A**) Cells were serum-starved for 24 hr, irradiated with UV light (55 mJ/cm^2) and harvested at the indicated times. Total cell lysates were prepared and subjected to Western blotting using specific antibodies. The bands are representative of results from three independent experiments. (**B**) HaCaT cells were pretreated with U0126(U) [ERK (MEK1) inhibitor; 10 μM], SP600125(SP) [JNK inhibitor; 10 μM], and SB203580(SB) [p38 inhibitor; 10 μM] for 1 hr, and then irradiated with UV. Irradiated cells were cultured for 48 hr and MMP-1 expression was determined by Western blotting. All experiments were performed in triplicate. Values shown are means ± SEM (n = 4), * $p<0.05$ versus the control, # $p<0.05$ versus UV-irradiated cells.

results suggest that $H(H_2O)_m$ inhibits UV-induced MMP-1 expression and that this inhibition may be mediated by a reduction in the level of phosphorylated c-Jun, which is known to be closely associated with UV-induced AP-1 activation. Because JNK is closely related to c-Jun phosphorylation and expression, these findings suggest that the inhibition of UV-induced phospho-cJun by $H(H_2O)_m$ may be mediated by inhibition of the activation of JNK.

$H(H_2O)_m$ reduced UV-induced ROS generation in HaCaT cells

UV causes generation of ROS and UV-triggered oxidative stress regulates a variety of cellular functions including MMP secretion and cytokine production [36,37,38,39]. It was proposed that antioxidants scavenging ROS can prevent skin photoaging. Therefore, we investigated whether $H(H_2O)_m$ may have an antioxidant effect. UV significantly increased ROS generation by 409.4±21.1% and $H(H_2O)_m$ significantly reduced this UV-induced ROS generation by 12.9±1.1%, compared with the UV-treated cells (Figure 6A). Also, in the result of DCF staining, we confirmed that $H(H_2O)_m$ has ROS scavenging effect against UV-induced ROS (Figure 6B).

$H(H_2O)_m$ decreased basal expressions of MMP-1, IL-6 and IL-1β in intrinsically aged human skin

Next, we investigated whether $H(H_2O)_m$ may have beneficial effects on intrinsically aged skin of the elderly subjects. The aged human buttock skin was treated with $H(H_2O)_m$ for 2 hr, and then skin was biopsied 24 hr post-treatment. By real-time RT-PCR analysis, we demonstrated that $H(H_2O)_m$ reduced the constitutive expressions of MMP-1, IL-6 and IL-1β mRNA, significantly (Figure 7A). However, the basal expression of type I procollagen mRNA was not changed by $H(H_2O)_m$ in aged skin. In addition, by immunohistochemical staining, we found that the basal level of MMP-1 protein expression in the aged skin was decreased by $H(H_2O)_m$ (Figure 7B).

$H(H_2O)_m$ increased basal expression of type I procollagen in photoaged facial skin and also reduced the basal expressions of MMP-1 and IL-6

Photoaged facial skin was treated with $H(H_2O)_m$ for 30 min/day for four consecutive days sequentially, and then 24 hr after the last treatment, skin was biopsied. Similar to data on intrinsic aging, MMP-1 and IL-6 mRNA levels were significantly decreased by 52.3±10.2 and 27.8±12.7%, respectively, by $H(H_2O)_m$ (Figure 7C). However, interestingly, in contrast to intrinsically aged skin, $H(H_2O)_m$ significantly increased basal expression of type I procollagen mRNA by 166.3±28.1%, compared with control fan-treated facial skin (Figure 7C). These results suggest that $H(H_2O)_m$ may modulate basal gene expression in aged and photoaged human skin.

Discussion

This study demonstrated that $H(H_2O)_m$ prevented UV-induced erythema and DNA damage in human skin and also inhibited UV-induced MMP-1, COX-2, IL-6 and IL-1β expressions significantly. Also, we found that $H(H_2O)_m$ exposure to human skin could modulate basal mRNA expressions of MMP-1, type I procollagen, COX-2, IL-1β and IL-6 in intrinsically aged and photoaged human skin. To our knowledge, this is the first report that an atmospheric gas component, such as $H(H_2O)_m$, could modulate

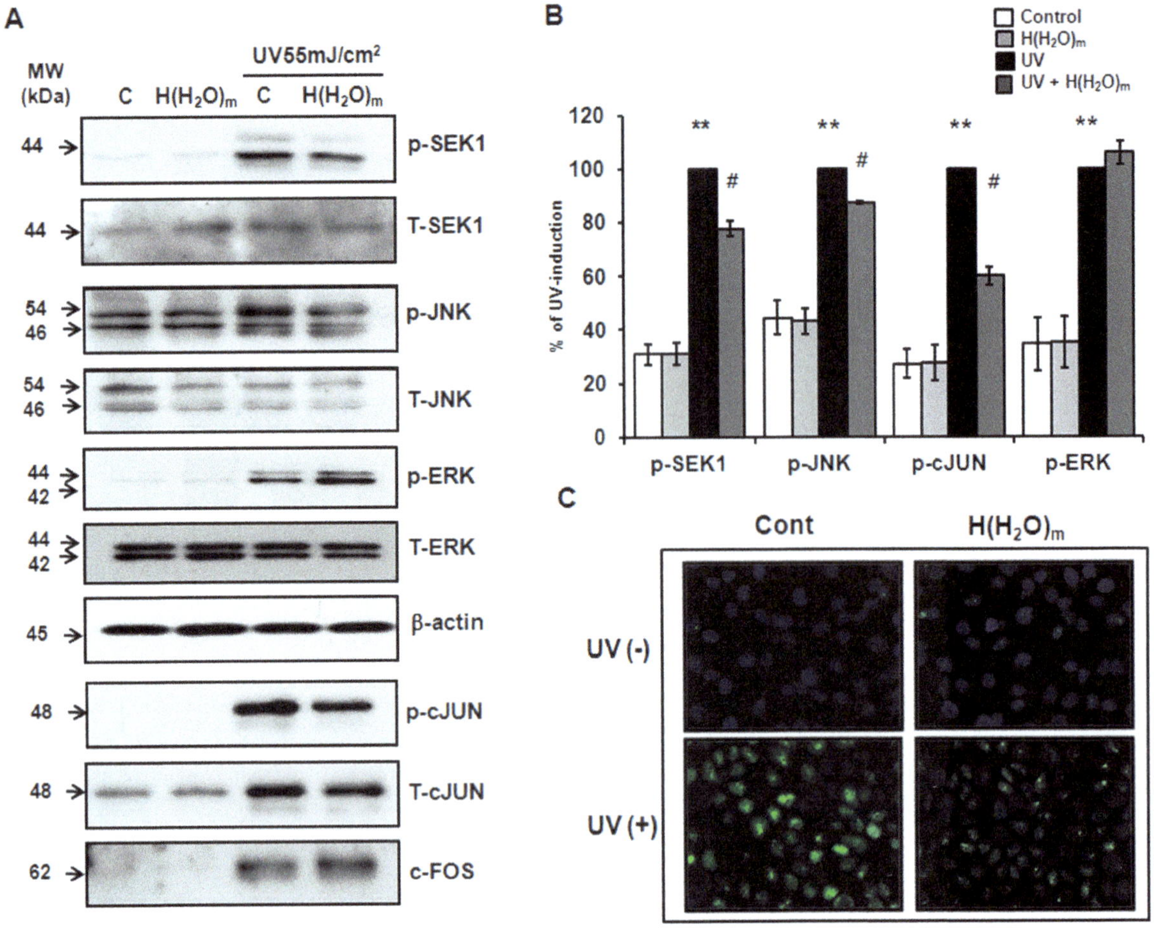

Figure 5. UV-induced SEK1/JNK activation and c-Jun phosphorylation are inhibited by $H(H_2O)_m$ treatment in HaCaT cells. (**A**) Cells were pre-treated with $H(H_2O)_m$ for 15 min, then irradiated with UV and post-treated with $H(H_2O)_m$ for 15 min in PBS. After incubation for 30 min, total cell lysates were prepared. Western blotting were performed using phospho-specific (p−) and total (T−) JNK, c-Jun, SEK1 and ERK antibodies. Level of β-actin was used as loading control. The bands are representative of results from three independent experiments. (**B**) Results are expressed as means ± SEM (n = 3), ** $p<0.01$ versus the control, # $p<0.05$ versus UV-irradiated cells. (**C**) Intracellular phospho-c-Jun levels in cells were visualized using a fluorescent microscope and the images presented are representative of the fluorescence levels observed in three separate experiments.

UV-induced skin responses and regulate basal gene expression in aged human skin. Since there are some reports that gas or air can penetrate or pass through the skin [40,41], we speculated that $H(H_2O)_m$ may penetrate the skin barrier and subsequently affect skin cells functions through an unknown mechanism.

UV-induced erythema is the most obvious of the photobiological responses evidenced by skin and a marker of tissue injury and inflammation [42,43]. DNA damage by UV exposure plays an essential part, and is the initial step, in skin cancer induction [44,45]. In our study, we determined that treatment of $H(H_2O)_m$ suppressed significantly UV-induced erythema response in human skin *in vivo*, and UV-induced thymidine dimer formation was also inhibited by $H(H_2O)_m$ in human skin. Moreover, the sunburn-reducing effect and DNA damage-inhibiting effect of $H(H_2O)_m$ may be in part due to its anti-inflammatory and anti-oxidant effects, based on the our results that $H(H_2O)_m$ inhibited UV-induced expression of COX-2 and inflammatory cytokines, including IL-6 and IL-1β, and reduced UV-induced ROS generation. Taken together, we propose that local application of $H(H_2O)_m$ can protect our skin from UV-induced inflammatory responses and DNA damages.

To understand the changes of signaling pathways caused by $H(H_2O)_m$ treatment leading to decreased expression of MMP-1 expression, we performed the experiments using human keratinocytes, HaCaT cells. MAPK is known to play an essential role in induction of MMP-1 expression by UV [46,47]. MAPKs activation is followed by an increase in the expression of c-Jun and c-Fos, which form the AP-1 complex. Transcription of several MMPs, including MMP-1, MMP-3 and MMP-9, is regulated by AP-1 [12], which is one of several transcriptional factors activated by UV [48]. Thus, increased AP-1 activity is responsible for the degradation of extracellular matrix proteins, such as collagen, by inducing MMPs. In human skin, UV-induced AP-1 transcriptional activity is determined by c-Jun expression, because c-Fos is expressed continuously [12,49]. Whereas c-Fos expression in young and aged skin is unaltered, c-Jun expression is higher in aged skin than in young skin [14]. In this study, we found that $H(H_2O)_m$ treatment inhibited UV-induced c-Jun phosphorylation, but c-Fos expression was not suppressed by $H(H_2O)_m$. Our results demonstrated that $H(H_2O)_m$ treatment inhibits UV-induced MMP-1 and that this inhibition may be mediated by a reduction in the level of phosphorylated SEK1/JNK and c-Jun, which are

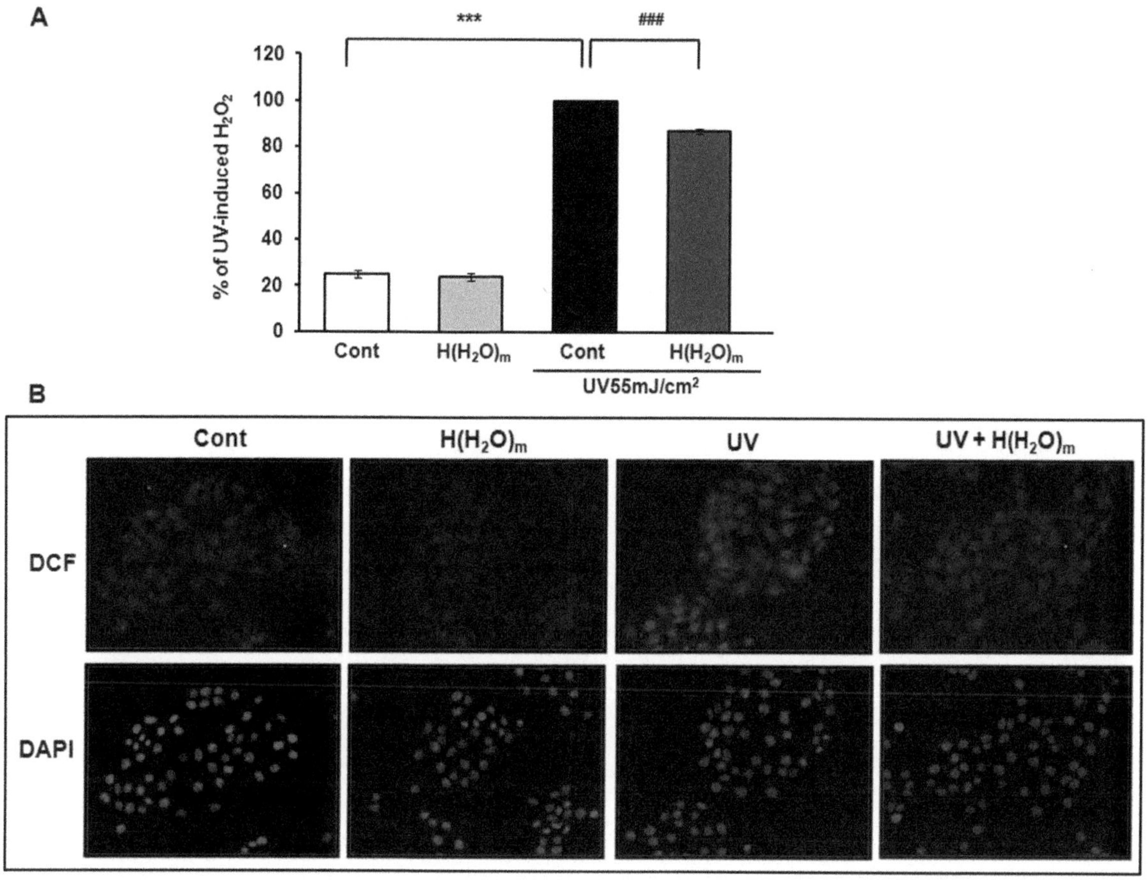

Figure 6. $H(H_2O)_m$ reduces UV-induced ROS production in HaCaT cells. (**A**) Cells were pre-treated with $H(H_2O)_m$ for 15 min, then irradiated with UV and post-treated with $H(H_2O)_m$ for 15 min in PBS. Subsequently, cells were treated with DCFDA (25 μM, freshly diluted in pre-warmed DMEM) for 30 min. Cells were then assayed using a fluorescence reader. Values shown are means ± SEM (n = 8), *** $p<0.001$ versus the control, ### $p<0.001$ versus UV-treated cells. (**B**) Intracellular H_2O_2 levels in HaCaT cells were visualized after DCF staining. The fluorescence intensity was visualized using a fluorescent microscope, and the images presented are representative of the fluorescence levels observed in three separate experiments. To normalize cell number, DAPI was used as a fluorescent marker for the nucleus.

known to be closely associated with UV-induced AP-1 activation in HaCaT cells.

On the other hand, UV is also known to activate NF-κB and regulate downstream NF-κB-dependent genes such as COX-2 and inflammatory cytokines [50,51]. In this study, $H(H_2O)_m$ treatment suppressed the expressions of UV-induced COX-2 and IL-6, but $H(H_2O)_m$ did not inhibit UV-induced NF-κB activation (data not shown). Therefore, our results suggest that the inhibition of UV-induced COX-2 and IL-6 by $H(H_2O)_m$ is not associated with NF-κB, and the exact action mechanism of $H(H_2O)_m$ remains to be investigated.

UV irradiation initiates the generation of ROS, which causes MMP-1 upregulation and the degradation of dermal collagen, possibly by activating the MAPK signaling pathway [52]. This mechanism predicts that a free radical scavenger might prevent UV-induced skin damage by inhibiting the induction of MMPs. Also, in the previous study, significant protective effects against OH radicals by $H(H_2O)_m$ in the air was observed in mammalian cells [32]. Cell death induced by an OH generator was suppressed by $H(H_2O)_m$ treatment [32]. In this study, we also found that $H(H_2O)_m$ inhibits UV-induced H_2O_2 generation, suggesting that the inhibition of UV-induced MMP-1 expression by $H(H_2O)_m$ may be associated with the inhibition of ROS production due to antioxidant effects of $H(H_2O)_m$ in HaCaT cells.

Although the typical appearance of photoaged and chronologically aged human skin can be readily distinguished, it has been reported that intrinsically aged and photoaged skin share important molecular features such as altered signal transduction pathways that promote MMP expression as well as decrease procollagen synthesis. This concordance of molecular mechanisms suggests that UV irradiation may accelerate many key aspects of the aging process in human skin [53,54]. In many studies, researchers have tried to develop new agents for the prevention of skin aging. The approaches to improve UV-induced skin damage in the aged skin could involve the use of antioxidant agents or potential sources of MMP-1 inhibitors and collagen-synthesis inducers, in addition to the administration of anti-inflammatory agents. Interestingly, this study demonstrated that $H(H_2O)_m$ treatment decreased basal MMP-1, COX-2, IL-6 mRNA expressions in intrinsically aged and photoaged human skin *in vivo*. In contrast to intrinsically aged skin, $H(H_2O)_m$ treatment increased basal expression of type I procollagen mRNA in photoaged facial skin. Therefore, we suggest that applying $H(H_2O)_m$ to the skin could be a new way to prevent UV-induced skin damage and slow aging of the skin. We also speculate that regulating atmospheric gas composition in a room or office may be an effective strategy to modulate skin functions.

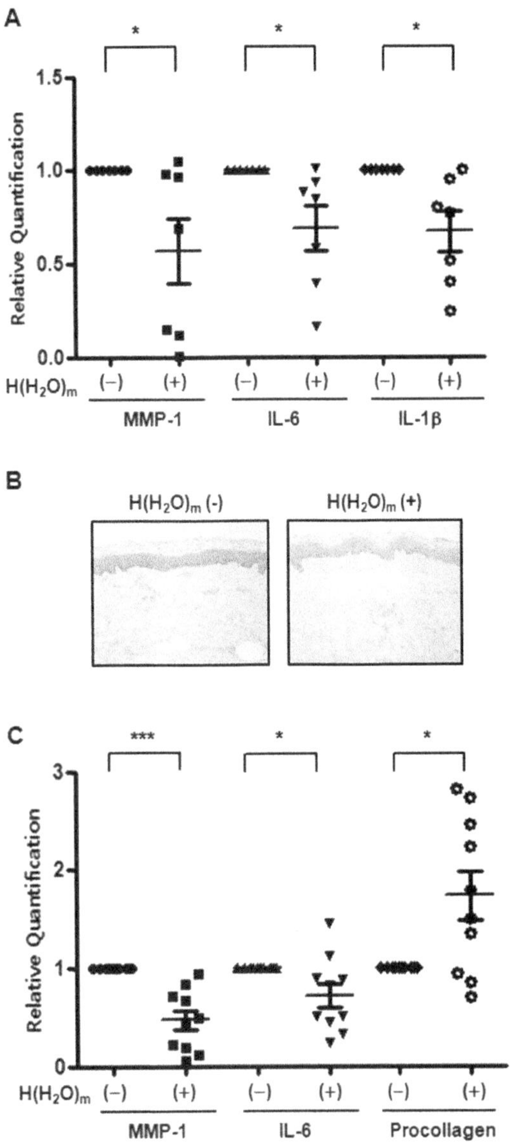

Figure 7. Basal expression of MMP-1, COX-2 and IL-6 are decreased by $H(H_2O)_m$ treatment in intrinsically aged human buttock skin and $H(H_2O)_m$ increases basal expression of type I procollagen expression in photoaged facial skin and also reduces the basal expressions of MMP-1 and IL-6. (**A**) Aged human buttock skin was topically treated with or without $H(H_2O)_m$ using a releasing device for 2 hr. MMP-1, COX-2 and IL-6 mRNA expressions were determined by real time RT-PCR. Results are shown as means ± SEM with scatter plots (n = 7), * $p<0.05$. (**B**) Immunohistochemical staining was performed using anti-human MMP-1 antibody. The figures shown are representative of seven subjects. (**C**) Aged human face skin was topically treated with or without $H(H_2O)_m$ for 30 min a day for 4 days. Type I procollagen, MMP-1 and IL-6 mRNA expressions were determined by real time RT-PCR. Results are expressed as means ± SEM with scatter plots (n = 10), * $p<0.05$, *** $p<0.001$.

Materials and Methods

Device Design

The developed device consists of a ceramic plate and a needle-shaped electrode with inner and outer electrodes as described previously [32]. When a pulse-shaped voltage is applied between the inner and outer electrodes of the plate, H^+ surrounded by water molecules, $H^+(H_2O)_m$ is generated as a positive ion (Figure S1, S2, S3). $H^+(H_2O)_m$ was measured by ion counter. It measured about $1{\sim}2\times10^6$ ions/cm^3 at 0.3 m distance. Then, the positive ion, $H^+(H_2O)_m$ is neutralized after combining with electrons from needle-shaped electrode and becomes atomic hydrogen surrounded by water molecules, $H(H_2O)_m$. $H^+(H_2O)_m$ after combining with electrons from needle-shaped electrode was less than 1×10^4 ions/cm^3, which is known to be normal level on the atmospheric pressure. This means most $H^+(H_2O)_m$ may be converted to $H(H_2O)_m$. The generation of atomic hydrogen in the device was detected by an optical spectroscopic method [32]. This device was manufactured by Samsung Electronics for the cell experiments and local application on human skin. The schematic experimental designs were showed in supporting information (Figure S1, S2, S3).

Cell culture, UV irradiation and $H(H_2O)_m$ treatment

Immortalized human keratinocyte HaCaT cells were grown in Dulbecco's modified eagle medium (DMEM) supplemented with 10% heat-inactivated fetal bovine serum (FBS), 2 mM glutamine, penicillin (100 U/ml) and streptomycin (100 µg/ml) in a 37°C humidified 5% CO_2 incubator. In all experiments, cells were cultured to 80% confluence and then starved in serum-free DMEM for 24 hr.

For cell experiments, the device was made as shown in figure S1. Briefly, the device releasing hydrogen atom ($H(H_2O)_m$) was installed in the top of a chamber. A fan was also installed in the chamber to aid the dispersion and circulation of the device-generated $H(H_2O)_m$. For control treatment, only a fan was installed in the chamber. The cells were pre-treated with $H(H_2O)_m$ for 15 min then irradiated with UV 55 mJ/cm^2 and post-treated with $H(H_2O)_m$ for 15 min in PBS. Philips TL20W/12RS fluorescent sun lamps (Einthoven, Netherlands) with an emission spectrum between 275 and 380 nm were used as the UV source [55]. The distribution of the power output of the lamps was 0.5% UVC (<280 nm), 56.7% UVB (280–320 nm), and 42.8% UVA (320–400 nm). And a Kodacel filter (TA401/407; Kodak, Rochester, NY) was used to remove wavelengths <290 nm (UVC). Therefore, in this experiment, used UV light includes UVA plus UVB, which we just commonly referred to as "UV". The UV strength was measured using a UV meter (Model 585100; Waldmann, Villingen-Schwenningen, Germany).

Local treatment of $H(H_2O)_m$ to human skin and UV irradiation

To investigate the effects of $H(H_2O)_m$ treatment on UV-induced skin damage in human skin *in vivo*, eleven young Koreans (mean age, 31.8 yr; age range, 24–47 yr), were irradiated by UV (1.5 MED). For human experiment, the device was made as shown in figure S2 and S3. Minimal erythema dose (MED) for each subject was determined 24 hr after irradiation of the buttock skin. MED ranged between 70 and 90 mJ/cm^2 for the skin of Koreans. The buttock skin was irradiated with UV and subsequently, treated with $H(H_2O)_m$ for 2 hr. Twenty-four hours post-irradiation, we measured UV-induced erythema using a DermaSpectrometer® (Cortex Technology, Hadsund, Denmark) and buttock skin was biopsied.

To investigate the effects of $H(H_2O)_m$ on intrinsically aged skin, buttock skin of the elderly subjects (seven Koreans; mean age, 73.1 yr; age range, 65–81 yr) were treated with $H(H_2O)_m$ for 2 hr. Twenty-four hours after $H(H_2O)_m$ treatment, buttock skin was biopsied.

To evaluate the effects of $H(H_2O)_m$ on the photoaged skin, photoaged facial skin (crow's feet area) of the elderly subjects (ten Koreans; mean age, 54.1 yr; age range, 45–62 yr) was topically treated with $H(H_2O)_m$ for 30 min a day for sequential four days. For control treatment, the other side of each photoaged facial skin of the volunteers was treated with only a fan. Twenty-four hours after the last treatment, facial skin was biopsied for real-time RT-PCR analysis. This study was conducted according to the Declaration of Helsinki Principles. All procedures received prior approval from the Institutional Review Board at Seoul National University Hospital and all subjects gave written informed consent.

Western blot analysis

To determine the amount of MMP-1 secreted into the culture media, equal aliquots of conditioned culture media from an equal number of cells were fractionated by 10% SDS PAGE, transferred to a Hybond ECL membrane (Amersham Biosciences, Buckinghamshire, England) and analyzed by Western blotting with a antibody against MMP-1 (Lab Frontier, Seoul, Korea) using enhanced chemiluminescence (Amersham Biosciences). To analyze MAPK activation, total cell lysates were prepared in a lysis buffer [25 mM Hepes (pH 7.7), 0.3 M NaCl, 1.5 mM $MgCl_2$, 0.2 mM ethylenediamine tetraacetic acid (EDTA), 0.1% Triton X-100, 0.5 mM dithiothreitol (DTT), 20 mM β-glycerolphosphate, 0.1 mM Na_3VO_4, 2 μg/ml leupeptin, 2 μg/ml aprotinin, 1 mM phenylmethylsulfonyl fluoride (PMSF), and a protease inhibitor cocktail tablet from Boehringer Mannheim (Indianapolis, IN)]. The protein concentrations were determined by Bradford assay using Bio-Rad Protein Assay reagents (Bio-Rad Laboratories, Hercules, CA). Equal amounts of protein samples were fractionated and transferred as described above and analyzed by Western blotting using phospho-specific antibodies against ERK1/2, JNK, and p38 MAPK (Cell Signaling Technology, Beverly, MA). As controls, the levels of the corresponding total MAPK were determined in the same samples using specific antibodies for ERK1/2, JNK and p38 MAPK (Cell Signaling Technology). Blotting proteins were visualized by enhanced chemiluminescence (Amersham, Buckinghamshire, England) and exposed to Kodak X-ray film. The band intensities were measured using Bio 1D software (Vilber Lourmat, Marne La Vallee, France).

Quantitative real-time RT-PCR

Total RNA was isolated using Trizol (Invitrogen, Carlsbad, CA) and 1 μg of total RNA was converted to cDNA using a First Strand cDNA Synthesis Kit (MBI Fermentas, Vilnius, Lithuania) according to the manufacturer's instructions. Quantitation of MMP-1, procollagen, COX-2, COX-1, IL-6, IL-1β and endogenous reference 36B4 cDNA was performed using a 7500 Real-time PCR System (Applied Biosystems, Foster City, CA). Data were analyzed using the 2(−Delta Delta C[T]) methods [56]. Data are expressed as the means ± SEM normalized to 36B4 and relative to the control sample. These experiments were carried out in triplicate.

Immunohistochemical staining

The frozen sections of 4 μm thickness were mounted onto silane coated slides (Dako, Glostrup, Denmark), then rehydrated in DW and endogenous peroxidase activity was quenched using 3% hydrogen peroxide for 10 min. The sections were then blocked with blocking solution (Zymed, San Francisco, CA) for 30 min, and washed and incubated with primary antibodies [anti-thymidine dimer antibody (Kamiya Co., Seattle, WA) or anti-MMP-1 antibody (R&D Systems, Minneapolis, MN)] in a humidified chamber at 4°C for 18 hr. After washing in PBS, they were incubated with biotinylated secondary antibody for 30 min, followed by horseradish-streptoavidin conjugate for 15 min. After a further washing in PBS, color was developed using AEC (3-amino-9-ethylcarbazole; Zymed).

Measurement of intracellular H_2O_2

Intracellular H_2O_2 levels were determined by measuring 2,7-dichlororofluorescein diacetate (DCFDA, Molecular Probes, Eugene, Oregon) fluorescence. HaCaT cells were cultured in DMEM until 80% confluent in 24-well plates, and starved with serum free DMEM for 24 h. Cells were pre-treated with $H(H_2O)_m$ m for 15 min, then irradiated with UV (55 mJ/cm^2) and post-treated with $H(H_2O)_m$ for 15 min in PBS. Subsequently, cells were treated with DCFDA (25 μM, freshly diluted in pre-warmed DMEM) for 30 min. Cells were then assayed using a fluorescence reader at an excitation wavelength of 488 nm and an emission wavelength of 515 nm. The fluorescence for DCF staining was detected at 485 nm/515 nm using a fluorescent microscope (Venox AHBT3/Q imaging system, Olympus, Tokyo, Japan). To normalize cell number, 4, 6-diamidino-2-phenylindole dihydrochloride hydrate (DAPI: 1 μg/ml, Molecular Probes) was used as a fluorescent marker for the nucleus with an excitation wavelength of 364 nm and an emission wavelength of 480 nm under a fluorescent microscope. The experiments were repeated at least three times per treatment.

Statistical analysis

Statistical analyses were performed using a Student's t-test. *p*-values of less than 0.05 were considered statistically significant.

Supporting Information

Figure S1 Schematic experimental design for the cell experiment.

Figure S2 Schematic experimental design for local application in human buttock skin.

Figure S3 Schematic experimental design for local application in aged human facial skin.

Author Contributions

Conceived and designed the experiments: MHS HN JHC. Performed the experiments: MHS YKK. Analyzed the data: MHS YKK JHC. Contributed reagents/materials/analysis tools: MHS HCK RP YKK. Wrote the paper: MHS JHC.

References

1. Smith WL, Meade EA, DeWitt DL (1994) Pharmacology of prostaglandin endoperoxide synthase isozymes-1 and -2. Ann N Y Acad Sci 714: 136–142.
2. Wlaschek M, Heinen G, Poswig A, Schwarz A, Krieg T, et al. (1994) UVA-induced autocrine stimulation of fibroblast-derived collagenase/MMP-1 by interrelated loops of interleukin-1 and interleukin-6. Photochem Photobiol 59: 550–556.
3. Kirnbauer R, Kock A, Neuner P, Forster E, Krutmann J, et al. (1991) Regulation of epidermal cell interleukin-6 production by UV light and corticosteroids. J Invest Dermatol 96: 484–489.
4. Konnikov N, Pincus SH, Dinarello CA (1989) Elevated plasma interleukin-1 levels in humans following ultraviolet light therapy for psoriasis. J Invest Dermatol 92: 235–239.

5. Ichihashi M, Ueda M, Budiyanto A, Bito T, Oka M, et al. (2003) UV-induced skin damage. Toxicology 189: 21–39.
6. Lavrovsky Y, Chatterjee B, Clark RA, Roy AK (2000) Role of redox-regulated transcription factors in inflammation, aging and age-related diseases. Exp Gerontol 35: 521–532.
7. Kim HJ, Jung KJ, Yu BP, Cho CG, Choi JS, et al. (2002) Modulation of redox-sensitive transcription factors by calorie restriction during aging. Mech Ageing Dev 123: 1589–1595.
8. Sarkar D, Fisher PB (2006) Molecular mechanisms of aging-associated inflammation. Cancer Lett 236: 13–23.
9. Kim MK, Chung SW, Kim DH, Kim JM, Lee EK, et al. (2010) Modulation of age-related NF-kappaB activation by dietary zingerone via MAPK pathway. Exp Gerontol 45: 419–426.
10. Fisher GJ, Voorhees JJ (1998) Molecular mechanisms of photoaging and its prevention by retinoic acid: ultraviolet irradiation induces MAP kinase signal transduction cascades that induce Ap-1-regulated matrix metalloproteinases that degrade human skin in vivo. J Investig Dermatol Symp Proc 3: 61–68.
11. Brenneisen P, Sies H, Scharffetter-Kochanek K (2002) Ultraviolet-B irradiation and matrix metalloproteinases: from induction via signaling to initial events. Ann N Y Acad Sci 973: 31–43.
12. Fisher GJ, Talwar HS, Lin J, Lin P, McPhillips F, et al. (1998) Retinoic acid inhibits induction of c-Jun protein by ultraviolet radiation that occurs subsequent to activation of mitogen-activated protein kinase pathways in human skin in vivo. J Clin Invest 101: 1432–1440.
13. Claret FX, Hibi M, Dhut S, Toda T, Karin M (1996) A new group of conserved coactivators that increase the specificity of AP-1 transcription factors. Nature 383: 453–457.
14. Chung JH, Kang S, Varani J, Lin J, Fisher GJ, et al. (2000) Decreased extracellular-signal-regulated kinase and increased stress-activated MAP kinase activities in aged human skin in vivo. J Invest Dermatol 115: 177–182.
15. Fisher GJ, Datta SC, Talwar HS, Wang ZQ, Varani J, et al. (1996) Molecular basis of sun-induced premature skin ageing and retinoid antagonism. Nature 379: 335–339.
16. Cooper SJ, Bowden GT (2007) Ultraviolet B regulation of transcription factor families: roles of nuclear factor-kappa B (NF-kappaB) and activator protein-1 (AP-1) in UVB-induced skin carcinogenesis. Curr Cancer Drug Targets 7: 325–334.
17. Kawaguchi Y, Tanaka H, Okada T, Konishi H, Takahashi M, et al. (1996) The effects of ultraviolet A and reactive oxygen species on the mRNA expression of 72-kDa type IV collagenase and its tissue inhibitor in cultured human dermal fibroblasts. Arch Dermatol Res 288: 39–44.
18. Wenk J, Brenneisen P, Meewes C, Wlaschek M, Peters T, et al. (2001) UV-induced oxidative stress and photoaging. Curr Probl Dermatol 29: 83–94.
19. Kitazawa M, Podda M, Thiele J, Traber MG, Iwasaki K, et al. (1997) Interactions between vitamin E homologues and ascorbate free radicals in murine skin homogenates irradiated with ultraviolet light. Photochem Photobiol 65: 355–365.
20. Scharffetter-Kochanek K, Wlaschek M, Brenneisen P, Schauen M, Blaudschun R, et al. (1997) UV-induced reactive oxygen species in photocarcinogenesis and photoaging. Biol Chem 378: 1247–1257.
21. Masaki H, Atsumi T, Sakurai H (1995) Detection of hydrogen peroxide and hydroxyl radicals in murine skin fibroblasts under UVB irradiation. Biochem Biophys Res Commun 206: 474–479.
22. Barber LA, Spandau DF, Rathman SC, Murphy RC, Johnson CA, et al. (1998) Expression of the platelet-activating factor receptor results in enhanced ultraviolet B radiation-induced apoptosis in a human epidermal cell line. J Biol Chem 273: 18891–18897.
23. Yasui H, Sakurai H (2000) Chemiluminescent detection and imaging of reactive oxygen species in live mouse skin exposed to UVA. Biochem Biophys Res Commun 269: 131–136.
24. Kang S, Chung JH, Lee JH, Fisher GJ, Wan YS, et al. (2003) Topical N-acetyl cysteine and genistein prevent ultraviolet-light-induced signaling that leads to photoaging in human skin in vivo. J Invest Dermatol 120: 835–841.
25. Quan T, Qin Z, Xia W, Shao Y, Voorhees JJ, et al. (2009) Matrix-degrading metalloproteinases in photoaging. J Investig Dermatol Symp Proc 14: 20–24.
26. Ohsawa I, Ishikawa M, Takahashi K, Watanabe M, Nishimaki K, et al. (2007) Hydrogen acts as a therapeutic antioxidant by selectively reducing cytotoxic oxygen radicals. Nat Med 13: 688–694.
27. Xie K, Yu Y, Zhang Z, Liu W, Pei Y, et al. (2010) Hydrogen gas improves survival rate and organ damage in zymosan-induced generalized inflammation model. Shock 34: 495–501.
28. Kawamura T, Huang CS, Tochigi N, Lee S, Shigemura N, et al. (2010) Inhaled hydrogen gas therapy for prevention of lung transplant-induced ischemia/reperfusion injury in rats. Transplantation 90: 1344–1351.
29. Lekic T, Manaenko A, Rolland W, Fathali N, Peterson M, et al. (2011) Protective effect of hydrogen gas therapy after germinal matrix hemorrhage in neonatal rats. Acta Neurochir Suppl 111: 237–241.
30. Huang CS, Kawamura T, Toyoda Y, Nakao A (2010) Recent advances in hydrogen research as a therapeutic medical gas. Free Radic Res 44: 971–982.
31. Fontanari P, Badier M, Guillot C, Tomei C, Burnet H, et al. (2000) Changes in maximal performance of inspiratory and skeletal muscles during and after the 7.1-MPa Hydra 10 record human dive. Eur J Appl Physiol 81: 325–328.
32. Hideo N, Rae-Eun P, Jun-Hyoun K, Inseon S, Junsang J, et al. (2007) Novel atmospheric pressure plasma device releasing atomic hydrogen: reduction of microbial-contaminants and OH radicals in the air. Journal of Physics D: Applied Physics 40: 501.
33. Lee Y, Kim H, Kim S, Shin MH, Kim YK, et al. (2009) Myeloid differentiation factor 88 regulates basal and UV-induced expressions of IL-6 and MMP-1 in human epidermal keratinocytes. J Invest Dermatol 129: 460–467.
34. Wang XY, Bi ZG (2006) UVB-irradiated human keratinocytes and interleukin-1alpha indirectly increase MAP kinase/AP-1 activation and MMP-1 production in UVA-irradiated dermal fibroblasts. Chin Med J (Engl) 119: 827–831.
35. Quan T, Qin Z, Xu Y, He T, Kang S, et al. (2010) Ultraviolet irradiation induces CYR61/CCN1, a mediator of collagen homeostasis, through activation of transcription factor AP-1 in human skin fibroblasts. J Invest Dermatol 130: 1697–1706.
36. Fisher GJ, Quan T, Purohit T, Shao Y, Cho MK, et al. (2009) Collagen fragmentation promotes oxidative stress and elevates matrix metalloproteinase-1 in fibroblasts in aged human skin. Am J Pathol 174: 101–114.
37. Briganti S, Picardo M (2003) Antioxidant activity, lipid peroxidation and skin diseases. What's new. J Eur Acad Dermatol Venereol 17: 663–669.
38. Kuhn M, Wolber R, Kolbe L, Schnorr O, Sies H (2006) Solar-simulated radiation induces secretion of IL-6 and production of isoprostanes in human skin in vivo. Arch Dermatol Res 297: 477–479.
39. Portugal-Cohen M, Soroka Y, Frusic-Zlotkin M, Verkhovsky L, Bregegere FM, et al. (2011) Skin organ culture as a model to study oxidative stress, inflammation and structural alterations associated with UVB-induced photodamage. Exp Dermatol 20: 749–755.
40. Wang SM, Shih TS, Huang YS, Chueh MR, Chou JS, et al. (2006) Evaluation of the effectiveness of personal protective equipment against occupational exposure to N,N-dimethylformamide. Journal of Hazardous Materials 138: 518–525.
41. Shih T-S, Kuo Y-C, Liang R-H, Liou S-H, Chang H-Y, et al. (2009) Assessment of airborne and dermal exposure to 2-ethoxyethyl acetate in an occupational environment. American Journal of Industrial Medicine 52: 654–661.
42. Berneburg M, Plettenberg H, Krutmann J (2000) Photoaging of human skin. Photodermatol Photoimmunol Photomed 16: 239–244.
43. Deliconstantinos G, Villiotou V, Stravrides JC (1995) Release by ultraviolet B (u.v.B) radiation of nitric oxide (NO) from human keratinocytes: a potential role for nitric oxide in erythema production. Br J Pharmacol 114: 1257–1265.
44. Burren R, Scaletta C, Frenk E, Panizzon RG, Applegate LA (1998) Sunlight and carcinogenesis: expression of p53 and pyrimidine dimers in human skin following UVA I, UVA I + II and solar simulating radiations. Int J Cancer 76: 201–206.
45. Katiyar SK, Perez A, Mukhtar H (2000) Green tea polyphenol treatment to human skin prevents formation of ultraviolet light B-induced pyrimidine dimers in DNA. Clin Cancer Res 6: 3864–3869.
46. Kim HH, Shin CM, Park CH, Kim KH, Cho KH, et al. (2005) Eicosapentaenoic acid inhibits UV-induced MMP-1 expression in human dermal fibroblasts. J Lipid Res 46: 1712–1720.
47. Yang B, Ji C, Kang J, Chen W, Bi Z, et al. (2009) Trans-Zeatin inhibits UVB-induced matrix metalloproteinase-1 expression via MAP kinase signaling in human skin fibroblasts. Int J Mol Med 23: 555–560.
48. Rittie L, Fisher GJ (2002) UV-light-induced signal cascades and skin aging. Ageing Res Rev 1: 705–720.
49. Quan T, He T, Voorhees JJ, Fisher GJ (2005) Ultraviolet irradiation induces Smad7 via induction of transcription factor AP-1 in human skin fibroblasts. J Biol Chem 280: 8079–8085.
50. Katiyar SK (2005) Silymarin and skin cancer prevention: anti-inflammatory, antioxidant and immunomodulatory effects (Review). Int J Oncol 26: 169–176.
51. Rundhaug JE, Fischer SM (2008) Cyclo-oxygenase-2 plays a critical role in UV-induced skin carcinogenesis. Photochem Photobiol 84: 322–329.
52. Shin MH, Rhie GE, Kim YK, Park CH, Cho KH, et al. (2005) H2O2 accumulation by catalase reduction changes MAP kinase signaling in aged human skin in vivo. J Invest Dermatol 125: 221–229.
53. Fisher GJ, Wang ZQ, Datta SC, Varani J, Kang S, et al. (1997) Pathophysiology of premature skin aging induced by ultraviolet light. N Engl J Med 337: 1419–1428.
54. Varani J, Warner RL, Gharaee-Kermani M, Phan SH, Kang S, et al. (2000) Vitamin A antagonizes decreased cell growth and elevated collagen-degrading matrix metalloproteinases and stimulates collagen accumulation in naturally aged human skin. J Invest Dermatol 114: 480–486.
55. Seo JY, Kim EK, Lee SH, Park KC, Kim KH, et al. (2003) Enhanced expression of cylooxygenase-2 by UV in aged human skin in vivo. Mech Ageing Dev 124: 903–910.
56. Livak KJ, Schmittgen TD (2001) Analysis of relative gene expression data using real-time quantitative PCR and the 2(-Delta Delta C(T)) Method. Methods 25: 402–408.

17

Photo-Oxidation Products of Skin Surface Squalene Mediate Metabolic and Inflammatory Responses to Solar UV in Human Keratinocytes

Vladimir Kostyuk[1,2], Alla Potapovich[1,2], Andrea Stancato[1], Chiara De Luca[1], Daniela Lulli[1], Saveria Pastore[1], Liudmila Korkina[1]*

1 Laboratory of Tissue Engineering & Skin Pathophysiology, Istituto Dermopatico dell'Immacolata (IDI IRCCS), Rome, Italy, **2** Biology Department, Belarus State University, Minsk, Belarus

Abstract

The study aimed to identify endogenous lipid mediators of metabolic and inflammatory responses of human keratinocytes to solar UV irradiation. Physiologically relevant doses of solar simulated UVA+UVB were applied to human skin surface lipids (SSL) or to primary cultures of normal human epidermal keratinocytes (NHEK). The decay of photo-sensitive lipid-soluble components, alpha-tocopherol, squalene (Sq), and cholesterol in SSL was analysed and products of squalene photo-oxidation (SqPx) were quantitatively isolated from irradiated SSL. When administered directly to NHEK, low-dose solar UVA+UVB induced time-dependent inflammatory and metabolic responses. To mimic UVA+UVB action, NHEK were exposed to intact or photo-oxidised SSL, Sq or SqPx, 4-hydroxy-2-nonenal (4-HNE), and the product of tryptophan photo-oxidation 6-formylindolo[3,2-b]carbazole (FICZ). FICZ activated exclusively metabolic responses characteristic for UV, i.e. the aryl hydrocarbon receptor (AhR) machinery and downstream *CYP1A1/CYP1B1* gene expression, while 4-HNE slightly stimulated inflammatory UV markers *IL-6, COX-2,* and *iNOS* genes. On contrast, SqPx induced the majority of metabolic and inflammatory responses characteristic for UVA+UVB, acting *via* AhR, EGFR, and G-protein-coupled arachidonic acid receptor (G2A).

Conclusions/Significance: Our findings indicate that Sq could be a primary sensor of solar UV irradiation in human SSL, and products of its photo-oxidation mediate/induce metabolic and inflammatory responses of keratinocytes to UVA+UVB, which could be relevant for skin inflammation in the sun-exposed oily skin.

Editor: Yoshiaki Tsuji, North Carolina State University, United States of America

Funding: This work was supported by the Italian Ministry for Health (Grant IDI IRCCS-2010). The funders had no role in study design, data collection and analysis, decision to publish, or preparation of the manuscript.

Competing Interests: The authors have declared that no competing interests exist.

* E-mail: l.korkina@idi.it

Introduction

Numerous mechanisms have been evolved in human skin to sense environmental stimuli and to mount adaptive responses in order to maintain homeostasis in the skin and protect the entire organism. The ultraviolet component of solar light consists of UVB and UVA parts, which differentially penetrate the skin barrier and thus affect prevalently epidermal (UVB) or dermal (UVA) skin cells and corresponding extracellular structures/molecules [1]. Skin surface lipids (SSL) play an important role for essential human skin functions such as mechanical and chemical barrier, thermoregulation, and photo-protection [1–3]. Laying on the surface of the skin, SSL are also exposed to the highest doses of UVA+UVB and they form the first-line defence against its potential danger. Major photo-protective components of SSL are α-tocopherol and squalene (2,6,10,15,19,23,-hexamethyl-2,6,10,14,18,22-tetracosahexaene, Sq), both working as sacrificing antioxidants, since they block photo-induced lipid peroxidation in cellular and acellular skin components, either by chain-breaking mechanism (α-tocopherol) [1], [4], [5] or by quenching singlet oxygen (Sq) [6]. Both are continuously produced by skin surface-open sebaceous glands to maintain their physiologically essential levels and substitute photo-destructed molecules [1–3]. Sq is the most abundant oxidisable component of SSL, its concentrations in adult human skin reaching up to 20%, while its levels are negligible in other organs [2], [7]. Upon action of environmental oxidants and microbial residents of the skin, fast oxidative degradation of Sq occurs giving rise to a wide spectrum of by-products, such as monohydroperoxides, epoxides, and aldehydes (Fig. 7A) [1], [2], [8]. Physiological doses of UVA oxidise Sq at much higher rates than UVB [1], [2]. The role of Sq and its oxidation products (SqPx) in skin photo-protection [9] and in the induction of inflammatory responses of keratinocytes in the context of acne pathogenesis [10] has been evaluated and recently reviewed in [2], [3].

The search of endogenous extracellular sensors of UV mediating its effects on skin cells has received growing interest in the last years. Products of tryptophan photo-oxidation, 6-formylindolo[3,2-b]carbazole (FICZ) in particular, were extensively studied and shown to mimic UVB in the induction of aryl hydrocarbon receptor (AhR)-controlled metabolic cascade in hepatocytes and HaCaT [11–13] , and of melanogenesis in melanocytes [14]. AhR is a cytosol-associated and ligand-activated receptor with transcription factor functions. Upon stimulation by a ligand, AhR liberates from its chaperon heat shock protein 90 (Hsp90), co-chaperon p23, and XAP-2 and moves to the nucleus, where it binds to its specific nuclear co-partner Arnt to acquire full binding capacity to the promoter of target genes, first of all *CYP1A1* and *CYP1B1*, to start the metabolic program [12], [13]. Over-expression of CYP1A1 and CYP1B1 enzymes has been detected in UVB exposed human skin [15]. As shown recently, the physiological role of AhR is not limited to the control of xenobiotic metabolism, but it extends to numerous cell functions such as breakdown of endogenous metabolites, proliferation, cell-to-cell contacts, immune and inflammatory responses, melanogenesis, and circadian rhythm [16], [17]. Among the endogenous AhR ligands known so far [18], [19], there are the products of tryptophan photo-oxidation [13], prostaglandins [20], bilirubin/biliverdin [21], and kinurenic acid [22], all of them present in the skin cells/cellular membranes.

Another UV-sensitive receptor is the epidermal growth factor receptor (EGFR), located on the cellular membrane of keratinocytes, which is a key regulator of numerous essential processes underlying skin development, homeostasis, stress responses, and repair [23–26]. 4-Hydroxy-2-nonenal (4-HNE), the final product of membrane-bound arachidonic acid photo-oxidation, appears to be a signalling molecule of UVB-induced EGFR nuclear translocation in keratinocytes [27–29], where the receptor physically or functionally interacts with other transcription factors with DNA-binding activity, including the signal transducer and activator of transcription 3 (*STAT3*). These events lead to the up-regulation of distinct genes controlling cell proliferation, DNA repair, as well as *COX-2* and *iNOS* [23]. Moreover, the cytoplasmic components of the EGFR system, the EGFR-ERK1/2 or EGFR-phosphoinositol-3-phosphate (PI3P)-protein kinase B (Akt1) pathways, are involved in the regulated expression of inflammatory chemokines in normal human keratinocytes [23], [25], [30], including CXCL8/IL-8, a chemokine sensitive to UV irradiation and reasonably involved in UV-induced granulocyte recruitment to the irradiated skin sites as well as in solar hyperkeratosis [25].

Upon skin exposure to UVB, both keratinocyte membranes and intercellular epidermal lipids containing linoleic acid are oxidised and 9-hydroxyoctadecadienoic acid (9-HODA) is formed. 9-HODA is a ligand for G-protein coupled arachidonic acid receptor (G2A) on the keratinocyte membrane [31]. G2A is a stress-inducible receptor for lisophosphatidylcholine and sphingosylphosphorylcholine [32] and for oxidized free fatty acids [31]. The 9-HODA-dependent activation of G2A leads to over-expression of pro-inflammatory cytokines-markers for UVB (IL-6, IL-8, and IL-1) [31], [33].

The major goal of the present study was the search for a first-line endogenous extracellular UV sensor(s) located in the outmost skin surface lipids (SSL). Here, we evaluated the role of Sq, a major photo-oxidisable component of SSL, in sensing solar UVA+UVB and transmitting their signal to underlying skin keratinocytes. We showed for the first time that photo-oxidised SqPx directly applied to primary human epidermal keratinocytes (NHEK) mimics the majority of UVA+UVB effects towards primary human epidermal keratinocytes (NHEK), by stimulating the AhR-controlled metabolic pathway and affecting EGFR- and G2A-connected inflammatory responses.

Materials and Methods

Ethics Statement

All experiments with human material (skin biopsies and skin surface lipids) were carried out in accord with Helsinki Declaration, the protocols were approved by Ethical Committee of Istituto Dermopatico dell'Immacolata, Rome, and the healthy adult donors signed the informed consent.

Skin surface lipid collection and analysis

SSL were obtained from sebum of 10 healthy adult male volunteers by non-invasive cup extraction method, by applying 10 ml diethyl ether on the upper dorsal skin with a glass cylinder with open ends (5.3 cm^2), allowing contact for 2 min. Then, the freshly collected SSL extracts were pooled, filtered, and evaporat-

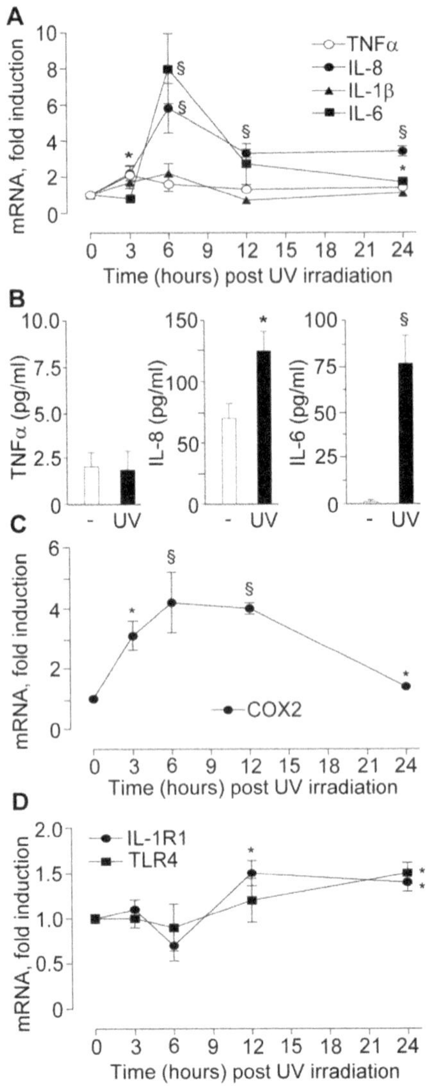

Figure 1. Inflammatory responses to UVA+UVB in normal human epidermal keratinocytes (NHEK). A. Time course of post-UV cytokine transcripts; **B.** TNFα, IL-6 and IL-8 proteins in the conditioned medium of sham-irradiated NHEK and 24 h post UVA+UVB irradiation (1.0+0.1 mJ/cm^2); **C.** Time course of post-UV *COX-2* transcript; **D.** Time course of post-UV *IL-1R1* and *TLR4* transcripts. *P<0.05 and §P<0.01*versus* sham-irradiated control.

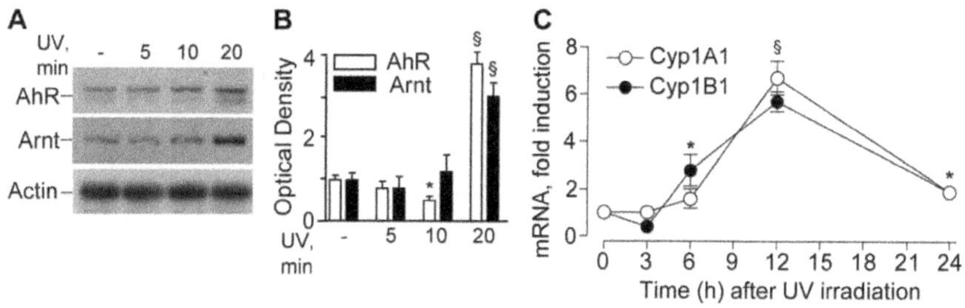

Figure 2. Time-dependent effects of UV irradiation on metabolic system in NHEK. A. Time-dependent effects on nuclear levels of AhR and Arnt post-UV irradiation. Actin was used as a loading control; **B.** Densitometry of western blot bands of AhR and Arnt in the nucleus; *P<0.05 and §P<0.01 *versus* untreated controls (-). **C.** Time-course of CYP1A1 and CYP1B1 transcripts post-irradiation; *P<0.05 and §P<0.01 *versus* untreated controls (0 h). Significance refers to both the transcripts at each time-point. The results are representative of three independent experiments.

ed under nitrogen flux [7]. SSL collection was performed during autumn-winter period to avoid effects of recent sun exposure. The SSL were derivatized at 80°C for 30 min by the addition of N,O-bis-(trimethylsylil)-trifluoroacetamide with 1% trimethylchlorosilane and analyzed by gas chromatography-mass spectrometry (GC-MS) on a SHIMADZU GC-17A/QP-5050, equipped with a J&W DB-1 capillary column (25 m×0,2 mm×0,33 μm). The following GC-MS parameters were used: 1 ml/min (helium) flux; split ratio, 1:10; injector temperature 250°C; detector temperature 270°C; temperature gradient: 100°C to 270°C in 33 min, peak detection method: selected ion monitoring technique [8]. All solvents, reagents, and standards of α-tocopherol, cholesterol, and squalene for GC-MS analysis were from Sigma-Aldrich (Milan, Italy).

Squalene isolation from skin surface lipids

Measured aliquots of SSL samples were separated by thin layer chromatography (TLC) with benzene/hexane (70/30) elution system, with commercial naïve and irradiated Sq (Sigma-Aldrich) as standards. The Sq fraction was extracted quantitatively with chloroform/methanol (2/1) from the silica spots of the SSL lane (Fig. S1), thoroughly filtered, evaporated and diluted in minimal quantity of methanol. To verify the purity of isolated Sq, the fraction was subjected to GC-MS analysis, and the typical spectrum (Fig. S2) showed more than 97% purity.

Cell cultures

Primary cultures of normal human epidermal keratinocytes (NHEK) were obtained from skin biopsies of healthy volunteers (n = 5) after their informed consent [30]. Keratinocytes were grown up to 60–80% confluence in serum-free medium, supplemented with hydrocortisone, EGF, insulin, epinephrine, transferrin, bovine pituitary extract, and gentamycin/amphotericin (KGM-Gold, Lonza, Walkersville, MD). In the 24 h preceding experiments, NHEK cultures were switched to supplement-depleted medium.

Irradiation of cells and skin surface lipids with solar simulated UVA and UVB

NHEK monolayer was exposed to low-dose UVA+UVB irradiation (time of irradiation 30 s, distance from cells 30 cm, dose UVA 1.0 J/cm^2+UVB 0.1 J/cm^2) produced by Solar Simulator (Dermalight Vario with filter A2, Dr. Hoehnle AG,

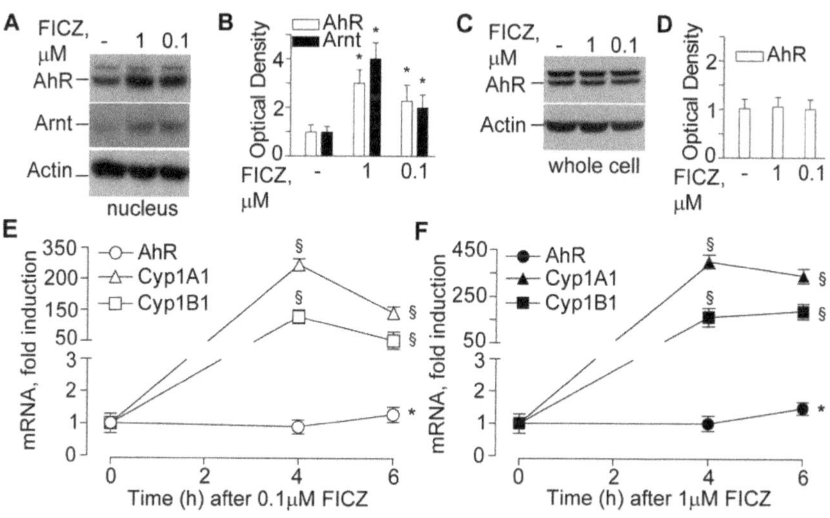

Figure 3. Effects of FICZ on metabolic system in NHEK. A. Western blots of nuclear AhR and Arnt after 30 min exposure to 0.1 or 1.0 μM FICZ. **B.** Densitometry of western blot bands. **C.** Western blots of total whole cell AhR after 30 min exposure to 0.1 or 1.0 μM FICZ. **D.** Densitometry of western blot bands. *P<0.05 and §P<0.01 *versus* untreated controls (-). Time-course of AhR, CypA1 and Cyp1B1 levels following treatment with 0.1 μM FICZ (**E**) and 1 μM FICZ (**F**). *P<0.05 and §P<0.01 *versus* untreated controls (0 h). The results are representative of three independent experiments.

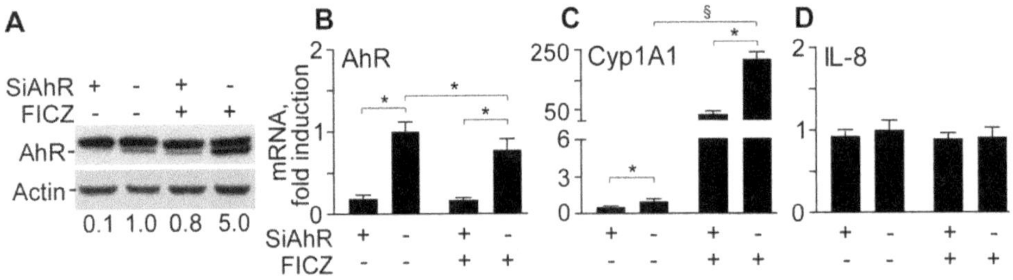

Figure 4. Effects of AhR silencing (SiAhR) on metabolic system and *IL-8* expression in NHEK. A. AhR levels in NHEK treated for 24 h with 1 μM FICZ. The treatment was started 48 h after initiation of RNA silencing of AhR (SiAhR) or mock (-). The mean values of the densitometry of AhR bands (three independent determinations) are reported. Levels of *AhR* (B), *Cyp1A1* (C) and *IL-8* (D) transcripts in NHEK treated for 24 h with 1 μM FICZ. *P<0.05 and §P<0.01.

UV Technology, Planegg, Germany) with emission spectrum from 280 nm and emission peak at 375 nm. The light effluence rate on the cell monolayer was 40 mW/cm^2.

In the *in vivo* experiments, dorsum skin of 10 healthy donors was exposed to the same UVA+UVB lamp (the distance 80 cm, irradiation time 30 min, dose UVA 30.0 J/cm^2+UVB 3.0 J/cm^2) and SSL were immediately collected and analyzed.

In the *ex vivo* experiments, dried-under-nitrogen SSL extracts (0,95 mg) were placed to glass Petri dishes (diameter 2 cm), and irradiated by the same UVA+UVB source (the distance from the bottom of dishes was 30 cm, irradiation time range 1–20 min, and dose range from UVA 1.0 J/cm^2+UVB 0.1 J/cm^2 to UVA 40.0 J/cm^2+UVB 4.0 J/cm^2). Immediately after irradiation, SSL extracts were dissolved in chloroform/methanol (2:1) with the addition of butylated hydroxyanisole to stop lipid peroxidation, and analyzed quantitatively for α-tocopherol, cholesterol, and squalene levels. Results of triplicate experiments were expressed as percent amount of α-tocopherol, squalene, or cholesterol in SSL as compared to non-irradiated controls. The same irradiation procedure was applied to commercial Sq, to use it as a reference standard of irradiated squalene for TLC and in the experiments with NHEK.

NHEK exposure to substances mediating UV effects

To simulate UV effects on AhR controlled metabolic pathways, 6-formylindolo[3,2-b]carbazole (FICZ, 0.1 μM and 1 μM, Biomol Research, Plymouth Meeting, CA), known to be an endogenous mediator of UV-induced signal transduction to AhR-driven machinery [11], [34], was added to NHEK cultures for 1 h.

In the experiments with 4-HNE (Cayman Chem, Ann Arbor, MI), reported to mediate UVB signaling to EGFR pathway in keratinocytes [27], [35], a 25 μM 4-HNE solution in DMSO or vehicle alone were added to NHEK. After 0.5–4 h of incubation, the conditioned medium was collected for further cytokine assay, while cells were processed for total lysate preparation and RNA isolation.

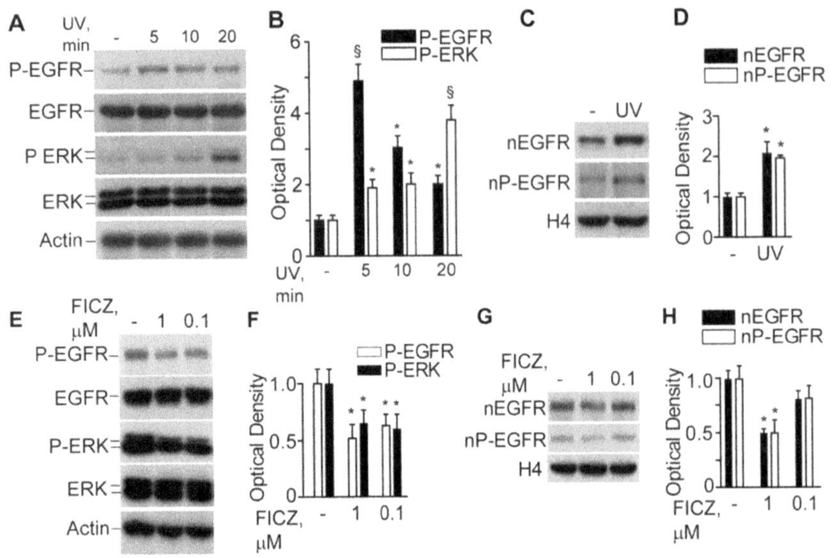

Figure 5. Effects of UV and FICZ on the EGFR signalling in NHEK. A. Western blot detection of the phosphorylated forms of EGFR (P-EGFR) and ERK (P-ERK) in total lysates of untreated NHEK (-) and post-UV irradiation; **B.** Densitometry of the bands. *P<0.05 and §P<0.01 *versus* untreated controls (-). **C.** Western blots of nuclear non-phosphorylated (nEGFR) and phosphorylated EGFR (nP-EGFR) before and 20 min after exposure to UV. Histone 4 (H4) was used as a loading control; **D.** Densitometry of nEGFR and nP-EGFR bands. *P<0.05 *versus* untreated control (-). **E.** Western blot detection of the phosphorylated forms of EGFR (P-EGFR) and ERK (P-ERK) in total lysates of untreated NHEK (-) and after 30 min exposure to 0.1 or 1.0 μM FICZ. **F.** Densitometry of the bands. *P<0.05 *versus* untreated control (-). **G.** Western blots of nuclear non-phosphorylated (nEGFR) and phosphorylated EGFR (nP-EGFR) after 30 min exposure to 0.1 or 1.0 μM FICZ; **H.** Densitometry of nEGFR and nP-EGFR bands. *P<0.05 *versus* untreated controls.

To elucidate possible SSL effects as sensors/mediators of solar UV signals to skin cells, NHEK cultures were exposed to the lipids normalized by the content of Sq, or SqPx isolated from *ex vivo* irradiated SSL, or SqPx-*in vivo* isolated from *in vivo* irradiated SSL (final concentrations of Sq, PxSq, or SqPx-*in vivo* were 1.0 μg/mL).

The effects of *tert*-butylperoxide and photo-oxidized linoleic acid (both from Sigma-Aldrich, Milan, Italy) were compared to the effects of photo-oxidized SSL and photo-oxidized Sq. *Tert*-butylperoxide was added to NHEK at two concentrations (0.1 mg/mL and 0.5 mg/mL). Linoleic acid was irradiated by UVA+UVB using the same protocol as for SSL, and the products of its photo-oxidation were added to NHEK at final concentrations 0.1 μg/mL and 0.4 μg/mL, the latter corresponds to the physiological ratio of squalene:linolenic acid % concentrations in SSL equal to 10:1 [2], [7]. The concentration of photo-oxidized linoleic acid 0.4 μg/mL corresponds to its 2 μM. The same molar concentration of PxSq was used in all experiments.

Transfection with AhR- specific small interference RNA

AhR was knocked-down by using a pool of four small interfering RNAs (siRNAs) provided by Euroclone (Milan, Italy) (ONTARGET*plus* SMARTpool, L-004990–00–0005). In parallel, a pool of four nontargeting siRNAs was used as negative control (ON-TARGET *plus* siCONTROL, D-001810–10–05). NHEK were incubated with a mixture of 50 nM SiRNA and 4 μL/mL INTERFERIN™ transfection reagent (Polyplus Transfection, Euroclone), according to the manufacturer's instructions. After 48 h incubation in starvation medium, SiRNA-transfected cells were exposed to FICZ for the indicated time interval. Cells were then lysed for protein extraction, or for RNA extraction.

Preparation of cell extracts and immunoblotting

Total non-phosphorylated and phosphorylated EGFR, ERK1/2, Akt1, and phosphorylated p65 subunit of NFκB were investigated in total cell lysates as previously described [36]. Anti-EGFR antibodies were from Santa Cruz, whereas anti-ERK, anti-Akt1, and anti-p65 NFκB antibodies were from Cell Signaling Technology (Beverly, MA).

NHEK were differentially lysed to obtain nucleic extracts according to [37]. The antibodies used for the detection of AhR, Arnt, non-phosphorylated and phosphorylated EGFR were from Santa Cruz Biotechnology, CA.

RNA isolation and quantitative real-time-PCR assay

Total RNA was isolated using the GenElute Mammalian Total RNA Kit (Sigma-Aldrich, Milan, Italy) and was reverse-transcribed using the iScript cDNA Synthesis Kit (Bio-Rad, Hercules, CA). cDNA was amplified with IQ SYBR green Supermix (Bio-Rad, Hercules, CA), using the MiniOpticon Real-Time PCR Detection System (Bio-Rad, Hercules, CA). Two housekeeping genes, ribosomal 18S and beta-actin were chosen as reference, and fold changes were calculated [38]. The primer sets were synthesized by Eurofins MWG Operon (Ebersberg, Germany):

β-actin fwd:5′-AATCTGGCACCACACCTTCTAC-3′; *β-actin* rev:5′-ATAGCACAGCCTGGATAGCAAC-3′; *18S* rRNA fwd:5′- TCCCCCAACTTCTTAGAGG-3′; *18S* rRNA rev:5′-GCTTATGACCCGCACTTAC-3′; *COX-2* frw:5′-TTCTCCTTGAAAGGACTTATGGGTAA-3′; *COX-2* rev:5′-AGAACTTGCATTGATGGTGACTGTTT-3′; *CYP1A1* frw:5′-CCTGGAGACCTTCCGGCACT-3′ ; *CYP1A1* rev:5′-AGACACAACGCCCCTTGGGG-3′ ;*CYP1B1* frw:5′-TGGTCTGTGAATCATGACCCAGTGA-3′; *CYP1B1* rev:5′-TCTTCGCCAATGCACCGCCT-3′; *G2A* frw: 5′-CGCACAGAGACAAAGTGGAA-3′; *G2A* rev: 5′-CTCATCTTCCCAAACGGAGA-3′; *IL1β* fwd:5′-TGGCTCATTTTCCCTCAAAAGTTG-3′; *IL1β* rev:5′-AGAAATCGTGAAATCCGAAGTCAAG-3′; *IL-6* fwd:5′-GTGTGAAAGCAGCAAAGAG-3′; *IL-6* rev:5′-

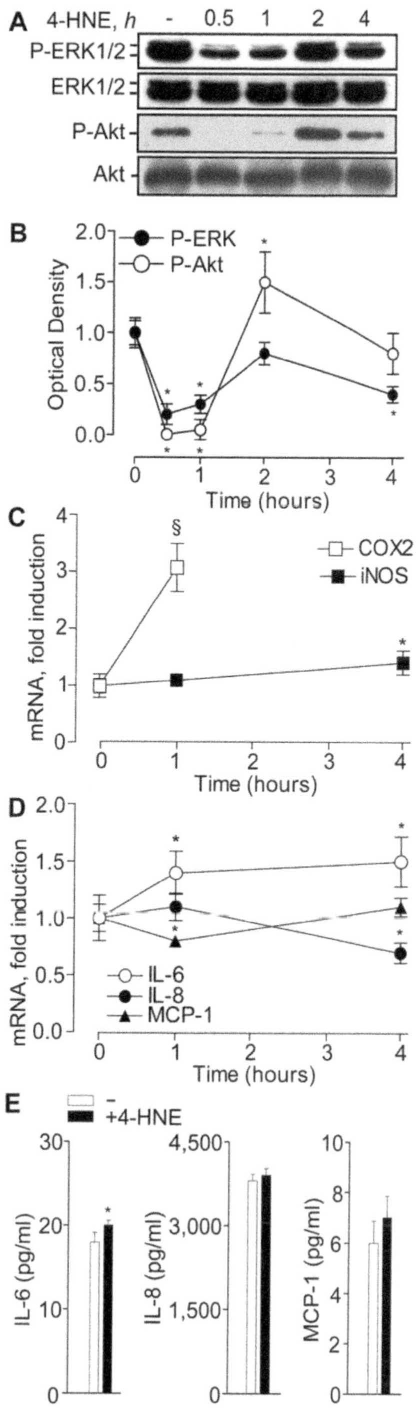

Figure 6. 4-hydroxy-2-nonenal (HNE) effects on signal transduction and expression of pro-inflammatory mediators in NHEK. Time-dependent effects of 25 μM HNE on ERK1/2 and Akt1 phosphorylation: **A**. Western blot and **B**. Densitometry of total cell extracts. Dynamics of HNE effects on COX-2 and iNOS (**C**) and pro-inflammatory cytokine (**D**) gene expression. Cytokine levels in the culture medium after 24 h treatment with 25 μM HNE (**E**). $^{*}P<0.05$ and $^{§}P<0.01$ *versus* untreated controls.

CTCCAAAAGACCAGTGATG-3′; *IL-8* frw:5′-GTCCTTGTT-CCACTGTGCCT-3′; *IL-8* rev:5′-GCTTCCACATGTCCTCA-CAA-3′; *IL-1R1* frw: 5′-CCAGAGGTCAGGAGTTCGAG-3′; *IL-1R1* rev: 5′-CCACCATGCCTAGCTCATTT-3′; *iNOS* fwd:5′- TACTCCACCAACAATGGCAA-3′; *iNOS* rev:5′-ATAGCGGATGAGCTGAGCAT-3′; *MCP1* frw:5′-AAGCA-GAAGTGGGTTCAGGA -3′; *MCP1* rev:5′-TAAAACAGGG-TGTCTGGGGA-3′; *MYD88* fwr: 5′-GAGCCTAACCATGT-CCCTGA-3′; *MYD88* rev: 5′-TGGGTCCTTTCCAGAGT-TTG-3′; *TLR4* fwd: 5′-AGTCCATCGTTTGGTTCTGG-3′; *TLR4* rev: 5′-CAATGGTCAAATTGCACAGG-3′; *TNFα* fwd:5′- TCCTTCAGACACCCTCAACC-3′; *TNFα* rev: 5′-AGGCCCCAGTTTGAATTCTT-3′.

Assays for inflammatory cytokine production by NHEK

The pro-inflammatory cytokines TNFα, IL-6, and IL-8 were measured in cell supernatants at 24 h post-irradiation or SqPx exposure, using BD OptEIA Elisa kits from BD Biosciences (San Diego, CA) [36].

Statistics

All measurements were done in triplicate, and data of at least three independent experiments were statistically evaluated. Statistical evaluation was carried out with the software package for Windows XP. Results were expressed as the mean ±SD. To evaluate the difference between experimental groups, the two-tailed Student's *t*-test was applied and P values<0.05 were considered to be significant.

Results

Physiological doses of solar simulated UVA+UVB induce inflammatory responses time dependently in NHEK

Exposure of NHEK to UVA+UVB led to time-dependent bell-shaped induction of genes encoding the pro-inflammatory cytokines *TNFα*, *IL-8*, and *IL-1β* and delayed induction of *IL-6* (Fig. 1A). Maximal although slight expression of *TNFα* and *IL-1β* was reached at 3 h, while the other pro-inflammatory cytokines were strongly and maximally expressed at 6 h. The protein level of TNFα did not change, whereas those of IL-8 and IL-6 were significantly increased in NHEK supernatants at 24 h post-irradiation (Fig. 1B). At 6 h, maximal expression of *COX-2* mRNA was observed (Fig. 1C). The mRNA expression of the two membrane receptors *TLR4* and *IL-1R1* was first temporarily suppressed and then, gradually increased up to 12–24 h (Fig. 1D).

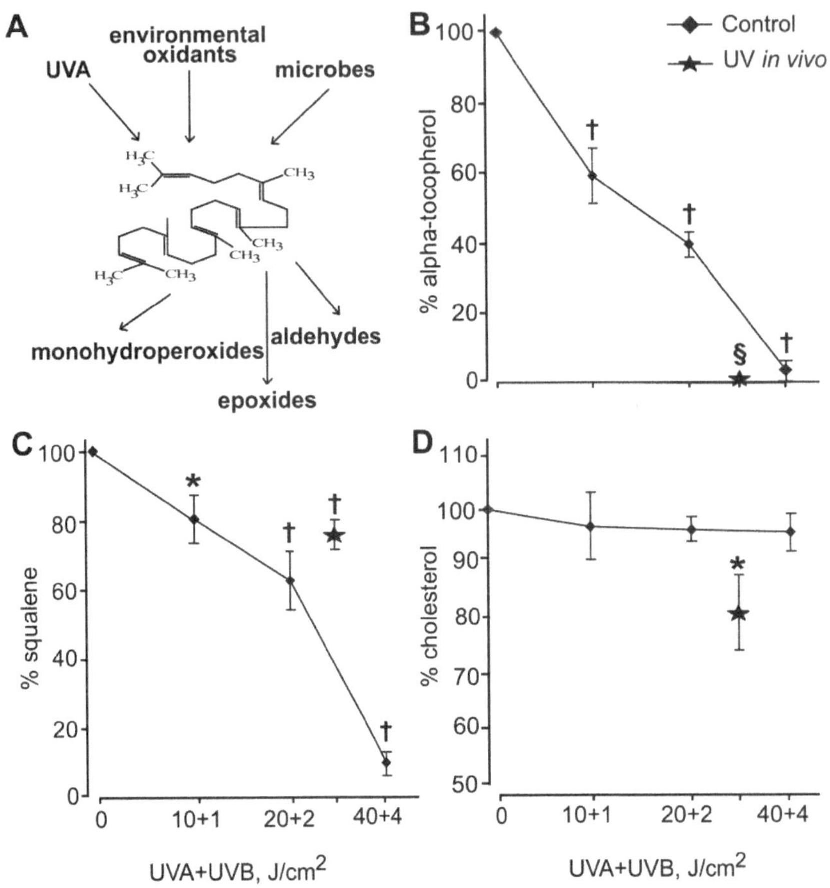

Figure 7. Degradation of UV-sensitive components of human skin surface lipids (SSL). SSL were *ex vivo* exposed to increasing doses of solar-simulated UV irradiation or *in vivo* exposed to cumulative dose of UVB+UVA = 3+30 J/cm^2. **A.** Scheme of SSL squalene oxidation; dose-dependent (UVA+UVB, J/cm^2) degradation of oxidisable SSL fractions **B.** Squalene; **C.** α-Tocopherol; **D.** Cholesterol. Stars represent results of *in vivo* exposure of healthy skin (n = 10) to solar-simulated UV light. *P<0.05 and †P<0.01 *versus* non-irradiated controls.

Physiological doses of solar simulated UVA+UVB activate AhR system and downstream cytochrome P450 isoforms CYP1A1 and CYP1B1

UVA+UVB irradiation stimulated AhR and Arnt nuclear translocation (Figs. 2A and 2B), an early event preceding the induction of *CYP1A1* and *CYP1B1* genes, which reached maximal levels 12h post-irradiation (Fig. 2C). AhR and Arnt nuclear translocation was significantly and dose-dependently triggered also by the product of tryptophan photo-oxidation FICZ (Figs. 3A and 3B). At the same time, total AhR protein level were not affected by FICZ (Figs. 3C and 3D), implying that the aromatic compound is an AhR ligand, which did not induce its *de novo* synthesis, but rather re-distributed the cytoplasmic receptor between nucleus and cytoplasm. Accordingly, both *CYP1A1* and *CYP1B1* were also strongly, dose-dependently up-regulated by FICZ, with maximal effect already achieved at 4 h (Figs. 3E and 3F). In addition, FICZ slightly but statistically significantly induced delayed *AhR* expression at 6 h (Figs. 3E and 3F). Upon AhR protein level knock-down by specific siRNA (Fig. 4A), both spontaneous and FICZ-associated AhR were dramatically down-regulated as expected (Fig. 4B), and correspondingly also CYP1A1 levels were remarkably reduced (Fig. 4C). Of note, constitutive IL-8 was not affected by AhR silencing or by the presence of FICZ (Fig. 4D). Similarly, FICZ did not perturb the expression of other pro-inflammatory genes, including TNFα, IL-6, and COX-2, the induction of which is characteristic of NHEK response to UV [33].

Physiological doses of solar-simulated UVA+UVB stimulate signal transduction through EGFR phosphorylation, downstream cytoplasmic signal transduction, and EGFR translocation to the nucleus

NHEK exposure to UV led to a rapid (5 min) and transient EGFR phosphorylation, while downstream ERK phosphorylation gradually increased up to 20 min post-irradiation when examined in total cell lysates (Figs. 5A and 5B). At 20 min post-irradiation, nuclear levels of both non-phosphorylated and phosphorylated EGFR were significantly increased (Figs. 5C and 5D). Conversely, exposure to FICZ did inhibit both EGFR and ERK in a dose-dependent fashion (Figs. 5E and 5F). Moreover, 1 μM FICZ significantly decreased nuclear levels of both non-phosphorylated and phosphorylated EGFR (Figs. 5G and 5H).

Exogenous 4-HNE dysregulates EGFR-connected signal transduction pathways time dependently, induces COX-2 expression but it only slightly affects pro-inflammatory cytokines and iNOS

We observed that a non-toxic dose of 4-HNE (25 μM), known to stimulate EGFR nuclear translocation and to mimic UVB effects on primary human keratinocyte cultures [29], inhibited downstream ERK and affected Akt1 phosphorylation in a biphasic fashion, with transient inhibition at 0.5 and 1 h, but stimulation at 2 h (Figs. 6A and 6B). With regard to inflammatory gene response, exposure to 4-HNE induced rapid and significant *COX-2* expression, slight and delayed *iNOX* (Fig. 6C), and durable although slight *IL-6* expression (Fig. 6D). None of the other EGFR-connected pro-inflammatory chemokines, *IL-8* or *MCP-1* or *IP-10* (data not shown), were affected by 4-HNE. Protein expression of IL-6, IL-8, and MCP-1 corresponded to their mRNA behaviour (Fig. 6E).

Squalene derivatives isolated from photo-oxidised skin surface lipids but not intact lipids/squalene induce UV-similar mRNA pattern of pro-inflammatory cytokines and receptors

Freshly collected SSL were exposed *ex vivo* to solar simulated low dose UVA+UVB irradiation for 5–20 min, and the content of UV-sensitive (α-tocopherol and Sq) and UV-insensitive (cholesterol) substances was monitored. *In vivo* skin irradiation with UVA+UVB (30+3 J/cm^2) also resulted in the degradation of photo-oxidisable components of SSL (Fig. 7B–7D).

Intact SSL, SSL irradiated *ex vivo* for 20 min (oxSSL), Sq isolated from intact SSL and from oxSSL (SqPx), and from *in vivo* irradiated SSL (SqPx-*in vivo*), as well as commercial Sq photo-irradiated for 20 min (Fig. S1), were normalised by Sq or SqPx content (1 μg/mL) and added to NHEK cultures. The purity of SqPx levels isolated from *ex vivo* or *in vivo* irradiated SSL was >99% (Fig. S2), and the levels of Sq or SqPx in SSL or oxSSL, respectively, ranged from 10 to 15%.

Fig. 8A shows that co-incubation of NHEK with intact SSL for 3 h practically did not affect gene expression of pro-inflammatory cytokines (*TNFα*, *IL-8*, and *MCP-1*) and only slightly induced *IL-6*. In addition, SSL did not exert any effect on *COX-2* (Fig. 8B) and *IL 1R1* mRNA, while it slightly down-regulated *G2A*, *TLR4* and its downstream co-activator *MYD88* (Fig. 8C). Sq isolated from intact SSL exhibited similar mode of action. On the other hand, oxSSL

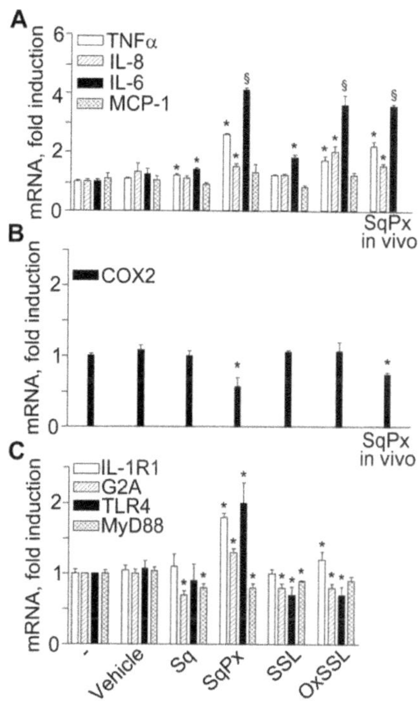

Figure 8. Effects of skin surface lipids on gene expression in NHEK. NHEK cultures were treated with skin surface lipids normalised by the content of squalene (Sq): intact freshly prepared skin surface lipids (SSL, with final Sq content 1 μg/mL), Sq isolated from the SSL (final content 1 μg/mL), SSL exposed to UVA+UVB for 20 min (oxSSL with final content of oxidised Sq (SqPx) 1 μg/mL), or PxSq isolated from oxSSL (final content of SqPx 1 μg/mL) or SqPx-*in vivo* isolated from the in vivo photo-exposed skin surface lipids (final content of SqPx-*in vivo* 1 μg/mL). The panels present fold of mRNA changes for pro-inflammatory cytokines (**A**), *COX-2* (**B**), and membrane receptors (**C**). *P<0.05 and §P<0.01 *versus* control treated with the vehicle for the lipids (0.1% methanol).

Table 1. Induction of inflammatory and metabolic genes (mRNA, fold of induction) by photo-oxidized commercial squalene and squalene from photo-oxidized human skin surface lipids (SSL).

Genes	Squalene isolated from photo-oxidized SSL	Photo-oxidized commercial squalene
TNF-alpha	2.5±0.10*	1.9±0.10*
IL-6	1.4±0.03*	1.6±0.06*
IL-8	1.5±0.12*	1.7±0.10*
CYP1A1	8.3±0.06†	4.2±0.26†

Commercial squalene or SSL were exposed to UVA+UVB irradiation (dose UVA = 20 J/cm^2 and UVB = 2 J/cm^2). Photo-exposed SSL were subjected to TLC and squalene containing spot was collected as per Materials and Methods. Squalene samples or 0.1% methanol (a vehicle for squalene) were added to NHEK cultures (final concentration - 1 µg/mL) for 3 h. Then, cells were thoroughly washed and RNA was isolated. Gene expression was determined by RT-PCR and results were expressed as a fold of induction versus vehicle. Three independent experiments were carried out and the mean values ±S.D. were calculated. *P<0.05 and †P<0.001.

up-regulated *TNFα*, *IL-6*, and *IL-8*, but it did not change *MCP-1* (Fig. 8A) or *COX-2* (Fig. 8B), *IL-1R1*, and *MYD88* expression, while it slightly inhibited *G2A* and *TLR4* (Fig. 8C). SqPx strongly up-regulated *TNFα*, *IL-6*, *IL-8*, *IL-1R1*, *G2A*, and *TLR4* (Fig. 8A and 8C), although it down-regulated *COX-2* and *MYD88* (Fig. 8B and 8C). SqPx-*in vivo* up-regulated *TNFα*, *IL-6*, *IL-8*, while down-regulating *COX-2* (Fig. 8A and 8B). The behaviour of commercial Sq upon UVA+UVB exposure was similar to SqPx (Table 1). It could be, however, noticed that photo-oxidized commercial Sq was less effective than Sq isolated from SSL exposed to the same dose of UVA+UVB. This could be explained by the fact that some lipids in SSL were co-oxidized with Sq thus accelerating its photo-oxidation. Also, trace amounts of transition metals, such as Fe and Cu, in SSL could catalyze photo-oxidation of Sq. Therefore, either more SSL squalene was photo-oxidized or deeper oxidation of SSL Sq (different oxidation metabolites) occurred as compared to pure squalene.

To evaluate whether hydroperoxides of photo-oxidized linoleic acid, which is a minor oxidizable component of human SSL [2], [7], could possess solar UV-mimicking effects similar to PxSq, photo-oxidized commercial linoleic acid was added to NHEK in physiologically relevant concentrations (0.1 and 0.4 µg/mL). Contrary to UV and PxSq, photo-oxidized linoleic acid inhibited *TNFα*, *IL-6*, *IL-8*, and *IL1R1*. Stimulation of *IL-8* expression occurred upon NHEK exposure to 0.4 µg/mL of photo-oxidized linoleic acid (Table 2). *Tert*-butyl hydroperoxide, a synthetic organic hydroperoxide traditionally used to model UVA effects on skin cells, at millimolar concentrations induced *TNFα*, *IL-8*, and *IL1R1* while suppressed *IL-6* (Table 2).

Skin surface lipids profoundly inhibit EGFR-ERK axis and activate AhR system, but exclusively SqPx up-regulates cytochrome P450 isoforms (CYP1A1 and CYP1B1)

All forms of skin surface lipids studied activated AhR translocation to the nucleus and the effect changed in the range: SqPx>SSL>oxSSL = Sq (Figs. 9A and 9B). Surprisingly, only SqPx and SqPx-*in vivo* up-regulated *CYP1A1* and *CYP1B1* genes, downstream targets for AhR (Fig. 9D). Both photo-oxidized linoleic acid and *tert*-butyl hydroperoxide significantly down-regulated *CYP1A1* and *CYP1B1* genes (Table 2). Several recent publications [34] have explained the initial transient inhibition of AhR nuclear translocation and *CYP1* expression by early transient activation of NFκB. Indeed, p65 phosphorylation was significantly induced only by oxSSL (Fig. 9C), while it did not stimulate *AhR* (Fig. 9B) or *CYP1* gene expression (Fig. 9D). The SSLs were also effective inhibitors of EGFR and ERK phosphorylation, SqPx being the strongest (Figs. 9A and 9C).

Discussion

Mechanisms of solar UV irradiation effects towards human skin have been the field of intense research mostly targeting UV-associated carcinogenesis and premature skin ageing [1], [5], [15], [38]. Based on the different capability of UVB and UVA light to penetrate in the epidermal and dermal layers, most of the studies

Table 2. Effects of photo-oxidized linoleic acid and *tert*-buthyl hydroperoxide (tBOOH) on the expression of solar UV-sensitive genes in cultivated primary human keratinocytes.

GENES	*TNFα*	*IL-6*	*IL-8*	*CYP1A1*	*CYP1B1*	*IL1R1*
SYSTEM						
Control	1.00±0.22	1.03±0.25	1.00±0.06	1.00±0.03	1.00±0.04	1.0±0.1
tBOOH, 0.1 mg/mL	14.70±0.36#	0.79±0.03	3.10±0.15&	0.01±0.00#	0.04±0.01#	1.40±0.03*
tBOOH, 0.5 mg/mL	25.60±0.85#	0.53±0.06	2.70±0.06&	0.01±0.00#	0.01±0.01#	1.30±0.06*
Photo-oxidized linoleic acid, 0.1 µg/mL	0.30±0.05*	0.61±0.01	0.40±0.06#	0.57±0.04#	0.81±0.02&	0.90±0.04
Photo-oxidized linoleic acid, 0.4 µg/mL	0.7±0.1	0.83±0.06	2.80±0.06#	0.20±0.02#	0.39±0.01&	0.70±0.00*

NHEK were incubated with photo-oxidized (see Materials and Methods) linoleic acid or with *tert*- butyl hydroperoxide (tBOOH) or with their vehicle methyl alcohol (0.02%, control) for 3 hours. Gene expression was determined by real-time PCR and results (fold of gene expression) are espressed as mean values ±S.D. of three independent experiments. *P<0.05, &P<0.01, and #P<0.001 versus control.

have been focused on the endogenous photo-receptors localised in the viable cellular compartments of the skin, such as DNA, urocanic acid, melanin precursors, porphyrins, tryptophan, dihydropyridins, etc. [2], [14], [39]. These cell-located molecules selectively absorb UV light within a distinct wavelength range and, in the presence of oxygen, initiate oxidative photo-reactions affecting cell signalling and enzymatic activities, which result in characteristic UV responses of the skin cells and UV-induced changes of extracellular skin matrix.

Lipid skin surface mantel represents the first-line protective barrier between solar UV and viable human skin structures: it directly and very effectively absorbs UVB and UVA rays [2], [5], inhibits free radical-driven lipid peroxidation (α-tocopherol and coenzyme Q_{10}) [1–4], and scavenges reactive oxygen species such as singlet oxygen (squalene) [6]. Here, we confirmed that at least two UV-sensitive SSL constituents, α-tocopherol and Sq, were dose-dependently degraded during exposure to solar-simulated UVA+UVB (Fig. 7).

The products of SSL photo-oxidation, such as Sq monohydroperoxides and epoxides (collectively, SqPx), aldehydes (Fig. 7A), and 9-HODA may easily diffuse in the skin depth reaching viable keratinocytes and melanocytes beneath *stratum corneum* [1], [2], thus exerting their UV-like biological effects. Indeed, SqPx was shown to induce melanocyte dendricity and melanogenesis [3] and IL-6 release from HaCaT [10]. Nuclear translocation of UVB-induced EGFR in primary human keratinocytes was mediated by 4-HNE [27], [35], and a UVB-like cytokine pattern was observed upon keratinocyte exposure to 9-HODA through UVB-like expression of *G2A* receptor [31]. Comparing data on direct UV-associated (Fig. 1) and photo-oxidised oxSSL- and SqPx-induced effects (Fig. 8) related to the expression of pro-inflammatory cytokines (*TNFα*, *IL-6*, *IL-8*, and *IL-1β*) or keratinocyte membrane receptors important for cytokine production (*IL-1R1* and *TLR4*), a striking similarity could be noticed. At the same time, the *TLR4* co-activator *MYD88*, essential for downstream gene transcription [25], [40] was down-regulated by the lipids. Also, in accord to published data on *G2A* up-regulation by UVB [31] , SqPx exerted similar action (Fig. 8C). Of importance, naive SSL collected from non-photoexposed human skin, as well as Sq isolated from these lipids were practically inactive, while SqPx alone induced the highest gene up-regulation as compared to the photo-oxidised lipid mixture oxSSL containing the same content of SqPx. We hypothesised that the complex mixture may also contain components such as linoleic acid with a mode of action opposite to SqPx. Characteristically, up-regulation of the secondary cytokine *IL-6* was slower upon irradiation than upon SqPx action (temporary down-regulation at 3 h in the latter case and a 4-fold up-regulation in the former), which suggests the necessity of UV-induced oxidative signalling molecules to start *IL-6* transcription [12]. With regard to induction of *COX-2*, another marker of UV response (Fig. 1C), exclusively SqPx exhibited opposite inhibiting action (Fig. 8B). *COX-2* [11], [23], [28], [29] as well as *iNOS* [23] expression is controlled by EGFR activation and nuclear translocation. In a good agreement with these data, solar-simulated UV induced fast (maximum at 5 min) EGFR phosphorylation (Figs. 5A and 5B), followed by downstream ERK phosphorylation (gradual increase until 20 min) and nuclear translocation of both EGFR and P-EGFR (Fig. 5C and 5D). Logically, time-dependent *COX-2* induction was observed. We hypothesised that inhibitory effects of SqPx and SqPx-*in vivo* towards COX-2 could be associated with inhibited phosphorylation (Fig. 9C), followed by inhibited nuclear translocation of EGFR. On contrast, very fast *COX-2* and *iNOS* induction was associated with NHEK exposure to non-toxic dosage of 4-HNE (Fig. 6C), able to mediate UVB-induced EGFR phosphorylation and translocation to the nucleus [28], [35]. Usually, *iNOS* up-regulation becomes detectable at 6 h post UV [41]. However, in the presence of the pre-formed redox mediator (4-HNE), a statistically significant difference was seen at 4 h. At the same time,

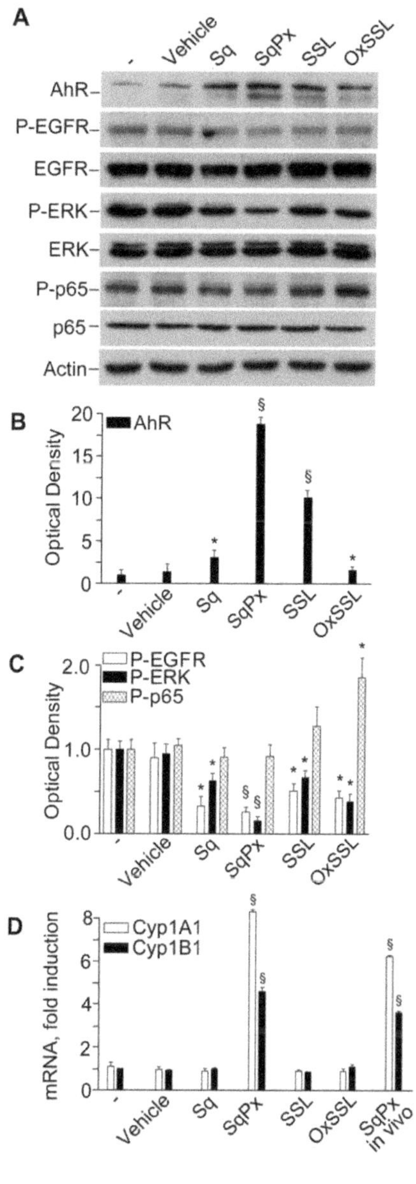

Figure 9. Effects of intact and UV-exposed skin surface lipids on signal transduction and AhR-CYP1 axis in NHEK. NHEK cultures were exposed to skin surface lipids normalised by the content of squalene (Sq): intact freshly prepared skin surface lipids (SSL, with final Sq content 1 μg/mL), Sq isolated from the SSL (final content 1 μg/mL), SSL exposed to UVA+UVB for 20 min (oxSSL with final content of oxidised Sq (PxSq) 1 μg/mL), or SqPx isolated from oxSSL (final content of SqPx 1 μg/mL), or SqPx-*in vivo* isolated from the in vivo photo-exposed skin surface lipids (final content of SqPx-*in vivo* 1 μg/mL). After 20 min of co-incubation, differential lysis was carried out, cytoplasmic and nuclear proteins extracted, and subjected to electrophoresis (**A**). Western blots were quantified by densitometry: (**B**) nuclear levels of AhR and (**C**) cytoplasmic levels of phosphorylated EGFR (P-EGFR), ERK (P-ERK), and the NFκB constituent p65 (P-p65). Transcripts of *CYP1A1* and *CYP1B1* were determined by RT-PCR at 3 h co-incubation (**D**). *$P<0.05$ and $^{\S}P<0.01$ *versus* control treated with the vehicle for the lipids (0.1% methanol).

4-HNE did not completely mimic UV in terms of inflammatory responses in NHEK, since it did not practically induce cytokines (Figs. 6D and 6E) while dramatically, although temporarily, inhibited ERK and Akt1 phosphorylation downstream EGFR (Figs. 6A and 6B).

The AhR has been suggested to be a light sensor in keratinocytes and melanocytes, since its transcriptional function and downstream CYP1 enzymes are activated by both visible and UV light, and mediated by endogenous high affinity AhR ligand FICZ, the tryptophan photo-product [11], [13], [14], [34]. Accordingly, in our hands solar-simulated UV time-dependently stimulated AhR machine (20 min, Figs. 2A and 2B), followed by CYP1A1 and CYP1B1 over-expression reaching maximum at 12 h (Fig. 2C). Similar events were induced by FICZ (Fig. 3) although maximal CYP1 expression was reached earlier (4 h). Experiments with AhR silencing showed that CYP1A1 expression was AhR-dependent (Figs. 4A and 4B), however, 1 μM FICZ slightly but significantly up-regulated AhR transcript at 6 h (Fig. 3D), but down-regulated this gene at 24 h (Fig. 4B), possibly due to negative feed-back mechanisms active in NHEK at this last time-point. Of utmost importance, we showed for the first time, that all the types of skin surface lipids studied induced nuclear translocation of AhR, although SqPx was the best, and oxSSL were the worst inducers (Figs. 9A and 9B). SqPx (approx. 1.5 μM) induced a much higher activation of AhR than FICZ (1 μM), therefore it can be regarded as a high affinity ligand for the receptor, as dioxin [13]. AhR activation resulted in an enhanced *CYP1A1/CYP1B1* expression only in the presence of SqPx (Fig. 9D). The strange co-incidence that both FICZ and SqPx also inhibited EGFR phosphorylation could be a hint on the possible involvement of EGFR in the mechanism of *CYP1A1/CYP1B1* induction. However, in our recent publication [36], we reported that resveratrol, being a strong inducer of AhR-CYP1 axis, did not suppress spontaneous or pro-inflammatory stimuli-induced EGFR phosphorylation. On these grounds, we concluded that EGFR pathway was not directly involved in the stimulation of classical AhR-CYP metabolic mechanism activated by both FICZ and SqPx. The induction of distinct inflammatory responses by SqPx could be EGFR-dependent in accord with previous publications [25], [30]. Repressed AhR and CYP1 in the presence of oxSSL corresponded to significantly activated NFκB (Fig. 9), probably induced by cholesterol oxidation products present in oxSSL [42–44]. Oxidative stress is known to induce NFκB pathway, whilst repressing AhR translocation and CYP1 transcription [34].

The AhR stimulation by UV initiates adaptive stress responses such as EGFR phosphorylation and internalization, and ERK phosphorylation (Figs. 5A–D) [11], *c-jun* induction [11] and cross talk with NFκB [34]. Redox regulation of UV-induced EGFR phosphorylation occurs due to oxidative inhibition of protein-tyrosine phosphatase activity [25], [28], and its nuclear translocation is controlled by 4-HNE [27], [28]. Phosphorylated EGFR binds cytoplasmic signal transduction proteins followed by activation of several pathways, such as phospholipase Cγ-protein kinase C, Ras-Raf-mitogen activated protein kinases, PI3K-Akt1, and STATs [23], [25], [30]. This complex UV-stimulated and EGFR-mediated molecular machine aims at adaptation to solar irradiation leading to cell survival and proliferation. Here, all chemical mediators of UV interaction with NHEK (FICZ, 4-HNE, and SqPx) profoundly inhibited spontaneous EGFR, ERK or Akt1 phosphorylation at 20 min. As it was previously shown by our group, deregulation of EGFR/ERK phosphorylation led to enhanced production of pro-inflammatory chemokines (IL-8, MCP-1, and IP-10) by NHEK [30], [33], [36]. Since the environmental contaminant benzo(a)pyrene [45] and plant-derived stilbenoids [36] induce redox-controlled IL-8 production *via* the AhR signalling pathway, we suggested the same mechanism for *IL-8* induction by SqPx and oxSSL (Fig. 8).

In general, a wide variety of lipid oxidation products such as 4-HNE [35], [42], cholesterol peroxides [44], enzymatically generated lipid hydroperoxides [46], and many others [43] have been considered endogenous signalling molecules for gene transcription. On these grounds, their roles in cell physiology and different human pathologies have been discussed. For the first time, we obtained convincing data that so far unidentified products of Sq photo-oxidation could also be regarded as lipid signalling molecules interacting with several transduction pathways in human keratinocytes. Of particular interest, Sq is present exclusively in the skin of humans, water apes, whales, otters, and other water mammals [47]. Its physiological role has been mainly discussed in terms of singlet oxygen scavenging, and thus photoprotection for the hairless human skin [2]. Our present data seem to open a new protective way of Sq action: the photo-oxidized metabolites of Sq are signalling molecules for keratinocytes, to mount adaptive/protective metabolic, proliferative, and inflammatory responses to the UV component of solar light. However, upon chronic exposure to UV or/and in the case of deregulated molecular pathways in the aged or pathological skin, photo-oxidized Sq may cause persistent inflammation and over-stimulated skin metabolism. These processes may well be further exaggerated in the oily skin, overproducing sebum Sq. Collectively, SqPx may be regarded as a novel molecular target for the prevention and treatment of UV-associated skin defects/pathologies, such as solar hyperkeratosis, acute and chronic inflammation, acne eruption, premature aging, and epidermal tumours. The exact mechanism and cellular specificity of SqPx action should be further elucidated.

Supporting Information

Figure S1 Thin layer chromatogram of the lipid fractions of SSL, performed with elution system as described in Materials and Methods. The squalene fraction is identified, and the width of the band isolated and extracted for experiments framed in the rectangle.

Figure S2 GC-MS total ion chromatogram (elution conditions as described in Materials and Methods section, scan mode) of squalene isolated from irradiated SSL, confirming the purity of the extracted band. SSL sample was derivatised by N,O-bis-(trimethylsylil)-trifluoroacetamide with 1% trimethylchlorosilane.

Acknowledgments

The authors are grateful to Dr. Paolo Fidanza for technical assistance.

Author Contributions

Conceived and designed the experiments: LK SP CDL. Performed the experiments: VK AP DL AS. Analyzed the data: LK SP CDL VK. Contributed reagents/materials/analysis tools: VK AP. Wrote the paper: LK SP.

References

1. Thiele JJ, Traber MG, Packer L (1998) Depletion of human stratum corneum vitamin E: an early and sensitive in vivo marker of UV induced photo-oxidation. J Invest Dermatol 110: 756–761.
2. De Luca C, Valacchi G (2010) Surface lipids as multifunctional mediators of skin responses to environmental stimuli. Mediators Inflamm doi: 10.1155/2010/321494.
3. Zouboulis CC, Baron JM, Bohm M, Kippenberger S, Kurzen H, et al. (2008) Frontiers in sebaceous gland biology and pathology. Exper Dermatol 17: 542–551.
4. Ekanayake-Mudiyanselage S, Hamburger M, Elsner P, Thiele JJ (2003) Ultraviolet A induces generation of squalene monohydroperoxide isomers in human sebum and skin surface lipids in vitro and in vivo. J Invest Dermatol 120: 915–922.
5. Thiele JJ, Barland CO, Ghadially R, Elias PM (2006) Permeability and antioxidant barriers in aged epidermis. In: *Skin Aging* edited by Gilchrest B and Krutmann J. Berlin-Heidelberg-New York: Springer, pp. 65–79.
6. Kohno Y, Egawa Y, Itoh S, Nagaoka S, Takahashi M, et al. (1995) Kinetic study of quenching reaction of singlet oxygen and scavenging reaction of free radical by squalene in n-butanol. Biochm Biophys Acta 1256: 52–56.
7. Passi S, Picardo M, Morrone A, De Luca C, Ippolito F (1991) Skin surface lipids in HIV sero-positive and HIV sero-negative patients affected with seborrheic dermatitis. J Dermatol Sci 2: 84–91.
8. Picardo M, Zompetta C, De Luca C, Amantea A, Faggioni A, et al. (1991) Squalene peroxides may contribute to ultraviolet light-induced immunological effects. Photodermatol Photoimmunol Photomed 8: 105–110.
9. Ryu A, Arakane C, Koide H, Nagano T (2009) Squalene as a target molecule in skin hyperpigmentation caused by singlet oxygen. Biol Pharm Bull 32: 1504–1509.
10. Ottaviani M, Alestas T, Flori E, Mastrofrancesco A, Zouboulis CC, et al. (2006) Peroxidated squalene induces the production of inflammatory mediators in HaCaT keratinocytes: a possible role in acne vulgaris. J Invest Dermatol 126: 2430–2437.
11. Fritsche E, Schafer C, Calles C, Bernsmann T, Bernshausen T, et al. (2007) Lightening up the UV response by identification of the arylhydrocarbon receptor as a cytoplasmic target for ultraviolet B radiation. Proc Nat Acad Sci USA 104, 8851–8856.
12. Rannug A (2010) The tryptophan photoproduct 6-formylindolo[3,2-b]carbazole helps genes jump. Proc Natl Acad Sci USA 107: 18239–18240.
13. Rannug A, Fritsche E (2006) The aryl hydrocarbon receptor and light. Biol Chem 387: 1149–1157.
14. Luecke S, Backlund M, Jux B, Esser C, Krutmann J, et al. (2010) Aryl hydrocarbon receptor (AHR), a novel regulator of human melanogenesis. Pigment Cell Melanoma Res 23: 828–833.
15. Katiyar SK, Matsui MS, Mukhtar H (2000) Uvtraviolet-B exposure of human skin induces cytochromes P450 1A1 and 1B1. J Invest Dermatol 114: 328–333.
16. Oesch-Bartolomowicz B, Oesch F (2009) Role of cAMP in mediating AHR signaling. Biochem Pharmacol 77. 627–641.
17. Vondracek J, Umannova L, Machala M (2011) Interactions of the aryl hydrocarbon receptor with inflammatory mediators: beyond CYP1A regulation. Curr Drug Metab 12: 89–103.
18. Nguyen LP, Bradfield CA (2008) The search for endogenous activators of aryl hydrocarbon receptor. Chem Res Toxicol 21: 102–116.
19. Stejskalova L, Dvorak Z, Pavek P (2011) Endogenous and exogenous ligands of aryl hydrocarbon receptor: current state of art. Curr Drug Metab 12: 198–212.
20. Seidel SD, Winters GM, Rogers WJ, Ziccardi MH, Keser B, et al. (2001) Activation of the Ah receptor signaling pathway by prostaglandins. J Biochem Mol Toxicol 15: 187–196.
21. Phelan D, Winter GM, Rogers WJ, Lam JC, Denison MS (1998) Activation of the Ah receptor signal transduction pathway by bilirubin and biliverdin. Arch Biochem Biophys 357: 155–163.
22. Di Natale BC, Murray IA, Schroeder JC, Flaveny CA, Lahoti TS, et al. (2010) Kinurenic acid is a potent endogenous aryl hydrocarbon receptor ligand that synergistically induces interleukin-6 in the presence of inflammatory signaling. J Biol Chem 285: 24388–24397.
23. Lin SY, Makino K, Matin A, Wen Y, Kwong KY, et al. (2001) Nuclear localization of EGF receptor and its potential new role as a transcription factor. Nat Cell Biol 3: 802–808.
24. Martinez-Carpio PA, Trelles MA (2010) Cutaneous epidermal growth factor receptor system following ultraviolet irradiation: exploring the role of molecular mechanisms. Photodermatol Photoimmunol Photomed 26: 250–256.
25. Pastore S, Mascia F, Mariani V, Girolomoni G (2008) The epidermal growth factor receptor system in skin repair and inflammation. J Invest Dermatol 128: 1365–1374.
26. Sutter CH, Yin H, Li Y, Mammen JS, Bodreddigari S, et al. (2009) EGF receptor signaling blocks aryl hydrocarbon receptor-mediated transcription and cell differentiation in human epidermal keratinocytes. Proc Natl Acad Sci USA 106: 4266–4271.
27. Liu W, Akhand AA, Kato M, Yokoyama I, Miyata T, et al. (1999) 4-hydroxynonenal triggers an epidermal growth factor-linked signal pathway for growth inhibition. J Cell Sci 112: 2409–2417.
28. Xu Y, Shao Y, Voorhees JJ, Fisher GJ (2006) Oxidative inhibition of receptor-type protein-tyrosine phosphatase k by ultraviolet irradiation activates epidermal growth factor receptor in human keratinocytes. J Biol Chem 281: 27389–27397.
29. Xu Y, Shao Y, Zhou J, Voorhees JJ, Fisher GJ (2009) Ultraviolet irradiation-induced epidermal growth factor receptor (EGFR) nuclear translocation in human keratinocytes. J Cell Biochem 107: 873–880.
30. Pastore S, Mascia F, Mariotti F, Dattilo C, Mariani V, et al. (2005) ERK1/2 regulates epidermal chemokine expression and skin inflammation. J Immunol 174: 5047–5056.
31. Hattori T, Obinata H, Ogawa A, Kishi M, Tatei K, et al. (2008) G2A plays proinflammatory roles in human keratinocytes under oxidative stress as a receptor for 9-hydroxyoctadecadienoic acid. J Invest Dermatol 128: 1123–1133.
32. Kabarowski JH, Zhu K, Le LQ, Witte ON, Xu Y (2001) Lysophosphtidylcholine as a ligand for the immunoregulatory receptor G2A. Science 293: 702–705.
33. Pastore S, Lulli D, Fidanza P, Potapovich AI, Kostyuk VA, et al. (2012) Plant polyphenols regulate chemokine expression and tissue repair in human keratinocytes through interaction with cytoplasmic and nuclear components of epidermal growth factor system. Antioxid Redox Signal 16: 314–328.
34. Luecke S, Wincent E, Backlund M, Rannug U, Rannug A (2010) Cytochrome P450 1A1 gene regulation by UVB involves crosstalk between the aryl hydrocarbon receptor and nuclear factor kB. Chem Biol Interact 184: 466–473.
35. Uchida K, Shiraishi M, Naito Y, Torii Y, Nakamura Y, et al. (1999) Activation of stress signaling pathways by the end product of lipid peroxidation. J Biol Chem 274: 2234–2242.
36. Potapovich AI, Lulli D, Fidanza P, Kostyuk VA, De Luca C, et al. (2011) Plant polyphenols differentially modulate inflammatory responses of human keratinocytes by interfering with activation of transcription factors NFkB and AhR and EGFR-ERK pathway. Toxicol Appl Pharmacol 255: 138–149.
37. Schreiber E, Matthias P, Muller MM, Schaffner W (1989) Rapid detection of octamer binding proteins with mini-extracts, prepared from a small number of cells. Nucl Acid Res 17: 6419–6424.
38. Livak KJ, Schmittgen TD (2001) Analysis of relative gene expression data using real-time quantitative PCR and the 2(-Delta Delta C(T)) method. Methods 25: 402–408.
39. Lamore SD, Azimian S, Horn D, Anglin BL, Cabello CM, et al. (2010) The malonyldialdehyde-derived fluorophore DHP-lysine is a potent sensitizer of UVA-induced photooxidative stress in human skin cells. J Photochem Photobiol B 101: 251–264.
40. McInturff JE, Modlin RL, Kim J (2005) The role of Toll-like receptors in the pathogenesis and treatment of dermatological diseases. J Invest Dermatol 125: 1–8.
41. Liu W, Wu S (2010) Differential roles of nitric oxide synthases in regulation of ultraviolet B light-induced apoptosis. Nitric Oxide 23: 199–205.
42. Leonarduzzi G, Robbesiyn F, Poli G (2004) Signaling kinases modulated by 4-hydroxynonenal. Free Rad Biol Med 37: 1694–1702.
43. Poli G, Leonarduzzi G, Biasi F, Chiarpotto E (2004) Oxidative stress and cell signalling. Curr Med Chem 11: 1163–1182.
44. Sottero B, Gamba P, Gargiulo S, Leonarduzzi G, Poli G (2009) Cholesterol oxidation products and disease: an emerging topic of interest in medicinal chemistry. Curr Med Chem 16: 685–705.
45. Tsuji G, Takahara M, Uchi H, Takeuchi S, Mitoma C, et al. (2011) An environmental contaminant, benzo(a) pyrene, induces oxidative stress-mediated interleukin-8 production in human keratinocytes via aryl hydrocarbon receptor signaling pathway. J Dermatol Sci 62: 42–49.
46. Brigelius-Flohè R, Flohè L (2011) Basic principles and emerging concepts in the redox control of transcription factors. Antioxid Redox Signal 15: 2335–2381.
47. Nicolaides N, Fu HC, Rice GR (1968) The skin surface lipids of man compared with those of eighteen species of animals. J Invest Dermatol 51: 83–89.

18

Gender Affects Skin Wound Healing in Plasminogen Deficient Mice

Birgitte Rønø[1,2], Lars Henning Engelholm[3], Leif Røge Lund[2], Andreas Hald[2,3,4]*

1 Center for Molecular Pathology, Department of Laboratory Medicine, Lund University, Malmo, Sweden, **2** Department of Cellular and Molecular Medicine, Faculty of Health Sciences, University of Copenhagen, Copenhagen, Denmark, **3** Finsen Laboratory, Rigshospitalet, Copenhagen, Denmark, **4** Biotech Research and Innovation Centre, University of Copenhagen, Copenhagen, Denmark

Abstract

The fibrinolytic activity of plasmin plays a fundamental role in resolution of blood clots and clearance of extravascular deposited fibrin in damaged tissues. These vital functions of plasmin are exploited by malignant cells to accelerate tumor growth and facilitate metastases. Mice lacking functional plasmin thus display decreased tumor growth in a variety of cancer models. Interestingly, this role of plasmin has, in regard to skin cancer, been shown to be restricted to male mice. It remains to be clarified whether gender also affects other phenotypic characteristics of plasmin deficiency or if this gender effect is restricted to skin cancer. To investigate this, we tested the effect of gender on plasmin dependent immune cell migration, accumulation of hepatic fibrin depositions, skin composition, and skin wound healing. Gender did not affect immune cell migration or hepatic fibrin accumulation in neither wildtype nor plasmin deficient mice, and the existing differences in skin composition between males and females were unaffected by plasmin deficiency. In contrast, gender had a marked effect on the ability of plasmin deficient mice to heal skin wounds, which was seen as an accelerated wound closure in female versus male plasmin deficient mice. Further studies showed that this gender effect could not be reversed by ovariectomy, suggesting that female sex-hormones did not mediate the accelerated skin wound healing in plasmin deficient female mice. Histological examination of healed wounds revealed larger amounts of fibrotic scars in the provisional matrix of plasmin deficient male mice compared to female mice. These fibrotic scars correlated to an obstruction of cell infiltration of the granulation tissue, which is a prerequisite for wound healing. In conclusion, the presented data show that the gender dependent effect of plasmin deficiency is tissue specific and may be secondary to already established differences between genders, such as skin thickness and composition.

Editor: Stefan Strack, University of Iowa, United States of America

Funding: The authors would like to acknowledge the following foundations for their financial support: The Lundbeck Foundation, The Danish Cancer Society, Cancerforskningsfonden af 1989, Ludvig og Franciska Andersens Legat, Dagmar Marshalls Foundation, Fabrikant Einar Willumsens Mindelegat, Aase og Ejnar Danielsens Fond. The funders had no role in study design, data collection and analysis, decision to publish, or preparation of the manuscript.

Competing Interests: The authors have declared that no competing interests exist.

* E-mail: ahald@finsenlab.dk

Introduction

The fibrinolytic activity of plasmin, the active form of the zymogen, plasminogen (Plg), is important for mucosal membrane maintenance and organ function. In humans, loss of plasmin dependent fibrinolysis leads to abnormal wound healing and development of pseudo membranes on mucosal tissues throughout the body. The gastrointestinal tract, respiratory system, and genitourinary tract are often strongly affected, which may ultimately lead to organ failure and increased morbidity. However, the most noticeable clinical syndrome in these patients is ligneous conjunctivitis represented by fibrin rich lesions on the eyelids, which may be resolved by local treatment with Plg [1,2]. Similarly, mice that harbor deficient Plg alleles ($Plg^{-/-}$) develop normally into adulthood but will eventually suffer from inflammatory lesions and ulcers throughout the gastrointestinal tract, lungs, and reproductive organs [3]. The progressive deformation of these organs results in organ dysfunction and wasting of the animals, which rarely live for more than 30 weeks. In addition to these syndromes, fibrin depositions, which are associated with infiltration of inflammatory cells, accumulate in the liver throughout the lifespan of $Plg^{-/-}$ mice [3,4]. Moreover, wound healing in humans with plasmin deficiency and in $Plg^{-/-}$ mice is severely retarded and associated with accumulation of fibrin in the provisional matrix [5,6]. Studies in mice have also shown that the initial recruitment of immune cells to an inflamed tissue is dependent on Plg [7], though the role of fibrin in this setting is not established and may vary according to choice of model. During the past decade, plasmin has been shown capable of activating matrix tethered growth factors and other extracellular proteases [8,9]. These functions may be important during the process of tissue reconstruction following chemical or physical damage as a result of e.g. chemotherapy [10]. During such processes, a large number of extracellular proteases are actively present, and some of these share, besides their expression pattern, also substrates [11,12]. Thus the specific contribution of individual proteases in the intricate system of extracellular proteolysis during a biological event is a challenge to identify [13,14].

Besides the important functions of plasmin in maintaining homeostasis and tissue integrity, plasmin and the Plg activation (PA) system also mediate pathological processes, such as tumor growth and cancer metastasis [15]. The mechanism linking the

PA-system to these malignant events varies according to the tissue of origin and to the metastatic site [15,16]. Depending on these factors, the function of the PA system has been shown to involve clearance of extracellular matrix, release/activation of tumor growth factors, and securing the patency of the tumor vasculature [15,17]. Recently, it was demonstrated that skin tumor growth in mice was retarded by the absence of plasmin driven fibrinolysis, which serves to clear tumor thrombosis and maintain a sufficient blood supply to the growing tumors [18]. Surprisingly, this effect of plasmin was restricted to male mice and thereby suggesting that $Plg^{-/-}$ female mice are not prone to the same decree of tumor thrombosis or can resolve fibrin clots by expressing fibrinolytic protease(s) besides plasmin. Alternatively, the endogenous differences in skin composition between genders could be responsible for the different effects of plasmin deficiency on skin tumor growth in male and female mice.

We here describe a systematic investigation of the phenotype of Plg deficiency in male and female mice, and reveal an effect of gender that is restricted to the skin. This gender effect could not be resolved by ovariectomy (OVX) thus suggesting that it is likely linked to variations in skin composition and less likely to a hormone dependent expression of a fibrinolytic protease.

Materials and Methods

Ethics Statement

All experimental animals were monitored daily by trained animal caretakers. Animals showing signs of distress were euthanized by cervical dislocation. All experiments were conducted according to institutional and national guidelines. The experiments performed in the current project were specifically approved by the Danish Animal Experiments Inspectorate (permit number 2010-561-1778). Following the experiments, animals were euthanized by anaesthetizing using hypnorm/dormicum (fentanyl 0.1 mg/ml, fluanison 5 mg/ml, midazolam 5 mg/ml) followed by perfusion, as described below.

Animal Breeding

Both FVB/n and C57Bl/6 mice were used for wound healing studies. Tissue libraries were derived from FVB/n mice [4]. The thioglycollate (TG) induced peritonitis experiments were performed in C57Bl/6 mice. The FVB/n $Plg^{-/-}$ mice and their littermate controls were generated by breeding heterozygous mice ($Plg^{-/+}$), that had been backcrossed into an FVB/n background for at least 30 generations (Panum Institute, Copenhagen, Denmark). C57Bl/6 $Plg^{-/+}$ mice were likewise backcrossed for at least 30 generations into the C57Bl/6 background. All mice were bred in the SPF facility at University of Copenhagen and during experimentation they were housed individually. Genotyping was performed as previously described [18] and following the experiments all used mice were regenotyped.

Ovariectomy

Mice of approximately five weeks of age were anaesthetized using hypnorm/dormicum and the ovaries were excised as previously described [18]. Briefly, the ventral skin and muscle tissue were cut with scissors and the ovaries resected and the wound suturated. Similar sham surgeries were performed in both male and female mice. One week following OVX, incisional wounding was performed as described below. At the termination of the experiment, successful OVX was confirmed by isolating and weighing the uteri.

Incisional Wounds

Six weeks old mice were used for incisional wound healing studies as described previously [4]. Briefly, mice were anaesthetized with hypnorm/dormicum and a 20 mm long full skin thickness incision was made along the dorsal midline. The mice were housed individually and wound lengths were measured every other day until healed, defined as complete wound closure and full restoration of the epidermis (termed reepithelialization). At this point, the mice were euthanized with hypnorm/dormicum and perfused with 10 ml phosphate buffered saline (PBS) followed by 10 ml of a 4% paraformaldehyde solution (PFA). Next, the wounded skin areas were isolated with scissors and the tissues were incubated overnight in 4% PFA and then transferred to 70% ethanol and kept at 4̊C until further processed and embedded in paraffin.

Thioglycollate Induced Peritonitis

Six weeks old mice were injected intraperitoneally (IP) with 1 ml of a 3.85% TG brew (Difco, BD, Denmark, Cat.# 243210), which had been incubated for at least four weeks at 4°C. After three days, the mice were anaesthetized with hypnorm/dormicum, the abdominal skin removed leaving behind the abdominal muscle tissue, and the mice were then injected IP with 4 ml PBS and gently shaken on a lab vibrator for 1 min. The lavage fluid was harvested and the cell concentration was defined using an automated cell counter (NucleoCounter NC-100, ChemoMetec, Allerød, Denmark).

Liver and Skin Samples

Liver and skin samples from naïve wildtype (Wt) and $Plg^{-/-}$ mice were derived from a tissue collection containing samples isolated from mice with an age of eight, 12 and 26 weeks [4].

Histology

Paraffin embedded tissues were sectioned, rehydrated and stained using a standard H&E staining protocol. For immunohistochemical detection of fibrin(ogen) and CD34, the following antibodies were used: rabbit-anti-mouse fibrin(ogen) [19] diluted 1:2000 and rat-anti CD34 (HyCult Biotech, Uden, the Netherlands, HM1015-3915M12) diluted 1:100, followed by incubation with a rabbit-anti-rat antibody (Dako, Glostrup, Denmark, K, E468) diluted 1:100. Chromogen staining was achieved using the $EnVision^{+}$ system (Dako, Glostrup, Denmark, K4003) in combination with NovaRED HRP substrate (VWR international, Herlev, Denmark, SK-4800). Stained sections were scanned using a motorized Olympus BX51 microscope with a 20X objective controlled by Visiopharm software (Visiopharm, Hørsholm, Denmark) or by a NanoZoomer-2.0HT (Hamamatsu, Denmark) using a 20X or 40X objective. In wound tissue, cell counting was performed in randomly selected areas either containing or devoid of fibrin. The average size of these regions of interest (ROIs) was 0.035 mm^2. The average thickness of the epidermis was derived from the area of the hyperplastic epidermis divided by the length. The combined area of fibrin rich lesions in the provisional matrix was determined using the staining analysis software VisiomorphDP, which is part of the Visiopharm software package (Visiopharm, Hørsholm, Denmark). In the liver, the degree of fibrin deposition was determined on one whole scanned tissue slide from each liver using VisiomorphDP (Visiopharm, Hørsholm, Denmark). Likewise, was the area of CD34 positive staining quantitated by use of VisiomorphDP on whole tissue slides scanned at 40X.

Statistical Analyses

Statistical analyses were performed using Two-way ANOVA, One-way ANOVA with a Newman-Keuls post test or with student's t-tests.

Results

Fibrin Accumulation in the Liver of Naïve Mice is Unaffected by Gender

Mice lacking functional Plg display large and disseminated fibrin rich lesions in the liver [3]. This pathological condition is also observed in mice with a deficient PA system [20] or in mice treated with PA inhibitors [21,22]. In order to investigate if gender affects the accumulation of fibrin rich lesions in unchallenged $Plg^{-/-}$ mice, we conducted a histological analysis of livers derived from a cohort of $Plg^{-/-}$ mice. Immunohistochemical staining revealed no signs of fibrin rich lesions in livers from Wt mice regardless of age (up to 26 weeks). However, in $Plg^{-/-}$ mice, fibrin rich lesions were evident already at an age of eight weeks. Computerized staining analysis revealed that the number, size and combined area of these lesions increased significantly up to the age of 26 weeks. However, when comparing livers from male and female $Plg^{-/-}$ mice it was evident that there were no differences between genders (Figure 1A). Together with previous reports stating that the plasma fibrinogen levels are constant between genders [18], these observations provide evidence that naïve $Plg^{-/-}$ female mice are just as incapable of clearing deposited fibrin in the liver as are $Plg^{-/-}$ male mice.

Both Male and Female Mice Depend on Plasminogen in the Acute Recruitment of Inflammatory Cells

The recruitment of inflammatory cells to the peritoneal cavity following an IP injection of a proinflammatory agent such as thioglycollate (TG) is known to depend on Plg [7]. Likewise has an obstructed PA system been shown to ameliorate the inflammatory response during chemically induced peritonitis [23]. This role of Plg has been ascribed to plasmin dependent matrix metalloproteinase (MMP)-9 activation and subsequent basement membrane degradation, which in turn allows inflammatory cells to migrate to the peritoneal cavity [8]. However, the possibility of a role for direct plasmin driven fibrinolysis in this process has yet to be addressed.

To test if the obstructed recruitment of inflammatory cells to the peritoneal cavity due to lack of Plg is gender dependent, we compared the response to IP injected TG in Wt and $Plg^{-/-}$ mice (C57Bl/6 backcrossed for at least 30 generations) of both genders totaling 26 mice. Three days after TG injection, Wt mice presented an almost tenfold increase in the concentration of cells in the peritoneal cavity. This response to TG was independent of gender. When comparing the response to TG in Wt and $Plg^{-/-}$ mice, a striking difference was observed, as the latter mice seemed completely unaffected by the administration of TG. This, however, was regardless of gender ($p = 0.8885$ for the difference between genders) (Figure 1B). The lack of a gender effect on the acute Plg-dependent recruitment of inflammatory cells does not support the notion that female mice may circumvent the lack of Plg by expressing other protease(s) with a similar repertoire of substrates.

Dysfunctional Skin wound Healing in $Plg^{-/-}$ Mice is Modulated by Gender

It has previously been demonstrated that Plg deficiency affects chemically induced skin tumor growth differently in male and female mice. Whereas Plg deficiency decreased tumor burden by 52% in male mice, biallelic Plg disruption did not affect the skin tumor burden in female mice compared to littermate control mice [18]. However, Plg deficiency has on other occasions been shown to affect biological events in female mice, involving substantial tissue remodeling, such as mammary gland involution [24,25]. Based on these reports and on the lack of gender effects on fibrin accumulation in the liver and on recruitment of inflammatory cells in $Plg^{-/-}$ mice, we speculated that gender only affected the phenotype of $Plg^{-/-}$ mice in terms of skin pathologies. As it has been thoroughly documented that skin wound healing is highly dependent on plasmin driven fibrinolysis [26], we compared the capacity of Wt and $Plg^{-/-}$ FVB mice of both genders to heal

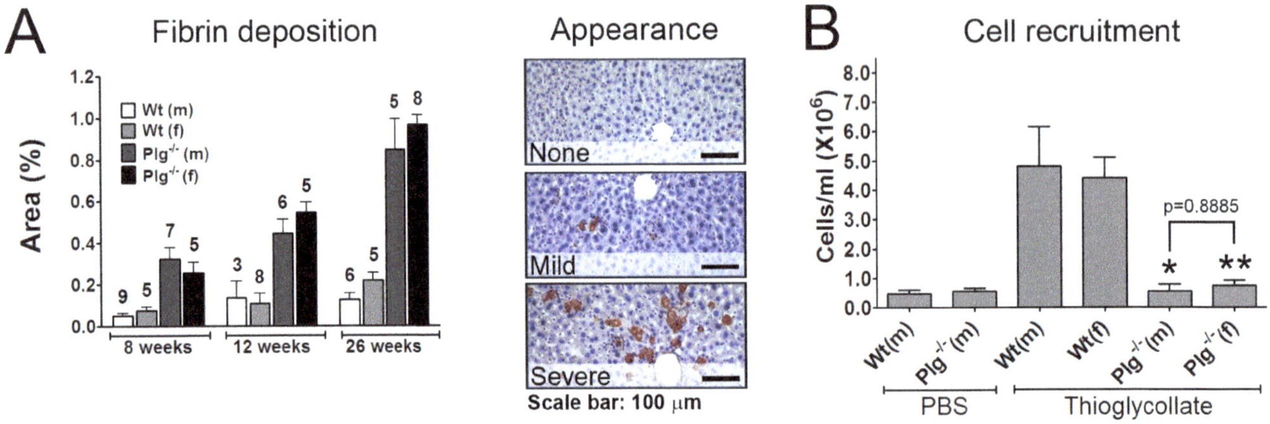

Figure 1. Deposition of fibrin in the liver and plasminogen dependent cell migration is unaffected by gender. The effect of gender on spontaneous fibrin deposition in the liver and recruitment of inflammatory cells was tested in $Plg^{-/-}$ mice. (A) The degree of fibrin deposition in the liver in $Plg^{-/-}$ mice and Wt controls of both genders was determined by computerized quantitative immunohistochemistry. The number of mice in each group is shown above each column. The difference between Wt and $Plg^{-/-}$ mice was significantly different at all time points ($p<0.01$), while there was no difference between genders. Representative liver stainings from mice with varying degrees of liver fibrin depositions are shown on the right. (B) The effect of Plg deficiency on Plg dependent inflammatory cell recruitment was tested by IP injections of TG and determining the concentration of cells in the peritoneal lavage fluid after three days. *, $p<0.05$; **, $p<0.01$ compared to TG treated Wt male and female mice. Data were analyzed with a one-way ANOVA and a Newman-Keuls post test. $n = 3–8$ in each group.

20 mm long incisional skin wounds on the back. No difference in the time to complete skin wound healing was observed between Wt male and female mice (17.7±0.66 and 16±0.62 days for males and females, respectively), while the time needed to complete wound healing in $Plg^{-/-}$ mice of both genders was markedly delayed compared to the Wt mice (Figure 2A–C,E). However, we also noted a distinct difference in wound healing between $Plg^{-/-}$ male and female mice. Already five days post wounding, $Plg^{-/-}$ female mice revealed faster wound healing than $Plg^{-/-}$ male mice. This trend was further emphasized from 20 days post wounding. Interestingly, as the wounds in the male and female $Plg^{-/-}$ mice were approximately 95% healed (75 days post wounding) no differences between the genders could be seen (Figure 2A–C). The healing time curves from $Plg^{-/-}$ male and $Plg^{-/-}$ female mice were significantly different ($p<0.0001$), while there were no differences in terms of average time to complete wound closure ($p = 0.2023$). These data suggested that it is not only skin tumor growth in $Plg^{-/-}$ mice that is affected by gender but also other types of tissue remodelling processes that takes place in the skin.

To further substantiate the concept of a gender dependent effect of Plg deficiency in terms of wound healing, a wound healing study similar to the one performed in FVB mice was performed in fully backcrossed C57Bl/6 mice (backcrossed for at least 30 generations). This experiment was carried out by independent research technicians that were unaware of the gender dependent phenotype observed in FVB mice. This experiment confirmed the existence of a gender dependent phenotype in relation to skin wound healing in $Plg^{-/-}$ mice. Indeed, the effect of gender was more pronounced in C57Bl/6 mice than in the corresponding FVB mice (Figure 2D). Noteworthy is that, in the applied wound healing model, both $Plg^{-/-}$ as well as the Wt control mice on the C57Bl/6 background heal much faster than the corresponding FVB mice. Pronounced differences between the FVB and C57Bl/6 mice strains lacking $Plg^{-/-}$ is also evident in regard to other phenotypic features, such as the development of rectal prolapses, which appear significantly faster in C57Bl/6 mice (unpublished results). Though C57Bl/6 mice with a dysfunctional PA-system also display fibrin depositions in the liver [22], a direct comparison of the liver pathology between $Plg^{-/-}$ FVB and C57Bl/6 mice has never been performed. Thus, the phenotype of Plg deficiency may very well be partly strain dependent.

Skin Thickness and Composition Differs between Genders but are Unaffected by Plasminogen Deficiency

The obtained data, suggesting that the ability of $Plg^{-/-}$ mice to execute tissue remodelling processes in the skin is affected by gender, prompted us to investigate if the known differences between the genders in terms of thickness of the dermal and hypodermal compartments were affected by Plg deficiency. For this purpose we analyzed normal skin samples from the previous mentioned cohort tissue collection [4]. We found, as expected, that naïve Wt male mice had thicker dermis and thinner subdermis than Wt female mice. Further studies revealed that these differences were not affected by Plg deficiency (Figure 3). Thus a differential gender effect of Plg deficiency on skin composition is not likely responsible for the gender differences observed with regard to skin wound healing in $Plg^{-/-}$ mice.

The Subtle Effect of Plasminogen Deficiency in Female Mice is not Augmented by Ovariectomy

Expression of distinct extracellular matrix proteases with a potential fibrinolytic activity may to some extent be regulated by sex-hormones. It can thus not be ruled out that female mice, during the process of skin wound healing, have the capacity to express fibrinolytic proteases, which can compensate for the lack of plasmin. To test this hypothesis we analyzed the effect of OVX on skin wound healing in Wt and $Plg^{-/-}$ mice.

As previously observed, we found no significant differences between Wt male and female mice in terms of wound healing.

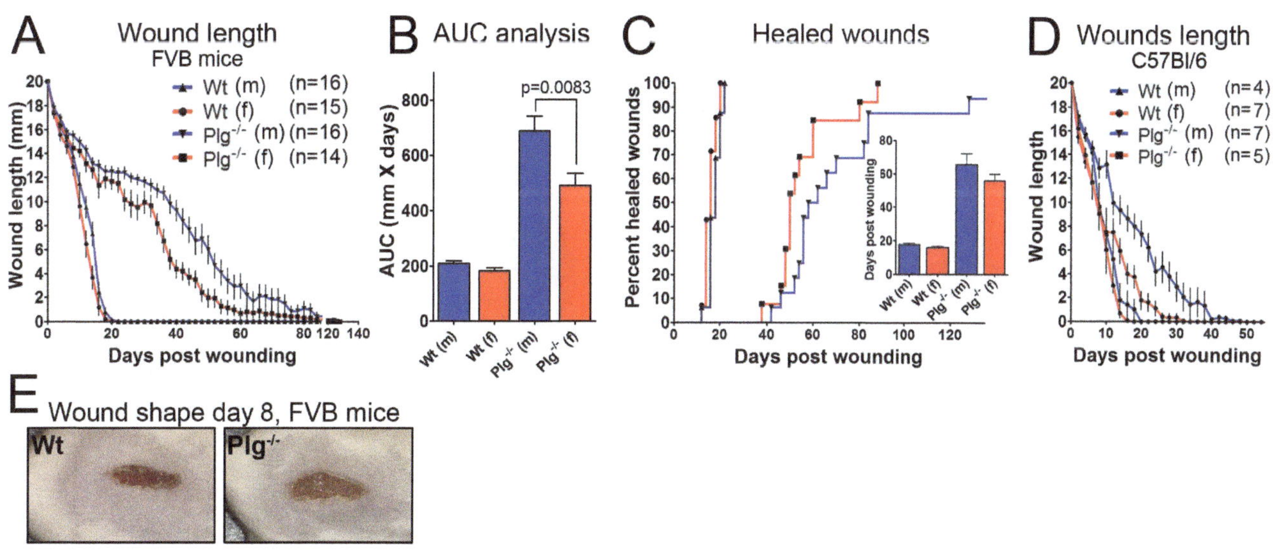

Figure 2. Skin wound healing in plasminogen deficient mice is affected by gender. Skin wound healing was tested by measuring time to complete reepithelialization of a 20 mm long full skin thickness incisional wound on the back. (A) The wound length in FVB mice was determined every other day using digital calipers. A substantial difference was observed between male and female $Plg^{-/-}$ mice ($p<0.0001$). (B) The area under the curve analysis revealed a significant difference between genders in the $Plg^{-/-}$ mice. (C) The fraction of fully reepithelialized wounds is presented as a function of time. The bar graph shows the average time to complete reepithelialization. (D) A wound healing study identical to the one carried out in FVB mice were performed in C57Bl/6 mice. Similar results were obtained in C57Bl/6 mice with a significant difference between wound healing times in male and female $Plg^{-/-}$ mice ($p = 0.01$). (E) Representative pictures of skin wounds in Wt and $Plg^{-/-}$ male mice eight days after the incision.

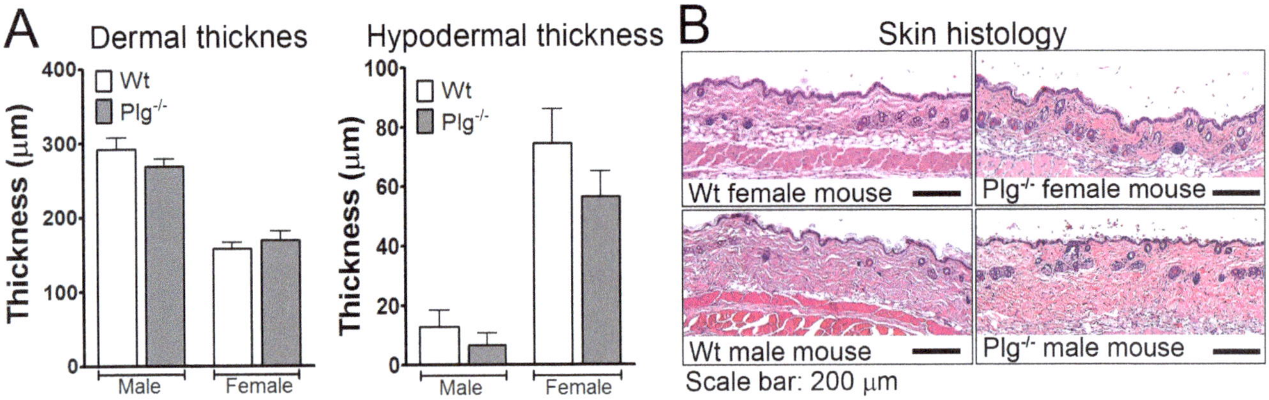

Figure 3. Plasminogen deficiency does not affect the structure of naïve skin. The effect of Plg deficiency on the known differences in skin histology between genders was investigated using back skin from naïve $Plg^{-/-}$ mice and Wt controls (8–12 weeks of age). n = 8–12 for each group. (A) The thickness of the dermis and hypodermis was determined by microscopy. (B) Representative skin sections from eight week old male and female mice.

Furthermore, in Wt mice, OVX did not significantly affect wound healing when compared to sham operated male and female mice. In $Plg^{-/-}$ mice, the gender differences in wound healing were still clearly evident despite sham and OVX surgeries. However, in contrast to Wt mice, OVX in $Plg^{-/-}$ mice led to a subtle delay in the initial phase of the wound healing process compared to both sham $Plg^{-/-}$ male and female mice. However, around day 30 post wounding, it was no longer possible to distinguish between sham and OVX $Plg^{-/-}$ female mice (Figure 4A,B), resulting in similar overall time to complete wound healing in the two groups (Figure 4C). Thus female sex-hormones may contribute in orchestrating the initial phase of wound healing, as suggested by others [27], but they do not seem to be responsible for the overall difference in wound healing between male and female $Plg^{-/-}$ mice.

Overt Differences between Genders in Epithelial Structure and Cell Invasion during Wound Healing

To further elucidate the impact of genders on wound healing in $Plg^{-/-}$ mice, we performed a histological analysis of reepithelialized wounds (skin biopsies were harvested within 24 hours of wound closure). The wounds all displayed a hyperplastic epidermis, which covered a dermal wound gap containing yet unresolved granulation tissue. The lengths of the hyperplastic epidermis and wound gap were similar in Wt male and female mice, while the thickness of the hyperplastic epidermis was increased in Wt females. Interestingly, the lengths of the hyperplastic epidermis and dermal wound gap were significantly longer in $Plg^{-/-}$ mice than in Wt mice, and furthermore, the lengths were 48% longer in $Plg^{-/-}$ male than in $Plg^{-/-}$ female mice (Figure 5A–F). These analyses show that, when wounds in $Plg^{-/-}$ mice are fully reepithelialized, the underlying matrix is only to a limited extend reconstructed, as previously described [11]. In contrast, wounds in

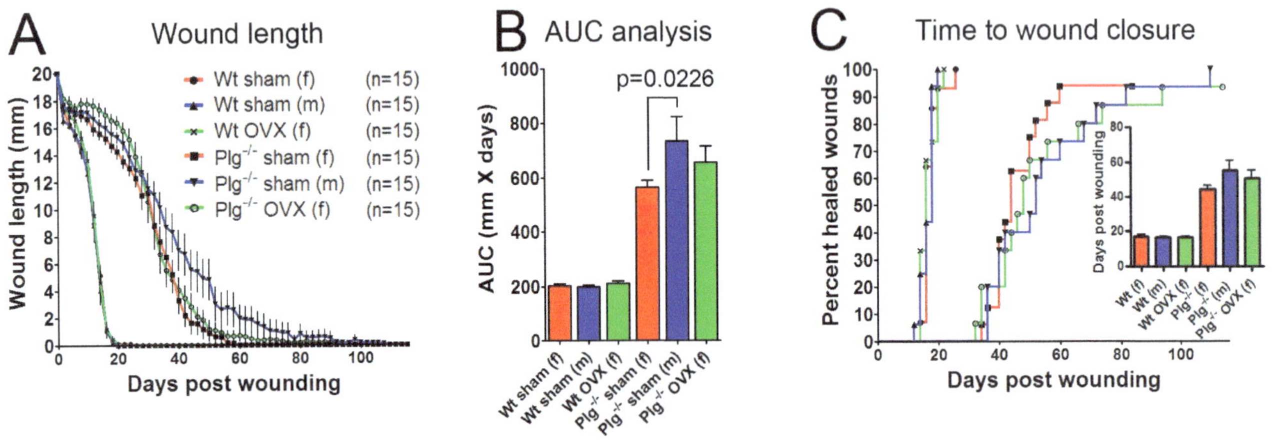

Figure 4. Ovariectomy does not induce a male like phenotype in plasminogen deficient female mice. A possible effect of ovarian derived hormones on skin wound healing in $Plg^{-/-}$ mice was tested by excision of the ovaries before a 20 mm full thickness incisional skin wound was made. (A) Wound lengths were measured using digital calipers every other day until completely healed. No statistical significant difference was found between the different groups belonging to Wt mice. The difference between sham operated male and female $Plg^{-/-}$ mice were statistically significant ($p<0.05$), while no significant difference was found between OVX operated $Plg^{-/-}$ mice and the sham operated $Plg^{-/-}$ mice. (B) An area under the curve analysis showed no significant effect of OVX in $Plg^{-/-}$ mice, while the difference between genders was significant. (C) The percentage of mice with completely reepithelialized wounds presented as a function of time. The bar graph shows the average time to complete reepithelialization.

Wt mice have much less granulation tissue (dermal wound gap) upon reepitheliazation despite the fact that reepithelialization happens much faster in Wt mice than in $Plg^{-/-}$ mice. Thus proliferation and migration of keratinocytes, which serves to reepithelialize wounds, seem less affected by Plg deficiency than does the rearrangement and contraction of the underlying granulation tissue.

A quantitative histological assessment of fibrin deposition and cell concentration in the reepithelialized wounds revealed that the combined area staining positive for fibrin in the provisional matrix in $Plg^{-/-}$ male mice was 62% higher than in $Plg^{-/-}$ female mice (no noteworthy fibrin depositions were found in Wt mice of either gender). Furthermore, the concentration of cells in the fibrin rich areas was decreased by almost 80% in comparison with areas not containing fibrin. In addition, the granulation tissue in $Plg^{-/-}$ female mice contained fewer cells than in $Plg^{-/-}$ male mice, both within and outside the fibrin rich areas (Figure 6A–I). The observed difference in the area of fibrin rich lesions, and thus cell concentration, in male and female $Plg^{-/-}$ mice could explain the gender dependent difference in wound healing time in $Plg^{-/-}$ mice.

The notion that deposited fibrin blocks the recruitment of cells to the granulation tissue at an early time point was further supported by analyses of 50% reepithelialized wound tissues harvested from $Plg^{-/-}$ mice, which revealed that the cellular infiltration of the granulation tissue with cells from the adjacent

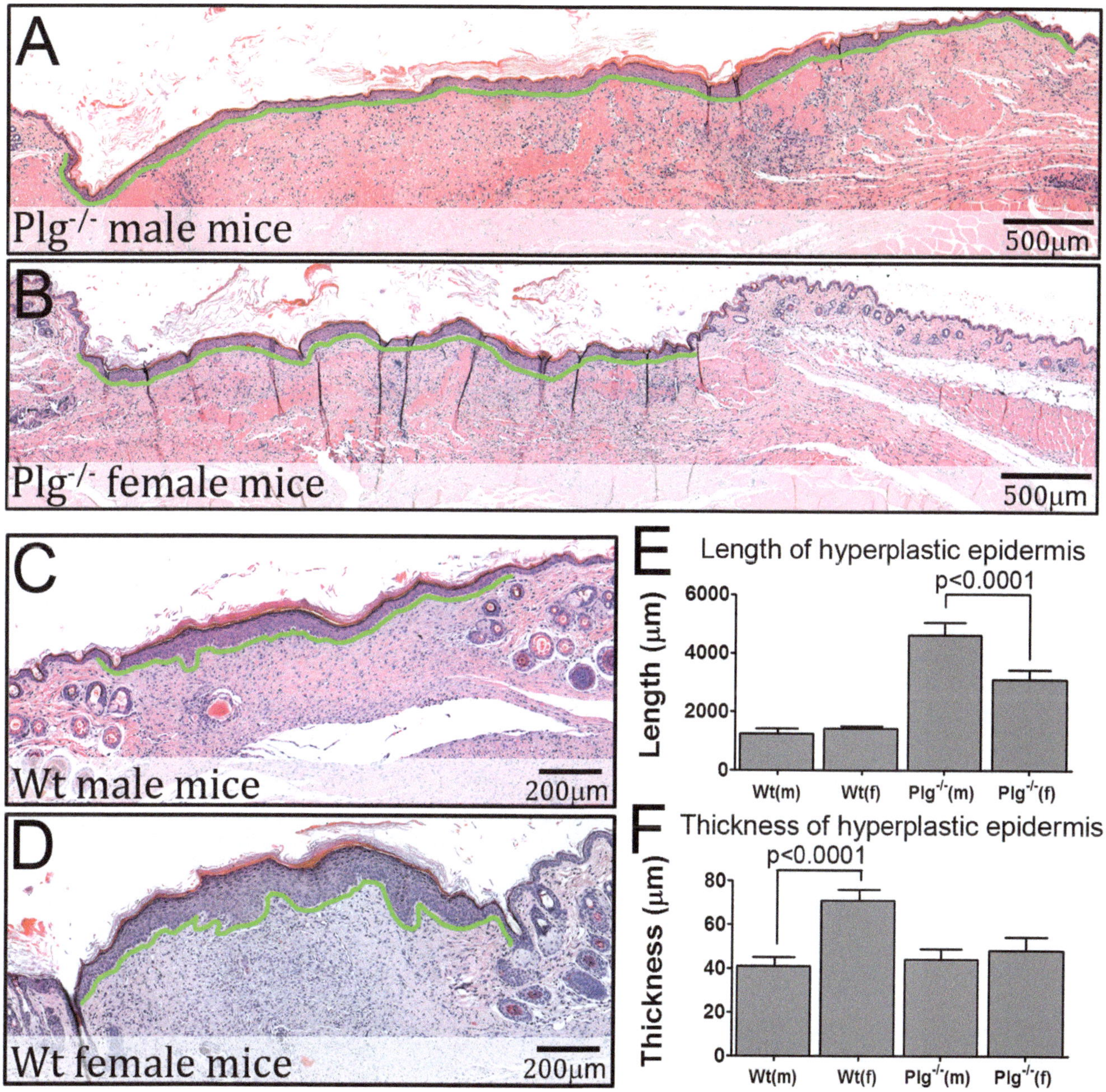

Figure 5. The length of the hyperplastic epidermis and dermal wound gap is affected by gender. Histological analysis of H&E stained sections from fully reepithelialized wounds. (A–D) representative sections of healed wounds from Wt and $Plg^{-/-}$ mice of both genders. The hyperplastic epidermis is underlined by green. (E & F) The length and average thickness of the hyperplastic epidermis. n = 9–11 for each group.

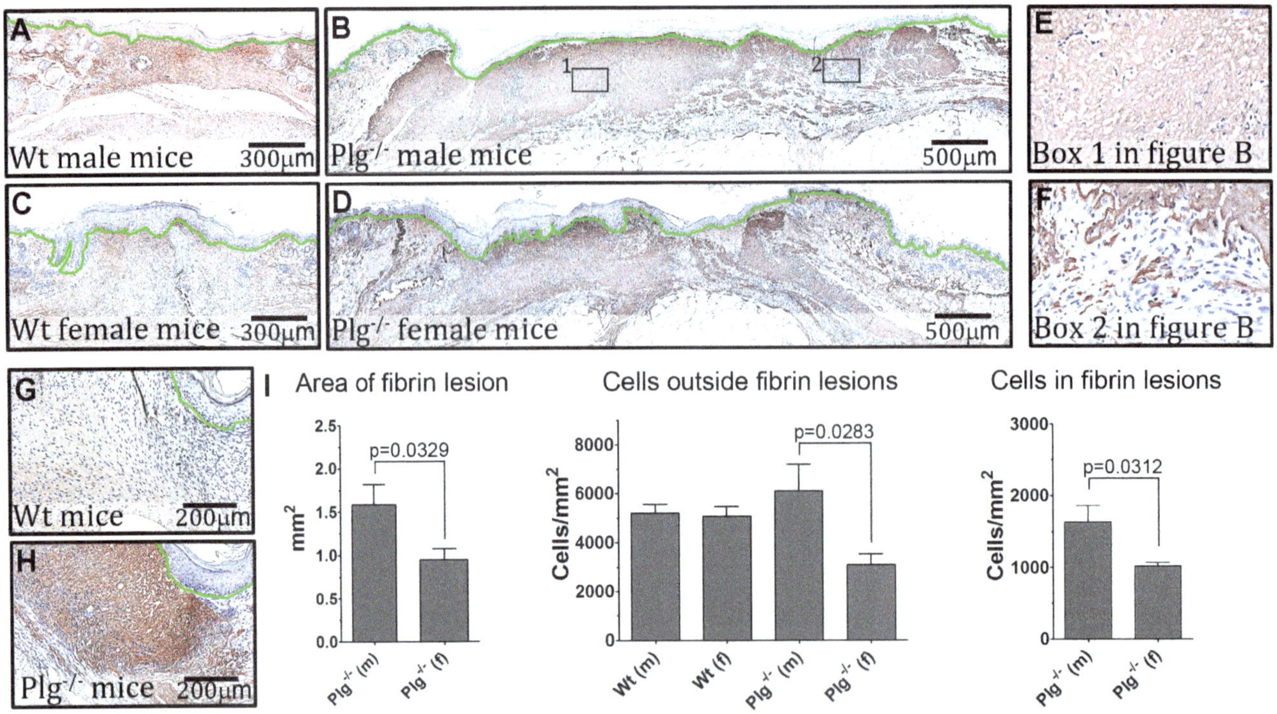

Figure 6. Decreased cell infiltration in fibrin rich areas of wound tissues. Fibrin(ogen) staining of skin wound sections. The epidermis is underlined by green, fibrin(ogen) is stained brown with NovaRED, and nuclei are stained blue with a hematoxylin counter stain. (A–D) representative stainings of wound tissues from Wt and Plg$^{-/-}$ mice of both genders. (E & F) enlarged micrographs of areas boxed in B. (G & H) sections from 50% healed wounds in the back skin of male mice, which show the area between the advancing keratinocytes and the underlying muscle tissue Note the lack of cells in this region in the Plg$^{-/-}$ mice. (I) quantifications of the total area of fibrin(ogen) positive lesions in the provisional matrix and quantifications of the number of cells within and outside this area. n = 9–11 for each group.

healthy skin was severely obstructed due to massive fibrin depositions (Figure 6G,H). This abolished recruitment of cells is most likely directly responsible for the lack of cells in the fibrin rich areas of the provisional matrix in the later fully reepithelialized wounds.

Wound healing is intimately associated with the generation of a vascular network throughout the granulation tissue. This process depends on the interaction between endothelial and matrix proteins as well as proteolytic matrix reorginization by MMPs and the PA system [28–30]. To investigate if vessel formation in skin wounds in Wt and Plg$^{-/-}$ mice were affected by gender, fully reepithelialized wounds stained for CD34 were scanned at 40X and subjected to computerized staining quantification. The combined area of CD34 positive vessels per μm wound tissue (defined by the presence of a hyperplastic epidermis) was compared. CD34 positive vessels were mainly observed within close distance to the epidermis in both Wt and Plg$^{-/-}$ mice of both genders and no overt differences were observed in terms of size or shape between these groups of mice (figure 7A–D). The quantification of the CD34 staining signal revealed no differences between genders, while there was a tendency of Plg$^{-/-}$ mice having decreased amounts of CD34 compared to Wt mice (Figure 7E).

Discussion

In the present study the effect of gender on the phenotype of Plg deficiency was illuminated. Three well described characteristics were assessed; spontaneous accumulation of fibrin in the liver, Plg dependent cell recruitment to the peritoneal cavity, and incisional skin wound healing. Among these, only skin wound healing in Plg$^{-/-}$ mice was affected by gender. Furthermore, the gender specific differences in naïve skin described in Wt mice were unaffected by Plg deficiency. Histological examination of healed wounds revealed that the combined area of fibrin rich lesions in the provisional matrix was larger in male Plg$^{-/-}$ mice than in female Plg$^{-/-}$ mice, and that these fibrin rich lesions contained far less cells than the surrounding wound matrix in both male and female mice. The difference in the area of fibrin rich lesions between genders correlated well to the differences in the length of the hyperplastic epidermis and amount of granulation tissue in healed wounds as well as to the measured difference in time to complete wound reepithelialization.

It is evident that the general phenotype of unchallenged Plg$^{-/-}$ mice is the same in males and females, though subtle differences may be observed [4]. The recent discovery of a gender dependent effect of Plg deficiency on chemically induced skin tumor growth was therefore highly surprising [18]. The mechanism underlying this gender effect has not been fully elucidated, but may relate to decreased fibrin depositions in the skin and/or tumor thrombosis [18], both of which may affect skin tumor growth. Additionally, it was shown that male and female mice contained the same amount of plasma fibrinogen throughout their lifespan [18], thus ruling out such a difference as being responsible for the gender effects on the Plg$^{-/-}$ phenotype. However, as spontaneous *in vivo* clot lysis, determined by intra-venous injections of radiolabeled fibrin clots, is remarkably reduced in Plg deficient mice compared to Wt mice [31], we cannot exclude that these differences may partly be accountable for the dissimilarities between the genders observed in Plg$^{-/-}$ mice. Yet, we find this questionable as identical levels of

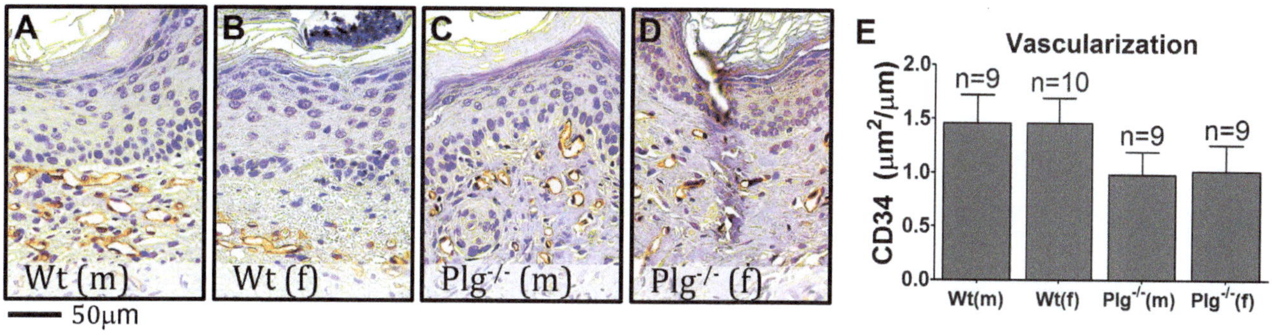

Figure 7. Gender does not affect the vessel concentration in fully reepithelialized wounds. CD34 stainings of fully reepithelialized wounds were performed to identify new vessels. (A–D) CD34 positive vessels were detected in the dermis proximal to the hyperplastic epidermis both in Wt and Plg$^{-/-}$ mice of both genders. (E) Computerized staining analysis on whole wound sections reveal that Plg$^{-/-}$ mice had a tendency to express less CD34 (area wise) than Wt mice while gender did not affect the level of CD34 staining.

fibrin depositions in the liver of male and female Plg$^{-/-}$ mice were observed, which not only suggests that the livers in male and female Plg$^{-/-}$ mice are equally degenerated over time, but also that a putative but insufficient extravascular fibrin clearance occurs at the same rate in both genders. Furthermore, the evident lack of a gender effect on the recruitment of immune cells to the peritoneal cavity in response to TG injections, suggests that males and females depend equally on plasmin activity to execute an inflammatory response. In accordance with these observations, Plg deficiency has not previously been reported to show a gender effect in macrophage recruitment [8], though experiments have been carried out in mice of both genders. Despite the hampered recruitment of immune cells in Plg$^{-/-}$ mice challenged with a proinflammatory agent, inflammatory reactions seem to be fully executed in some chronic pathological settings, such as in the development of inflammatory colon lesions and skin tumors [4,18], while ameliorated in other models [32].

In contrast to fibrin deposition in the liver and immune cell recruitment, we found that incisional skin wound healing in Plg$^{-/-}$ mice was highly dependent on gender. The intricate process of wound healing involves fibrin clearance, which likely facilitates the recruitment of cells into the granulation tissue and/or keratinocyte migration [5,26]. Besides increased activity of the PA-system during wound healing processes, zymographic studies on wound tissue have also revealed a transient increase in the activity of MMPs [33,34]. These alterations in the proteolytic environment may be driven by protease expression both by dermal fibroblasts and the leading edge keratinocytes [35–37]. Plasmin has been shown to cleave and thus activate other extracellular proteases important for wound healing [38] and it may thus be speculated that plasmin in this way facilitate wound healing by a fibrinolysis independent manner. Additionally, it has been suggested that other proteases besides plasmin may contribute to fibrin clearance during tissue remodeling. This has been tested by using mice deficient in Plg in addition to specific members of the MMP family, including MMP2, MMP9, or MMP13 [4,12,34,39]. Among these MMP13 deficiency induced a marked delay in wound healing in Plg$^{-/-}$ mice but not to the extent observed when treating Plg$^{-/-}$ mice with the broad spectrum MMP inhibitor Galardin [12,19,27]. Thus, several proteases may act in concert to degrade fibrin in the wound matrix. Taking the expression pattern and the multitude of possible functions of plasmin(ogen) into account, the delayed wound healing in Plg$^{-/-}$ mice may very well be directly linked to obstructed cell recruitment or keratinocyte migration. In the current study, we found, that reepithelialized skin wounds in Plg$^{-/-}$ mice still contained large dermal wound gaps, which was significantly larger than that observed in Wt mice. This observation suggests that epidermal wound closure may be less affected by Plg deficiency than reconstruction of the underlying dermal compartment.

Concerning the role of female sex hormones on cutaneous wound healing, it was noted that during the first four weeks post wounding, OVX of Plg$^{-/-}$ mice induced a subtle but statistically significant delay in wound closure compared to sham operated female Plg$^{-/-}$ mice. We speculate, that the enhanced effect of OVX on wound healing in Plg$^{-/-}$ mice compared to Wt mice may relate to specific events during the healing process. Skin wound healing can be divided into several and partially overlapping phases. Following the initial event of coagulation and haemostasis, neutrophils are recruited to the wound site followed by macrophages, which phagocytose remaining neutrophils and secrete tissue growth factors that activate keratinocytes and fibroblasts [40]. Estrogen has previously been shown to modulate the inflammatory response during wound healing through an estrogen dependent down-regulation of the macrophage migration inhibitory factor (MMIF) [27]. The observed delay in the initial phase of wound healing in OVX operated Plg$^{-/-}$ mice in the current study could be related to an additive or synergistic effect of Plg deficiency and depletion of female sex hormones on macrophage migration and activation [41], possibly involving disturbed MIFF activity [27]. As mentioned skin wound healing depends on plasmin driven fibrinolysis but other proteases with fibrinolytic activity seem to take part of the fibrin degradation process in Plg$^{-/-}$ mice [12]. The expression of some of the candidate fibrinolytic proteases e.g. the MT1-MMP [42] have been shown to be regulated by estrogen [43] and could thus be involved in the reduced dependency of Plg in female mice during skin wound healing.

Of notice is that we did not observe any gender dependent difference between sham and OVX operated Wt mice with regard to wound healing. This observation is contradicted by previous reports stating a role for estrogen/estrogen receptor β interaction in cutaneous wound healing [44]. The different outcome of the current study and the one presented by Campbell et al. 2010, may stem from fundamental differences in the model setup (e.g. wound size, age of mice, time between OVX surgery and wounding) or choice of mice strain i.e. FVB/n vs. C57Bl/6 mice, two strains, which in this report has been shown to differ significantly in terms of healing time. Both Wt and Plg$^{-/-}$ C57Bl/6 healed faster than the corresponding FVB mice, thus indicating major differences in either skin composition per se or in one or more of the distinct phases of the wound healing process.

Additional explicatory factors may relate to endogenous differences between male and female mice in skin properties, such as skin strength and mechanical features. In the current study we therefore performed analyses of unchallenged skin biopsies from Wt and Plg deficient male and female mice. In line with other reports, we demonstrated inherent gender differences in normal skin histology. Although these differences were not affected by Plg deficiency, they might affect wound healing in $Plg^{-/-}$ mice. In male mice we observed larger dermal thickness compared to female mice, a parameter that has been reported to be under the influence of male hormones [45]. A direct relationship between dermal thickness and collagen content, and thereby skin strength/mechanical resistance, has been suggested [46]. In relation to skin injury the expression of collagen is markedly increased in fibroblasts in the dermis. This is followed by an extensive remodeling phase, in which the collagen content is degraded by the coordinated action of several collagenolytic proteases, whose expression and activation have been reported to depend on plasmin [47]. Thus, disruption of Plg may have an impact on these processes.

Our data showing that the combined area of fibrin rich lesions in the provisional matrix was significantly lower in $Plg^{-/-}$ female mice compared to $Plg^{-/-}$ male mice could simply be a reflection of the fact that the overall thickness of the skin is smaller in females [45] and that the dermal wound gap in reepithelialized wounds in $Plg^{-/-}$ female mice is smaller than in the corresponding males. However, it is conceivable that the decreased level of fibrin deposition in $Plg^{-/-}$ female mice is secondary to an accelerated fibrinolytic process in comparison with male mice. Interestingly, the differences in dermal fibrin levels between male and female $Plg^{-/-}$ mice did not seem to result in differences within vessel density of the fully healed wounds. However, disregarding gender $Plg^{-/-}$ mice did tend to have fewer CD34 positive vessels underneath the hyperplastic epidermis compared to Wt mice. As extracellular proteases mediate angiogenic processes and that angiogenesis is important for skin wound healing [28–30] one of the factors responsible for delayed wound healing in $Plg^{-/-}$ mice may indeed be partly related to hampered angiogenesis.

In conclusion, the presented data show that the effect of Plg deficiency is both gender and tissue specific. The results further suggest that the observed differences in wound healing between male and female $Plg^{-/-}$ mice is not solely related to sex-hormones, though the lack of female sex-hormones, induced by OVX, affected wound healing in female $Plg^{-/-}$ mice to some extent. It is possible that the endogenous differences in skin histology between genders are responsible for the varying effect of Plg deficiency on wound healing, which would explain why the gender effect is restricted to the skin.

Acknowledgments

We would like to thank Simone Gress Hansen, Anne Vive, and Lotte Frederiksen for technical assistance. We acknowledge the Department of Experimental Medicine, University of Copenhagen for breeding and housing of the experimental animals.

Author Contributions

Conceived and designed the experiments: AH BR LRL. Performed the experiments: AH BR. Analyzed the data: AH. Contributed reagents/materials/analysis tools: LRL LHE. Wrote the paper: AH.

References

1. Schuster V, Hugle B, Tefs K (2007) Plasminogen deficiency. J Thromb Haemost 5: 2315–2322.
2. Mehta R, Shapiro AD (2008) Plasminogen deficiency. Haemophilia 14: 1261–1268.
3. Bugge TH, Flick MJ, Daugherty CC, Degen JL (1995) Plasminogen deficiency causes severe thrombosis but is compatible with development and reproduction. Genes Dev 9: 794–807.
4. Hald A, Rono B, Melander MC, Ding M, Holck S, et al. (2011) MMP9 is protective against lethal inflammatory mass lesions in the mouse colon. Dis Model Mech 4: 212–227.
5. Romer J, Bugge TH, Pyke C, Lund LR, Flick MJ, et al. (1996) Impaired wound healing in mice with a disrupted plasminogen gene. Nat Med 2: 287–292.
6. Schuster V, Seregard S (2003) Ligneous conjunctivitis. Surv Ophthalmol 48: 369–388.
7. Ploplis VA, French EL, Carmeliet P, Collen D, Plow EF (1998) Plasminogen deficiency differentially affects recruitment of inflammatory cell populations in mice. Blood 91: 2005–2009.
8. Gong Y, Hart E, Shchurin A, Hoover-Plow J (2008) Inflammatory macrophage migration requires MMP-9 activation by plasminogen in mice. J Clin Invest 118: 3012–3024.
9. McColl BK, Baldwin ME, Roufail S, Freeman C, Moritz RL, et al. (2003) Plasmin activates the lymphangiogenic growth factors VEGF-C and VEGF-D. J Exp Med 198: 863–868.
10. Heissig B, Lund LR, Akiyama H, Ohki M, Morita Y, et al. (2007) The plasminogen fibrinolytic pathway is required for hematopoietic regeneration. Cell Stem Cell 1: 658–670.
11. Lund LR, Green KA, Stoop AA, Ploug M, Almholt K, et al. (2006) Plasminogen activation independent of uPA and tPA maintains wound healing in gene-deficient mice. EMBO J 25: 2686–2697.
12. Lund LR, Romer J, Bugge TH, Nielsen BS, Frandsen TL, et al. (1999) Functional overlap between two classes of matrix-degrading proteases in wound healing. EMBO J 18: 4645–4656.
13. Egeblad M, Werb Z (2002) New functions for the matrix metalloproteinases in cancer progression. Nat Rev Cancer 2: 161–174.
14. Hald A, Rono B, Lund LR, Egerod KL (2012) LPS counter regulates RNA expression of extracellular proteases and their inhibitors in murine macrophages. Mediators Inflamm 2012: 157894.
15. McMahon B, Kwaan HC (2008) The plasminogen activator system and cancer. Pathophysiol Haemost Thromb 36: 184–194.
16. Dano K, Behrendt N, Hoyer-Hansen G, Johnsen M, Lund LR, et al. (2005) Plasminogen activation and cancer. Thromb Haemost 93: 676–681.
17. Palumbo JS, Talmage KE, Liu H, La Jeunesse CM, Witte DP, et al. (2003) Plasminogen supports tumor growth through a fibrinogen-dependent mechanism linked to vascular patency. Blood 102: 2819–2827.
18. Hald A, Eickhardt H, Maerkedahl RB, Feldborg CW, Egerod KL, et al. (2012) Plasmin-driven fibrinolysis facilitates skin tumor growth in a gender-dependent manner. FASEB J.
19. Green KA, Almholt K, Ploug M, Rono B, Castellino FJ, et al. (2008) Profibrinolytic effects of metalloproteinases during skin wound healing in the absence of plasminogen. J Invest Dermatol 128: 2092–2101.
20. Bugge TH, Flick MJ, Danton MJ, Daugherty CC, Romer J, et al. (1996) Urokinase-type plasminogen activator is effective in fibrin clearance in the absence of its receptor or tissue-type plasminogen activator. Proc Natl Acad Sci U S A 93: 5899–5904.
21. Jogi A, Pass J, Hoyer-Hansen G, Lund LR, Nielsen BS, et al. (2007) Systemic administration of anti-urokinase plasminogen activator receptor monoclonal antibodies induces hepatic fibrin deposition in tissue-type plasminogen activator deficient mice. J Thromb Haemost 5: 1936–1944.
22. Lund IK, Jogi A, Rono B, Rasch MG, Lund LR, et al. (2008) Antibody-mediated targeting of the urokinase-type plasminogen activator proteolytic function neutralizes fibrinolysis in vivo. J Biol Chem 283: 32506–32515.
23. Larmann J, Frenzel T, Hahnenkamp A, Herzog C, Lorenz A, et al. (2010) In vivo fluorescence-mediated tomography for quantification of urokinase receptor-dependent leukocyte trafficking in inflammation. Anesthesiology 113: 610–618.
24. Lund LR, Bjorn SF, Sternlicht MD, Nielsen BS, Solberg H, et al. (2000) Lactational competence and involution of the mouse mammary gland require plasminogen. Development 127: 4481–4492.
25. Green KA, Nielsen BS, Castellino FJ, Romer J, Lund LR (2006) Lack of plasminogen leads to milk stasis and premature mammary gland involution during lactation. Dev Biol 299: 164–175.
26. Bugge TH, Kombrinck KW, Flick MJ, Daugherty CC, Danton MJ, et al. (1996) Loss of fibrinogen rescues mice from the pleiotropic effects of plasminogen deficiency. Cell 87: 709–719.
27. Ashcroft GS, Mills SJ, Lei K, Gibbons L, Jeong MJ, et al. (2003) Estrogen modulates cutaneous wound healing by downregulating macrophage migration inhibitory factor. J Clin Invest 111: 1309–1318.
28. Feng X, Clark RA, Galanakis D, Tonnesen MG (1999) Fibrin and collagen differentially regulate human dermal microvascular endothelial cell integrins:

stabilization of alphav/beta3 mRNA by fibrin1. J Invest Dermatol 113: 913–919.
29. Hattori N, Mochizuki S, Kishi K, Nakajima T, Takaishi H, et al. (2009) MMP-13 plays a role in keratinocyte migration, angiogenesis, and contraction in mouse skin wound healing. Am J Pathol 175: 533–546.
30. Binder BR, Mihaly J, Prager GW (2007) uPAR-uPA-PAI-1 interactions and signaling: a vascular biologist's view. Thromb Haemost 97: 336–342.
31. Ploplis VA, Carmeliet P, Vazirzadeh S, Van Vlaenderen I, Moons L, et al. (1995) Effects of disruption of the plasminogen gene on thrombosis, growth, and health in mice. Circulation 92: 2585–2593.
32. Swaisgood CM, French EL, Noga C, Simon RH, Ploplis VA (2000) The development of bleomycin-induced pulmonary fibrosis in mice deficient for components of the fibrinolytic system. Am J Pathol 157: 177–187.
33. Arumugam S, Jang YC, Chen-Jensen C, Gibran NS, Isik FF (1999) Temporal activity of plasminogen activators and matrix metalloproteinases during cutaneous wound repair. Surgery 125: 587–593.
34. Frossing S, Rono B, Hald A, Romer J, Lund LR (2010) Skin wound healing in MMP2-deficient and MMP2/plasminogen double-deficient mice. Exp Dermatol 19: e234–240.
35. Bator JM, Cohen RL, Chambers DA (1998) Hydrocortisone regulates the dynamics of plasminogen activator and plasminogen activator inhibitor expression in cultured murine keratinocytes. Exp Cell Res 242: 110–119.
36. Island E, Wu H, Warburton D, Anderson K, Tuan TL (1999) Developmental differences in the expression and modulation of extracellular matrix proteases and inhibitors in mouse skin fibroblasts. Wound Repair Regen 7: 467–476.
37. Weckroth M, Vaheri A, Virolainen S, Saarialho-Kere U, Jahkola T, et al. (2004) Epithelial tissue-type plasminogen activator expression, unlike that of urokinase, its receptor, and plasminogen activator inhibitor-1, is increased in chronic venous ulcers. Br J Dermatol 151: 1189–1196.
38. Murphy G, Stanton H, Cowell S, Butler G, Knauper V, et al. (1999) Mechanisms for pro matrix metalloproteinase activation. APMIS 107: 38–44.
39. Juncker-Jensen A, Lund LR (2011) Phenotypic overlap between MMP-13 and the plasminogen activation system during wound healing in mice. PLoS One 6: e16954.
40. Velnar T, Bailey T, Smrkolj V (2009) The wound healing process: an overview of the cellular and molecular mechanisms. J Int Med Res 37: 1528–1542.
41. Gilliver SC (2010) Sex steroids as inflammatory regulators. J Steroid Biochem Mol Biol 120: 105–115.
42. Hotary KB, Yana I, Sabeh F, Li XY, Holmbeck K, et al. (2002) Matrix metalloproteinases (MMPs) regulate fibrin-invasive activity via MT1-MMP-dependent and -independent processes. J Exp Med 195: 295–308.
43. Grandas OH, Mountain DH, Kirkpatrick SS, Cassada DC, Stevens SL, et al. (2009) Regulation of vascular smooth muscle cell expression and function of matrix metalloproteinases is mediated by estrogen and progesterone exposure. J Vasc Surg 49: 185–191.
44. Campbell L, Emmerson E, Davies F, Gilliver SC, Krust A, et al. (2010) Estrogen promotes cutaneous wound healing via estrogen receptor beta independent of its antiinflammatory activities. J Exp Med 207: 1825–1833.
45. Azzi L, El-Alfy M, Martel C, Labrie F (2005) Gender differences in mouse skin morphology and specific effects of sex steroids and dehydroepiandrosterone. J Invest Dermatol 124: 22–27.
46. Shuster S, Black MM, McVitie E (1975) The influence of age and sex on skin thickness, skin collagen and density. Br J Dermatol 93: 639–643.
47. Pins GD, Collins-Pavao ME, Van De Water L, Yarmush ML, Morgan JR (2000) Plasmin triggers rapid contraction and degradation of fibroblast-populated collagen lattices. J Invest Dermatol 114: 647–653.

19

Humanized Mouse Model of Skin Inflammation Is Characterized by Disturbed Keratinocyte Differentiation and Influx of IL-17A Producing T Cells

Vivian L. de Oliveira[1], Romy R. M. C. Keijsers[1,2], Peter C. M. van de Kerkhof[2], Marieke M. B. Seyger[2], Esther Fasse[1], Lars Svensson[4], Markus Latta[4], Hanne Norsgaard[5], Tord Labuda[5], Pieter Hupkens[3], Piet E. J. van Erp[2], Irma Joosten[1], Hans J. P. M. Koenen[1]*

1 Laboratory of Medical Immunology, Department of Laboratory Medicine, Radboud University Nijmegen Medical Centre, Nijmegen, The Netherlands, **2** Dermatology Department, Radboud University Nijmegen Medical Centre, Nijmegen, The Netherlands, **3** Department of Plastic Surgery Radboud University Nijmegen Medical Centre, Nijmegen, The Netherlands, **4** Department of Disease Pharmacology, LEO Pharma, Ballerup, Denmark, **5** Department of Molecular Biomedicine, LEO Pharma, Ballerup, Denmark

Abstract

Humanized mouse models offer a challenging possibility to study human cell function *in vivo*. In the huPBL-SCID-huSkin allograft model human skin is transplanted onto immunodeficient mice and allowed to heal. Thereafter allogeneic human peripheral blood mononuclear cells are infused intra peritoneally to induce T cell mediated inflammation and microvessel destruction of the human skin. This model has great potential for *in vivo* study of human immune cells in (skin) inflammatory processes and for preclinical screening of systemically administered immunomodulating agents. Here we studied the inflammatory skin response of human keratinocytes and human T cells and the concomitant systemic human T cell response. As new findings in the inflamed human skin of the huPBL-SCID-huSkin model we here identified: 1. Parameters of dermal pathology that enable precise quantification of the local skin inflammatory response exemplified by acanthosis, increased expression of human β-defensin-2, Elafin, K16, Ki67 and reduced expression of K10 by microscopy and immunohistochemistry. 2. Induction of human cytokines and chemokines using quantitative real-time PCR. 3. Influx of inflammation associated IL-17A-producing human CD4+ and CD8+ T cells as well as immunoregulatory CD4+Foxp3+ cells using immunohistochemistry and -fluorescence, suggesting that active immune regulation is taking place locally in the inflamed skin. 4. Systemic responses that revealed activated and proliferating human CD4+ and CD8+ T cells that acquired homing marker expression of CD62L and CLA. Finally, we demonstrated the value of the newly identified parameters by showing significant changes upon systemic treatment with the T cell inhibitory agents cyclosporine-A and rapamycin. In summary, here we equipped the huPBL-SCID-huSkin humanized mouse model with relevant tools not only to quantify the inflammatory dermal response, but also to monitor the peripheral immune status. This combined approach will gain our understanding of the dermal immunopathology in humans and benefit the development of novel therapeutics for controlling inflammatory skin diseases.

Editor: T. Mark Doherty, Statens Serum Institute, Denmark

Funding: Part of this work was supported by a research grant from the VanderEs Research Foundation and other part was supported by a research grant from LEO Pharma A/S. The funders had no role in study design, data collection, decision to publish, or preparation of the manuscript. However, they have been involved in a few sample analyses and data discussions in addition to manuscript reviewing.

Competing Interests: Svensson L, Latta M, Norsgaard H, and Labuda T are all employees at LEO Pharma A/S.

* E-mail: h.koenen@labgk.umcn.nl

Introduction

The *in vivo* study of human biological processes is severely limited by ethical and technical constraints. An attractive relevant alternative is the use of humanized mice or "mouse-human chimaeras". Humanized mice are immunodeficient mice that are engrafted with human tissue or cells, such as hematopoietic stem cells (HSCs) or peripheral blood mononuclear cells (PBMC). Humanized mice offer a valuable tool in pre-clinical drug testing in translational medicine and investigations of human biology in areas like cancer, (auto-) inflammation/immunity, infectious diseases and immunotherapy [1,2].

Several humanized mouse models have been described to study T cell mediated skin diseases [3–7]. In these models, healthy human skin, diseased-prone skin or bioengineered skin is transplanted onto immunodeficient mice, allowed to become vascularized and heal, and in some of these models human immune cells are infused that will reconstitute the recipient with human immune cells to induce skin inflammation [5,6]. Although all these models have advantages and disadvantages their application to drug discovery and for the development of cellular therapies has already proven to be fruitful [8–11].

To study the local inflammatory as well as the systemic human T cell response *in vivo* we focused on the human peripheral blood lymphocyte reconstituted severe combined immunodeficient mouse (SCID) human skin allograft model (huPBL-SCID-huSkin model) initially described by Pober's group [5,6]. In this model human skin is transplanted on to immunodeficient SCID/beige mice, and since these recipients lack functional mature T and B cells and have impaired NK cell- and macrophage function [12,13], human skin is revascularized and accepted. After healing of the human skin, allogeneic human PBMC are infused intra peritoneally (ip), resulting within 2–3 weeks in microvascular cell injury and human T cell infiltration of the human skin [5,6]. This model is of particular interest to study the local pathology of skin inflammation. For this purpose it is crucial to be able to quantify the cutaneous inflammatory response by clinical relevant parameters associated with dermal inflammation, such as inflammation-associated deregulated expression of keratinocyte differentiation markers and characterization and enumeration of skin infiltrating human lymphocytes. This information has not previously been published regarding this model.

Most studies on inflammation in humanized mouse models focus on the local site of inflammation. A caveat in these humanized mouse models is the study of the systemic immunological response, which besides the local site of inflammation is crucial in the generation and regulation of the immune program (e.g, effector Thelper Th1, Th2, Th17, or regulating suppressor Treg). Important steps in mounting a T cell immune response include T cell activation, differentiation and expansion in the draining lymph nodes. Activated T cells leave the lymph node via the efferent lymphatics and enter the circulation through the lymph-vascular system and depending on their homing imprint the cells migrate into tissues or colonize other immune compartments [14,15]. Moreover, inflammatory skin diseases, such as moderate to severe psoriasis, are traditionally treated with systemic medication such as methotrexate, retinoids, and cyclosporine A and more recently with biologicals such as anti-TNF or anti-p40 therapy. This systemic treatment will not only influence the local skin immune response, but will also interfere systemically with T cell activation, differentiation, expansion and homing. At present, little Information is available on the effects of systemic medication of immune modulating agents and their effects on the systemic immune response in humanized mouse models. This information is crucial to identify treatment-related systemic biomarkers for immunomonitoring of patients undergoing clinical trials.

In the present study, both local human skin inflammatory processes as well as systemic human CD4+ and CD8+ T cell responses in the huPBL-SCID-huSkin model were studied. As new findings in this model we identified relevant markers of human dermal pathology such as aberrant expression of hBD2, Elafin, K10 and K16, enabling quantification of the local skin inflammatory response by keratinocytes, markers for T cell mediated responses in the skin, as well as, chemokine and cytokine induction and analysis of IL-17A-producing and Foxp3+ T cells. Also, we determined markers that enable quantitative analysis of systemic immune activation responses. Human skin inflammation was paralleled by the presence of CD4+Foxp3+ T cells, suggesting that immune regulatory pathways are serving to limit human tissue inflammation. Unraveling these pathways of human cells in this *in vivo* model will undoubtedly offer novel therapeutic strategies for controlling autoimmune tissue responses.

Results

Acanthosis and aberrant epidermal marker expression of hBD2, Elafin, K10 and K16 in the inflamed human skin in the huPBL-SCID-huSkin allograft model

Here we set out to define and quantify clinical relevant dermal parameters in the inflamed human skin the huPBL-SCID-huSkin allograft model as initially described by Pober's group [5,6]. The model in brief, after grafting and healing of human skin onto immunodeficient SCID beige recipients, allogeneic human PBMC are infused intra peritoneally (i.p.), which results in microvessel destruction and human T cell influx of the human skin graft [5,6].

Using histological microscopic examination of the human skin (**Fig. 1A**) we demonstrated hyperkeratosis (thickened keratinized upper layer), parakeratosis (nucleated keratinocytes in the cornified layer), acantosis (abnormal epidermal thickening, 155,1$\pm$10,6 vs 315,9$\pm$39,4 µm; PBS vs huPBMC, resp, $p<0{,}01$)(**Fig. 1B**), exocytosis (lymphocytes in the epidermis), spongiosys (intercellular edema between the keratinocytes and elongated rete ridges (fingerlike epidermal projections into the dermis) such as often observed in psoriatic lesions (**Fig. 1A**).

Using immunohistochemistry we quantitatively demonstrated that the changes in skin morphology were paralleled by a significant induction of keratinocyte associated inflammatory markers such as human β-defensin-2 (hBD2; 12,5$\pm$2,1 vs 31,7$\pm$10,9, $p<0{,}01$), Elafin (22,4$\pm$2,5 vs 43,0$\pm$14,7, $p<0{,}05$) and the hyper-proliferative marker keratin-16 (K16; 11,3$\pm$1,0 vs 38,6$\pm$12,5, $p<0{,}01$) , and down regulation of normal supra-basal keratin-10 (K10; 59,3$\pm$1,6 vs 11,6$\pm$4,9, $p<0{,}01$) (**Fig. 1C**).

Up-regulation of Ki67 expression by the keratinocytes indicated the presence of an increased number of dividing cells in the epidermis, which supports ongoing epidermal hyper-proliferation (**Fig. 1D**). Normal supra-basal K10 expression was found in the human skin transplants in the absence of PBMC infusion, indicating that the transplant procedure did not disturb normal supra-basal K10 expression (**Fig. 1C**).

In summary, as a new finding we defined deregulated epidermal marker expression of hBD2, Elafin, K10, K16 and Ki67 in the inflamed human skin of the huPBL-SCID-huSkin model that can be employed to analyze the local inflammatory skin response in quantitative way.

Human T cell infiltration and detection of human chemokines and cytokines in the inflamed human skin

Next to the epidermal changes described above, we found mononuclear cell infiltrates, including human CD3+ T cells, with a diffuse distribution throughout the human skin, but not in the mouse skin (**Fig. 2A+B**). Control mice that were transplanted with human skin and which received PBS instead of huPBMC showed no evidence of inflammation in either epidermis or dermis (**Fig. 1A**).

Inflammation of lymphocytes is regulated by pro-inflammatory cytokines and chemokines that attract these immune cells. To assess if human cytokines and chemokines might be involved in the development of skin inflammation in the huPBL-SCID/skin allograft model we determined gene expression levels in the skin grafts using quantitative real time PCR (qPCR). To this end the human skin grafts were removed 21 days after infusion of PBMC, at this time point clear inflammation hallmarks were observed by histology and immunohistochemistry (**Fig. 1,2A**). From the centre of the human skin grafts 4 mm punch biopsies were taken and subsequently prepared for qPCR analysis. A clear increase in gene

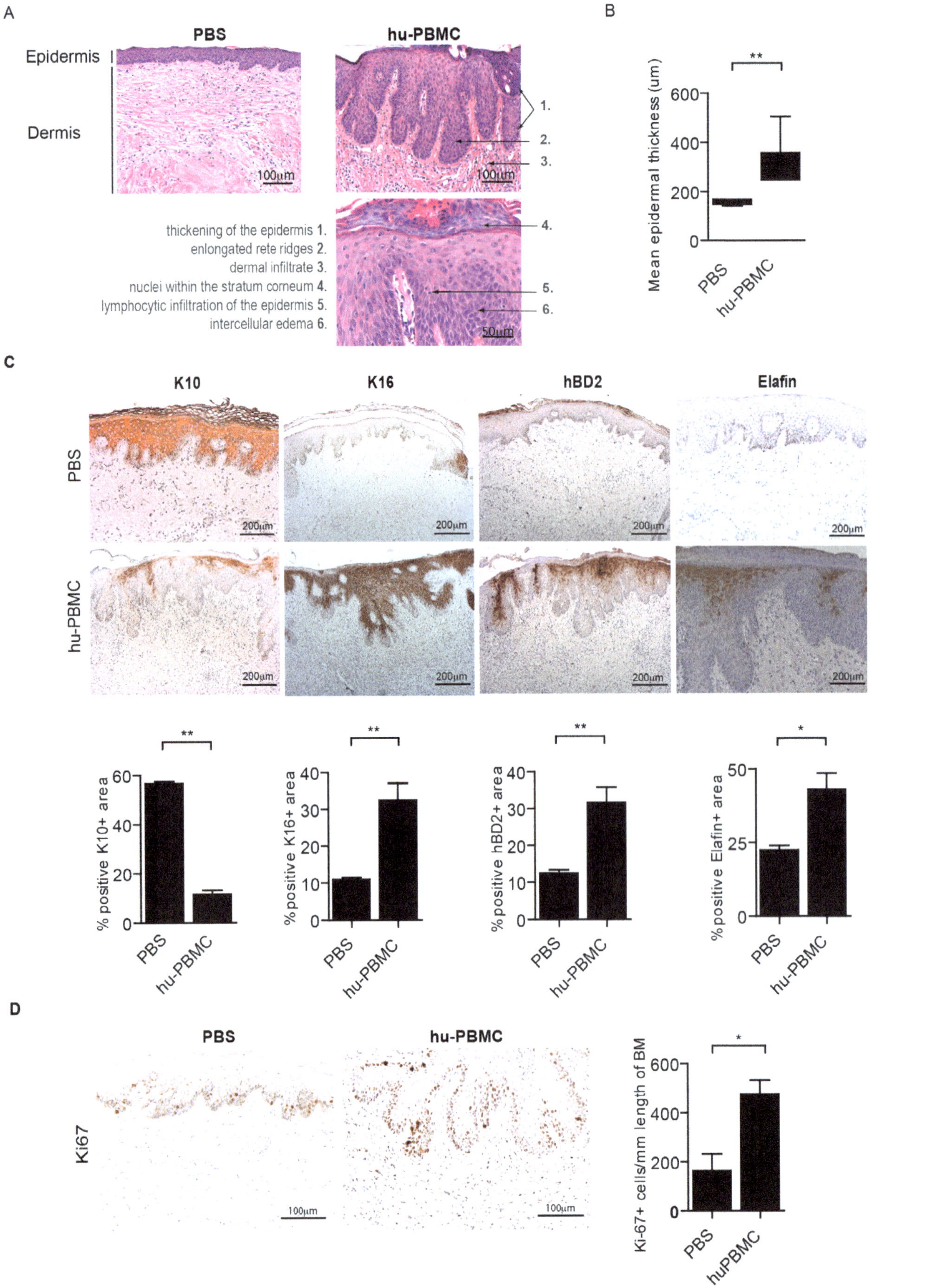

A
PBS
hu-PBMC
Epidermis
Dermis
100µm
100µm
1.
2.
3.
4.
5.
6.
50µm
thickening of the epidermis 1.
enlongated rete ridges 2.
dermal infiltrate 3.
nuclei within the stratum corneum 4.
lymphocytic infiltration of the epidermis 5.
intercellular edema 6.
B
Mean epidermal thickness (um)
**
600
400
200
0
PBS
hu-PBMC
C
K10
K16
hBD2
Elafin
PBS
hu-PBMC
200µm
% positive K10+ area
% positive K16+ area
% positive hBD2+ area
% positive Elafin+ area
D
PBS
hu-PBMC
Ki67
100µm
Ki-67+ cells/mm length of BM
PBS
huPBMC

Figure 1. Acanthosis and aberrant epidermal marker expression of hBD2, Elafin, K10 and K16 in the inflamed human skin of the huPBL-SCID-hu Skin allograft model. A. Histology (H&E staining) of human skin grafts from SCID beige mice 21 days after infusion (i.p.) of huPBMC. Representative photographs are shown after PBS (left photograph) and huPBMC infusion (right photograph). Photograph shows increased epidermal thickness (acanthosis) and elongated fingerlike epidermal projections into the dermis (rete ridges) and large lymphocyte infiltration after huPBMC infusion. Abnormal presence of nuclei in the stratum corneum (parakeratosis) and infiltration of lymphocytes in the epidermis (exocytosis) (bottom-right photograph). 20×, 20×, 40× magnifications respectively. **B.** Quantitative microscopic histological analysis of the epidermal thickness (μm) of human skin grafts following infusion of PBS and huPBMC. Mean±SEM are shown for n = 3 and 6 upon PBS and huPBMC infusion resp. **C.** Immunohistochemistry of K10, K16, hBD2 and Elafin (brown) in human skin grafts from SCID beige mice 21 days after infusion (i.p.) of PBS (top panels) or huPBMC (lower panels). Photograpsh show representative examples, summarized data are given in the figures. Mean±SEM percentages of the area positive for the indicated markers is shown for n = 3 and 5–8 upon PBS and huPBMC infusion resp. 10× magnification. **D.** Ki-67 expression (brown) in the stratum basale of the epidermis. The insert shows a higher magnification. A representative example of n = 12 is shown. 20× magnification. Graphs show summarized data of Ki67+ cells/mm length of basement membrane after PBS or huPBMC infusion in human skin biopsies (mean±SEM, of n = 4 and 6, resp.).

expression of the proinflammatory human cytokines IL1B, IL6 and IL8 was observed in the PBMC-injected skin compared to the PBS-treated controls (**Fig. 2B**). Also, we found increased gene expression of the human chemokines CXCL1, CXCL10 and CCL5, as well as DEFB4, the gene encoding the antimicrobial peptide human beta defensin-2 (hBD2) which was recently demonstrated to attract CCR6 expressing cells [16]. mRNA levels of human cytokines exclusively or predominantly expressed by immune cells were close to or below the detection limit in either some of the PBS-injected controls (e.g. IFNγ which is clearly induced in the treated skin) or in both treated and control skin samples (such as IL12B, IL23A, IL17A, IL22 and IL20)

Infiltration of CD4+ and CD8+ IL-17A-producing T cells and CD4+ Foxp3-expressing T cells in the inflamed human skin

Next, we further characterized the mononuclear cell infiltrate in the skin by immunohistochemistry, and focused our analysis on quantification of human CD4+ and CD8+ T cells. As reported previously on the huPBL-SCID/skin allograft model [5,6] the human skin contained both CD4+ and CD8+ T cells (**Fig. 3A**). CD4+ T cell infiltrates were predominantly present within the dermis (296,56±86,52 vs 954,68±35,9 cells/mm^2, PBS vs huPBMC, respectively, p<0,01), while CD8+ T cells were present in both dermis (245,42±10,3 vs 1162,85±107,8 cells/mm^2 p<0,05) and epidermis (296,6±86,5 vs 954,7±309,4 cells/mm^2 p<0,05) (**Fig. 3B**).

The cytokine interleukin 17A, which amongst other cell types is produced by T cells, has strong pro-inflammatory potential and has been clearly associated with psoriasis [17–19], and it also contributes to the pathology of atopic dermatitis [20,21]. Therefore, we analyzed the *in vivo* potential of the human CD4+ and CD8+ T cells to produce IL-17A in this huPBL/SCID model. IL-17A-producing cells were clearly present in the dermis, at the basal layer and also in the epidermis (**Fig. 3C**); both human CD4+/IL-17A+ and CD8+/IL-17A+ (41.95±12.38 and 27.8±5.97 cells/mm2, resp.) were observed (**Fig. 3D**). Next to these IL-17 -producing T cells, also CD3 negative IL-17-producing cells were observed. Mast cells and neutrophils are known for their IL-17A producing potential [22]. Here, we could clearly demonstrate that in the inflamed human skin human IL-17 production was associated with tryptase+ human mast cells, while we could not demonstrate IL-17+ elastase+ human neutrophils (**Fig. 3E**). We could not demonstrate IL-17A in the serum of the mice 3 weeks after infusion of huPBMC (data not shown), which suggests that IL-17 plays a predominant role in the local inflammatory skin response.

As opposed to pro-inflammatory cells, anti-inflammatory cells are needed to regulate the immune response. CD4+ regulatory T cells that express the transcription factor Foxp3 are renowned for their immunosuppressive potential and control of proinflammatory T cells. Therefore we analyzed the presence of human Foxp3+ cells in the human skin of the huPBL-SCID-huSkin model. CD4+ Foxp3+ cells were mainly present at the basal layer (**Fig. 3F**).

Taken together, inflammation of the human skin transplant of the huPBL-SCID-huSkin model is characterized by aberrant epidermal differentiation, presence of human cytokines and chemokines and influx of CD4+ and CD8+ T cells and mast cells that are able to produce the proinflammatory cytokine IL-17 as well as the presence of putative anti-inflammatory Foxp3 expressing CD4+ T cells.

Local human skin inflammation in the huPBL-SCID-huSkin model is paralleled by systemic CD4 and CD8 T cell activation, proliferation and acquisition of homing markers

In addition to the analysis of the local inflammatory response in the human skin, we studied the systemic response of the CD4+ and CD8+ T cells in the huPBL-SCID-huSkin model. Mice were transplanted with human skin that was allowed to heal for 3 weeks and subsequently inoculated with 150×10^6 human PBMC (i.p.) as describe above. After 3 weeks the CD4+ and CD8+ T cells were enumerated in peripheral blood, spleen and lymph nodes, and these cells were analyzed for cell division status, activation and homing marker expression using flowcytometry.

Anti-human CD45 monoclonal antibody was used to detect human lymphocytes in the humanized mice. CD45-expressing CD4+ and CD8+ T cells were observed in the peripheral blood, spleen and lymph nodes of the huPBL-SCID-huSkin model (**Fig. 4A**). In the peripheral blood equal percentages of CD4+ (42,3±5,5%) and CD8+ (48,5±7,6%) T cells were found (**Fig. 4A**), whereas in the lymph nodes CD4+ T cells (58,9±3,7%) were more predominant as compared to CD8+ T cells (27,7±3,9%)(**Fig. 4B**). Although less clear, the spleen seemed to contain more CD8+ (55,0±6,9%) than CD4+ T cells (30,2±2,0%) (**Fig. 4B**).

The majority of human T cells present in spleen, lymph nodes and peripheral blood expressed the memory marker CD45RO (**Fig. 4C,D**). Given that the inoculated huPBMC population pre-infusion contained about 60% CD45RA expressing T cells (**Fig. 4D**), which is indicative for the presence of naïve T cells, this suggests that the naïve T cells became activated *in vivo*. The presence of an allogeneic human skin transplant was required to induce this activated phenotype *in vivo*, as in the absence of a human skin transplant higher number of naïve CD45RA+ were observed spleen and lymph nodes (**Fig. 4C**). Irrespective of whether human skin was grafted, in peripheral blood we found similar percentages (>90%) of CD45RO+ cells (**Fig. 4C**). It should however be emphasized that higher absolute CD45RO+ numbers were found when a skin transplant was present (approx.

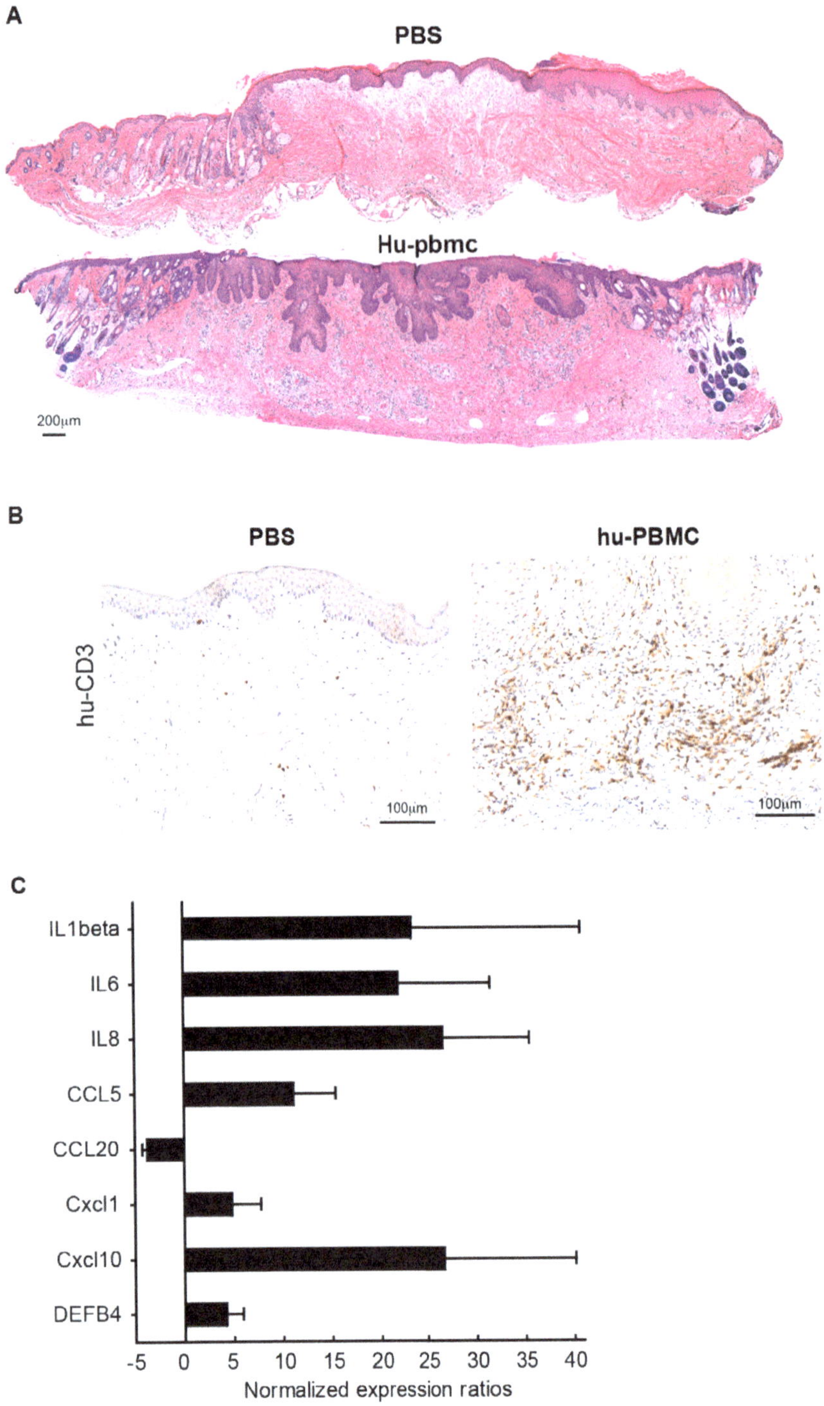

Figure 2. Induction of human chemokines and cytokines and influx of human T cells in the dermis and in the epidermis of huPBL-SCID-hu Skin allograft model. A. Images show representative panoramic overviews (H&E staining) of human skin grafts from SCID beige mice 21 days after infusion (i.p.) of PBS (top) or huPBMC (below). Note that human epidermis is thicker than the mouse epidermis (present in the left edge of the specimen in the top image and in both edges in the bottom image) and in contrast with human skin, mouse skin has closely spaced hair folicules troughout the epidermis. Images were composed using PTGui software (New House Internet Services B.V.; http://www.ptgui.com/). **B.** Immunohistochemistry of human CD3+ (brown) T cell infiltration in the human dermis and epidermis, 21 days after infusion of huPBMC. Representative example of n = 12 are shown. 20× magnification. **C.** Gene expression analysis using quantitative real-timePCR of human cytokine and chemokine transcripts in the human skin 21 days after infusion of huPBMC. Figure shows fold increase in cytokine and chemokine mRNA expression levels after huPBMC infusion as compared to PBS infusion (n = 5 and 3; huPBMC and PBS resp.).

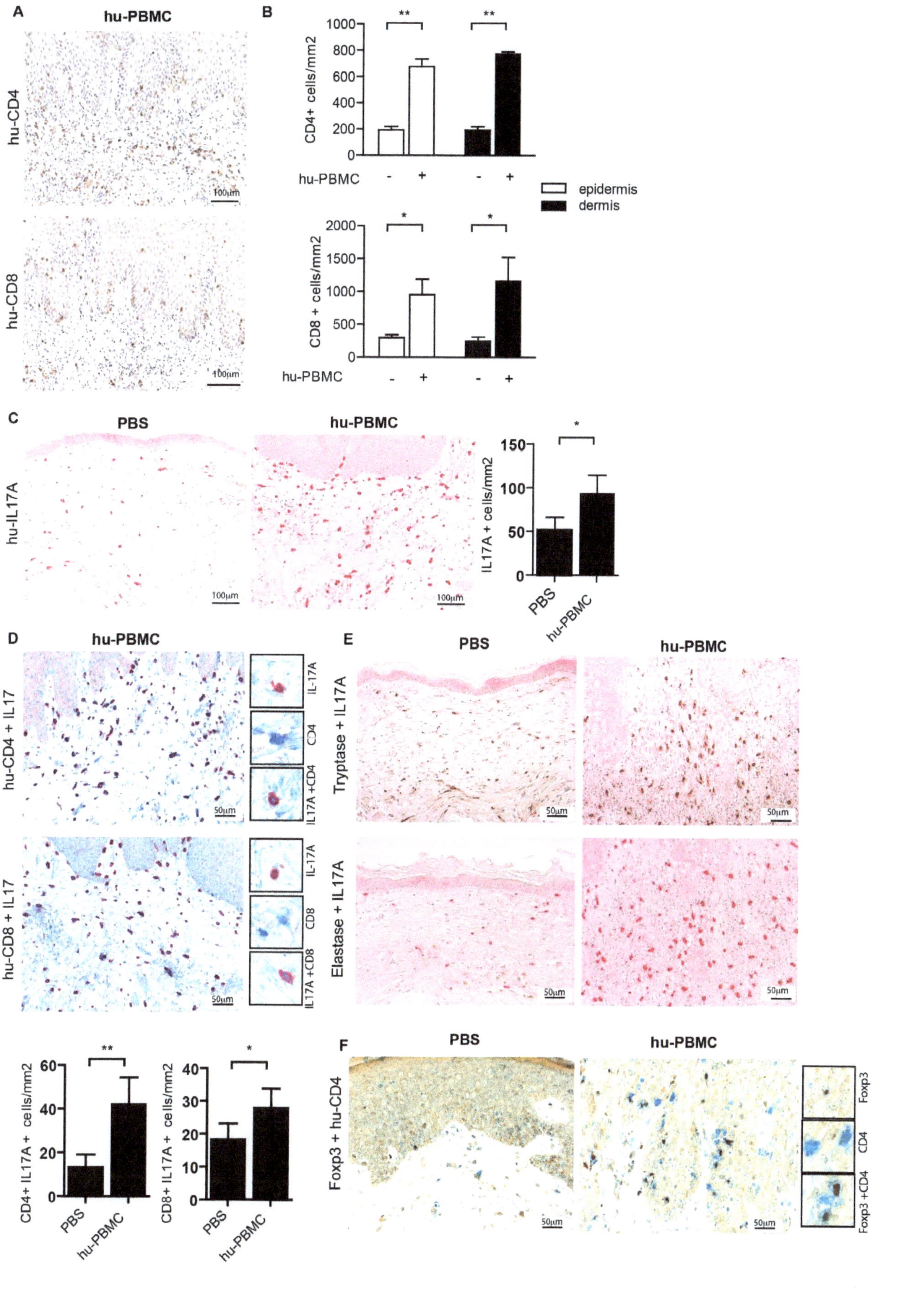
A
hu-PBMC
hu-CD4
hu-CD8
100µm
B
CD4+ cells/mm2
1000
800
600
400
200
0
**
hu-PBMC
- + - +
epidermis
dermis
CD8 + cells/mm2
2000
1500
1000
500
0
*
C
PBS
hu-PBMC
hu-IL17A
IL17A + cells/mm2
150
100
50
0
PBS
hu-PBMC
D
hu-PBMC
hu-CD4 + IL17
hu-CD8 + IL17
IL-17A
CD4
IL17A +CD4
CD8
IL17A +CD8
50µm
CD4+ IL17A + cells/mm2
60
40
20
0
CD8+ IL17A + cells/mm2
40
30
20
10
0
E
PBS
hu-PBMC
Tryptase + IL17A
Elastase + IL17A
F
Foxp3 + hu-CD4
Foxp3
Foxp3 +CD4

Figure 3. Infiltration of human IL-17A-producing T cells and CD4+ Foxp3-expressing T cells in the inflamed human skin in the SCID/skin allograft mouse model. A. Immunohistochemistry of human CD4 (brown, top) and CD8 (brown, bottom) expression in human skin grafts from SCID beige mice 21 days after infusion or huPBMC. Photographs show representative examples. 20× magnification. **B.** Summarized data of figure A. showing mean±SEM CD4 (top) or CD8 (bottom) positive cells/mm^2 of n = 4 and 10 upon PBS and huPBMC infusion resp in the epidermis (white bars) and dermis (black bars). **C.** Immunohistochemistry of human IL-17A expression in human skin grafts from SCID beige mice 21 days after infusion of PBS (left) or huPBMC (right). Photographs show representative examples of n = 6 (huPBMCs) n = 3 (controls). 20× magnification. Graph shows summarized data of IL-17A positive cells/mm^2 following PBS or huPBMC infusion in the human skin biopsies (mean±SEM, of n = 4 and 10). **D.** Immunohistochemistry of coexpression of human CD4 (blue) and IL-17A (red, top) and CD8 (blue) and IL-17A (red, bottom) in human skin grafts from SCID beige mice 21 days after infusion of huPBMC (20× magnification). Inserts show a higher magnification (40×) of single CD4/CD8 and IL-17A staining and CD4/IL-17A or CD8/IL-17A co-staining. . Photographs show representative examples of n = 6. **E.** Immunohistochemistry of IL-17A (red) in human mastcell tryptase (brown) and granulocyte elastase (brown) in human skin biopsies from SCID beige mice 21 days after infusion of PBS (left) or huPBMC (right). Photographs show representative examples of n = 6 (huPBMCs) n = 3 (controls). 20× magnification. **F.** Immunohistochemistry of co-expression of human Foxp3 (brown) and CD4 (blue) in human skin grafts from SCID beige mice 21 days after infusion of PBS (left) or huPBMC (right) (40× magnification). Inserts show a higher magnification (63×) of single Foxp3 and CD4+ staining and Foxp3/CD4 co-staining. Photographs show representative examples of n = 6 (huPBMCs) n = 3 (controls).

5×10^4 vs. 1×10^2 CD45RO+ cells in 20 µl *retro-orbital blood samples* after human skin transplantation vs. no transplantation, resp.) In peripheral blood, and spleen we found proliferating human CD4+ and CD8+ cells, as indicated by Ki67 staining (**Fig. 4E,F**). Interestingly, we observed that the presence of a human skin graft led to the induction of cutaneous lymphocyte associated antigen (CLA) expression on peripheral CD3+ T cells (**Fig. 4G,H**). This was not the case for the lymph node homing marker CD62L (**Fig. 4G,H**). It appeared that in particular CD8+ T cells had acquired CLA expression which was observed in both peripheral blood cells and spleen, but not in the case of lymph nodes (**Fig. 4I,J**). This indicates that the human skin can instruct homing receptor expression of the inoculated human cells in this humanized mouse model. Moreover, we found that more CD4+ T cells as compared to CD8+ T cells in the peripheral blood expressed the lymph node homing marker CD62L (**Fig. 4I,J**).

In summary, the flowcytometric analysis of human CD4+ and CD8+ T cells in peripheral blood and lymphoid organs in the huPBL-SCID-huSkin humanized mouse enables the study of the immune status and homing of human T cells *in vivo*. This together with the study of the local inflammatory response, as described above, empowers the huPBL-SCID-huSkin model as an important tool in the development and preclinical evaluation of novel systemic immunomodulating agents.

Cyclosporin-A and rapamycin prevent human T cell mediated skin inflammation and systemic activation and proliferation of the human T cells

Next, we studied the value of the above mentioned newly identified parameters in the huPBL-SCID-huSkin allograft model by analyzing the effect of systemic treatment with the T cell inhibitory agents cyclosporine-A and rapamycin. We used the combination of Cyclosporine (CsA) and Rapamycin (Rapa), which has previously been demonstrated to decrease the extent of mononuclear cell infiltration and reduce the degree of microvessel injury in a huPBL-SCID-huSkin model [6]. Administration of CsA (0,4 mg/kg/day) was started at the day of inoculation with the huPBMC. Co-administration of Rapa (0,4 mg/kg/day) was initiated at day 7 and given on alternate days until the end of the immunosuppressive treatment.

Macroscopic evaluation 21 days after inoculation with huPBMC indicated that treatment with CsA and Rapa reduce visible signs of inflammation; the skin graft looked healthier and less inflamed, as indicated by a reduction in erythema, scaling and skin thickness (**Fig. 5A**). Histological analysis revealed that the epidermal thickening, elongated rete ridge formation and mononuclear cell infiltrates induced in this humanized mouse model was effectively inhibited by combined CsA and Rapa treatment (**Fig. 5B**). Quantitative microscopic analysis clearly demonstrated a significant reduction in epidermal thickening by CsA and Rap treatment (315,9±68,2 vs 135,4±45,1 µm, no treatment vs CsA+Rapa, resp, $p<0,05$)(**Fig. 5B**). Immunohistochemistry revealed that the aberrant epidermal differentiation, as indicated by the increased hBD2 and Elafin expression, and dysregulated K10/K16 expression, in the human skin were significantly inhibited following CsA and Rapa treatment (hBD2; 40,2±2,9 vs 12,2±5,2, Elafin; 24±2 vs 14,4±4,K10; 18,9±3,4 vs 43,6±6,8, K16; 73,3±4,7 vs 17,8±10% positive area, no treatment vs CsA+Rapa, resp, $p<0,05$) (**Fig. 5C,D**). As expected, the number of CD4+ and CD8+ T cells in the human dermis (CD4; 783,5±38,8 vs 251,1±42,9, CD8; 1162,9±716,3 vs 71,3±38,4 cells/mm^2, no treatment vs CsA+Rapa, resp, $p<0,05$ and $p<0,01$) and epidermis (CD4; 605,8±76,6 vs 296,6±35,6, CD8; 1232,5±648,4 vs 183,9,9±10,7 cells/mm^2, both $p<0,01$) were significantly reduced by the immunosuppressive treatment (**Fig. 5E,F**). Interestingly, the numbers of IL-17A-producing T cells were also substantially inhibited (**Fig. 5G**). CsA+Rapa treatment resulted in a substantial reduction of Foxp3+ cells in both the human skin graft and spleen (data not shown).

Next, using flowcytometry, we analyzed the effect of CsA and Rapa treatment on the systemic immune response. We found that following CsA and Rapa treatment the number of human CD4+ and CD8+ T cells was reduced in peripheral blood of the mice (CD4+, $6,66\times10^5\pm6,08\times10^3$ vs $1,47\times10^5\pm2,78\times10^4$ and CD8+, $5,78\times10^5\pm5,51\times10^3$ vs $1,96\times10^5\pm1,00\times10^5$ total cell numbers, no treatment vs CsA+Rapa, resp. ($p<0,01$) **Fig. 6A**).

Moreover, after CsA and Rapa treatment the number of proliferating (Ki67 expressing) (**Fig. 6B**) and activated/differentiated (CD45RO expressing) (**Fig. 6C**) human CD4+ and CD8+ T cells in the peripheral blood was substantially decreased.

Discussion

In our current work we further advanced the huPBL-SCID-huSkin allograft model initially described Pober's group [5,6] for studying local skin inflammation, by identifying new local (skin) – as well as systemic parameters that turn this model into an even more powerful tool to study human skin immunopathology *in vivo*. A good understanding of the human skin immunopathology is crucial in the development of novel therapeutics for the treatment of (auto) inflammatory skin diseases.

Although the major focus of the huPBL-SCID-huSkin allograft model is on skin immune pathology, we also directed our attention on the systemic immune response of the human PBMC. We here demonstrate systemic proliferation, activation, and induction of homing marker acquisition by human T cells. This was prevented by systemic treatment with the immunosuppressive agents CsA

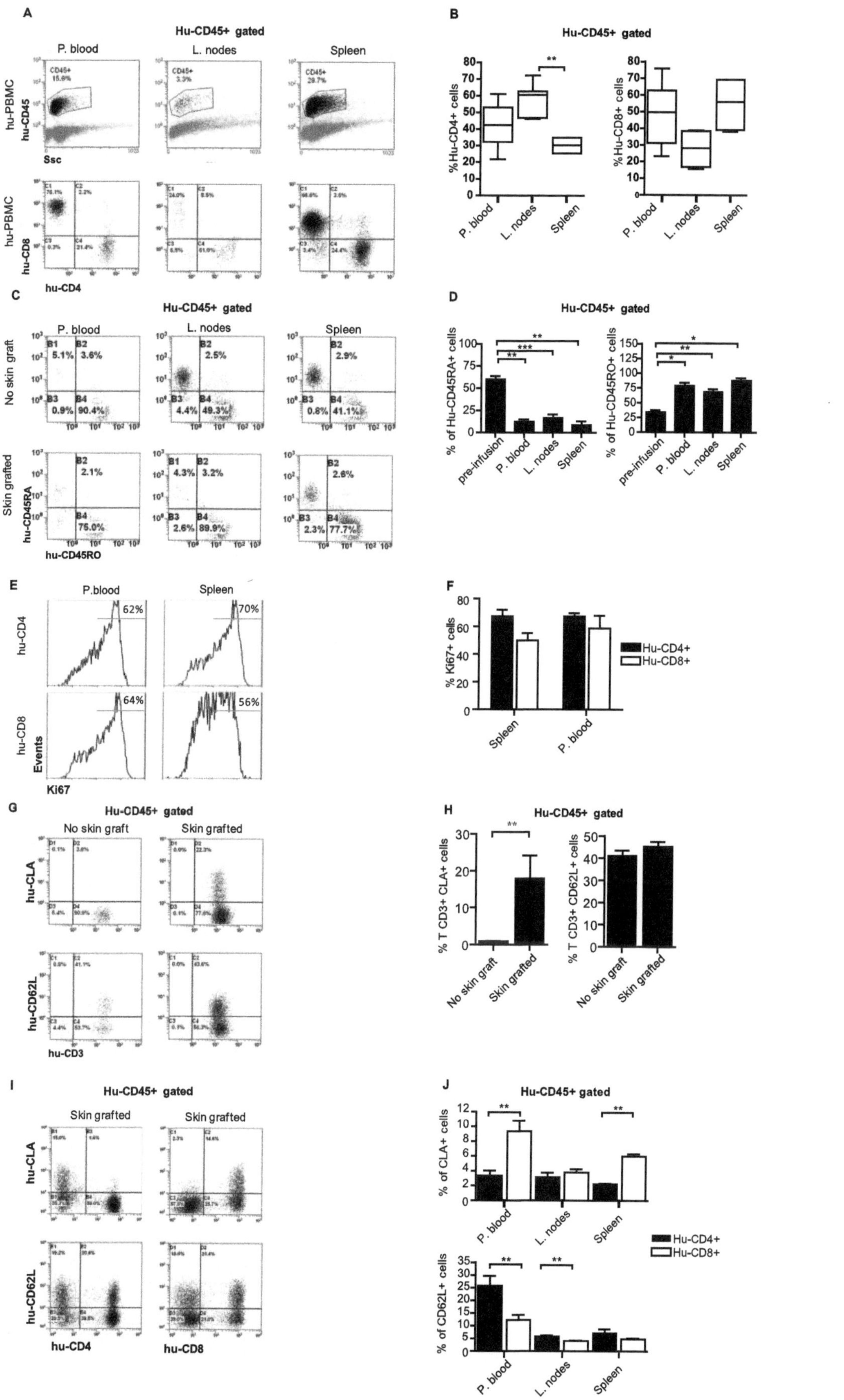
A
Hu-CD45+ gated
P. blood
L. nodes
Spleen
hu-PBMC
hu-CD45
Ssc
hu-CD8
hu-CD4
B
Hu-CD45+ gated
%Hu-CD4+ cells
%Hu-CD8+ cells
P. blood
L. nodes
Spleen
C
Hu-CD45+ gated
No skin graft
Skin grafted
hu-CD45RA
hu-CD45RO
B1 5.1%
B2 3.6%
B3 0.9%
B4 90.4%
B2 2.5%
B3 4.4%
B4 49.3%
B2 2.9%
B3 0.8%
B4 41.1%
B2 2.1%
B4 75.0%
B1 4.3%
B2 3.2%
B3 2.6%
B4 89.9%
B2 2.6%
B3 2.3%
B4 77.7%
D
Hu-CD45+ gated
% of Hu-CD45RA+ cells
% of Hu-CD45RO+ cells
pre-infusion
E
P.blood
Spleen
hu-CD4
hu-CD8
Events
Ki67
62%
70%
64%
56%
F
% Ki67+ cells
Hu-CD4+
Hu-CD8+
G
Hu-CD45+ gated
No skin graft
Skin grafted
hu-CLA
hu-CD62L
hu-CD3
H
Hu-CD45+ gated
% T CD3+ CLA+ cells
% T CD3+ CD62L+ cells
No skin graft
Skin grafted
I
Hu-CD45+ gated
Skin grafted
Skin grafted
hu-CLA
hu-CD62L
hu-CD4
hu-CD8
J
Hu-CD45+ gated
% of CLA+ cells
% of CD62L+ cells
Hu-CD4+
Hu-CD8+

Figure 4. Systemic human CD4 and CD8 T cell activation, proliferation and acquisition of homing markers in the SCID/skin allograft mouse model. A. Flowcytometry showing side scatter (SSC, X-axis) and CD45 expression (Y-axis) (top panel) and CD4 (X-axis) and CD8 (Y-axis) expression (lower panel) in peripheral blood and lymph node and spleen cell suspensions 21 days after infusion or huPBMC. Representative dotplots are shown (n = 4–7). CD4/CD8 expression is shown after gating on huCD45+ cells. In case of PBS infusion hardly any human CD45+ lymphocytes was detected (data not shown). **B.** Summarized flowcytometry data of human CD4+ and CD8+ cells upon huPBMC infusion as shown in A. (n = 6). **C.** Flowcytometry of human CD45RO+ (X-axis) and CD45RA+ (Y-axis) cell populations in peripheral blood and lymph node and spleen cell suspensions 21 days after infusion of huPBMC in SCID beige mice that either lacked (top panel) or were previously grafted with human skin (lower panel) Representative dotplots gated on huCD45+ cells are shown. **D.** Summarized flowcytometry data of CD45RO+ and CD45RA+ cells upon huPBMC infusion in SCID beige mice that were grafted with human skin as shown in C. (n = 6). **E.** Flowcytometry of Ki67 expression in CD4+ (top panel) and CD8+ (lower panel) human T cells in peripheral blood (left) and spleen (right). **F.** Summarized flowcytometry data of Ki67 expression in CD4+ and CD8+ human T cells as shown in E. (n = 6). **G.** Flowcytometry of CLA (top panel) and CD62L (lower panel) expression on human CD3+ cells populations in peripheral blood, 21 days after infusion of huPBMC in SCID beige mice that either lacked (right panel) or were previously grafted with human skin (right panel) Representative dotplots gated on huCD45+ cells are shown. **H.** Summarized flowcytometry data of CLA and CD62L expression on human CD3+ cells as shown in G. (n = 4–5). **I.** Flowcytometry of CLA (top panel) and CD62L (lower panel) expression on human CD4+ (left) and CD8+ (right) cells in peripheral blood, 21 days after infusion of huPBMC in SCID beige mice that previously grafted with human skin. Representative dotplots gated on huCD45+ cells are shown. **J.** Summarized flowcytometry data of CLA and CD62L expression on human CD4+ and CD8+ cells as shown in peripheral blood, lymph nodes and spleen. (n = 4–5).

and Rapa. Systemic analysis of the immune response in this preclinical humanized model is important for two reasons. First, the induction of a local T cell immune response is a multistep phenomenon taking place locally at the affected skin site (antigen recognition), in the draining lymph nodes (antigen presentation, T cell activation, differentiation, expansion) and peripheral blood (migration of activated T cells to the affected site and to other lymph nodes) [14]. Second, during the last decade there is an increasing use of systemic agents, like anti-inflammatory drugs or biologicals, to treat severe inflammatory skin diseases [23] [24]. At present, little Information is available on the effects of systemic medication of immune modulating agents and their effects on the systemic immune response in humanized mouse models. This information is crucial to identify treatment-related systemic biomarkers for immunomonitoring of patients undergoing clinical trials. For analysis of the systemic human immune response in the huPBL-SCID-huSkin model, peripheral blood samples containing relatively few cells can be used to analyze the effects of an anti-inflammatory drug by multi-color flowcytometry over time.

In the huPBL-SCID-huSkin model we observed that the presence of the human skin graft instructs CLA expression on a fraction of the peripheral human CD8+ T cells. This suggests that migration of T cells from skin or skin draining lymph nodes to the periphery is taking place. In mice it has been demonstrated that memory/effector phenotype T cells migrated from the skin to the draining lymph nodes in the steady state conditions, and this process was increased during a cutaneous immune response [25]. Early in a primary cutaneous immune response, proliferating T cells were released from the skin-draining lymph nodes and migrated via the circulation to antigen free lymph nodes that drain other tissues [26]. This migration of dividing T cells from the skin draining lymph nodes might explain the presence of human dividing Ki67+ T cells that we identify in the peripheral blood and spleen in the huPBL-SCID-huSkin model. Little is known about the migratory capacity of human T cells *in vivo*, the huPBL-SCID-huSkin model will be a helpful tool in improving our understanding in this respect.

IL-17-producing CD4+ T cells, designated Th17 cells, are important in the protection against extracellular pathogens, but Th17 cells are also associated with inflammatory and autoimmune conditions in humans [27]. IL-17 is a cytokine that acts as a potent proinflammatory mediator by increasing chemokine production to recruit monocytes and neutrophils to the site of inflammation. Immunity mediated by Th17 cells is particularly important at epithelial and mucosal surfaces [28]. IL-17-producing T cells appear to be important in the pathogenesis of psoriasis; Th17 cells have been demonstrated by both immunohistochemistry and flowcytometry in psoriatic lesions [17,18]. Furthermore, a recent phase-II clinical study with a human antibody to IL-17A (AIN457, secukinumab) in psoriasis patients showed promising results supporting a role for Th17 in the pathophysiology of psoriasis [19]. Also in the early stages of atopic dermatitis IL-17-producing cells seem to contribute to the pathology of the disease [20,21]. In the inflamed skin of the huPBL-SCID-huSkin model we observed the presence of IL-17A-producing CD4+ and CD8+ cells. Although Th17 cells, which are classically defined as CD4+ IL-17-producing cells, previously has received the major focus, it has recently been established that also CD8+ IL-17-producing cells contribute to inflammatory skin disorders including psoriasis [29,30].

Regulatory T cells are important in the control of immune homeostasis and tolerance [31]. In particular CD4+ regulatory T cells expressing the Treg master transcription factor Foxp3 were extensively studied over the last decade. Skin resident CD4+ Foxp3+ Treg were identified in mice and men [25,32]. In mice, skin resident CD4+Foxp3+ Treg suppress inflammation and appear to migrate from the skin to the draining lymph nodes under steady state conditions. During a cutaneous immune response migration of Treg was increased [25,32]. Moreover, Treg that migrated from the skin returned to the skin upon skin antigen exposure [25]. In normal human skin under steady state conditions between 5 and 10% of the skin resident T cells are CD3+/FOXP3+ Treg [33] and proliferation of CD4+/Foxp3+ Treg was induced after a cutaneous challenge [34]. Together these data suggest that Treg circulate between blood, skin, and lymphoid tissues and that local Treg proliferation takes place in order to regulate peripheral skin immune responses. In the affected human skin of the huPBL-SCID-huSkin model, we now demonstrate the presence of human CD4+Foxp3+ T cells in the dermis of the human skin, which suggests active immune regulation in the inflamed human skin of this humanized mouse model. A possible reason why Foxp3+ Treg in this model do no inhibit the IL-17A production by CD4+ and CD8+ T cells might be explained by the fact that Treg can become unstable under proinflammatory conditions and lose suppressor function and even gain pro-inflammatory characteristics, resulting in an increased inflammatory response [35]. Also human Treg have this propensity to convert into proinflammatory cytokine secreting cells, in particular when activated under proinflammatory conditions [36].

We studied gene expression levels of cytokines and chemokines by quantitative real-time PCR in the affected human skin of the mice 3 weeks after the inoculation with PBMC when inflammation of the human skin was established. We found an increase in gene expression of human IL1B, IL6, IL8, CXCL1, CXCL10, CCL5

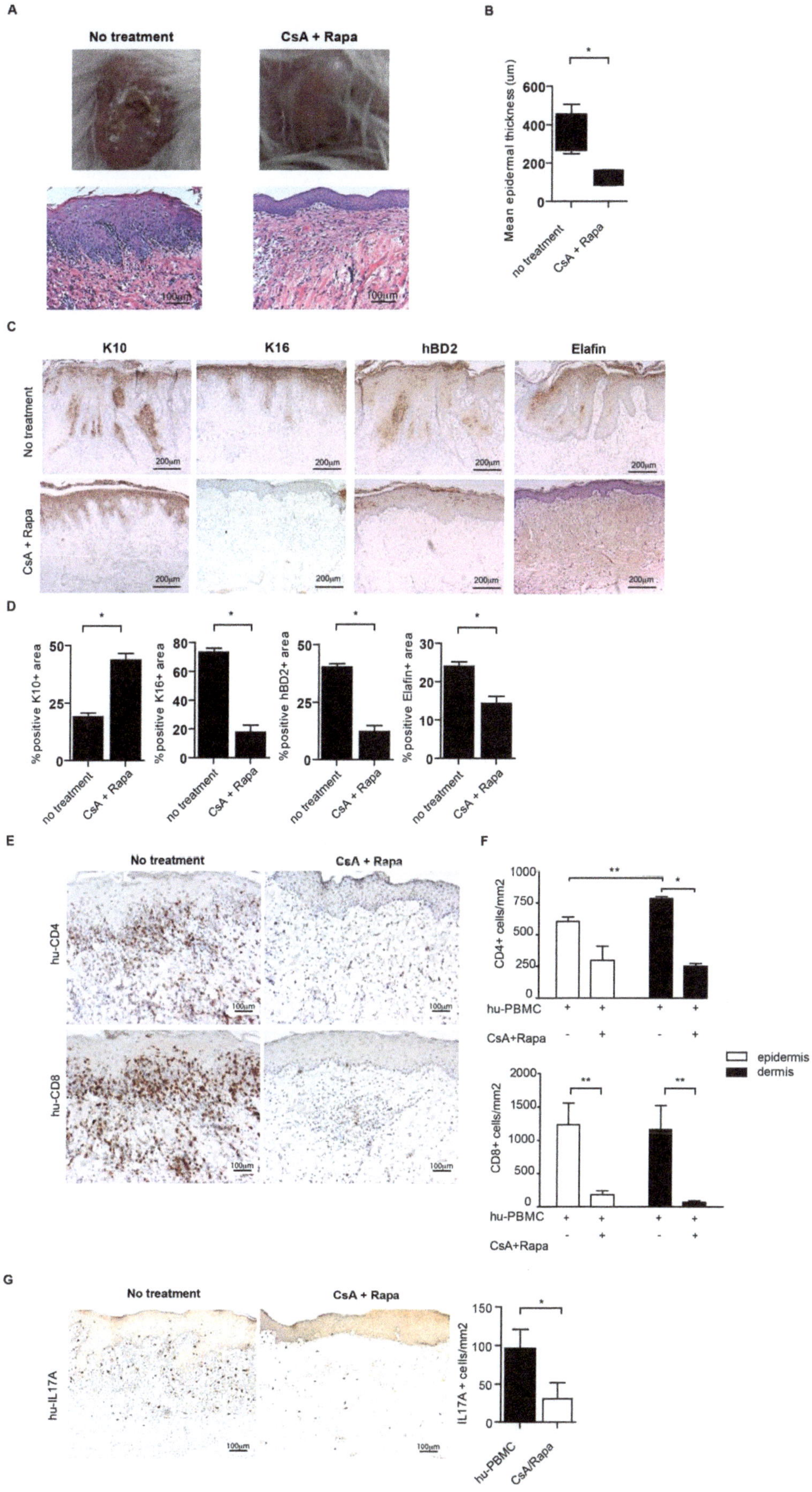
A
No treatment
CsA + Rapa
100µm
B
Mean epidermal thickness (um)
600
400
200
0
no treatment
CsA + Rapa
C
K10
K16
hBD2
Elafin
No treatment
CsA + Rapa
200µm
D
% positive K10+ area
% positive K16+ area
% positive hBD2+ area
% positive Elafin+ area
E
No treatment
CsA + Rapa
hu-CD4
hu-CD8
100µm
F
CD4+ cells/mm2
CD8+ cells/mm2
hu-PBMC
CsA+Rapa
epidermis
dermis
G
No treatment
CsA + Rapa
hu-IL17A
IL17A + cells/mm2
hu-PBMC
CsA/Rapa

Figure 5. Cyclosporin-A and rapamycin treatment restores aberrant human epidermal differentiation marker expression and prevents infiltration of inflammation associated IL-17A producing human T cells of the human skin in the huPBL-SCID/skin allograft mouse model. A. Macroscopic (top panel) and histological (H&E) (lower panel) appearance of human skin graft from SCID beige mice 21 days after infusion of huPBMC with no treatment (left panel) and treatment with CsA and Rapa (right panel). **B.** Quantitative microscopic histological analysis of the epidermal thickness (µm) of skin grafts following infusion of huPBMC with or without CsA and Rapa. Mean±SEM are shown for n = 3 and 5 upon PBS and huPBMC infusion resp. 20× magnification. **C.** Immunohistochemistry of K10, K16, hBD2 and Elafin in human skin grafts from SCID beige mice 21 days after infusion (i.p.) of huPBMC without (top panel) and with CsA and Rapa treatment (lower panel). Representative examples are show. 10× magnification. **D.** Summarized data represented in C are given in the figures. Mean±SEM percentages of the area positive for the indicated markers is shown for n = 3 and 4–6 upon no treatment and treatment with CsA and Rapa, resp. **E.** Immunohistochemistry of CD4 (top panel) and CD8 (lower panel) in human skin grafts from SCID beige mice 21 days after infusion (i.p.) of huPBMC without (left panel) and with CsA and Rapa treatment (right panel). Representative examples are show. 20× magnification. **F.** Summarized data represented in E. are given in the figures. Mean±SEM percentages of CD4 (top) and CD8 (bottom) positive cells is shown for n = 3 and 4–5 upon no treatment and treatment with CsA and Rapa, resp. **G.** Immunohistochemistry of IL-17A (brown) (representative examples of n = 5 are shown) 10× magnification. Graph shows summarized data of IL-17A positive cells/mm^2 present in human skin biopsies following infusion of huPBMC in the absence or presence of Rap/CsA resp. (mean±SEM, of n = 3 and 4–5).

and DEFB4. The upregulation of DEFB4 correlated with the increased protein levels of hBD2 found by immunohistochemistry. Besides the chemokines and cytokines presented in figure 2C, we analyzed a number of other relevant cytokines that might play a role in skin inflammation (such as IL12, IL23, IL17, and IL22). Gene expression levels of these cytokines, arising from immune cells, were close to or below the detection limit. The reason for this is probably related to the fact that we have been analyzing gene expression at a late time point when overt inflammation was taken place (3 weeks after infusion of human PBMC) combined with the low levels of immune cells compared to keratinocytes in the skin biopsy. Future studies are needed to reveal time-kinetics of gene expression.

In the humanized inflammatory skin model that we here present, we showed differential expression of epidermal pathology-related proteins such as increased human β-defensin-2, Elafin, Keratin 16 (K16), and Ki67 levels, and reduced expression of Keratin 10 (K10). Most chronic inflammatory skin diseases are characterized by increased proliferation of keratinocytes, resulting in epidermal thickening (acanthosis). Proliferating keratinocytes are further characterized by upregulation of the proliferation marker Ki67. The proliferative response is further accompanied by a shift in keratin expression in the supra-epidermal layers. K16 is upregulated, while K10 is downregulated in keratinocytes. K16 expression, which is not expressed in healthy epidermis, was first explained as the specific result of hyperproliferation. However, more recent studies show K16 expression to be a marker of general trauma and stress of the skin ([37,38]. Elafin and hBD-2 are anti-microbial peptide/proteins secreted by keratinocytes, they constitute part of the innate immune defense and participate in skin protection against invading microorganisms [39]. Elafin and hBD-2 are not present in healthy human epidermis, but they are highly induced under chronic inflammatory conditions of the skin (eg. psoriasis) and in case of skin barrier disruption [40–43]. The proinflammatory cytokine IL-17A can induces the expression of hBD2 in keratinocytes [44–46]. Next to its antimicrobial activity, hBD2 acts as pro-inflammatory chemoattractant for immune cells such as T-cells, dendritic cells, mast cells and neutrophils [47]. The upregulation of these anti-microbial peptides in our model is most likely the result of the influx of activated T cells and other immune cells and points to involvement of the innate immune system and impaired skin barrier function.

Psoriasis is a highly prevalent T cell mediated chronic inflammatory skin disease, which has both environmental and genetic causes to its etiology [48,49]. The multi factorial and complex pathophysiology of the disease results in disturbed communication between cells of the immune system and epidermal cells, leading to abnormal differentiation and hyper-proliferation of keratinocytes [50]. Recently it emerged that the disease is strongly associated with IL-23 [51] and IL-17-producing T helper cells [17–19]. Psoriatic plaque lesions are histologically characterized by an increase in epidermal thickness, caused by disturbed keratinocyte differentiation and hyper proliferation (acanthosis), elongated epidermal rete ridges and influx of immune

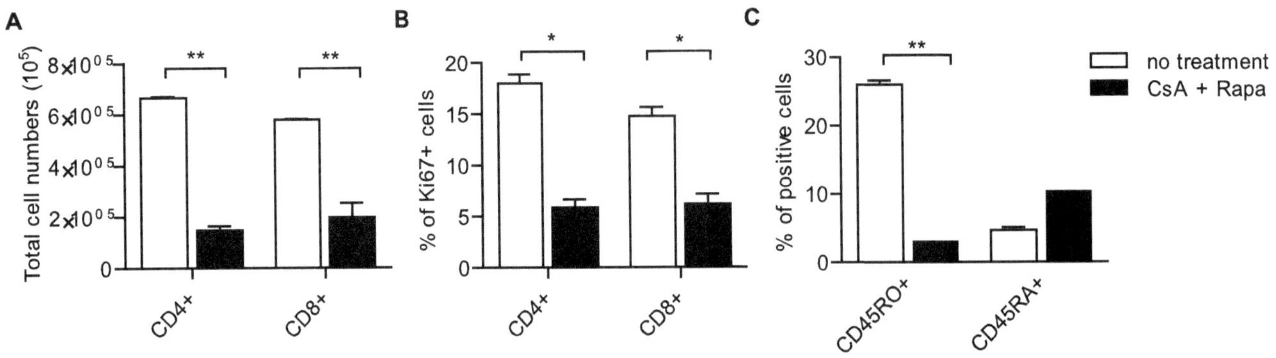

Figure 6. Cyclosporin-A and rapamycin treatment prevents systemic activation and proliferation of human CD4+ and CD8+ T cells in the huPBL-SCID/skin allograft mouse model. A. Enumeration of CD4+ and CD8+ cell populations by flowcytometry in peripheral blood 21 days after infusion of huPBMC without (white bars) or with CsA (black bars) and Rapa. Summarized flowcytometry data are presented (n = 6). **B.** Flowcytometry of Ki67 in human CD4+ of CD8+ cells in peripheral blood 21 days after infusion of huPBMC without (white bars) or with CsA and Rapa (black bars). Summarized data of n = 6 are shown. **C.** Flowcytometry of CD45RO and CD45RA expression on human CD3+ T cells in peripheral blood after infusion of huPBMC without (white bars) or with CsA and Rapa (black bars). Summarized data of n = 6 are shown.

cells among which many T cells [50]. Clinically these alterations are represented by scaling, plaque thickening, and erythema [50]. At the molecular level, a regenerative epidermal differentiation program is induced that includes expression of genes such as Keratin 16 (K16), elafin, psoriasin and β-defensin-2 (hBD-2), and because differentiation is impaired keratinocytes loose expression of normal supra-basal keratin-10 (K10) [52–55] and increase expression of Ki67 in basal keratinocytes [50]. The association of psoriasis and hBD-2 induction [52] has recently been further substantiated by demonstrating increased β-defensin copy numbers in psoriasis patients [42].

In the inflamed human skin of the huPBL-SCID-huSkin model we here demonstrate that the skin inflammatory phenotype resembles human plaque-type psoriasis at multiple levels; macroscopically we found erythema and skin thickening, microscopically using histology we demonstrated acanthosis, parakeratosis and psoriasis like rete ridges, and by immunohistochemistry we found increased expression of hBD-2, elafin, K16 and Ki67 and reduced K10 expression. Moreover, we detected CLA expressing human CD8+ T cells in the peripheral blood of the huPBL-SCID-huSkin model. The presence of CLA-expressing CD8+ T cells in the peripheral blood of psoriasis patients is a hallmark of the disease [56,57]. Most of the huPBMC-induced changes were significantly inhibited or completely prevented after CsA and Rapamycin treatment. Together these findings suggest that the huPBL-SCID-huSkin model is of potential interest to study the pathology of psoriasis at the level of skin and immune biology.

In conclusion, employing the huPBL-SCID-huSkin allograft model of human skin inflammation combined with the local and systemic markers for human cells that we here identified enable preclinical evaluation of novel immuno-modulating agents and cell-based therapy. Also, it will contribute to our understanding of inflammatory and regulatory processes by human T cells and keratinocytes in the pathology of skin inflammatory disorders *in vivo*.

Materials and Methods

Mice

Female B17.B6-*Prkdc*^{scid}*Lyst* ^{bg}/Crl (SCID/beige) mice, 6–8 weeks old, were purchased from Charles River Breeding Laboratories and housed in the SPF facility of the Central Animal Laboratory of the RUNMC. All the animal experimental procedures were in accordance with the international welfare guidelines taking in consideration the 3Rs (Refinement, Reduction, Replacement) and approved by the institutional ethical animal care committee of the Radboud University Nijmegen (number 2008167).

Humanized mouse model; huPBL-SCID-hu Skin allograft model

The huPBL-SCID-hu Skin allograft model used in our study is with slight adaptations based on the model described by Murray et al. [5]. Superficial human skin, 600 to 700 µm thick, was harvested using a dermatome and kept in culture medium with penicillin/streptavidin at 4°C and within max. 30 hours transplanted onto the back of SCID/beige mice. Abdominal skin from healthy individuals was obtained from elective surgeries through the RUNMC Department of Plastic Surgery. After healing of the human skin (21 days), 150×10^6 ficoll density gradient isolated (Lymphoprep; Nycomed-Pharma AS, Oslo, Norway) human peripheral blood mononuclear cells (huPBMC), obtained from buffy coats of blood donors, purchased from Sanquin Blood Bank, Nijmegen, The Netherlands, were infused intra peritoneally (i.p) in a volume of 0.8 ml PBS. Mice were killed at the end of the experiment and tissues of interest were collected.

The use of human skin and peripheral blood were approved and in accordance with the regulations set by the Medical Ethical Committees for human research of the RUNMC. Human skin and buffy coats from healthy donors, who gave written informed consent for scientific use of the human materials. Buffy coats were purchased from Sanquin Blood Bank, Nijmegen, The Netherlands

Drug treatment

Cyclosporine-A (Sandimmune, Novartis®) was administered at a concentration of 0.4 mg/kg/day s.c. via mini-osmotic pump (pumping rate was 1 µl/h , reservoir volume 200 µl). The control group was implanted with a mini-osmotic pump filled with PBS. Rapamycin was injected intraperitoneally (i.p.) at a dose of 0.4 mg/kg body weight in a volume of 100 µL PBS at alternating days, starting 7 days after the infusion of huPBMC.

Histology & Immunohistochemistry

Human skin grafts were fixed in neutral buffered 4% formalin (Mallinckrodt Baker, Inc Deventer, The Netherlands) for 4 hours, processed and embedded in paraffin. Sections (6 µm) were stained with hematoxilin eosin (HE) or processed for immunohistochemical staining.

Keratinocyte differentiation was analyzed using primary, antibodies directed against: Elafin (rabbit 92-1), hBD-2 (ab9871, Peprotech, London,UK), K10 (RKSE60, Eurodiagnostica) and K16 (LL025, Novocastra Laboratories, Newcastle upon Tyne,UK). Cell division was studied using antibodies against Ki67 (MiB-1, Dako cytomation). To enumerate CD4+ and CD8+ T cells antibodies against CD4 (BC/F6, Santa Cruz Biotechnology, Santa Cruz, CA) and CD8 (144B, Dako Cytomation) were used. IL-17 production was detected using polyclonal goat IL-17A antibody (R&D-systems). To detect Foxp3 expression anti-FoxP3 (PCH101) was used. To detect the presence of human neutrophils and mast cells, antibodies against human neutrophil elastase (NP57; Dako) or human mast cell tryptase (AA1; Dako) were used. Antibody stainings were visualized using the Dako Cytomation EnVision+system-HRP (ABC) kit (DAKO, Glostrup, Copenhagen, Denmark) combined with 3,3′-diaminobenzidine tetrahydrochloride (DAB, brown) (Sigma-Aldrich, St. Louis, USA) or using that Labeled Streptavidin Biotin method (Universal LSAB Kit/AP; Dako) combined with either Permanent Red (Dako) or 5-Bromo-4-Chloro-3-Indolyl Phosphate/Nitro Blue Tetrazolium (BCIP/NBT) (Dako).

Sections were photographed using a microscope (Axiokop2 MOT; Zeiss, Sliedrecht, the Netherlands), digital camera (Axiocam MRc5; Zeiss) and AxioVision software (Zeiss).

Image analysis of immunohistochemistry

To enumerate huCD4+ and huCD8+ cells, representative pictures were made at 10× magnification. A representative region of interest (ROI) was drawn from the lowest epidermal papilla till 300 µm dept into the dermis. Cell quantification was performed by setting a threshold and relating this to a number of cells per mm^2. For evaluation of number of CD4+ and CD8+ IL-17A-secreting cells, double positively stained cells were counted manually in CD4 CD8 infiltrated areas of the tissues and the numbers were reported per mm^2. Ki67+ cells were counted manually and related to the length of basement membrane (BM). For quantification of hBD-2, Elafin, K10 and K16 positive cells, photographs were made at 10× magnification. The total epidermal area and K10 or K16 positive area was measured in the ROI (epidermal compartment). Epidermal differentiation was defined as: % K10 or K16 positive epidermal area. Each photo was analyzed using ImageJ software (NIH, http://rsb.info.nih.gov/ij).

Determination of epidermal thickness

Histologic assessment of the grafts was performed by light microscopy both before and after transplantation of human skin. The mean epidermal thickness was calculated using the program Visiopharm Integrator System (VIS) (Visiopharm, Hørsholm, Denmark) as epidermal area divided by epidermal surface length.

Flowcytometry

Mesenteric/peripheral lymph nodes and spleen were processed to obtain a single cell suspension. Retro-orbital blood samples were collected and lymphocytes were isolated by density gradient centrifugation. For cell surface staining, the following conjugated mAbs were used: anti-CD45 PE (Beckman-Coulter), anti-CD3 PE (Beckman-Coulter), anti-CD4 PE-Cy7 (SFCI12T4D11, Beckman-Coulter), anti-CD8 PE-Cy5(B9.11 , Beckman-Coulter), anti-CD62L (DREG56, Beckman-Coulter) anti-CD45RA FITC (HI100, BD), anti-CD45RO ECD (UCHL1, Beckman-Coulter) and anti-CLA FITC (HECA-452, BD). Intracellular Foxp3 staining was performed after fixation and permeabilization of the cells as indicated by the supplier (Ebioscience). Cell samples were measured on a 5 color FC500 flowcytometer (Beckman-Coulter), and the data were analyzed using CXP software (Beckman-Coulter).

Gene expression analysis

Tissues were homogenized using a TissueLyser (Qiagen). RNA was extracted using the RNeasy Lipid Tissue Mini Kit (Qiagen) and reverse-transcribed by use of the High-Capacity cDNA Reverse Transcription Kit (Applied Biosystems). The samples were amplified by quantitative real-time PCR using Applied Biosystems validated gene expression assays and PRISM7900HT sequence detection system (SDS 2.3). Expression of GAPDH was used for normalization and fold changes calculated by the comparative Ct method.

Gene expression assay ID: IL1B-Hs00174097_m1, IL6-Hs00985639_m1, IL8-Hs00174103_m1, CCL5-Hs00174575_m1, CCL20-Hs00171125_m1, CXCL1-Hs00236937_m1, CXCL10-Hs00171042_m1, DEFB4-Hs00823638_m1, IFNG-Hs00174143_m1, IL12B-Hs00233688_m1, IL23A-Hs00372324_m1, IL17A-Hs00174383_m1, IL22-Hs00220924_m1, IL20-Hs00218888_m1, GAPDH-Hs99999905_m1.

Statistics

The results were analyzed by a two-tailed Mann Whitney t test using GraphPad Prism software. *, P value<0.05; **, P value<0.01; ***, P value<0.001.

Acknowledgments

We thank all the personnel involved in collecting human skin samples at the plastic surgery department and biotechnicians at the central animal facility (CDL) of the RUNMC, Nijmegen for expert assistance in animal experiments and care.

Author Contributions

Conceived and designed the experiments: VLO IJ HJPMK. Performed the experiments: VLO HN EF RRMCK. Analyzed the data: VLO HJPMK PEvE LS MMBS. Contributed reagents/materials/analysis tools: PH PCMvdK ML TL. Wrote the paper: VLO HJPMK IJ.

References

1. Shultz LD, Ishikawa F, Greiner DL (2007) Humanized mice in translational biomedical research. Nat Rev Immunol 7: 118–130.
2. Legrand N, Ploss A, Balling R, Becker PD, Borsotti C, et al. (2009) Humanized mice for modeling human infectious disease: challenges, progress, and outlook. Cell Host Microbe 6: 5–9.
3. Nickoloff BJ, Wrone-Smith T (1999) Injection of pre-psoriatic skin with CD4+ T cells induces psoriasis. Am J Pathol 155: 145–158.
4. Wrone-Smith T, Nickoloff BJ (1996) Dermal injection of immunocytes induces psoriasis. J Clin Invest 98: 1878–1887.
5. Murray AG, Petzelbauer P, Hughes CC, Costa J, Askenase P, et al. (1994) Human T-cell-mediated destruction of allogeneic dermal microvessels in a severe combined immunodeficient mouse. Proc Natl Acad Sci U S A 91: 9146–9150.
6. Murray AG, Schechner JS, Epperson DE, Sultan P, McNiff JM, et al. (1998) Dermal microvascular injury in the human peripheral blood lymphocyte reconstituted-severe combined immunodeficient (HuPBL-SCID) mouse/skin allograft model is T cell mediated and inhibited by a combination of cyclosporine and rapamycin. Am J Pathol 153: 627–638.
7. Guerrero-Aspizua S, Garcia M, Murillas R, Retamosa L, Illera N, et al. (2010) Development of a bioengineered skin-humanized mouse model for psoriasis: dissecting epidermal-lymphocyte interacting pathways. Am J Pathol 177: 3112–3124.
8. Igney FH, Asadullah K, Zollner TM (2004) Techniques: species' finest blend–humanized mouse models in inflammatory skin disease research. Trends Pharmacol Sci 25: 543–549.
9. Sagoo P, Ali N, Garg G, Nestle FO, Lechler RI, et al. (2011) Human regulatory T cells with alloantigen specificity are more potent inhibitors of alloimmune skin graft damage than polyclonal regulatory T cells. Sci Transl Med 3: 83ra42.
10. Feng G, Nadig SN, Backdahl L, Beck S, Francis RS, et al. (2011) Functional regulatory T cells produced by inhibiting cyclic nucleotide phosphodiesterase type 3 prevent allograft rejection. Sci Transl Med 3: 83ra40.
11. Issa F, Hester J, Goto R, Nadig SN, Goodacre TE, et al. (2010) Ex vivo-expanded human regulatory T cells prevent the rejection of skin allografts in a humanized mouse model. Transplantation 90: 1321–1327.
12. Mosier DE, Stell KL, Gulizia RJ, Torbett BE, Gilmore GL (1993) Homozygous scid/scid;beige/beige mice have low levels of spontaneous or neonatal T cell-induced B cell generation. J Exp Med 177: 191–194.
13. Takizawa Y, Saida T, Tokuda Y, Dohi S, Wang YL, et al. (1997) New immunodeficient (nude-scid, beige-scid) mice as excellent recipients of human skin grafts containing intraepidermal neoplasms. Arch Dermatol Res 289: 213–218.
14. Clark RA (2010) Skin-resident T cells: the ups and downs of on site immunity. J Invest Dermatol 130: 362–370.
15. Tomura M, Itoh K, Kanagawa O (2010) Naive CD4+ T lymphocytes circulate through lymphoid organs to interact with endogenous antigens and upregulate their function. J Immunol 184: 4646–4653.
16. Rohrl J, Yang D, Oppenheim JJ, Hehlgans T (2010) Specific binding and chemotactic activity of mBD4 and its functional orthologue hBD2 to CCR6-expressing cells. J Biol Chem 285: 7028–7034.
17. Wilson NJ, Boniface K, Chan JR, McKenzie BS, Blumenschein WM, et al. (2007) Development, cytokine profile and function of human interleukin 17-producing helper T cells. Nat Immunol 8: 950–957.
18. Lowes MA, Kikuchi T, Fuentes-Duculan J, Cardinale I, Zaba LC, et al. (2008) Psoriasis vulgaris lesions contain discrete populations of Th1 and Th17 T cells. J Invest Dermatol 128: 1207–1211.
19. Hueber W, Patel DD, Dryja T, Wright AM, Koroleva I, et al. (2010) Effects of AIN457, a fully human antibody to interleukin-17A, on psoriasis, rheumatoid arthritis, and uveitis. Sci Transl Med 2: 52ra72.
20. Koga C, Kabashima K, Shiraishi N, Kobayashi M, Tokura Y (2008) Possible pathogenic role of Th17 cells for atopic dermatitis. J Invest Dermatol 128: 2625–2630.
21. Di CA, Di MP, Nestle FO (2008) A role for Th17 cells in the immunopathogenesis of atopic dermatitis? J Invest Dermatol 128: 2569–2571.
22. Cua DJ, Tato CM (2010) Innate IL-17-producing cells: the sentinels of the immune system. Nat Rev Immunol 10: 479–489.
23. Paul C, Ortonne JP (2011) Use of conventional systemic treatments in psoriasis: systematic review and expert opinion of a panel of dermatologists. J Eur Acad Dermatol Venereol 25 Suppl 2: 1.
24. Griffiths CE, Strober BE, van de KP, Ho V, Fidelus-Gort R, et al. (2010) Comparison of ustekinumab etanercept for moderate-to-severe psoriasis. N Engl J Med 362: 118–128.
25. Tomura M, Honda T, Tanizaki H, Otsuka A, Egawa G, et al. (2010) Activated regulatory T cells are the major T cell type emigrating from the skin during a cutaneous immune response in mice. J Clin Invest 120: 883–893.

26. Liu L, Fuhlbrigge RC, Karibian K, Tian T, Kupper TS (2006) Dynamic programming of CD8+ T cell trafficking after live viral immunization. Immunity 25: 511–520.
27. Tesmer LA, Lundy SK, Sarkar S, Fox DA (2008) Th17 cells in human disease. Immunol Rev 223: 87–113.
28. Miossec P, Korn T, Kuchroo VK (2009) Interleukin-17 and type 17 helper T cells. N Engl J Med 361: 888–898.
29. Ortega C, Fernandez A, Carrillo JM, Romero P, Molina IJ, et al. (2009) IL-17-producing CD8+ T lymphocytes from psoriasis skin plaques are cytotoxic effector cells that secrete Th17-related cytokines. J Leukoc Biol 86: 435–443.
30. Clark RA, Chong BF, Mirchandani N, Yamanaka K, Murphy GF, et al. (2006) A novel method for the isolation of skin resident T cells from normal and diseased human skin. J Invest Dermatol 126: 1059–1070.
31. Sakaguchi S (2000) Regulatory T cells: key controllers of immunologic self-tolerance. Cell 101: 455–458.
32. Dudda JC, Perdue N, Bachtanian E, Campbell DJ (2008) Foxp3+ regulatory T cells maintain immune homeostasis in the skin. J Exp Med 205: 1559–1565.
33. Clark RA, Kupper TS (2007) IL-15 and dermal fibroblasts induce proliferation of natural regulatory T cells isolated from human skin. Blood 109: 194–202.
34. Vukmanovic-Stejic M, Agius E, Booth N, Dunne PJ, Lacy KE, et al. (2008) The kinetics of CD4+Foxp3+ T cell accumulation during a human cutaneous antigen-specific memory response in vivo. J Clin Invest 118: 3639–3650.
35. Zhou X, Bailey-Bucktrout SL, Jeker LT, Penaranda C, Martinez-Llordella M, et al. (2009) Instability of the transcription factor Foxp3 leads to the generation of pathogenic memory T cells in vivo. Nat Immunol 10: 1000–1007.
36. Koenen HJ, Smeets RL, Vink PM, van RE, Boots AM, et al. (2008) Human CD25highFoxp3pos regulatory T cells differentiate into IL-17-producing cells. Blood 112: 2340–2352.
37. Paladini RD, Takahashi K, Bravo NS, Coulombe PA (1996) Onset of re-epithelialization after skin injury correlates with a reorganization of keratin filaments in wound edge keratinocytes: defining a potential role for keratin 16. J Cell Biol 132: 381–397.
38. Franssen ME, Boezeman JB, van de Kerkhof PC, Van Erp PE (2004) Monitoring hyperproliferative disorders in human skin: flow cytometry of changing cytokeratin expression. Cytometry B Clin Cytom 57: 32–39.
39. Gallo RL, Huttner KM (1998) Antimicrobial peptides: an emerging concept in cutaneous biology. J Invest Dermatol 111: 739–743.
40. Schalkwijk J, van V, I, Alkemade JA, de Jongh GJ (1993) Immunohistochemical localization of SKALP/elafin in psoriatic epidermis. J Invest Dermatol 100: 390–393.
41. Alkemade JA, Molhuizen HO, Ponec M, Kempenaar JA, Zeeuwen PL, et al. (1994) SKALP/elafin is an inducible proteinase inhibitor in human epidermal keratinocytes. J Cell Sci 107 (Pt 8): 2335–2342.
42. Hollox EJ, Huffmeier U, Zeeuwen PL, Palla R, Lascorz J, et al. (2008) Psoriasis is associated with increased beta-defensin genomic copy number. Nat Genet 40: 23–25.
43. Kamsteeg M, Jansen PA, van Vlijmen-Willems IM, Van Erp PE, Rodijk-Olthuis D, et al. (2010) Molecular diagnostics of psoriasis, atopic dermatitis, allergic contact dermatitis and irritant contact dermatitis. Br J Dermatol 162: 568–578.
44. Liang SC, Tan XY, Luxenberg DP, Karim R, Dunussi-Joannopoulos K, et al. (2006) Interleukin (IL)-22 and IL-17 are coexpressed by Th17 cells and cooperatively enhance expression of antimicrobial peptides. J Exp Med 203: 2271–2279.
45. Nograles KE, Zaba LC, Guttman-Yassky E, Fuentes-Duculan J, Suarez-Farinas M, et al. (2008) Th17 cytokines interleukin (IL)-17 and IL-22 modulate distinct inflammatory and keratinocyte-response pathways. Br J Dermatol 159: 1092–1102.
46. Peric M, Koglin S, Kim SM, Morizane S, Besch R, et al. (2008) IL-17A enhances vitamin D3-induced expression of cathelicidin antimicrobial peptide in human keratinocytes. J Immunol 181: 8504–8512.
47. Lai Y, Gallo RL (2009) AMPed up immunity: how antimicrobial peptides have multiple roles in immune defense. Trends Immunol 30: 131–141.
48. Nestle FO, Kaplan DH, Barker J (2009) Psoriasis. N Engl J Med 361: 496–509.
49. Mueller W, Herrmann B (1979) Cyclosporin A for psoriasis. N Engl J Med 301: 555.
50. Schon MP, Boehncke WH (2005) Psoriasis. N Engl J Med 352: 1899–1912.
51. Nair RP, Duffin KC, Helms C, Ding J, Stuart PE, et al. (2009) Genome-wide scan reveals association of psoriasis with IL-23 and NF-kappaB pathways. Nat Genet 41: 199–204.
52. Ong PY, Ohtake T, Brandt C, Strickland I, Boguniewicz M, et al. (2002) Endogenous antimicrobial peptides and skin infections in atopic dermatitis. N Engl J Med 347: 1151–1160.
53. Nonomura K, Yamanishi K, Yasuno H, Nara K, Hirose S (1994) Up-regulation of elafin/SKALP gene expression in psoriatic epidermis. J Invest Dermatol 103: 88–91.
54. de Jongh GJ, Zeeuwen PL, Kucharekova M, Pfundt R, van d V, et al. (2005) High expression levels of keratinocyte antimicrobial proteins in psoriasis compared with atopic dermatitis. J Invest Dermatol 125: 1163–1173.
55. Zaba LC, Cardinale I, Gilleaudeau P, Sullivan-Whalen M, Suarez-Farinas M, et al. (2007) Amelioration of epidermal hyperplasia by TNF inhibition is associated with reduced Th17 responses. J Exp Med 204: 3183–3194.
56. Sigmundsdottir H, Gudjonsson JE, Jonsdottir I, Ludviksson BR, Valdimarsson H (2001) The frequency of CLA+ CD8+ T cells in the blood of psoriasis patients correlates closely with the severity of their disease. Clin Exp Immunol 126: 365–369.
57. Langewouters AM, Bovenschen HJ, de Jong EM, Van Erp PE, van de Kerkhof PC (2007) The effect of topical corticosteroids in combination with alefacept on circulating T-cell subsets in psoriasis. J Dermatolog Treat 18: 279–285.

Selective Ablation of Ctip2/Bcl11b in Epidermal Keratinocytes Triggers Atopic Dermatitis-Like Skin Inflammatory Responses in Adult Mice

Zhixing Wang[1], Ling-juan Zhang[1], Gunjan Guha[1], Shan Li[1], Kateryna Kyrylkova[1], Chrissa Kioussi[1,2], Mark Leid[1,2,3], Gitali Ganguli-Indra[1,2], Arup K. Indra[1,2,3,4]*

1 Department of Pharmaceutical Sciences, College of Pharmacy, Oregon State University, Corvallis, Oregon, United States of America, **2** Molecular Cell Biology Program, Oregon State University, Corvallis, Oregon, United States of America, **3** Environmental Health Science Center, Oregon State University, Corvallis, Oregon, United States of America, **4** Department of Dermatology, Oregon Health and Science University, Portland, Oregon, United States of America

Abstract

Background: Ctip2 is crucial for epidermal homeostasis and protective barrier formation in developing mouse embryos. Selective ablation of Ctip2 in epidermis leads to increased transepidermal water loss (TEWL), impaired epidermal proliferation, terminal differentiation, as well as altered lipid composition during development. However, little is known about the role of Ctip2 in skin homeostasis in adult mice.

Methodology/Principal Findings: To study the role of Ctip2 in adult skin homeostasis, we utilized Ctip2$^{ep-/-}$ mouse model in which Ctip2 is selectively deleted in epidermal keratinocytes. Measurement of TEWL, followed by histological, immunohistochemical, and RT-qPCR analyses revealed an important role of Ctip2 in barrier maintenance and in regulating adult skin homeostasis. We demonstrated that keratinocytic ablation of Ctip2 leads to atopic dermatitis (AD)-like skin inflammation, characterized by alopecia, pruritus and scaling, as well as extensive infiltration of immune cells including T lymphocytes, mast cells, and eosinophils. We observed increased expression of T-helper 2 (Th2)-type cytokines and chemokines in the mutant skin, as well as systemic immune responses that share similarity with human AD patients. Furthermore, we discovered that thymic stromal lymphopoietin (TSLP) expression was significantly upregulated in the mutant epidermis as early as postnatal day 1 and ChIP assay revealed that TSLP is likely a direct transcriptional target of Ctip2 in epidermal keratinocytes.

Conclusions/Significance: Our data demonstrated a cell-autonomous role of Ctip2 in barrier maintenance and epidermal homeostasis in adult mice skin. We discovered a crucial non-cell autonomous role of keratinocytic Ctip2 in suppressing skin inflammatory responses by regulating the expression of Th2-type cytokines. It is likely that the epidermal hyperproliferation in the Ctip2-lacking epidermis may be secondary to the compensatory response of the adult epidermis that is defective in barrier functions. Our results establish an initiating role of epidermal TSLP in AD pathogenesis via a novel repressive regulatory mechanism enforced by Ctip2.

Editor: Michel Simon, CNRS-University of Toulouse, France

Funding: These studies were supported by grant 5R01AR056008-03 (AI) from the National Institutes of Health, an Oregon Health and Science University Medical Research Foundation grant (AI), and a National Institute of Environmental Health Sciences center grant (ES00210) to Environmental Health Sciences Center, Oregon State University. The funders had no role in study design, data collection and analysis, decision to publish, or preparation of the manuscript.

Competing Interests: The authors have declared that no competing interests exist.

* E-mail: arup.indra@oregonstate.edu

These authors contributed equally to this work.

Introduction

Mammalian skin forms the first defense barrier in the body for protecting against physical injuries, ultraviolet radiation, bacterial infections as well as excessive loss of water [1]. The most abundant cell type in epidermis is keratinocytes, which forms four layers: basal, spinous, granular and stratum corneum [1,2]. Atopic dermatitis (AD) is a chronic, inflammatory disease of the skin that starts at early childhood. AD patients are genetically predisposes to the disease, which has a prevalence of 10%–20% in children and 1%–3% in adults [3,4]. Clinical features of AD include skin xerosis, pruritus and eczematoid skin lesions [4]. AD is characterized by both skin barrier deficiencies and immunological responses [5]. In AD, a defective skin barrier is thought to permit the penetration of allergens and induces the interactions of the allergens with immune cells, promoting the subsequent release of pro-inflammatory cytokines and chemokines and elevation of IgE level [6].

The molecular pathways involved in AD pathogenesis remain unclear. There have been many reports on the connections between atopic dermatitis and Th2 inflammatory pathways [4,7,8]. Pro-Th2 cytokines, such as IL-4, IL-13, IL-5, and IL10, are elevated in AD patients [7]. One possible candidate that has been linked to the initiation of inflammatory responses in AD and other allergic diseases is thymic stromal lymphopoietin (TSLP), a member of the hematopoietic cytokine family. It is expressed at a low level primarily by epithelial cells, including keratinocytes, upregulated in acute and chronic AD lesions and responsible for activating cutaneous DCs, endowing them with the capacity to polarize $CD4^+$ T cells toward a Th2 cell allergic response [9–12]. TSLP signals through a heterodimeric receptor formed by TSLP receptor (TSLPR) as well as IL-7 receptor alpha (IL7Rα) [9]. Mice that are deficient of nuclear receptors (NRs) retinoid X receptor α (RXRα), vitamin D receptor (VDR) or Notch1 in epidermal keratinocytes, exhibit epidermal permeability barrier (EPB) defects, express elevated levels of TSLP in skin, and subsequently develop AD-like phenotypes [10,12–14].

Chicken ovalbumin upstream promoter transcription factor (COUP-TF) interacting protein 2 (Ctip2), also known as Bcl11b, is a C_2H_2 zinc finger protein that is crucial in the development of central nervous and immune system [15–18]. In T cells and neuroblastoma cells, Ctip2 appears to function predominantly as a transcription repressor. Ctip2 interacts indirectly with histone deacetylases (HDACs) within the context of the Nucleosome Remodeling and Deacetylation (NuRD) or SIRT1 complexes [16,19,20]. Ctip2 also acts as a transcriptional activator in a promoter-dependent manner in stimulated thymocytes [21,22]. Ctip2 is also expressed in human and mouse adult epidermis [23,24]. Studies with mice harboring germline deletion and epidermal specific ablation of Ctip2 revealed its critical role(s) in epidermal proliferation and terminal differentiation, as well as barrier formation during mouse embryonic development in both cell autonomous and non-cell autonomous ways [25]. Ctip2 was shown to be an important regulator of epidermal homeostasis and barrier formation by interacting with the promoter regions of many genes involved in epidermal development such as EGFR and Notch1 and in skin lipid metabolism such as eLox3, Gba2 and Lass2 ([26], Wang et al., 2012, in press). Since Ctip2-null mice die at birth, the function(s) of keratinocytic Ctip2 in adult mice EPB maintenance as well as in epidermal homeostasis is unknown.

Here we report a novel role of Ctip2 in maintenance of adult epidermal homeostasis and in skin inflammation by selective Cre-recombinase mediated ablation of Ctip2 gene in epidermal keratinocytes of mice skin [27,28]. We show that ablation of Ctip2 in mice epidermal keratinocytes during development results in impaired EPB maintenance, increased epidermal hyperplasia and a severe form of AD-like skin inflammation of adult skin that becomes disseminated with progression of the disease, all of which are very similar to AD in humans. Our present data indicates that keratinocytic Ctip2 plays a crucial role in triggering skin inflammatory responses by regulating the expression of genes encoding Th2-type cytokines in adult mouse skin. These results presented herein establish an initiating role of epidermal TSLP in AD pathogenesis and demonstrate a key anti-inflammatory role of Ctip2, which strongly represses TSLP expression in wild-type skin.

Results

Selective ablation of Ctip2 in epidermal keratinocytes leads to altered epidermal proliferation, differentiation and spontaneous dermatitis in adult skin

The function of Ctip2 in adult mice skin homeostasis was characterized using $Ctip2^{ep-/-}$ mice that selectively lacked Ctip2 in epidermal keratinocytes by Cre-recombinase mediated deletion of Ctip2 gene in keratinocytes using K14-Cre deleter mice [27,28]. At approximately 8–10 weeks after birth, 67% $Ctip2^{ep-/-}$ mice (n = 18) developed dry and scaly skin and 17% mutant mice also developed spontaneous lesions on the dorsal skin at the same age, which were absent in wildtype (WT) mice (Fig. 1A). The severity of all of these abnormalities worsened with age (Figure 1A). By 4 months of age, almost all the mutants (89%, n = 18) developed spontaneous dermatitis that occurred predominantly on the dorsal skin, in the neck region, and on the face (Figure 1A). Furthermore, progressive alopecia was evident in most of the 4 month-old $Ctip2^{ep-/-}$ mice (~85%) (Figure 1A). We hypothesized that the skin lesions observed in the mutant mice could be due to impaired function of the skin barrier. To test this hypothesis, trans-epidermal water loss (TEWL) was measured in wildtype and $Ctip2^{ep-/-}$ mice skin. Interestingly, the mutant mice showed increased TEWL as early as 2 weeks of age, and the values were ~10-fold higher than wildtype mice at 4 months of age (Figure 1B; note that 2 M and 4 M TEWL were measured on lesional skin sites). At 4 M, TEWL of nonlesional mutant skin was a third of the TEWL of lesional skin, but it was still 3.5-fold higher than WT controls (Figure S1B). Histological analysis of hematoxylin- and eosin- (H&E) stained skin sections revealed significant epidermal hyperplasia in $Ctip2^{ep-/-}$ mice as early as 2 weeks of age (Figures 1C and S1A).

In order to determine if increased epidermal hyperplasia could be due to altered keratinocyte proliferation, immunohistochemical (IHC) analyses for proliferation marker Ki67 and keratin 14 (K14) were performed on control and mutant skin (Figures 1D and S1C–D). The percentage of Ki67-positive cells was significantly higher in $Ctip2^{ep-/-}$ epidermis compared to the wildtype littermates at all time-points (Figure 1D, S1C). Similarly, the expression level of K14 in the mutant epidermis was prominently increased in $Ctip2^{ep-/-}$ mice at 2 and 4 months of age (Figure S1D). Expression levels of the early differentiation marker K10 were not significantly different between wildtype and $Ctip2^{ep-/-}$ mice (Figure S1E). Expression of terminal differentiation marker filaggrin was reduced in 1-week-old mutant epidermis (Figure S1F); however, the decrease of its expression was transient, as filaggrin expression became similar between WT and in $Ctip2^{ep-/-}$ mice at later timepoints from 2 weeks to 4 months (Figure 1E, S1F G). The expression of loricrin was similar between wildtype and $Ctip2^{ep-/-}$ mice at all timepoints (Figure 1F). These results indicate that selective, somatic ablation of Ctip2 in epidermal keratinocytes leads to increased epidermal proliferation and unaltered terminal differentiation during adulthood. Altogether, results suggest that adult $Ctip2^{ep-/-}$ mice exhibited impaired barrier functions and developed spontaneous dermatitis that further aggravated with age.

Increased infiltration of inflammatory cells in adult $Ctip2^{ep-/-}$ mice skin

Dermal infiltrates were notable in $Ctip2^{ep-/-}$ mice starting around 2 months of age, as revealed by histological analyses (Figure 1C). Combined eosinophil and mast cell (C.E.M.) staining revealed increased eosinophils in the dermis of $Ctip2^{ep-/-}$ mutant skin around 1 month of age, while mast cells were most numerous in the mutant dermis around 2 months of age (Figures 2A and S2A). Besides the early induction of eosinophil and mast cells, IHC staining for T lymphocytes revealed a two-fold increase in $CD3^+$ T cells mainly at later timepoint in the skin of 4 month-old $Ctip2^{ep-/-}$ mice compared to the wild-type skin (Figures 2B and C). A similar late increase in the number of $CD4^+$ T cells was observed in 4 month-old mutant skin compared to the wildtype skin (Figure 2D–E). The number of F4/80+ macrophages in the dermis was significantly higher in $Ctip2^{ep-/-}$ mice skin at 4 months of age (Figure 3A–B). IHC staining using anti-Ly6g antibody showed significantly increased number of neutrophils in the dermis of 4

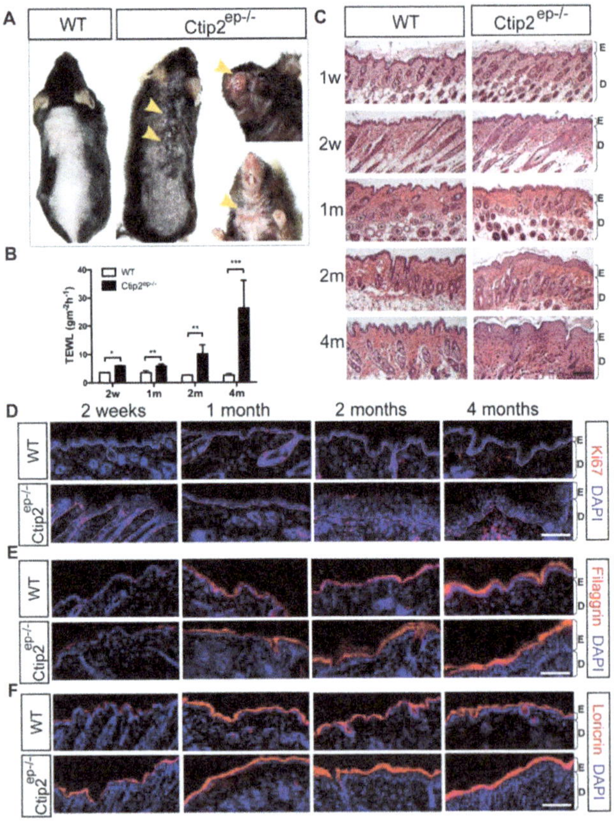

Figure 1. Ctip2$^{ep-/-}$ mice develop a chronic skin lesions and enhanced epidermal proliferation and differentiation. (**A**) Gross morphology of 4 months old wildtype (WT) and Ctip2$^{ep-/-}$ mice. The yellow arrowheads indicate lesion and alopecia of Ctip2$^{ep-/-}$ mice in the back, face and neck, to be compared with the normal appearance in a wildtype mouse. (**B**) Measurement of trans-epidermal water loss (TEWL) from dorsal skin of wildtype and Ctip2$^{ep-/-}$ mice at different time points. Statistical analyses were performed by student's unpaired t-test using GraphPad Prism software; ** P<0.01, *** P<0.001. (**C**) Hemotoxylin & Eosin stained 5 μm thick paraffin sections from dorsal skin of WT and Ctip2$^{ep-/-}$ mice at 1 week (1W), 2 weeks (2w), 1month (1 m), 2 months (2 m) and 4 months (4 m). Immunohistochemical staining of dorsal skin biopsies from WT and Ctip2$^{ep-/-}$ mice was performed with antibodies directed against (**D**) Ki67, (**E**) Filaggrin and (**F**) Loricrin (all in red). All sections were counterstained with DAPI (blue). Scale bar: 100 μm. Epidermis (E) and dermis (D) are indicated.

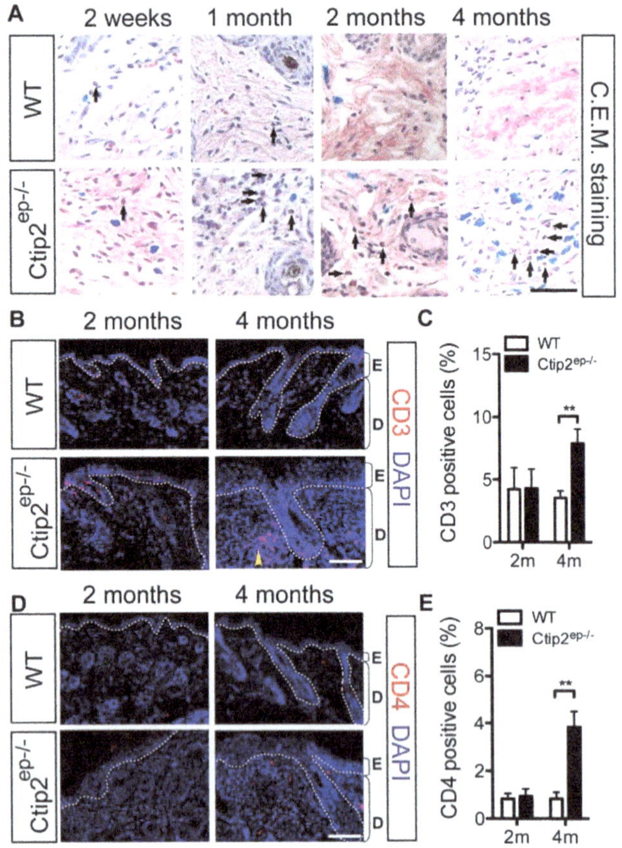

Figure 2. Characterization of inflammatory cell infiltrates in dorsal skin of WT and in Ctip2$^{ep-/-}$ adult mice. (**A**) Combined eosinophil and mast cell (C.E.M) staining for eosinophils (pink) and mast cells (blue). Black arrows point to eosinophils. Scale bar: 50 μm. (**B**) Immunohistochemical staining of dorsal skin biopsies from WT and Ctip2$^{ep-/-}$ mice were performed with specific antibodies against CD3 (red). Yellow arrowhead indicates dermal infiltrates of CD3+ cells. Scale bar: 100 μm. (**C**) Percent CD3+ T cells at 2 m and 4 m. (**D**) Immunostaining of CD4+ T cells (red) in WT and mutant mice. Scale bar: 100 μm. (**E**) Percent CD4+ T cells at 2 m and 4 m. All sections were counterstained with DAPI (blue). Statistical analyses were performed by student's unpaired t-test using GraphPad Prism software; ** P<0.005.

months old mutant skin (Figure 3C and D). Similarly, staining with anti-CD11b antibodies revealed significantly increased number of infiltrating monocytes, in the 4 months old mutant dermis compared to the wild-type dermis (Figure 3E–F). In addition, CD45^{+} leukocyte infiltration was observed in one month-old Ctip2$^{ep-/-}$ mice skin, but this resolved by 4 months of age (Figure S2B–C). Expression of CD11c positive antigen for dendritic cells was similar between wildtype and Ctip2$^{ep-/-}$ mice skin (Figure S2D). Taken together, these results demonstrate an increased inflammatory response in Ctip2$^{ep-/-}$ skin that progressively increased with time.

Preferential induction of Th2-type cytokines and chemokines in adult Ctip2$^{ep-/-}$ skin

Upregulated expression of cytokines and chemokines play a crucial role in inflammatory skin diseases [7,29]. Differential expression profiles of cytokines and/or chemokines orchestrate and determine the type and outcome of inflammatory responses in mouse and human skin. We next determined if expression of pro-inflammatory cytokines/chemokines were dysregulated in mutant skin. RT-qPCR analyses revealed a preferential induction of Th2-type cytokines, including TSLP, CCL17, IL13, IL4, IL6, and IL10 in mutant skin (Figures 4A–E and S3A). In contrast, expression of Th1-type (IL1α, IL2, IL12a/b; Figure S3B–E) was reduced and that of Th17-type (IL17a, IL18 and IL23; Figure S3F–H) cytokines was not induced in mutant skin.

Time course analyses also revealed several distinct induction patterns of cytokines and chemokines in the mutant skin. Chemokine CCL17 is one of known downstream genes whose expression can be stimulated by TSLP [30]. CCL17 and IL13 transcripts were significantly induced in the mutant skin at around 1 week and 2 weeks after birth, respectively. Induction of these two genes was transient, peaking at 1 month, followed by a decrease of expression during later time points (2–4 months; Figure 4B and C). In contrast to these early and transient inductions, we observed a strong, late induction of cytokines IL4 and IL6 and chemokines CCL3 and CXCL2 in the mutant skin (Figure 4D–E, S3L–M). We

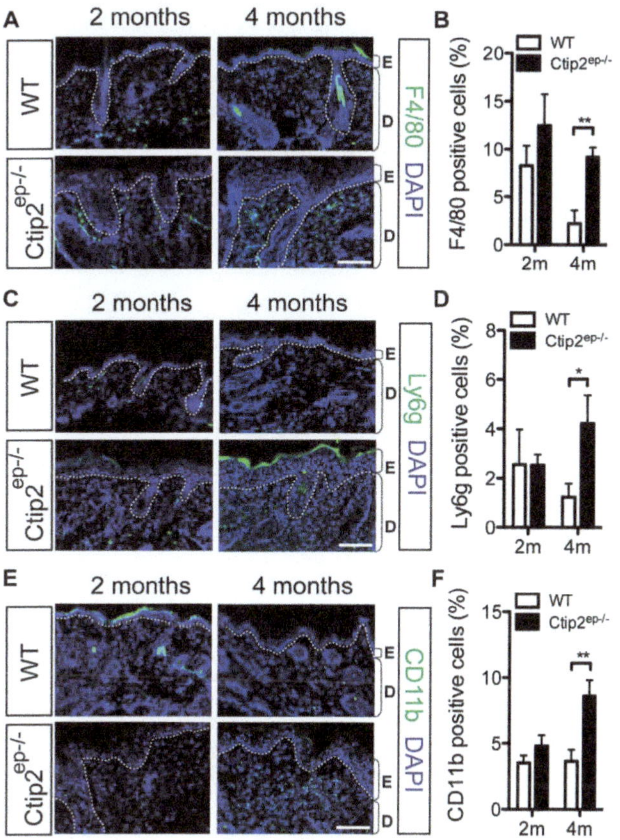

Figure 3. Increased inflammatory cell infiltrate in Ctip2$^{ep-/-}$ adult mice. (**A**) Immunohistochemical staining of dorsal skin biopsies from WT and Ctip2$^{ep-/-}$ mice were performed with specific antibodies against F4/80 (green) to detect macrophage/dendritic cells. (**B**) Percent F4/80 positive cells at 2 m and 4 m. (**C**) Immunostaining of neutrophils (green) using anti-Ly6g antibody in WT and mutant mice skin. (**D**) Percent Ly6g positive cells at 2 m and 4 m. (**E**) Immunostaining of monocytes/macrophages (green) with anti-CD11b antibody in WT and mutant mice skin. (**F**) Percent CD11b positive cells at 2 m and 4 m. All sections were counterstained with DAPI (blue). Scale bar (A, C, and E): 100 µm. Statistical analyses were performed by student's unpaired t-test using GraphPad Prism software; * $P<0.05$, ** $P<0.005$.

also observed a late onset of induction of Th1-type cytokines, including TNFα and IFNγ, at 4 months of age (Figure S3N–O).

TSLP, a master initiator of Th2 inflammatory responses, was induced ~30-fold at postnatal day 1 (P1), and we observed a ~200-fold induction at P7 compared to control skin [31]. Expression of TSLP remained significantly high at all later time points (~1000-fold induction between 1 month to 4 months after birth; Figure 4A). Interestingly, the high level of TSLP expression was observed predominantly in the mutant epidermis, whereas TSLP transcripts were barely detectable in the dermal layer of the mutant skin (Figure 4F). Immunohistochemistry analyses revealed that TSLP protein was barely detectable and restricted to differentiating layers of epidermis in WT skin, whereas TSLP protein was strongly upregulated throughout the epidermis including basal proliferative cells and differentiating keratinocytes in the mutant skin (Figure S4A). These data provide strong evidence that TSLP may be an initial triggering cytokine that is induced in the absence of Ctip2 in the epidermis. Altogether, these results suggest that deletion of Ctip2 in the epidermis leads to an increased inflammatory response, which is characterized by a Th2-type cytokine/chemokine profile.

TSLP is a direct target of Ctip2 in epidermal keratinocytes

Recent studies have revealed that ablation of RXRα and RXRβ in adult murine keratinocytes leads to an AD-like phenotype triggered by induction of TSLP [13].Similarly, TSLP is also elevated in Notch signaling-deficient keratinocytes (deficient in either Notch1/2 or recombining binding protein suppressor of hairless (RBP-j) [12,13,32]. Thus, it is possible that Ctip2 regulates TSLP expression via the nuclear receptor or Notch signaling pathways in epidermis. To test that, we determined the expression of key players in both the Notch and RXR signaling pathways, including Notch1, Notch2, RBP-j, RXRα and RXRβ. Expression of the corresponding transcripts was not affected by loss of Ctip2 in the epidermis at both one and four months after birth (Figure S5A–D, data not shown). Similarly, epidermal protein levels of Notch1 and RXRα were comparable between wildtype and mutants at all time-points, suggesting an alternative mechanism of Ctip2-mediated regulation of TSLP expression in the adult murine skin (Figure S5E–F).

In order to determine if Ctip2 directly regulates TSLP expression in murine keratinocytes, we conducted chromatin immunoprecipitation (ChIP) assays on neonatal mouse epidermal extracts. Multiple primer sets were designed from the proximal (−200 bp) and distal (−1 kb) promoter regions relative to the transcriptional start site of TSLP to determine the possible interaction of Ctip2 with TSLP. We observed that Ctip2 interacted with the distal but not the proximal region of TSLP promoter, suggesting Ctip2 may directly repress TSLP transcription in mouse keratinocytes (Figure 4G). Hence, ablation of Ctip2 in epidermal keratinocytes could lead to upregulation of TSLP expression due a derepression mechanism.

Systemic inflammatory responses in older Ctip2$^{ep-/-}$ mice

We hypothesized that chronic skin inflammation developed in Ctip2$^{ep-/-}$ mice may trigger systemic immune responses in the mutant skin. To test that we determined blood plasma concentrations of IgE as well as various Th2-type cytokines/chemokines (IL-4, IL-13, CCL17 and TSLP) and Th1-type cytokine TNFα from 1-month and 4-months-old mice by ELISA (Figure 5A–F). Plasma level for all of the tested Th2 cytokines, were observed to be higher in both 1-month and 4-month old mutant mice (Figure 5A–E), including IL4 and the related IL-13 (Figure 5A, B), CCL17 (Figure 5C) and TSLP (Figure 5D). In contrast, plasma level of Th1 cytokine TNFα was higher only at 4-month but not in 1-month old mutant mice (Figure 5E). While circulating IgE levels were elevated in both wild-type and mutant mice at four months of age, IgE levels in mutant mice were 2.5 times greater than those in wildtype mice (Fig. 5F).

Ctip2$^{ep-/-}$ mice exhibited inguinal lymphadenopathy and smaller convoluted thymus at four months of age (Figure 5G, data not shown). The mutant mice displayed progressive splenomegaly starting from one month of age, with a 2-fold increase in spleen weight at the age of four months (Figure 5G–H). Histological studies of the spleens revealed an increased cell infiltration in the 4-month-old mutant spleen in comparison with wildtype (Figure S6 A, D, G, J). 4 month-old Ctip2$^{ep-/-}$ mice exhibited increased eosinophil infiltration in the spleen and lymph node compared with wildtype (Figure S6, B, E, H, K). Very few mast cells were observed in both wildtype and mutant mice spleens and the number of mast cells was larger in the lymph node, indistinguishable between 4 month-old wildtype and mutant mice (Figure S6,

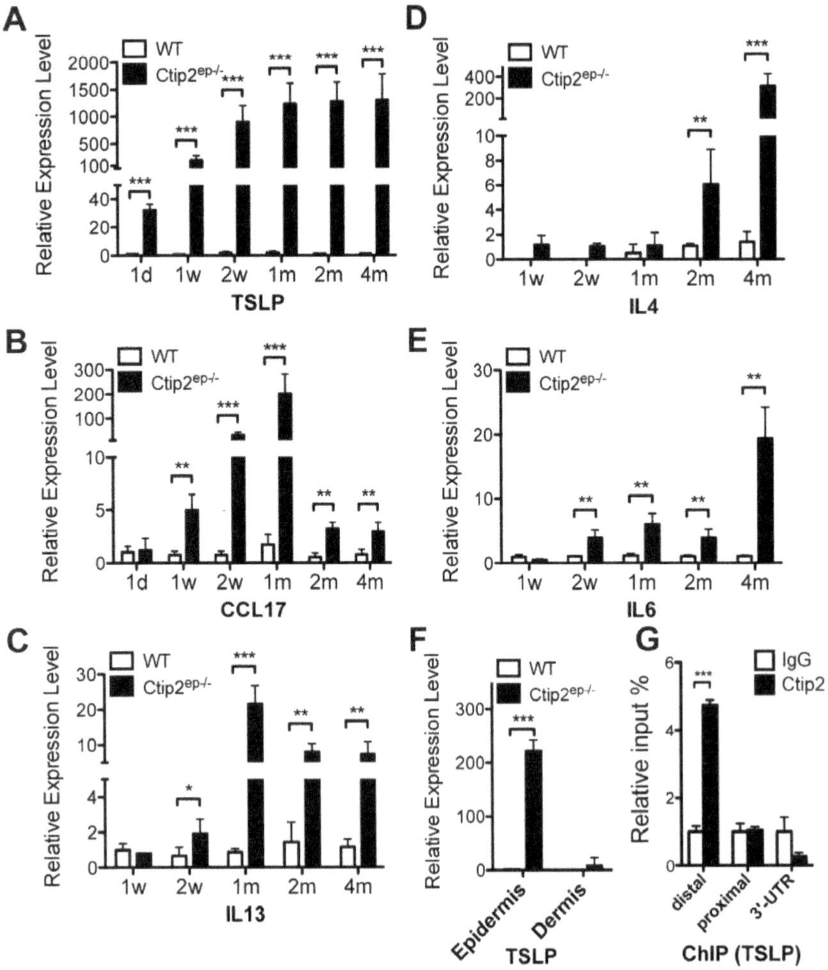

Figure 4. Th2-dependent cytokine and chemokine expression levels in WT and Ctip2$^{ep-/-}$ skin. (**A–F**) Quantitative RT-PCR (RT-qPCR) analyses of cytokines and chemokines in the dorsal skin of 1day, 1 week, 2 weeks, 1month, 2 months and 4 months old WT and mutant mice using specific primers as indicated in Table S1. Relative mRNA expression levels of (**A**) TSLP, (**B**) CCL17, (**C**) IL13, (**D**) IL4, and (**E**) IL6 in Ctip2$^{ep-/-}$ skin was compared to wildtype (WT) skin (set as 1.0). (**F**) RT-qPCR analyses of TSLP mRNA levels in separated epidermis and dermis from tail skin. All values represent relative transcript level after normalization with HPRT transcripts. (**G**) Chromatin immunoprecipitation (ChIP) assay was performed on freshly isolated neonatal mouse skin keratinocytes using anti-Ctip2 antibody and results were analyzed by qPCR using primers indicated in Table S1. Rat IgG was used as a control. Ctip2 was recruited to the distal promoter regions of TSLP. Statistical analyses were performed by student's unpaired t-test using GraphPad Prism software; * $P<0.05$, ** $P<0.01$, *** $P<0.001$.

C, F, I, L). These results clearly indicate that Ctip2$^{ep-/-}$ mice display a systemic immune response that may be primarily driven by TSLP expression from keratinocytes.

Discussion

Epidermal keratinocytes have long been suspected to play a crucial role in initiating and directing the immune response in inflammatory skin diseases, such as AD. In the present report we have shown that skin of adult Ctip2$^{ep-/-}$ mice, with an epidermal-specific deletion of the gene encoding Ctip2, display histological and cellular features that are typical of human AD. First, Ctip2$^{ep-/-}$ mice develop skin lesions, alopecia and pruritus, which are major clinical features in patients afflicted with AD [4,33,34]. Second, Ctip2$^{ep-/-}$ mice exhibit epidermal hyperplasia that is characterized by increased epidermal proliferation, similar to what has been observed in AD patients [2]. Third, the skin of Ctip2$^{ep-/-}$ mice is characterized by a dramatic upregulation of Th2-type cytokines and chemokines, including TSLP, CCL17, IL13 and IL4, all of which were induced early in Ctip2$^{ep-/-}$ epidermis, and are crucially involved in the initiation of pathogenesis in human AD [3,7,35]. Finally, Ctip2$^{ep-/-}$ adult mice exhibit Th2-like systemic immune syndrome that is similar to that found in most AD patients [36]. Based on the above phenotypic spectrum of Ctip2$^{ep-/-}$ adult mice, it appears that this line may serve as a useful model for the study of human AD.

During development, selective ablation of Ctip2 in the epidermis reduced epidermal proliferation and impaired terminal differentiation of keratinocytes [25]. Isolated Ctip2-null keratinocytes also exhibit severe proliferation and differentiation defects in culture [26]. To our surprise, in the postnatal stages, a hyperplastic epidermis and a significantly higher percentage of Ki67-positive cells were observed in the Ctip2$^{ep-/-}$ skin as early as 1 week after birth (Figure 1). Elevated proliferation could be secondary to impaired epidermal barrier functions caused by Ctip2 ablation. Previous studies have established that hyperproliferation and acanthosis (thickened epidermis) are compensatory responses and secondary to impaired epidermal barrier [37–40]. It is also

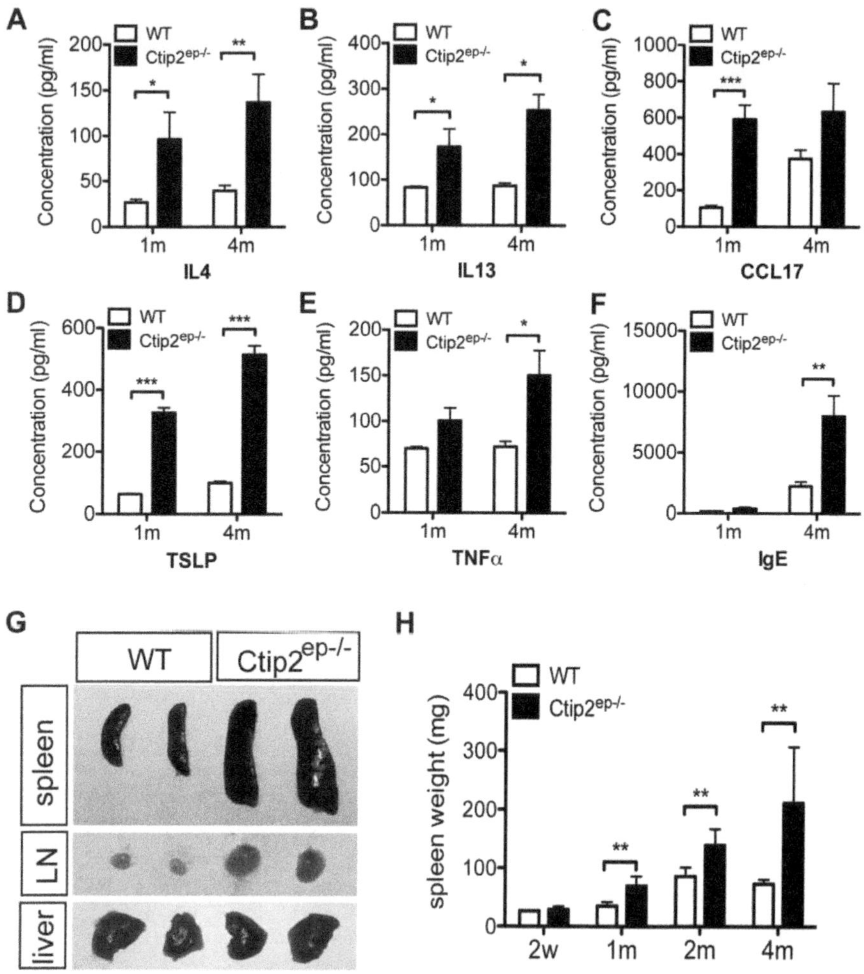

Figure 5. Systemic immunological abnormalities in Ctip2$^{ep-/-}$ adult mice. Serum concentration of (**A**) IL4, (**B**) IL13, (**C**) CCL17, (**D**) TSLP, (**E**) TNFα and (**F**) IgE was measured by ELISA. (**G**) Gross morphological comparison of spleen, lymph node (LN) and liver in 4-months-old WT and Ctip2$^{ep-/-}$ mice. (**H**) Spleen weight of WT and Ctip2$^{ep-/-}$ mice at different months of age is indicated. Statistical analyses were performed by student's unpaired t-test using GraphPad Prism software; * P<0.05, ** P<0.01, *** P<0.005.

possible that impaired skin barrier in Ctip2$^{ep-/-}$ mice skin could be partially due to deficiency in tight junctions. That possibility was ruled out since immuno-histochemical staining of dorsal skin exhibited no significant difference in tight junction protein expression including beta-catenin, E-cadherin, claudin-1 and claudin-4 between wildtype and mutant mice (Figure S4B–E).

A number of candidate genes have been identified in association with AD, however, many of these linkages have been called into question due to insufficiently powered studies and/or heterogeneity of the disease [33,34]. In independent studies, several genes such as Filaggrin (FLG), trans-acting T-cell-specific transcription factor (GATA3) and IL4 has been reported to be involved in AD pathogenesis [41]. FLG deficiency alone decreases stratum corneum hydration and leads to increased TEWL, and has been correlated with AD in the highest number of studies [41,42]. It is worth mentioning that skin barrier deficiency has also been reported in AD patients without FLG mutation(s) or loss of expression [43] suggesting existence of different subtypes of AD in humans. We have shown previously that Ctip2 deficiency is associated with impaired terminal differentiation and decreased FLG expression during development [25]. Indeed, we have observed a ~50% reduction of FLG expression in the epidermis of Ctip2$^{ep-/-}$ skin compared to that of wildtype littermates around 1 week of age (Figure S1F). However, no significant difference in level of FLG expression was observed between the wildtype and mutant epidermis at later timpoints from 2 weeks to 4 months of age, possibly due to a compensatory upregulation of other related factors such as Ctip1 (Figure 1E). The lack of loss-of-FLG expression observed in Ctip2$^{ep-/-}$ mice at later stages indicates possible involvement of other factors to modulate barrier integrity.

It appears that during adulthood, the requirement of Ctip2 for epidermal proliferation and differentiation is compensated by upregulation of a Ctip2-independent growth pathway. The increase of epidermal proliferation may also be secondary to the inflammatory phenotype together with defects in barrier function. The role of Th2 cytokines in AD skin lesion is to promote the recruitment, proliferation and development of Th2-type immune cells to lesional site, whereas their direct roles in keratinocyte proliferation still remain largely unknown. Activation of TSLP signaling in dendritic cells and T cells is known to activate multiple growth pathways, including STATs, Src kinases, PI3K and ERK1/2 [44–48]. It is possible that inflammatory cytokines, such as TSLP may contribute to the hyperproliferative response of Ctip2$^{ep-/-}$ adult epidermis.

TSLP, a keratinocyte-derived triad of cytokines, has been studied intensively recently in the pathogenesis of allergic inflammation and subsequent development of AD and other immune disorder [31,49,50]. It is recognized as the master switch for AD and other atopic diseases, such as asthma, as it plays a critical role to induce the Th2-type allergic inflammation in AD pathogenesis [31]. Keratinocyte-derived TSLP participates in the inflammatory cascade by activation of other immune cells, such as dendritic cells and mast cells, and subsequent stimulation of release of Th2-related cytokines/chemokines from these immune cells, eventually initiate inflammatory a Th2 lymphocyte response [9,49,51]. In the present study, we have observed that TSLP was the earliest known cytokine induced in Ctip2$^{ep-/-}$ mice and this induction was maintained in the mutants at all postnatal stages of development. The induction of TSLP was mainly restricted to the epidermis, which correlates well with epithelial cells of the keratinocyte lineage as major producers of TSLP in AD patients (see Figures 4F and S4A) [49]. Hence, induction of TSLP in Ctip2 mutant keratinocytes could be a trigger factor that initiates and directs the Th2-type inflammatory cascade observed in Ctip2$^{ep-/-}$ skin.

Transgenic mice over-expressing TSLP in keratinocytes develop AD-like symptoms, indicating that TSLP expression is sufficient to initiate AD-like inflammatory responses [50]. Therefore, it remains critical to address upstream triggers of TSLP expression and how TSLP is regulated before and during AD pathogenesis. Putative NF-κB response element has been detected in the mouse and human TSLP gene promoter and NF-κB regulated mouse and human TSLP gene expression in presence of inflammatory cytokines *in vitro* [13,14,52–54]. Putative AP-1 transcription factor binding motif was also detected on the promoter region of human TSLP gene [13,14,52–54]. Similarly, nuclear receptor (NR) RXR directly repressed TSLP transcription through the binding of RXR-VDR and RXR-RARγ heterodimer containing co-repressor complexes to the mouse TSLP promoter [13,14,52–54]. Previous studies have also identified presence of putative VDREs (DR3) and RAREs (DR2 and DR1) upstream of the human TSLP promoter [14]. Since we have observed Ctip2 recruitment around that region on the mTSLP promoter, it is possible that NRs and Ctip2 could be a part of the same transcriptional complex to regulate TSLP gene expression in mouse keratinocytes. However, additional recruitment of Ctip2 along with NRs on the further distal region of mouse TSLP gene promoter cannot be ruled out. Here, we have identified a novel transcriptional regulatory mechanism(s) of negative regulation of TSLP expression by Ctip2 in mouse epidermis. Ctip2 appears to interact directly with and repress expression of the TSLP promoter.

We have demonstrated a predominant upregulation of Th2 cytokines in the Ctip2$^{ep-/-}$ skin at all timepoints, but a late surge of Th1 cytokines, including IFNγ and TNFα, was also observed in the mutant skin at 4 months (Figure S3N-O). Indeed, it has been demonstrated that Th2- and Th1 type cytokines both contribute to different stages of the development of skin lesions in AD patients [29]. Th2-cell subsets are specifically activated during the initiation phase, followed by the Th1-cell subset to maintain the persistence of the chronic inflammatory response. Our work confirms that Th2- and Th1-type immune responses are not mutually exclusive, especially at the chronic phage of the inflammatory disease. The interaction between different Th-cell subsets at the chronic stage may be a fruitful area for future investigation of AD pathogenesis.

Systemic immune response related to elevated expression of IL-4, IL13, CCL17 and IgE, observed in Ctip2$^{ep-/-}$ mice is evidently Th2 cell-dependent and humoral in nature. IL-4, for example, induces differentiation of CD4$^+$ T-cells into Th2 cells, and also inhibits production of Th1 cells [55]. Th2 cells secrete IL-13, which together with IL-4, initiates a B lymphocyte-directed, humoral response [55]. IL-4 also upregulates MHC class II expression and induces B-cell class switching to IgE [56]. Furthermore, TSLP stimulation of naïve CD4$^+$ T-cells induces a specialized Th2 polarization, which results in production of downstream Th2-associated pro-inflammatory cytokines, such as IL-13, which carry out humoral immune processes [30]. Simultaneously, CCL17 is known to attract Th2 cells, thereby favoring humoral responses [57]. In summary, inflammation due to selective Ctip2 ablation in mice epidermis is not restricted to the site of deletion; rather Ctip2$^{ep-/-}$ mice show a chronic secondary Th2-dependent humoral systemic inflammatory response that could possibly lead to inflammation of airway and pulmonary epithelium and asthma.

Our group has previously shown that Ctip2 expression was increased in samples from AD and ACD patients, and here we also show an increase of Ctip2 expression in the epidermis of another known mouse AD model (RXRα$^{ep-/-}$; Figure S7A–B) [24]. Based on our study here, we hypothesize that induction of Ctip2 during AD progression may have a protective role, which is to suppress the inflammatory response by inhibiting TSLP expression. In contrast, the elevated proliferation in the Ctip2$^{ep-/-}$ mice epidermis is likely due to compensatory responses and secondary to impaired epidermal barrier functions. Additional studies to determine TSLP level in AD and ACD patients with elevated Ctip2 expression will be useful to validate our hypothesis.

In summary, our study reveals a novel role(s) of keratinocytic Ctip2 in epidermal barrier maintenance and homeostasis, and inflammation in adult mice. Ctip2 clearly modulates AD-like responses within the skin, as well as systemic inflammatory responses. TSLP was strongly induced in Ctip2$^{ep-/-}$ epidermis and likely causes increased dendritic cells infiltration into lymph nodes, in which these cells interact with CD4$^+$ T cells to produce Th-2 inflammatory cytokines. Subsequently, other immune cells such as macrophages, leukocytes, mast cells and eosinophils could be attracted and recruited to the site of skin inflammation, which become disseminated, leading to elevated circulating levels of inflammatory mediators. This study identifies a new mediator, Ctip2, which may be implicated in the etiology of AD. However, several issues need to be resolved in the future. For example, it is presently unclear if a defective skin barrier precedes inflammation and enhanced cellular proliferation in the early stages of AD development. Second, the contributory role of TSLP in AD and the mechanistic basis of regulation of TSLP gene expression in mouse and human keratinocytes have not been fully elucidated. Finally, the role of Ctip1 in AD development in presence or absence of Ctip2 could shed further lights in AD pathogenesis and identify new avenues for therapeutic intervention. Our study highlights a central role of epidermal keratinocytes in initiating and shaping the immune response during the pathogenesis of AD-like skin diseases in mice.

Materials and Methods

Mice

The function of Ctip2 in adult mice skin homeostasis was characterized using Ctip2$^{ep-/-}$ mice that selectively lacked Ctip2 in epidermal keratinocytes after Cre-recombinase mediated deletion of Ctip2 gene in keratinocytes using K14-Cre deleter mice [25,27,28]. Ctip2 floxed mice (Ctip2 $^{L2/L2}$, wildtype) were used as controls [25,28]. 8 to 10 mice from multiple litters were used in each group at each time point. Mice were maintained in a temperature/humidity-controlled facility with a 12-hour light/dark cycle. Animal protocol was approved by Oregon State University Institutional Animal Care and Use Committee (IACUC), under permit number 4300.

Transepidermal water loss (TEWL) measurement

Transepidermal water loss was measured using the calibrated Tewameter TM300 with Multi Probe Adapter (CK electronic GmbH, Köln, Germany) in accordance with manufacture operating instructions. Data was expressed in g/m^2 h, and represents the mean ± S.E.M. for 8 independent animals (10 measurements each animal) of each genotype. Statistical analysis was performed using Graphpad Prism software with student's unpaired t-test.

Histological analysis

Skin biopsies were fixed in 4% paraformaldehyde overnight and embedded in paraffin blocks. 5 mm paraffin sections were sectioned using a Leica RM2255 microtome (Bannockburn, IL). Hematoxylin and eosin staining was performed according to general protocols [58].

Combined eosinophil/mast cell stain (C.E.M) was performed using a commercial kit according to the manufacturer's protocol (American MasterTech, Lodi, CA). Briefly, slides were deparaffinized with xylene and hydrated through alcohols. After washed in running tap water, slides were placed in astra blue staining solution for 30 minutes and rinsed in tap water. Slides were put in vital new red staining solution for another 30 minutes and rinsed with tap water. After that, slides were placed in modified Mayer's hematoxylin for 15–30 seconds and rinsed again with tap water for 2 minutes. Finally, dehydration of slides was performed with 3 changes of absolute alcohol and xylene before mounting. Mast cells showed bright blue color while eosinophils were red. Nuclei were stained blue.

Toluidine blue staining was performed as described [13]. Toluidine blue working solution was prepared by mixing 5 ml 1% toluidine blue EtOH solution (Sigma-Aldrich, St. Louis, MO) with 45 ml 1% sodium chloride (pH 2.3). Slides were deparaffinized and hydrated in distilled water. Sections were stained with toluidine blue working solution (pH 2.0–2.5) for 2–3 minutes before washed in 3 changes of distilled water. Slides were dehydrated through alcohols and xylenes and mounted with resinous mounting medium.

Immunohistochemistry

IHC staining of paraffin and frozen sections was described previously [58,59]. In brief, paraffin sections were deparaffinized and antigen retrieval was performed with pH 6.0 citrate buffer and 95–100°C for 20 minutes and cooled down. For frozen sections, slides were fixed with cold acetone for 20 minutes and allowed for air dry. Slides were washed with 0.1% PBST and blocked with 10% normal goat serum (Vector Laboratories, Builingame, CA) for 30 minutes before incubated with primary antibodies overnight at 4°C. Fluorescently labeled secondary antibodies were applied to slides for an hour at room temperature. Nuclei were visualized with DAPI. After the final washes, slides were dehydrated and mounted. Images were captured at ×20 magnification using a Carl Zeiss Axio Imager Z1 fluorescent microscope and AxioCam camera. Data were analyzed and quantified using Adobe Photoshop and ImageJ software. Multiple IHC fields were randomly chosen and 10–15 such fields per slide were counted independently in a double-blinded manner. All experiments in each category were repeated in triplicates.

The concentrations of antibodies used were as follows: Ki67 (Abcam, Cambridge, MA, 1:500), K14 (Abcam, 1:1000), K10 (Abcam, 1:1000), Filaggrin (Abcam, 1:1000), Loricrin (Abcam, 1:500), F4/80 (Biolegend, San Diego, CA, 1:250), CD11b (Abcam, 1:100), CD45 (Abcam, 1:500), Ly6g (Abcam, 1:250), CD11c (BD Pharmingen, San Jose, CA, 1:100), RXRα (Santa Cruz Biotechnology, Santa Cruz, CA, 1:1000), Notch1 (Cell Signaling technology, Danvers, MA, 1:500), Ctip2 (Abcam, 1:300), Claudin4 (Abcam, 1:50), Claudin1 (Abcam, 1:100), E-cadherin (Cell Signaling, Danvers, MA, 1:200), b-Catenin (Cell Signaling, 1:50), TSLP (Invitrogen, 1:100), Cy3 goat anti rabbit (Jackson ImmunoResearch Laboratories Inc., West Grove, PA, 1:500), Cy3 goat anti rat (Jackson ImmunoResearch, 1:500), Cy2 goat anti rat (Jackson ImmunoResearch, 1:500), Cy3 goat anti mouse (Jackson ImmunoResearch, 1:1000).

RT-qPCR

RNA extraction and cDNA preparation were performed as described [60]. Real-time PCR was performed on an ABI 7500 Real-Time PCR system using SYBR Green methodology using specific sets of primers as indicated in Table S1 [60,61]. Relative gene expression analysis of the RT-qPCR data was performed using HPRT as an internal control. All assays were performed in triplicates.

ELISA

ELISA kits for detecting mouse IL-4, IL-13, TNFα and TSLP were obtained from eBioscience, Inc. (San Diego, CA, USA). Mouse IgE ELISA kit was procured from Bethyl Laboratories, Inc. (Montgomery, TX, USA), while CCL17 immunoassay kit was purchased from R&D Systems, Inc. (Minneapolis, MN, USA).

1-month and 4-month-old mice (6 wildtypes and 6 Ctip2$^{ep-/-}$ from each age group) were selected for studying secondary systemic response to Ctip2$^{ep-/-}$ genotype. Blood plasma was isolated from the mice following the method of Argmann and Auwerx [62]. ELISA was performed for estimation of the levels of IL-4, IL-13, IgE, CCL17, TNFα and TSLP using kits following the respective manufacturer's instructions. All samples were assayed in triplicates.

Chromatin immunoprecipitation (ChIP)

ChIP assay was performed according to Hyter *et al.*, 2010 with minor modifications [63]. Briefly, mouse epidermal keratinocytes from 1-day postnatal wildtype mice skin were isolated and fixed in 1% formaldehyde. Cell lysate from 3×10^6 keratinocytes (each ChIP) were obtained after incubation with hypotonic buffer (10 mM Tris/HCl, pH 7.5, 10 mM NaCl, 3 mM $MgCl_2$ and 0.5% NP40). Nuclei were suspended in ChIP sonication buffer (50 mM Hepes, pH 7.9, 150 mM NaCl, 1 mM EDTA, 1% Triton X-100, 0.1% SDS, 0.1% sodium deoxycholate) with 0.2% SDS. Nuclei were sonicated and immunoprecipitated with 2 µg anti-Ctip2 antibody (Abcam, Cambridge, MA) overnight at 4°C. Rat IgG was used as a control. 25 ml pre-equilibrated protein G beads (Invitrogen, Carlsbad, CA) were added to each ChIP and incubated for four hours at 4°C. After washing twice with ChIP sonication buffer, buffer A (50 mM Hepes, 500 mM NaCl, 1 mM EDTA, 1% Triton X-100, 0.1% SDS and 0.1% sodium deoxycholate), buffer B (20 mM Tris/HCl, pH 8.0, 1 mM EDTA, 250 mM LiCl, 0.5% NP40 and 0.5% sodium deoxycholate) and once with TE buffer, DNA was uncrosslinked at 65°C overnight and purified by QIAquick PCR Purification Kit (Qiagen, Germantown, MD). All the buffers used in the study were added with PMSF and protease inhibitors before use. DNA was amplified using ABI-7500 Real-time PCR machine with specific primers indicated in Table S1. Primers were designed from proximal (−200 bp) and distal (−1 kb) promoter regions of TSLP to study the possible interaction between Ctip2 and TSLP, and primers selected from 3′-UTR region was used as a control.

Western blotting

Protein was extracted from mouse epidermis and western blotting was performed according to previous reports using specific antibodies against filaggrin (Abcam,1:1000) and loricrin (Abcam, 1:1000) [58]. Western blotting represents the results from three separate experiments performed in triplicate.

Statistics

Statistical significance of differences between groups was analyzed using GraphPad Prism software using student's unpaired *t*-test. All statistical analyses were performed in a double-blinded manner.

Supporting Information

Figure S1 Characterization of epidermal proliferation and differentiation in Ctip2$^{ep-/-}$ mice. (**A**) Measurement of epidermal thickness of WT and Ctip2$^{ep-/-}$ mice skin. (**B**) Measurement of trans-epidermal water loss (TEWL) from dorsal skin of wildtype, lesional Ctip2$^{ep-/-}$ mice and non-lesional Ctip2$^{ep-/-}$ mice at 4 month. (**C**) Epidermal percent Ki67 positive cells in dorsal skin sections of WT and mutant mice. Statistical analyses were performed by student's unpaired t-test using GraphPad Prism software; * P<0.05, ** P<0.005, *** P<0.0001. Immunohistochemical staining of dorsal skin biopsies from WT and Ctip2$^{ep-/-}$ mice was performed with antibodies directed against (**D**) K14 and (**E**) K10 (all in red). All sections were counterstained with DAPI (blue). Scale bar (in D and E): 100 μm. Epidermis (E) and dermis (D) are indicated. (**F**) Quantitative RT-PCR (RT-qPCR) analyses of filaggrin in the dorsal skin of 1-week and 2-week- old wild type (WT) and Ctip2$^{ep-/-}$ mice using specific primers as indicated in Table S1. ** P<0.005. All values represent relative transcript level after normalization with HPRT transcripts. (**G**) Immunoblotting analysis of filaggrin (FLG) and loricrin (LOR) in the skin of 2-week and 4-month-old wild type (WT) and Ctip2$^{ep-/-}$ mice. β-actin is used as an internal control. Statistical analyses were performed by student's unpaired t-test using GraphPad Prism software; ** P<0.01, *** P<0.001.

Figure S2 Characterization of inflammatory cell infiltrates in dorsal skin of WT and Ctip2$^{ep-/-}$ adult mice. (**A**) Toluidine blue stained dorsal paraffin skin sections of WT and Ctip2$^{ep-/-}$ mice. Mast cells stain intensive blue color. Scale bar: 100 μm. (**B**) Immunohistochemical staining of dorsal skin biopsies with antibody against CD45 (green). Scale bar: 100 μm. (**C**) Percent CD45 positive cells in the dermis of WT and mutant skin. Statistical analyses were performed by student's unpaired t-test using GraphPad Prism software; * P<0.05. Scale bar: 100 μm. (**D**) Immunohistochemical staining of CD11c (red) in dorsal skin of WT and Ctip2$^{ep-/-}$ mice. Scale bar: 50 μm. All sections (in B & D) were counterstained with DAPI (blue).

Figure S3 Relative expression levels of cytokines and chemokines in WT and Ctip2$^{ep-/-}$ skin. The expression level of (**A**) IL10, (**B**) IL1α, (**C**) IL2, (**D**) IL12a, (**E**) IL12b, (**F**) IL17a, (**G**) IL18, (**H**) IL23, (**I**) CCL20, (**J**) CCL22, (**K**) CXCL10, (**L**) CCL3, (**M**) CXCL2, (**N**) IFNγ and (**O**) TNFα was studied with RT-qPCR in 1-month and 4-month-old wildtype and Ctip2$^{ep-/-}$ dorsal skin. Values represent relative transcript level after normalization with HPRT transcripts. Statistical analyses were performed by student's unpaired t-test using GraphPad Prism software; * P<0.05, ** P<0.01, *** P<0.001.

Figure S4 Characterization of TSLP and tight junction proteins in dorsal skin of 1-month and 4-month-old WT and in Ctip2$^{ep-/-}$ adult mice. Immunohistochemical staining of dorsal skin biopsies from WT and Ctip2$^{ep-/-}$ mice were performed with specific antibodies against (**A**) TSLP; (**B**) β-catenin, (**C**) E-cadherin; (**D**) Claudin-1 and (**E**) Claudin-4 (all in red). All sections were counterstained with DAPI (blue). Scale bar: 100 μm.

Figure S5 Relative expression levels of RXRα and genes involved in Notch signaling pathway. The expression level of (**A**) Notch1, (**B**) Notch2, (**C**) Rbp-j and (**D**) RXRα was studied with RT-qPCR in 1-month and 4-month-old wildtype and Ctip2$^{ep-/-}$ dorsal skin. Values represent relative transcript level after normalization with GAPDH transcripts. Statistical analyses were performed by student's unpaired t-test using GraphPad Prism software. (E) Immunohistochemical staining of dorsal skin biopsies with antibody against Notch1 (red) and (F) RXRα (red). Scale bar: 100 μm. All sections (in E & F) were counterstained with DAPI (blue).

Figure S6 Immunological abnormalities of spleen and lymph node in Ctip2$^{ep-/-}$ adult mice. (**A, D**) Hemotoxylin & Eosin stained 5 μm thick paraffin sections from spleen of WT and Ctip2$^{ep-/-}$ mice at 4 m. (**B, C, E, F**) C.E.M staining for eosinophils (pink) and mast cells (blue) in 4 month-old mice spleen sections. (**G, J**) Hemotoxylin & Eosin stained 5 μm thick paraffin sections of WT and Ctip2$^{ep-/-}$ mice lymph node at 4 m. (**H, I, K, L**) C.E.M staining for eosinophils (pink) and mast cells (blue) in 4 month-old mice lymph node. Black arrows point to eosinophils. Scale bar: 50 μm.

Figure S7 Expression of Ctip2 in RXRα$^{ep-/-}$ mouse model. (**A**) Immunohistochemical staining of dorsal skin biopsies with antibody against Ctip2 (red). Sections were counterstained with DAPI (blue). NE, normal epidermis; HPE, hyperfroliferative epidermis. Scale bar: 100 μm. (**B**) Bar graph indicates the percentage of Ctip2 positive cells in the dorsal skin of normal epidermis (NE) from the wildtype (WT) and the hyperproliferative epidermis (HPE) form RXRα$^{ep-/-}$ mice. Statistical analyses were performed by student's unpaired t-test using GraphPad Prism software; ** P<0.01. All experiments were performed in triplicates.

Table S1 List of primers used for RT-qPCR.

Acknowledgments

We would like to thank Xiaobo Liang for technical assistance including mouse colony maintenance and Shreya Bhattacharya for re-validation of the ChIP experiments. We also thank Drs. Mark Zabriskie and Gary DeLander of College of Pharmacy, Oregon State University for continuous support and encouragement.

Author Contributions

Conceived and designed the experiments: AKI GGI ML. Performed the experiments: ZW LZ GG SL. Analyzed the data: AKI GGI ML ZW LZ GG KK. Contributed reagents/materials/analysis tools: AKI GGI CK ML. Wrote the paper: ZW LZ AKI GGI ML.

References

1. Fuchs E, Raghavan S (2002) Getting under the skin of epidermal morphogenesis. Nat Rev Genet 3: 199–209.
2. Proksch E, Brandner JM, Jensen JM (2008) The skin: an indispensable barrier. Exp Dermatol 17(12): 1063–1072. Available: http://www.ncbi.nlm.nih.gov/pubmed/19043850. Accessed 2012 Nov 23.
3. Tokura Y (2010) Extrinsic and intrinsic types of atopic dermatitis. Journal of Dermatological Science 58: 1–7. doi:10.1016/j.jdermsci.2010.02.008.
4. Leung DY, Bieber T (2003) Atopic dermatitis. The Lancet 361: 151–160. doi:10.1016/S0140-6736(03)12193-9.
5. Scharschmidt TC, Segre JA (2008) Modeling atopic dermatitis with increasingly complex mouse models. J Invest Dermatol 128: 1061–1064. doi:10.1038/sj.jid.5701201.
6. Cork MJ, Danby SG, Vasilopoulos Y, Hadgraft J, Lane ME, et al. (2009) Epidermal Barrier Dysfunction in Atopic Dermatitis. Journal of Investigative Dermatology 129: 1892–1908. doi:10.1038/jid.2009.133.
7. B. Brandt E, Sivaprasad U (2011) Th2 Cytokines and Atopic Dermatitis. Journal of Clinical & Cellular Immunology 02. Available:http://www.omicsonline.org/2155-9899/2155-9899-2-110.digital/2155-9899-2-110.html. Accessed 2012 Mar 9.
8. Biedermann T, Röcken M, Carballido JM (2004) TH1 and TH2 lymphocyte development and regulation of TH cell-mediated immune responses of the skin. J Investig Dermatol Symp Proc 9: 5–14. doi:10.1111/j.1087-0024.2004.00829.x.
9. Comeau MR, Ziegler SF (2010) The influence of TSLP on the allergic response. Mucosal Immunol 3: 138–147. doi:10.1038/mi.2009.134.
10. Ziegler SF (2010) The role of thymic stromal lymphopoietin (TSLP) in allergic disorders. Current Opinion in Immunology 22: 795–799. doi:10.1016/j.coi.2010.10.020.
11. Kashyap M, Rochman Y, Spolski R, Samsel L, Leonard WJ (2011) Thymic stromal lymphopoietin is produced by dendritic cells. J Immunol 187: 1207–1211. doi:10.4049/jimmunol.1100355.
12. Demehri S, Liu Z, Lee J, Lin M-H, Crosby SD, et al. (2008) Notch-Deficient Skin Induces a Lethal Systemic B-Lymphoproliferative Disorder by Secreting TSLP, a Sentinel for Epidermal Integrity. PLoS Biology 6: e123. doi:10.1371/journal.pbio.0060123.
13. Li M (2005) Retinoid X receptor ablation in adult mouse keratinocytes generates an atopic dermatitis triggered by thymic stromal lymphopoietin. Proceedings of the National Academy of Sciences 102: 14795–14800. doi:10.1073/pnas.0507385102.
14. Li M (2006) Topical vitamin D3 and low-calcemic analogs induce thymic stromal lymphopoietin in mouse keratinocytes and trigger an atopic dermatitis. Proceedings of the National Academy of Sciences 103: 11736–11741. doi:10.1073/pnas.0604575103.
15. Avram D, Fields A, Pretty On Top K, Nevrivy DJ, Ishmael JE, et al. (2000) Isolation of a novel family of C(2)H(2) zinc finger proteins implicated in transcriptional repression mediated by chicken ovalbumin upstream promoter transcription factor (COUP-TF) orphan nuclear receptors. J Biol Chem 275: 10315–10322.
16. Topark-Ngarm A, Golonzhka O, Peterson VJ, Barrett B, Martinez B, et al. (2006) CTIP2 associates with the NuRD complex on the promoter of p57KIP2, a newly identified CTIP2 target gene. J Biol Chem 281: 32272–32283.
17. Arlotta P, Molyneaux BJ, Chen J, Inoue J, Kominami R, et al. (2005) Neuronal Subtype-Specific Genes that Control Corticospinal Motor Neuron Development In Vivo. Neuron 45: 207–221. doi:10.1016/j.neuron.2004.12.036.
18. Kastner P, Chan S, Vogel WK, Zhang L-J, Topark-Ngarm A, et al. (2010) Bcl11b represses a mature T-cell gene expression program in immature CD4(+)CD8(+) thymocytes. Eur J Immunol 40: 2143–2154. doi:10.1002/eji.200940258.
19. Cismasiu VB, Adamo K, Gecewicz J, Duque J, Lin Q, et al. (2005) BCL11B functionally associates with the NuRD complex in T lymphocytes to repress targeted promoter. Oncogene 24: 6753–6764. doi:10.1038/sj.onc.1208904.
20. Senawong T, Peterson VJ, Avram D, Shepherd DM, Frye RA, et al. (2003) Involvement of the histone deacetylase SIRT1 in chicken ovalbumin upstream promoter transcription factor (COUP-TF)-interacting protein 2-mediated transcriptional repression. J Biol Chem 278: 43041–43050. doi:10.1074/jbc.M307477200.
21. Kastner P, Chan S, Vogel WK, Zhang L-J, Topark-Ngarm A, et al. (2010) Bcl11b represses a mature T-cell gene expression program in immature CD4(+)CD8(+) thymocytes. Eur J Immunol 40: 2143–2154. doi:10.1002/eji.200940258.
22. Zhang L-J, Vogel WK, Liu X, Topark-Ngarm A, Arbogast BL, et al. (2012) Coordinated Regulation of Transcription Factor Bcl11b Activity in Thymocytes by the Mitogen-activated Protein Kinase (MAPK) Pathways and Protein Sumoylation. J Biol Chem 287: 26971–26988. doi:10.1074/jbc.M112.344176.
23. Golonzhka O, Leid M, Indra G, Indra AK (2007) Expression of COUP-TF-interacting protein 2 (CTIP2) in mouse skin during development and in adulthood. Gene Expr Patterns 7: 754–760.
24. Ganguli-Indra G, Liang X, Hyter S, Leid M, Hanifin J, et al. (2009) Expression of COUP-TF-interacting protein 2 (CTIP2) in human atopic dermatitis and allergic contact dermatitis skin. Experimental Dermatology 18: 994–996. doi:10.1111/j.1600-0625.2009.00876.x.
25. Golonzhka O, Liang X, Messaddeq N, Bornert J-M, Campbell AL, et al. (2008) Dual Role of COUP-TF-Interacting Protein 2 in Epidermal Homeostasis and Permeability Barrier Formation. J Investig Dermatol 129: 1459–1470. doi:10.1038/jid.2008.392.
26. Zhang L-J, Bhattacharya S, Leid M, Ganguli-Indra G, Indra AK (2012) Ctip2 is a dynamic regulator of epidermal proliferation and differentiation by integrating EGFR and Notch signaling. J Cell Sci. doi:10.1242/jcs.108969.
27. Dassule HR, Lewis P, Bei M, Maas R, McMahon AP (2000) Sonic hedgehog regulates growth and morphogenesis of the tooth. Development 127: 4775–4785.
28. Indra AK, Warot X, Brocard J, Bornert JM, Xiao JH, et al. (1999) Temporally-controlled site-specific mutagenesis in the basal layer of the epidermis: comparison of the recombinase activity of the tamoxifen-inducible Cre-ER(T) and Cre-ER(T2) recombinases. Nucleic Acids Res 27: 4324–4327.
29. Grewe M, Bruijnzeel-Koomen CA, Schöpf E, Thepen T, Langeveld-Wildschut AG, et al. (1998) A role for Th1 and Th2 cells in the immunopathogenesis of atopic dermatitis. Immunol Today 19: 359–361.
30. Ziegler SF, Artis D (2010) Sensing the outside world: TSLP regulates barrier immunity. Nature Immunology 11. 289–293. doi:10.1038/ni.1852.
31. Liu Y-J (2006) Thymic stromal lymphopoietin: master switch for allergic inflammation. J Exp Med 203: 269–273. doi:10.1084/jem.20051745.
32. Dumortier A, Durham A-D, Di Piazza M, Vauclair S, Koch U, et al. (2010) Atopic Dermatitis-Like Disease and Associated Lethal Myeloproliferative Disorder Arise from Loss of Notch Signaling in the Murine Skin. PLoS ONE 5: e9258. doi:10.1371/journal.pone.0009258.
33. Boguniewicz M, Leung DYM (2011) Atopic dermatitis: a disease of altered skin barrier and immune dysregulation. Immunol Rev 242: 233–246. doi:10.1111/j.1600-065X.2011.01027.x.
34. Dubrac S, Schmuth M, Ebner S (2010) Atopic dermatitis: the role of Langerhans cells in disease pathogenesis. Immunology and Cell Biology 88: 400–409. doi:10.1038/icb.2010.33.
35. Novak N, Leung DY (2011) Advances in atopic dermatitis. Current Opinion in Immunology 23: 778–783. doi:10.1016/j.coi.2011.09.007.
36. Spergel J (2003) Atopic dermatitis and the atopic march. Journal of Allergy and Clinical Immunology 112: S118–S127. doi:10.1016/j.jaci.2003.09.033.
37. Proksch E, Feingold KR, Man MQ, Elias PM (1991) Barrier function regulates epidermal DNA synthesis. Journal of Clinical Investigation 87: 1668–1673. doi:10.1172/JCI115183.
38. Segre JA, Bauer C, Fuchs E (1999) Klf4 is a transcription factor required for establishing the barrier function of the skin. Nat Genet 22: 356–360. doi:10.1038/11926.
39. Matsuki M, Yamashita F, Ishida-Yamamoto A, Yamada K, Kinoshita C, et al. (1998) Defective stratum corneum and early neonatal death in mice lacking the gene for transglutaminase 1 (keratinocyte transglutaminase). Proc Natl Acad Sci USA 95: 1044–1049.
40. de Guzman Strong C, Wertz PW, Wang C, Yang F, Meltzer PS, et al. (2006) Lipid defect underlies selective skin barrier impairment of an epidermal-specific deletion of Gata-3. J Cell Biol 175: 661–670.
41. Barnes KC (2010) An update on the genetics of atopic dermatitis: Scratching the surface in 2009. Journal of Allergy and Clinical Immunology 125: 16–29.e11. doi:10.1016/j.jaci.2009.11.008.
42. Palmer CNA, Irvine AD, Terron-Kwiatkowski A, Zhao Y, Liao H, et al. (2006) Common loss-of-function variants of the epidermal barrier protein filaggrin are a major predisposing factor for atopic dermatitis. Nat Genet 38: 441–446. doi:10.1038/ng1767.
43. Jakasa I, Koster ES, Calkoen F, McLean WHI, Campbell LE, et al. (2010) Skin Barrier Function in Healthy Subjects and Patients with Atopic Dermatitis in Relation to Filaggrin Loss-of-Function Mutations. Journal of Investigative Dermatology 131: 540–542. doi:10.1038/jid.2010.307.
44. Wong CK, Hu S, Cheung PFY, Lam CWK (2010) Thymic stromal lymphopoietin induces chemotactic and prosurvival effects in eosinophils: implications in allergic inflammation. Am J Respir Cell Mol Biol 43: 305–315. doi:10.1165/rcmb.2009-0168OC.
45. Reche PA, Soumelis V, Gorman DM, Clifford T, Liu Mr, et al. (2001) Human thymic stromal lymphopoietin preferentially stimulates myeloid cells. J Immunol 167: 336–343.
46. Quentmeier H, Drexler HG, Fleckenstein D, Zaborski M, Armstrong A, et al. (2001) Cloning of human thymic stromal lymphopoietin (TSLP) and signaling mechanisms leading to proliferation. Leukemia 15: 1286–1292.
47. Sebastian K, Borowski A, Kuepper M, Friedrich K (2008) Signal transduction around thymic stromal lymphopoietin (TSLP) in atopic asthma. Cell Commun Signal 6: 5. doi:10.1186/1478-811X-6-5.

48. Tasian SK, Doral MY, Borowitz MJ, Wood BL, Chen I-M, et al. (2012) Aberrant STAT5 and PI3K/mTOR pathway signaling occurs in human CRLF2-rearranged B-precursor acute lymphoblastic leukemia. Blood 120: 833–842. doi:10.1182/blood-2011-12-389932.
49. Soumelis V, Reche PA, Kanzler H, Yuan W, Edward G, et al. (2002) Human epithelial cells trigger dendritic cell–mediated allergic inflammation by producing TSLP. Nature Immunology. Available:http://www.nature.com/doifinder/10.1038/ni805. Accessed 2012 Mar 27.
50. Yoo J (2005) Spontaneous atopic dermatitis in mice expressing an inducible thymic stromal lymphopoietin transgene specifically in the skin. Journal of Experimental Medicine 202: 541–549. doi:10.1084/jem.20041503.
51. Liu Y (2009) Chapter 1 TSLP in Epithelial Cell and Dendritic Cell Cross Talk. Advances in Immunology. Elsevier, Vol. 101. pp. 1–25. Available:http://linkinghub.elsevier.com/retrieve/pii/S0065277608010018. Accessed 2012 Apr 30.
52. Lee H-C, Ziegler SF (2007) Inducible expression of the proallergic cytokine thymic stromal lymphopoietin in airway epithelial cells is controlled by NF B. Proceedings of the National Academy of Sciences 104: 914–919. doi:10.1073/pnas.0607305104.
53. Takai T (2012) TSLP expression: cellular sources, triggers, and regulatory mechanisms. Allergol Int 61: 3–17. doi:10.2332/allergolint.11-RAI-0395.
54. Lee H-C, Headley MB, Iseki M, Ikuta K, Ziegler SF (2008) Cutting edge: Inhibition of NF-kappaB-mediated TSLP expression by retinoid X receptor. J Immunol 181: 5189–5193.
55. Abbas AK, Murphy KM, Sher A (1996) Functional diversity of helper T lymphocytes. Nature 383: 787–793. doi:10.1038/383787a0.
56. van Vliet E, Uhrberg M, Stein C, Gleichmann E (1993) MHC control of IL-4-dependent enhancement of B cell Ia expression and Ig class switching in mice treated with mercuric chloride. Int Arch Allergy Immunol 101: 392–401.
57. Nakayama T, Hieshima K, Nagakubo D, Sato E, Nakayama M, et al. (2004) Selective induction of Th2-attracting chemokines CCL17 and CCL22 in human B cells by latent membrane protein 1 of Epstein-Barr virus. J Virol 78: 1665–1674.
58. Wang Z, Coleman DJ, Bajaj G, Liang X, Ganguli-Indra G, et al. (2011) RXRα ablation in epidermal keratinocytes enhances UVR-induced DNA damage, apoptosis, and proliferation of keratinocytes and melanocytes. J Invest Dermatol 131: 177–187. doi:10.1038/jid.2010.290.
59. Liang X, Bhattacharya S, Bajaj G, Guha G, Wang Z, et al. (2012) Delayed Cutaneous Wound Healing and Aberrant Expression of Hair Follicle Stem Cell Markers in Mice Selectively Lacking Ctip2 in Epidermis. PLoS ONE 7: e29999. doi:10.1371/journal.pone.0029999.
60. Indra AK, Mohan WS, Frontini M, Scheer E, Messaddeq N, et al. (2005) TAF10 is required for the establishment of skin barrier function in foetal, but not in adult mouse epidermis. Dev Biol 285: 28–37.
61. Indra AK, Dupe V, Bornert JM, Messaddeq N, Yaniv M, et al. (2005) Temporally controlled targeted somatic mutagenesis in embryonic surface ectoderm and fetal epidermal keratinocytes unveils two distinct developmental functions of BRG1 in limb morphogenesis and skin barrier formation. Development 132: 4533–4544.
62. Argmann CA, Auwerx J (2006) Collection of blood and plasma from the mouse. Curr Protoc Mol Biol Chapter 29: Unit 29A.3. doi:10.1002/0471142727.mb29a03s75.
63. Hyter S, Bajaj G, Liang X, Barbacid M, Ganguli-Indra G, et al. (2010) Loss of nuclear receptor RXRα in epidermal keratinocytes promotes the formation of Cdk4-activated invasive melanomas. Pigment Cell Melanoma Res 23: 635–648. doi:10.1111/j.1755-148X.2010.00732.x.

Permissions

All chapters in this book were first published in PLOS ONE, by The Public Library of Science; hereby published with permission under the Creative Commons Attribution License or equivalent. Every chapter published in this book has been scrutinized by our experts. Their significance has been extensively debated. The topics covered herein carry significant findings which will fuel the growth of the discipline. They may even be implemented as practical applications or may be referred to as a beginning point for another development.

The contributors of this book come from diverse backgrounds, making this book a truly international effort. This book will bring forth new frontiers with its revolutionizing research information and detailed analysis of the nascent developments around the world.

We would like to thank all the contributing authors for lending their expertise to make the book truly unique. They have played a crucial role in the development of this book. Without their invaluable contributions this book wouldn't have been possible. They have made vital efforts to compile up to date information on the varied aspects of this subject to make this book a valuable addition to the collection of many professionals and students.

This book was conceptualized with the vision of imparting up-to-date information and advanced data in this field. To ensure the same, a matchless editorial board was set up. Every individual on the board went through rigorous rounds of assessment to prove their worth. After which they invested a large part of their time researching and compiling the most relevant data for our readers.

The editorial board has been involved in producing this book since its inception. They have spent rigorous hours researching and exploring the diverse topics which have resulted in the successful publishing of this book. They have passed on their knowledge of decades through this book. To expedite this challenging task, the publisher supported the team at every step. A small team of assistant editors was also appointed to further simplify the editing procedure and attain best results for the readers.

Apart from the editorial board, the designing team has also invested a significant amount of their time in understanding the subject and creating the most relevant covers. They scrutinized every image to scout for the most suitable representation of the subject and create an appropriate cover for the book.

The publishing team has been an ardent support to the editorial, designing and production team. Their endless efforts to recruit the best for this project, has resulted in the accomplishment of this book. They are a veteran in the field of academics and their pool of knowledge is as vast as their experience in printing. Their expertise and guidance has proved useful at every step. Their uncompromising quality standards have made this book an exceptional effort. Their encouragement from time to time has been an inspiration for everyone.

The publisher and the editorial board hope that this book will prove to be a valuable piece of knowledge for researchers, students, practitioners and scholars across the globe.

List of Contributors

Dror Avni
Laboratory of Molecular Cell Biology, Center for Cancer Research and Department of Internal Medicine C, Sheba Medical Center, Tel Hashomer, Israel

Camila Avivi, Corine Mardoukh, Iris Barshack and Sylvie Polak-Charcon
Institute of Pathology Sheba Medical Center, Tel Hashomer, Israel
Department of Dermatology Sheba Medical Center, Tel Hashomer, Israel

Aviv Barzilai and Felix Pavlotsky
Department of Dermatology Sheba Medical Center, Tel Hashomer, Israel

Ariel Tessone and Arie Orenstein
Department of Plastic and Reconstructive Surgery and Burns Sheba Medical Center, Tel Hashomer, Israel

Ben Gradus and Eran Hornstein
Department of Molecular Genetics Weizmann Institute of Science, Rehovot, Israel

Galya Lerman and Yechezkel Sidi
Laboratory of Molecular Cell Biology, Center for Cancer Research and Department of Internal Medicine C, Sheba Medical Center, Tel Hashomer, Israel
Sackler School of Medicine, Tel Aviv University, Tel Aviv, Israel

Zhong Zheng, Kevin S. Lee, Xinli Zhang, Calvin Nguyen, Chingyun Hsu, Todd Matthew Rackohn, Maxwell Murphy and Kang Ting
Dental and Craniofacial Research Institute and Section of Orthodontics, School of Dentistry, University of California Los Angeles, Los Angeles, California, United States of America

Joyce Z. Wang
Department of Emergency Medicine, State University of New York Downstate/Kings Country Hospital Center, New York, New York, United States of America

Dwarak Reddy Enjamuri
Department of Psychobiology, University of California Los Angeles, Los Angeles, California, United States of America

Chia Soo
UCLA and Orthopaedic Hospital Department of Orthopaedic Surgery and the Orthopaedic Hospital Research Center, University of California Los Angeles, Los Angeles, California, United States of America
Division of Plastic and Reconstructive Surgery, Department of Surgery, School of Medicine, University of California Los Angeles, Los Angeles, California, United States of America

Xiaoqian Ye and Zhuan Bian
The State Key Laboratory Breeding Base of Basic Science of Stomatology (Hubei-MOST) and Key Laboratory of Oral Biomedicine Ministry of Education, School and
Hospital of Stomatology, Wuhan University, Wuhan, Hubei, China

Huali Fan
The Second General Department, Hangzhou Stomatology Hospital, Hangzhou, Zhejiang, China

Wei Yin
The State Key Laboratory Breeding Base of Basic Science of Stomatology (Hubei-MOST) and Key Laboratory of Oral Biomedicine Ministry of Education, School and
Hospital of Stomatology, Wuhan University, Wuhan, Hubei, China
Department of Endodontics and Periodontics, College of Stomatology, Dalian Medical University, Dalian, Liaoning, China

Ariadna Mendoza-Naranjo, Peter Cormie, Antonio E. Serrano, Chiuhui Mary Wang, Christopher Thrasivoulou, Kieran T. Power and David L. Becker
Department of Cell and Developmental Biology, University College London, London, United Kingdom

Rebecca Hu, Shay O'Neill, Alexis White and Anthony R. J. Phillips
CoDa Therapeutics, Auckland, New Zealand

Thomas Serena
Newbridge Medical Research Corp, Warren, Pennsylvania, United States of America

Kosuke Miyauchi, Yasutaka Motomura and Yoshie Suzuki
Laboratory for Signal Network, Research Center for Allergy and Immunology, RIKEN Yokohama Institute, Yokohama, Kanagawa, Japan

Naoko Ozaki and Shinobu Suzuki
Department of Molecular and Cellular Biology, Kobe Pharma Research Institute, Nippon Boehringer Ingelheim Co., Ltd., Kobe, Hyogo, Japan

Akihiko Yoshimura
Department of Microbiology and Immunology, Keio University School of Medicine, Tokyo, Japan

Daniel Cua
Schering-Plough Biopharma, Palo Alto, California, United States

Ayako Uto-Konomi
Laboratory for Signal Network, Research Center for Allergy and Immunology, RIKEN Yokohama Institute, Yokohama, Kanagawa, Japan
Department of Molecular and Cellular Biology, Kobe Pharma Research Institute, Nippon Boehringer Ingelheim Co., Ltd., Kobe, Hyogo, Japan

Masato Kubo
Laboratory for Signal Network, Research Center for Allergy and Immunology, RIKEN Yokohama Institute, Yokohama, Kanagawa, Japan
Division of Molecular Pathology, Research Institute for Biological Science, Tokyo University of Science, Noda, Chiba, Japan

Weihui Li
Martinos Center for Biomedical Imaging, Massachusetts General Hospital, Charlestown, Massachusetts, United States of America

Andrew C. Ahn
Martinos Center for Biomedical Imaging, Massachusetts General Hospital, Charlestown, Massachusetts, United States of America
Division of General Medicine and Primary Care, Beth Israel Deaconess Medical Center, Boston, Massachusetts, United States of America

Zhihui Zhu and Jinrong Peng
Key Laboratory for Molecular Animal Nutrition, Ministry of Education, College of Animal Sciences, Zhejiang University, Hangzhou, China

Jun Chen
College of Life Sciences, Zhejiang University, Hangzhou, China

Jing-Wei Xiong
Institute of Molecular Medicine, Peking University, Beijing, China

Nannie Bangsgaard and Lone Skov
Department of Dermato-allergology, Copenhagen University Hospital Gentofte, Hellerup, Denmark

Mischa Houtkamp, Danita H. Schuurhuis and Paul W. H. I. Parren
Genmab, Utrecht, The Netherlands

Ole Baadsgaard
Genmab, Copenhagen, Denmark

Hans W. M. Niessen
Department of Pathology and Cardiac Surgery, VU University Medical Centre, Amsterdam, The Netherlands

Shin Kumadaki, Chika Higashi, Makoto Ozawa, Mikihiko Shinozaki, Yutaka Kato, Koutarou Hoshida, Satomi Kikuchi, Yoshihisa Nakano and Shoji Furusako
Discovery Research, Mochida Pharmaceutical Company Limited, Shizuoka, Japan

Yoshihiro Ogawa
Department of Molecular Endocrinology and Metabolism, Graduate School of Medical and Dental Sciences, Tokyo Medical and Dental University, Tokyo, Japan

Naoto Tsuda
Discovery Research, Mochida Pharmaceutical Company Limited, Shizuoka, Japan
Department of Molecular Endocrinology and Metabolism, Graduate School of
Medical and Dental Sciences, Tokyo Medical and Dental University, Tokyo, Japan

Neera Tewari-Singh, Anil K. Jain and Rajesh Agarwal
Department of Pharmaceutical Sciences, Skaggs School of Pharmacy and Pharmaceutical Sciences, University of Colorado Denver, Aurora, Colorado, United States of America

David J. Orlicky
Department of Pathology, School of Medicine, University of Colorado Denver, Aurora, Colorado, United States of America

Carl W. White
Department of Pediatrics, School of Medicine, University of Colorado Denver, Aurora, Colorado, United States of America

Urszula Lipinska, Katleen Hermans, Lieve Meulemans and Freddy Haesebrouck
Department of Pathology, Bacteriology and Avian Diseases, Faculty of Veterinary Medicine, Ghent University, Merelbeke, Belgium

Luc Duchateau
Department of Physiology and Biometry, Faculty of Veterinary Medicine, Ghent University, Merelbeke, Belgium

Cedric Badiou
Centre National de Référence des Staphylocoques, Université Lyon 1, Lyon, France
INSERM U851, IFR128, Lyon, France

Oana Dumitrescu, Jerome Etienne and Gerard Lina
Centre National de Référence des Staphylocoques, Université Lyon 1, Lyon, France
INSERM U851, IFR128, Lyon, France
Hospices Civils de Lyon, Lyon, France

Mikiro Takaishi and Shigetoshi Sano
Department of Dermatology, Kochi Medical School, Kochi University, Nankoku, Japan

Shota Tokuoka
Pharmacology Department, Drug Research Center, Kaken Pharmaceutical Co., Ltd., Kyoto, Japan

Kenji Sato
Department of Dermatology, Kochi Medical School, Kochi University, Nankoku, Japan
Pharmacology Department, Drug Research Center, Kaken Pharmaceutical Co., Ltd., Kyoto, Japan

Leanne M. Johnson-Huang, Judilyn Fuentes-Duculan, Irma Cardinale, Kathleen M. Bonifacio, Nicholas Gulati and Hiroshi Mitsui
Laboratory for Investigative Dermatology, The Rockefeller University, New York City, New York, United States of America

Kristine E. Nograles, Mayte Suárez-Fariñas and James G. Krueger
Laboratory for Investigative Dermatology, The Rockefeller University, New York City, New York, United States of America
Center for Clinical and Translational Science, The Rockefeller University, New York City, New York, United States of America

Andrea Chiricozzi
Laboratory for Investigative Dermatology, The Rockefeller University, New York City, New York, United States of America
Center for Clinical and Translational Science, The Rockefeller University, New York City, New York, United States of America
Department of Dermatology, University of Rome "Tor Vergata", Rome, Italy

Emma Guttman-Yassky
Laboratory for Investigative Dermatology, The Rockefeller University, New York City, New York, United States of America
Center for Clinical and Translational Science, The Rockefeller University, New York City, New York, United States of America
Department of Dermatology, Mount Sinai School of Medicine, New York City, New York, United States of America

Ashley W. Seifert, James R. Monaghan and Malcolm Maden
Department of Biology, University of Florida, Gainesville, Florida, United States of America

S. Randal Voss
Department of Biology, University of Kentucky, Lexington, Kentucky, United States of America
Spinal Cord and Brain Injury Research Center, University of Kentucky, Lexington, Kentucky, United States of America

Boris Dufournet
Clinical Pharmacology Unit, Inserm CIC03, Grenoble University Hospital, Grenoble, France

Marcin Hellmann
Clinical Pharmacology Unit, Inserm CIC03, Grenoble University Hospital, Grenoble, France
Joseph Fourier University, Grenoble, France

Claire Arnaud, Diane Godin-Ribuot and Christophe Ribuot
Laboratoire HP2 - U1042, Inserm, Grenoble, France
Joseph Fourier University, Grenoble, France

Jean Boutonnat
Joseph Fourier University, Grenoble, France
TIMC UMRCNRS 5525, Grenoble, France

Matthieu Roustit, Claire Millet and Jean-Luc Cracowski
Clinical Pharmacology Unit, Inserm CIC03, Grenoble University Hospital, Grenoble, France
Laboratoire HP2 - U1042, Inserm, Grenoble, France
Joseph Fourier University, Grenoble, France

Sophie Blaise
Laboratoire HP2 - U1042, Inserm, Grenoble, France
Joseph Fourier University, Grenoble, France
Vascular Medicine Department, Grenoble University Hospital, Grenoble, France

Raeeun Park, Hideo Nojima and Hyung-Chel Kim
R&D Team, Samsung Electronics CO., LTD, Suwon, Korea

Mi Hee Shin, Yeon Kyung Kim and Jin Ho Chung
Department of Dermatology, Seoul National University College of Medicine, Seoul, Korea
Laboratory of Cutaneous Aging Research, Biomedical Research Institute, Seoul National University Hospital, Seoul, Korea
Institute of Human-Environment Interface Biology, Medical Research Center, Seoul National University, Seoul, Korea

Andrea Stancato, Chiara De Luca, Daniela Lulli, Saveria Pastore and Liudmila Korkina
Laboratory of Tissue Engineering & Skin Pathophysiology, Istituto Dermopatico dell'Immacolata (IDI IRCCS), Rome, Italy

Vladimir Kostyuk and Alla Potapovich
Laboratory of Tissue Engineering & Skin Pathophysiology, Istituto Dermopatico dell'Immacolata (IDI IRCCS), Rome, Italy
Biology Department, Belarus State University, Minsk, Belarus

Leif Røge Lund
Department of Cellular and Molecular Medicine, Faculty of Health Sciences, University of Copenhagen, Copenhagen, Denmark

Lars Henning Engelholm
Finsen Laboratory, Rigshospitalet, Copenhagen, Denmark

Birgitte Rønø
Center for Molecular Pathology, Department of Laboratory Medicine, Lund University, Malmo, Sweden
Department of Cellular and Molecular Medicine, Faculty of Health Sciences, University of Copenhagen, Copenhagen, Denmark

Andreas Hald
Department of Cellular and Molecular Medicine, Faculty of Health Sciences, University of Copenhagen, Copenhagen, Denmark
Finsen Laboratory, Rigshospitalet, Copenhagen, Denmark
Biotech Research and Innovation Centre, University of Copenhagen, Copenhagen, Denmark

Vivian L. de Oliveira, Esther Fasse, Irma Joosten and Hans J. P. M. Koenen
Laboratory of Medical Immunology, Department of Laboratory Medicine, Radboud University Nijmegen Medical Centre, Nijmegen, The Netherlands

Peter C. M. van de Kerkhof, Marieke M. B. Seyger and Piet E. J. van Erp
Dermatology Department, Radboud University Nijmegen Medical Centre, Nijmegen, The Netherlands

Pieter Hupkens
Department of Plastic Surgery Radboud University Nijmegen Medical Centre, Nijmegen, The Netherlands

Lars Svensson and Markus Latta
Department of Disease Pharmacology, LEO Pharma, Ballerup, Denmark

Hanne Norsgaard and Tord Labuda
Department of Molecular Biomedicine, LEO Pharma, Ballerup, Denmark

Romy R. M. C. Keijsers
Laboratory of Medical Immunology, Department of Laboratory Medicine, Radboud University Nijmegen Medical Centre, Nijmegen, The Netherlands
Dermatology Department, Radboud University Nijmegen Medical Centre, Nijmegen, The Netherlands

Zhixing Wang, Ling-juan Zhang, Gunjan Guha, Shan Li and Kateryna Kyrylkova
Department of Pharmaceutical Sciences, College of Pharmacy, Oregon State University, Corvallis, Oregon, United States of America

Chrissa Kioussi and Gitali Ganguli-Indra
Department of Pharmaceutical Sciences, College of Pharmacy, Oregon State University, Corvallis, Oregon, United States of America
Molecular Cell Biology Program, Oregon State University, Corvallis, Oregon, United States of America

Mark Leid
Department of Pharmaceutical Sciences, College of Pharmacy, Oregon State University, Corvallis, Oregon, United States of America
Molecular Cell Biology Program, Oregon State University, Corvallis, Oregon, United States of America
Environmental Health Science Center, Oregon State University, Corvallis, Oregon, United States of America

Arup K. Indra
Department of Pharmaceutical Sciences, College of Pharmacy, Oregon State University, Corvallis, Oregon, United States of America
Molecular Cell Biology Program, Oregon State University, Corvallis, Oregon, United States of America
Environmental Health Science Center, Oregon State University, Corvallis, Oregon, United States of America
Department of Dermatology, Oregon Health and Science University, Portland, Oregon, United States of America

Index